THE CIBA COLLECTION
OF MEDICAL ILLUSTRATIONS

Volume 6

Kidneys, Ureters, and Urinary Bladder

A compilation of paintings depicting anatomy and
embryology, physiology, pathology, pathophysiology,
and clinical features and treatment of diseases

Prepared by

Frank H. Netter, M.D.

Edited by

Robert K. Shapter, M.D., C.M.

Fredrick F. Yonkman, M.D., Ph.D.
Editor Emeritus

With a foreword by
E. Lovell Becker, M.D.
Professor of Medicine
Cornell University Medical College

Commissioned and published by

C I B A

Other published volumes of
THE CIBA COLLECTION OF MEDICAL ILLUSTRATIONS
Prepared by
Frank H. Netter, M.D.

Nervous System
Reproductive System
Upper Digestive Tract
Lower Digestive Tract
Liver, Biliary Tract and Pancreas
Endocrine System and Selected Metabolic Diseases
Heart
Respiratory System

See page 295 for additional information

Color slides of all illustrations contained in this book are available from CIBA Medical Education Division, 556 Morris Avenue, Summit, N.J. 07901.

First Printing 1973
Second Printing 1975
Third Printing 1979

ISBN 0-914168-08-8
Library of Congress Catalogue No. 53-2151

Printed in U.S.A.

Color Engraving: Embassy Photo Engraving Co., Inc., New York, N.Y.
Offset Conversion: The Case-Hoyt Corporation, Rochester, N.Y.
Text Typography: Cooper & Beatty, Limited, Toronto, Ontario
Illustration Typography: Cesareo Studio, Elmsford, N.Y.
Printing: The Case-Hoyt Corporation, Rochester, N.Y.

An Unusual Man

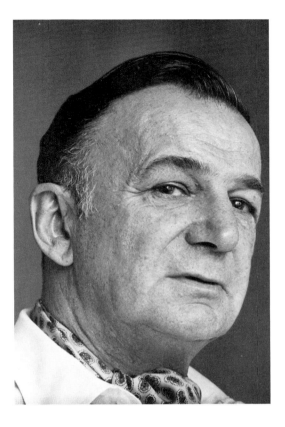

When you first meet Frank Netter, you are a little surprised. You expect a man who has devoted a lifetime to painting such magnificent medical art to be outgoing, talkative, bursting with ideas. Instead, Frank Netter is quiet, reserved, almost reticent. To carry the conversation, you appear to do all the talking; he speaks little, listens a lot. Slowly, you realize that the greatest talent of this world famous physician-artist is neither medical nor artistic. For Frank H. Netter, M.D. is perhaps the world's greatest interpreter and communicator of medical knowledge through the medium of art. To interpret he must understand, to understand he must absorb information, and so he listens.

As a means of communication, art is as old as civilization. Long before human beings created the written word they left their messages on the walls of caves. Throughout history, art has been one form of expression capable of traversing the barriers of language, culture, and time in order to communicate. An artist who chooses to use brush and canvas leaves a part of his inner self in the medium. His message may be simple, direct, obvious, and reach many, or it may be complex, hidden, obscure, and touch only a few.

When young Frank Netter studied at the Sorbonne, he was very much an artist. His canvases were the expressions of his essence. When young Dr. Netter savored the beauty of the East River and the Brooklyn skyline from a window of Bellevue Hospital, the artist's love of form and color and life guided his spirit. With the skill and talent of an artist his hands expressed what his eyes saw and his soul felt, and when he finished, a part of him lay infused in the oils on the canvas. When, as a practicing physician in New York, the still young Dr. Netter painted a memorable series of paintings capturing events in the education of a physician, the artist was still very much at work. The paintings individually communicated joy, sadness, nostalgia, pathos, and inspiration. There was added, though, another dimension—realism—bold, factual, blunt realism. Patients were very much patients and artistic license was not taken for the sake of emotional impact.

Those paintings, a curious blend of great artistic sensitivity in a setting of stark clinical realism, document the true turning point in Frank Netter's life. Previously, the artist Netter wrestled with the physician Netter for his time and talents. He had been the artist who had become the physician, the physician who had been part-time artist, but before that series of paintings never really both at once.

During the next few pre-World War II years Frank Netter evolved into a new breed of man, unlike any before him, capable of portraying the clinical scene with the skill of the artist and the coolness of the surgeon. If important to the clinical setting, a patient's emotional reactions to illness and suffering would command the viewer's attention, but the viewer would never be lured into an emotional association with the scene. Artistic license might be taken with shadows and highlights to make a medical point; time might be compressed to show the dynamic continuance of clinical disease, but always the message was clear. Always the clinical detachment, the hallmark of medical objectivity, remained. Accuracy was never compromised for effect.

Frank Netter maintains a tremendous mental pace. In 25 years he has produced in excess of 2,300 paintings, a rate which means a new painting every four days, day in, day out, week after week, month after month. Each painting is detailed, thorough, accurate. Each is researched, planned, sketched, checked, rethought, and painted for the sole purpose of transmitting thoughts. Each communicates a vast amount of data, and uniquely stands alone; it needs no previous or subsequent paintings to support it. Yet each painting is a part of the overall scheme conceived years ago to portray the total world of medical science, organ by organ, system by system.

Not even Dr. Netter is capable of knowing all there is to know about the human body. Where once he relied on personal reading and literature research as sources of knowledge for a painting, now the emphasis is on direct contact with a recognized expert in a particular field. The consultant speaks, Netter listens, and Netter becomes the extension of the mind of the consultant.

The process is repeated continuously. Throughout the world there exists a group of distinguished leaders in medicine and the biologic sciences who are the collaborators and consultants to Dr. Netter and the CIBA COLLECTION. United by the common goals of learning, teaching, and research, this geographically scattered group has one additional bond of unity—its association with Frank H. Netter, M.D., the dean of a university without walls, the teacher who listens.

ROBERT K. SHAPTER, M.D., C.M.

Kidneys, Ureters, and Urinary Bladder

Associate Editors:
E. Lovell Becker, M.D.
Jacob Churg, M.D.

Subeditors:
Louis L. Bergmann, M.D.
H. O. Heinemann, M.D.
Robert M. Kark, M.D., F.R.C.P.
Johannes A. G. Rhodin, M.D., Ph.D.

Foreword

Renal disease respects no one; it is found in newborns, the young, and the elderly. It is seen in both sexes, in all socioeconomic groups, and in every geographic area of the world. There are diseases affecting the kidneys which are more prevalent in some areas than in others; there are some diseases which affect one sex more than another, but no one is free from the threat of renal disease.

The first observations of diseases of the kidney are probably lost in the unrecorded past. The Greeks had been aware of edema (hydrops) and Hippocrates made several references to the clinical features of kidney disease.[1] In his writings Hippocrates mentions acute nephritis:

in cases of pain in the back and chest, the passing of bloody urine turning into anuria indicates a distressing illness ending fatally.

Further, he comments on uremia:

patients who suffer from drowsiness, showing twitching of the hands and sleepiness, are of bad color and liable to oedema, while the pulse is sluggish and parts under the eyes swollen.

He also refers to albuminuria:

bubbles appearing on the surface of the urine indicate disease of the kidneys and a prolonged illness.

Probably the first description of kidney disease in western literature was that of William of Salicet (Guglielmo Salicetti) who was Professor of Medicine at Bologna from 1269 to 1274. His description was probably based on ancient or Arabic sources rather than on personal observation:[2]

the signs of hardness in the kidneys are that the quantity of urine is diminished, there is heaviness in the kidneys and of the spine with some pain, and the belly begins to swell up after a time and dropsy is produced.

Following these early descriptions, there was a long period during the Middle Ages in which uroscopy was popular, but knowledge of kidney disease advanced only a very little during the ensuing centuries. Many observers recognized the association of uremia and urine output. Further, there were many references to coagulable urine, even the association of dropsy with coagulable urine. However, it was not until the contributions of Richard Bright (1789-1858) that we have a foundation for our knowledge of renal disease. Bright's observations were the basis for the method of careful clinicopathologic correlation which was to be the cornerstone of 19th century investigational methods in medicine. Bright observed:[3]

there are other appearances to which I think too little attention has heretofore been paid.

He also noted those evidences of organic disease which occasionally present themselves in the structure of the kidney:

I have never yet examined the body of a patient dying with dropsy attended with coagulable urine in whom some obvious derangement was not discovered in the kidney.

After Bright's early observations, a wealth of material was published dealing primarily with clinical observations. Advancement of the knowledge and understanding of renal disease was not spectacular. Physiologists were adding greatly to our knowledge of the kidney, and interest in morbid anatomy was stimulated and catapulted forward by the development of the technic for percutaneous renal biopsy. Further, the physiologists from the schools of Homer Smith, D. D. Van Slyke, E. K. Marshall, Robert Pitts, and James Shannon made contributions which, in their own right, were of major significance. More importantly, these scientists stimulated an entire generation of physicians to carry on the work and delve further into the mysteries of normal as well as altered physiology and pathology.

Within the past 20 years we have come to view a patient diagnosed as having kidney disease with an attitude of hope rather than defeat. Previously, little was known about the various types of kidney disease, and diagnosis was limited to either glomerulonephritis or pyelonephritis. Today, literally hundreds of diseases can be diagnosed and in many cases treated.

The refinement of technics of microscopy also added greatly to our knowledge of renal disease. The greater use of electron and fluorescent microscopy allowed further delineation of diseases. Technics for detection and diagnosis have been refined.

Two innovators in the study of the kidney are William Kolff and John Merrill. Dr. Kolff's experimental work with the artificial kidney in occupied Holland during World War II led to the use of dialysis as an accepted form of therapy; in the past 15 years, the use of peritoneal dialysis and hemodialysis has moved from the laboratory to the bedside.

In 1953 in Boston, Dr. Merrill first undertook the now famous kidney transplantation on twins. His technic has been developed to the point that now thousands upon thousands of patients who have had kidney transplants lead nearly normal lives.

The artificial kidney and transplantation are two approaches to therapy for renal disease which are not mutually exclusive. For example, in 1970 in the United States approximately 1,100 new patients were placed on chronic intermittent dialysis, and over 900 transplant operations were performed.

Because of this awe-inspiring explosion of knowledge, technic, and capability in the field of renal disease, the CIBA Pharmaceutical Company wished that the next volume in THE CIBA COLLECTION OF MEDICAL ILLUSTRATIONS series would be devoted to renal disease and encompass all of the available information on this important subject.

Realizing that kidney disease involves every specialty of medicine including surgery, internal medicine, pediatrics, pathology, physiology, radiology, and many others, the editors knew they were faced with an overwhelming task. All of the contributors recognized the good fortune of having the opportunity to work with Dr. Frank Netter. His artistic talent, delving approach to problems, scientific acumen, and uncanny ability to obtain data from his colleagues made this volume a reality. Those of us who had the pleasure of working with Dr. Netter were constantly impressed by his grasp of the problems, situations, and points we wished to portray. This volume of THE CIBA COLLECTION OF MEDICAL ILLUSTRATIONS represents the combined efforts of numerous physicians and scientists throughout the world.

What then is the future? The horizons of medicine are constantly being extended by the magnificent achievements of the imaginative, interested, and dedicated scientific community. In the future, physiologists will tell us more and more about the normal functioning of the kidney and the alterations found in renal disease. Pathologists, who have added so much to the understanding and classification of renal disease, will contribute even more with the utilization of newer, more refined methods. Similarly, radiologists and nephrologists will enlarge the understanding of renal disease in both children and adults. Technics which are now acceptable for the management of patients with end-stage renal disease (*i.e.*, dialysis and transplantation), will be even further refined. In the foreseeable future, the dialysis machines will be made smaller and more efficient. The problem of transplant rejection will be overcome. The challenge of better technics of detection and diagnosis, and more efficacious drug therapy, however, will remain. Infection of the kidney, renal hypertension, and immunology of the kidney must be better understood.

It is with a true sense of appreciation that the medical profession expresses its gratitude to Dr. Frank Netter for his magnificent documentation of the present state of the art of nephrology.

E. LOVELL BECKER, M.D.

---

[1] Chadwick, J and Mann, WN: *The Medical Works of Hippocrates*, Blackwell, Oxford, 1950

[2] Salicetti, G: *Liver in Scientia Medicinali*, Johannus Petrus de Ferratis, Placentiae, Chap. 140, 1476, in Garrison, FH: *An Introduction to the History of Medicine*, 4th ed., W. B. Saunders Company, Philadelphia, 1929

[3] Bright, R: *Tubular view of the morbid appearances in 100 cases with albuminous urine*, Guy's Hosp. Rep. 1:380, 1836

Contributors and Consultants

The artist, editor, and publishers express their appreciation to the following authorities for their generous collaboration:

E. Lovell Becker, M.D.
Professor of Medicine, Cornell University
Medical College, New York, N.Y.

Louis L. Bergmann, M.D.
Professor of Anatomy, New York Medical
College, Valhalla, N.Y.

G. M. Berlyne, M.D., F.R.C.P.
Director, Department of Nephrology,
Central Negev Hospital;
Professor, Faculty of Natural Sciences,
University of Negev, Beersheva, Israel

D. A. K. Black, M.D., F.R.C.P.
Professor of Medicine, University of Manchester;
Physician, Manchester Royal Infirmary,
Manchester, England

Claus Brun, M.D.
Director, Department of Clinical Chemistry and
Nephropathology, Kommunehospitalet,
Copenhagen, Denmark

Richard E. Buenger, M.D.
Professor and Chairman, Department of
Diagnostic Radiology,
Rush-Presbyterian-St. Luke's Medical Center,
Chicago, Ill.

Paul J. Cannon, M.D.
Associate Professor of Medicine, Columbia
University College of Physicians and Surgeons;
Associate Attending Physician,
Columbia Presbyterian Medical Center,
New York, N.Y.

Jacob Churg, M.D.
Professor of Pathology and Chief, Division
of Renal Pathology, Mount Sinai School
of Medicine of The City University of
New York, New York, N.Y.

Fredric L. Coe, M.D.
Director, Renal Division, Michael Reese
Hospital and Medical Center; Assistant
Professor, Department of Medicine, The
University of Chicago, The Pritzker School
of Medicine, Chicago, Ill.

Alan S. Cohen, M.D.
Conrad Wesselhoeft Professor of Medicine,
Boston University School of Medicine;
Director, Boston University Medical Services,
Boston City Hospital; Head, Arthritis and
Connective Tissue Disease Section,
Boston University Medical Center,
Boston, Mass.

Gustave J. Dammin, M.D.
Elsie T. Friedman Professor of Pathology,
Harvard Medical School;
Pathologist-in-Chief, Peter Bent
Brigham Hospital, Boston, Mass.

Michael E. DeBakey, M.D.
President and Chairman, Department of
Surgery, Baylor College of Medicine;
Director, Cardiovascular Research and
Training Center, The Methodist Hospital,
Houston, Texas

Thomas Doxiadis, M.D.
Consulting Internist, Evangelismos Hospital,
Athens, Greece; Visiting Professor,
University of California,
Los Angeles, Calif.

John L. Duffy, M.D.
Associate Chairman, Department of
Pathology and Laboratories, Nassau
County Medical Center, East Meadow, N.Y.;
Associate Professor of Pathology,
Health Sciences Center, State University
of New York, Stony Brook, N.Y.

David P. Earle, M.D.
Professor and Chairman, Department of
Medicine, Northwestern University
Medical School, Chicago, Ill.

Edwin R. Fisher, M.D.
Director of Laboratories, Shadyside Hospital;
Professor of Pathology,
University of Pittsburgh, Pittsburgh, Pa.

Gerhard Giebisch, M.D.
Chairman, Department of Physiology,
Yale University School of Medicine,
New Haven, Conn.

Marvin Goldstein, M.D.
Associate Professor of Medicine,
Mount Sinai School of Medicine of The City
University of New York, New York, N.Y.

Albert S. Gordon, Ph.D.
Professor of Biology and Director,
Laboratory of Experimental Hematology,
Department of Biology, Graduate School
of Arts and Sciences, New York University,
New York, N.Y.

Carl W. Gottschalk, M.D.
Kenan Professor of Medicine and
Physiology and Career Investigator,
American Heart Association, Department
of Medicine, University of North Carolina
School of Medicine, Chapel Hill, N.C.

Edith Grishman, M.D.
Assistant Professor of Pathology,
Mount Sinai School of Medicine of The
City University of New York, New York, N.Y.;
Associate Attending Pathologist,
The Mount Sinai Hospital Services,
City Hospital Center, Elmhurst, N.Y.

H. O. Heinemann, M.D.
Associate Professor of Medicine,
Cornell University Medical College,
New York, N.Y.

Robert M. Kark, M.D., F.R.C.P.
Professor of Medicine, Rush Medical College;
Attending Physician,
Rush-Presbyterian-St. Luke's Medical Center,
Chicago, Ill.

Paul Kimmelstiel, M.D. (Deceased)
Distinguished Professor of Pathology,
University of Oklahoma Medical Center,
Oklahoma City, Okla.

J. Stauffer Lehman, Jr., M.D., M.P.H.
Assistant Professor of Tropical Public Health,
Department of Tropical Public Health,
Harvard School of Public Health,
Boston, Mass.

Hermann Mattenheimer, M.D.
Professor of Biochemistry, Rush Medical
College, Rush-Presbyterian-St. Luke's
Medical Center, Chicago, Ill.

Willy Mautner, M.D.
Associate Professor of Pathology,
Mount Sinai School of Medicine of The City
University of New York, New York, N.Y.

Robert T. McCluskey, M.D.
S. Burt Wolbach Professor of Pathology,
Harvard Medical School; Pathologist-in-Chief,
Children's Hospital Medical Center,
Boston, Mass.

John P. Merrill, M.D.
Professor of Medicine, Harvard Medical School;
Director, Cardiorenal Section,
Peter Bent Brigham Hospital, Boston, Mass.

G. A. G. Mitchell, O.B.E., T.D., M.B.,
Ch.M., D.Sc., F.R.C.S.
Hon. Alumnus, The University, Louvain, Belgium;
Chevalier (1st Cl.) Order of the Dannebrog;
Professor of Anatomy and Director
of Anatomical Laboratories,
The University, Manchester, England

F. K. Mostofi, M.D.
Chief, Genitourinary Pathology Branch and
Chief, General and Special Pathology,
Division D, Armed Forces Institute of Pathology;
Clinical Professor of Pathology,
Georgetown University School of Medicine,
Washington, D.C.; Assistant Professor of
Pathology, Johns Hopkins University
School of Medicine, Baltimore, Md.

Steen Olsen, M.D.
Professor of Pathology, University of Århus;
Director, University Institute of Pathology,
Kommunehospitalet, Århus, Denmark

Solomon Papper, M.D.
Chairman of Medicine, General Rose
Memorial Hospital; Professor of Medicine,
University of Colorado Medical Center,
Denver, Colo.

Suresh K. Patel, M.D.
Director, Section of Urologic Radiology,
Department of Diagnostic Radiology,
Rush-Presbyterian-St. Luke's Hospital,
Chicago, Ill.

Conrad L. Pirani, M.D.
Professor of Pathology and Director of
the Renal Pathology Laboratory, Columbia
University College of Physicians and
Surgeons, New York, N.Y.; formerly
Chairman, Department of Pathology,
Michael Reese Hospital and Medical Center;
formerly Professor of Pathology, The University
of Chicago, The Pritzker School of Medicine,
Chicago, Ill.

Theodore N. Pullman, M.D.
Professor of Medicine, Department of
Medicine, The University of Chicago,
The Pritzker School of Medicine,
Chicago, Ill.

Johannes A. G. Rhodin, M.D., Ph.D.
Professor and Chairman, Department of
Anatomy, New York Medical College,
Valhalla, N.Y.

J. U. Schlegel, M.D.
Professor and Chairman, Section of Urology,
Department of Surgery, Tulane University
School of Medicine, New Orleans, La.

George E. Schreiner, M.D.
Professor of Medicine and Director,
Nephrology Division, Department of Medicine,
Georgetown University School of Medicine,
Washington, D.C.;
Chairman, Medical Advisory Board,
National Kidney Foundation;
Past President, American Society of Nephrology

Gerald S. Spear, M.D.
Associate Professor of Pathology,
Johns Hopkins University School of Medicine,
Baltimore, Md.

Maurice B. Strauss, M.D.
Professor of Medicine and Associate Dean,
Tufts University School of Medicine,
Boston, Mass.

Yasunosuke Suzuki, M.D.
Research Associate Professor,
Division of Renal Pathology, Department of
Pathology, Mount Sinai School of Medicine
of The City University of New York,
New York, N.Y.

Carlos A. Vaamonde, M.D.
Associate Professor of Medicine,
University of Miami School of Medicine;
Chief, Nephrology Section, Miami
Veterans Administration Hospital,
Miami, Fla.

Victor Vertes, M.D.
Director, Division of Medicine,
Mount Sinai Hospital of Cleveland;
Professor of Medicine, Case Western Reserve
University School of Medicine, Cleveland, Ohio

Howard G. Worthen, M.D., Ph.D.
Professor of Pediatrics, The University
of Texas Southwestern Medical School,
Dallas, Texas.

Introduction

It is now more than 25 years since I began preparing the series of volumes entitled THE CIBA COLLECTION OF MEDICAL ILLUSTRATIONS. As originally conceived, the series was to depict, system by system, the anatomy, embryology, physiology, pathology, pathologic physiology, and pertinent clinical features of diseases of the entire human organism. As I progressed through the volumes, I continually postponed the day when I would attempt to portray the kidneys and urinary tract. Since so much progress was being made in the study of these organs and their disorders, I hoped that the discrepancies in our knowledge would be rectified, the inconsistencies in our theories clarified, and the differences in our interpretations and opinions resolved. Miraculously, through the persistent endeavors of many brilliant and devoted researchers, clinicians, and surgeons throughout the world, this took place.

Nevertheless, when the day came to begin this volume, I found that, because of the tremendous progress, my task had become not easier and simpler, but more difficult and involved. With each discovery, new vistas of exploration had appeared; with each clarification, new avenues of investigation had opened. Indeed, progress in clinical nephrology often necessitated reevaluation of formerly established concepts. Even renal anatomy, once thought of as a static subject, had been completely restudied to provide the more precise comprehension of nephron structure, organization, and blood supply needed for better understanding of normal and abnormal kidney function.

Technology had also progressed. For example, the electron microscope had not only greatly enlarged our knowledge of renal structure and pathology, but it had also improved our visualization of the underlying processes in many renal disorders. The whole field of dialysis had opened and kidney transplantation had become a practical reality. New renal function tests had been devised and new technics for urine examination developed. The field of renal radiology had greatly expanded and radioactive scanning had been utilized as a valuable diagnostic tool.

This incredible progress as well as the clinical aspects of the many renal and urinary tract disorders required illustration. In this volume, I have included a number of illustrative flow charts depicting the common clinical course of renal diseases such as acute and chronic glomerulonephritis. In my efforts to portray the kidney, I found I could not consider either it or nephrology as an isolated study because kidney function is intimately related to function of other organ systems, and to bodily function in general. The circulatory, endocrine, and metabolic systems are particularly involved, and progress in the study of these fields has meant progress in nephrology. It was necessary to consider kidney function and kidney disease in relation to such topics as hypertension, renin, angiotensin, aldosterone, other cortical hormones, pituitary hormones, parathyroid function, inborn metabolic errors, immunologic factors, homeostasis, and water and electrolyte balance.

The task with which I was faced was thus truly formidable. Its accomplishment was only made possible by the gracious and devoted help of the many distinguished collaborators and consultants who are credited individually on other pages of this volume. I wish to express here my sincere appreciation for their help and for the time which they gave me despite their busy schedules, as well as to express my admiration for their knowledge and wisdom. I especially thank Dr. E. Lovell "Stretch" Becker and Dr. Jacob "Jack" Churg. They guided me through this project, and their devotion to it was a source of stimulation. The close cooperation of the editor, Dr. Robert K. Shapter, who took over in "midstream" from Dr. Fredrick Yonkman, was most gratifying. There were many others who lightened the burden of this endeavor in various ways, but foremost among these was Miss Louise Stemmle, production editor.

Underlying the creation of this and the other volumes of this series has been the vision, understanding, and unreserved backing of CIBA Pharmaceutical Company and its executives who have given me so free a hand in this work.

FRANK H. NETTER, M.D.

Preface

It is difficult to understand why an organ as intriguing as the kidney has remained so little understood until recently, while other but no more vital organs occupied the center stage of medicine and biology. Perhaps it was because the kidneys and urinary tract have neither a counterpart to a Starling's law to mystify and beckon students, nor a wallerian-type degeneration to allow precise definition of morphology. Instead, when viewed superficially the kidney appears to be an organ of monotonously similar structures. The dynamic nature of this remarkable organ—its ability to constantly adapt to the changing internal body environment, its unique role in maintaining body fluid, electrolyte, and acid-base homeostasis—has only been appreciated in recent years.

Twenty-five years ago, when the first CIBA COLLECTION OF MEDICAL ILLUSTRATIONS appeared, the word *nephrologist* could not be found in many medical dictionaries although *cardiologist* and *neurologist* were defined with accuracy. Even as late as 1966 a prestigious text of physiology devoted more than six times as much space to the circulation as it did to "the excretion of urine."

The understanding of cellular morphology gained with the electron microscope, the technics of immunofluorescence, the use of experimental models, and an understanding of physics have helped unravel the true meaning of the kidney in the economy of life. This new knowledge of the pathophysiology of renal disease, combined with the conventional and traditional approaches to the patient and the use of newer diagnostic technics, has enhanced our understanding of this remarkable organ; nephrology has emerged as a discipline as dynamic as the kidney itself.

It must be remembered, though, that today's knowledge is but a transition from the "excretion of urine" to the events of tomorrow. In fact, the rapidity with which our knowledge of the kidney is changing makes it extremely difficult to assemble even a conventional textbook of the kidney which is current when published. With Volume 6, this problem of being up-to-date was compounded by the fact that the immense amount of artwork alone required four years of Dr. Netter's time. One way we have attempted to solve this problem was to have our consultants and collaborators, whenever possible, review their texts while the book was in final (pre-press) assembly stages. However, we were not always successful. For instance, the determination of renal vein renin levels has become more feasible and may well replace the older, split-function tests. Even now, an issue of CIBA CLINICAL SYMPOSIA which discusses renin and renal vein renin levels is under preparation.

Volume 6 of THE CIBA COLLECTION OF MEDICAL ILLUSTRATIONS represents, in many ways, a transition from the old to the new. During the four years that it has been under development many unforeseen changes delayed production. Were it not for the perseverance of Dr. Netter and the continual faith and stamina of the Associate Editors, Dr. E. Lovell Becker and Dr. Jacob Churg, this book might never have come into being.

The work on this volume began in mid-1968 while Dr. Fredrick F. Yonkman (Fritz, to many) was Editor of the CIBA COLLECTION. The original planning and much of the preliminary "spadework" in organization and text editing was done by Dr. Yonkman. However, halfway through preparation, this distinguished editor, who was well past retirement, wished to take a long deserved rest and devote his time to his wife and family, his home in Massachusetts, and his duties as a member of the Board of Trustees of Hope College in Holland, Michigan. He asked me to assume the duties of Editor. Neither he nor I foresaw the difficulties which lay ahead in such a change, and it is a tribute to Dr. Netter, Dr. Becker, and Dr. Churg, especially, and to the consultants and collaborators, as well, that they displayed the patience to wait for me to familiarize myself with the project. We lost considerable momentum during this transitional period and the life of the book was sustained primarily by these able and devoted men.

It is impossible to give credit to all the dedicated men of medicine and science who have in one way or another contributed to this work. Apart from the unnamed hundreds who have influenced Dr. Netter and me, and who have contributed basic research data to nephrology and allied disciplines, there are the associates of our contributors and consultants who have helped in so many ways. In particular, four Subeditors (a terminology which fails to describe adequately their true contribution to this book) deserve special mention. Drs. Johannes A. G. Rhodin and Louis L. Bergmann were responsible as Subeditors for Section I, Anatomy, Structure, and Embryology, Dr. H. O. Heinemann for Section II, Renal Physiology, and Dr. Robert M. Kark for Section III, Diagnostic Technics.

Also, we wish to thank those scientists whose assistance is gratefully acknowledged throughout the text. We are specifically indebted to Dr. Marshall for his clarification of the technic illustrated on page 240, and to Dr. Lapides for his technic, depicted on page 81. In addition, the immunofluorescent preparations furnished by Dr. McCluskey, the microscopic slides by Drs. Williams and Berlyne, the arteriogram by Dr. Robin Watson, and the photomicrograph by Dr. Mostofi (see pages 136, 140, 156, and 181 respectively) are appreciated. Also, we would like to thank the following authors and their publishers for their aid in preparing the following:

Pages 41 and 42—Graphs modified from Pitts[1]
Page 63—Top modified from Rector[2]
Page 158—Modified from Goldblatt
Page 171—Table I modified from Becker[3]
 Table II modified from Schreiner[4]

As if the described changes were not sufficient, the actual production of Volume 6 of the CIBA COLLECTION also represents a transition from the old to the new. This book is the first of the series to be printed by offset, although in the original planning the book began as a letterpress production. We have also introduced modern typography and a new overall appearance which builds upon the tradition established in the preceding books of the series. For the first time in the CIBA COLLECTION, computer-controlled photocomposition has been used, allowing us to make last minute changes with relative impunity. Importantly, this book is printed on a new, whiter, nonglare stock which eliminates the annoying reflections of the older, glossy paper. These changes in production methods required the close cooperation of many people, some of whom have become involved with THE CIBA COLLECTION OF MEDICAL ILLUSTRATIONS for the first time. The cooperation of numerous people on the staffs of Cooper & Beatty, Limited, The Case-Hoyt Corporation, and Cesareo Studio helped ease the CIBA COLLECTION through a difficult period of transition, and the earlier work of Embassy Photo Engraving Co., Inc. in preparing the letterpress engravings must not go unmentioned.

Within the CIBA organization change was also evident for, during the development of this book, the company merged with a former competitor to become CIBA-GEIGY Corporation. Thus, my gratitude to the members of the publication team who also worked with dedication to bring this book through a most difficult time is expressed with the knowledge that more than extra effort was necessary. I am particularly indebted to Mr. Melvin F. Jacolow, Miss Louise Stemmle, Mrs. Helen Sward, and Mrs. Edith Van Allen.

My sincere appreciation is also extended to our editorial and indexing consultants. The copy editing of earlier manuscripts by Mrs. Anne Clark of Destin, Florida is thankfully acknowledged, as is the assistance of Mrs. Kim Richman of New York City for her manuscript editing of the later texts in this volume. I am also especially grateful to Mrs. Julia Stair of Kingston, Massachusetts for her competent work in compiling the index in record time and for her help in proofreading.

Finally, an editor should always say a few words about style and consistency. Throughout we have used Nomina Anatomica as our guide, but the astute reader may find that Nomina Anatomica has not been rigorously followed, either because of personal preference on the part of a contributor, Dr. Netter, or one of the editors. In the interest of good communication, we have attempted to maintain a consistency of style, but undoubtedly the keen-eyed reader will find those imperfections which mar the work of any human.

ROBERT K. SHAPTER, M.D., C.M.

[1] Pitts, RF: *Physiology of the Kidney and Body Fluids*, 2nd ed., Year Book Medical Publishers, Inc., Chicago, 1968 (used with permission of copyright owner)

[2] Rector, FC: *Role of the kidney in the homeostatic control of hydrogen ion concentration in body fluids* in *Proceedings of the XXIII International Congress of Physiological Science*, Tokyo, Excerpta Medica International Congress Series No. 87, 1965

[3] Becker, EL, Editor: *Structural Basis of Renal Disease*, Hoeber Medical Division, Harper and Row, New York, 1968

[4] Schreiner, GE: *Toxic nephropathy. Adverse renal effects caused by drugs and chemicals*, J.A.M.A. 191:145, 1965

Contents

Section I

Anatomy, Structure, and Embryology

Frank H. Netter, M.D.

in collaboration with

Louis L. Bergmann, M.D. and Johannes A. G. Rhodin, M.D., Ph.D.   *Plates 1–24*

G. A. G. Mitchell, O.B.E., T.D., M.B., Ch.M., D.Sc., F.R.C.S.   *Plates 25–27*

J. U. Schlegel, M.D.   *Plate 33*

Yasunosuke Suzuki, M.D.   *Plates 28–32*

Anatomic Relations of the Kidney

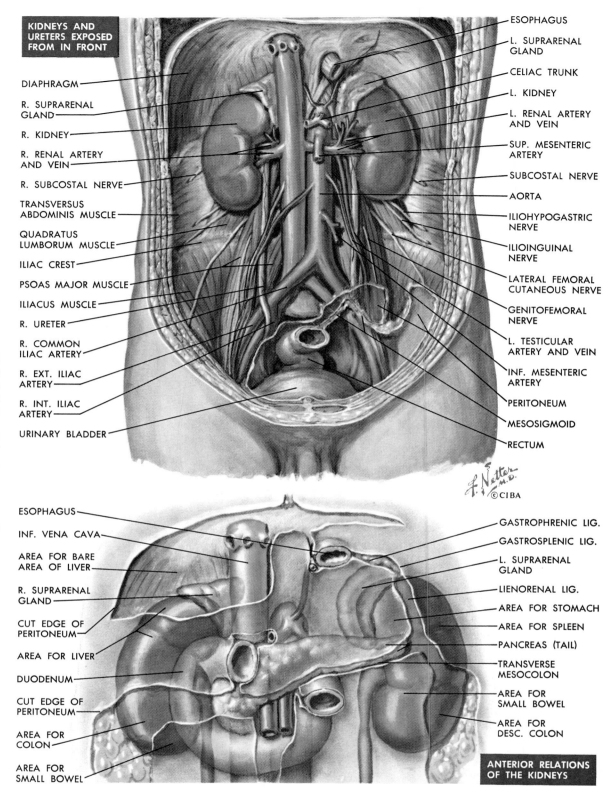

KIDNEYS AND URETERS EXPOSED FROM IN FRONT

DIAPHRAGM

R. SUPRARENAL GLAND

R. KIDNEY

R. RENAL ARTERY AND VEIN

R. SUBCOSTAL NERVE

TRANSVERSUS ABDOMINIS MUSCLE

QUADRATUS LUMBORUM MUSCLE

ILIAC CREST

PSOAS MAJOR MUSCLE

ILIACUS MUSCLE

R. URETER

R. COMMON ILIAC ARTERY

R. EXT. ILIAC ARTERY

R. INT. ILIAC ARTERY

URINARY BLADDER

ESOPHAGUS

L. SUPRARENAL GLAND

CELIAC TRUNK

L. KIDNEY

L. RENAL ARTERY AND VEIN

SUP. MESENTERIC ARTERY

SUBCOSTAL NERVE

AORTA

ILIOHYPOGASTRIC NERVE

ILIOINGUINAL NERVE

LATERAL FEMORAL CUTANEOUS NERVE

GENITOFEMORAL NERVE

L. TESTICULAR ARTERY AND VEIN

INF. MESENTERIC ARTERY

PERITONEUM

MESOSIGMOID

RECTUM

ESOPHAGUS

INF. VENA CAVA

AREA FOR BARE AREA OF LIVER

R. SUPRARENAL GLAND

CUT EDGE OF PERITONEUM

AREA FOR LIVER

DUODENUM

CUT EDGE OF PERITONEUM

AREA FOR COLON

AREA FOR SMALL BOWEL

GASTROPHRENIC LIG.

GASTROSPLENIC LIG.

L. SUPRARENAL GLAND

LIENORENAL LIG.

AREA FOR STOMACH

AREA FOR SPLEEN

PANCREAS (TAIL)

TRANSVERSE MESOCOLON

AREA FOR SMALL BOWEL

AREA FOR DESC. COLON

ANTERIOR RELATIONS OF THE KIDNEYS

The kidneys are a pair of specialized organs located retroperitoneally in the lumbar region. Each kidney is reddish brown in color in the fresh state and is characteristically shaped. The lateral edge is convex while the medial border is concave with a marked depression or notch called the hilus. In the adult, each kidney is about 11 cm long, 2.5 cm thick, 5 cm wide, and weighs between 120 and 170 grams.

Position and Movement

Usually the left kidney lies 1 to 2 cm higher than the right. When the patient is in the supine position, the superior pole of the left kidney is at the level of the twelfth thoracic vertebra while the inferior pole is at the level of the third lumbar vertebra, or between 2.5 and 5 cm superior to the iliac crest. On deep inspiration, or when the patient is in the erect position, both kidneys may descend to, or near, the iliac crest and occasionally lower. If the patient is in a recumbent, head down position, the kidneys can ascend slightly, the left as far as the tenth intercostal space, the right to the eleventh intercostal space.

Because the kidneys are in close anatomic relation to the muscles of the posterior abdominal wall, the oblique course of the psoas muscle causes slight lateral displacement of the lower pole of each kidney. Therefore, if the left kidney is positioned higher than the right, it will be closer to the midline.

The aorta lies anterior to the vertebral column, about 2.5 cm from the left kidney. The inferior vena cava is to the right of and slightly anterior to the aorta and so almost touches the right kidney. Between the two kidneys, in intimate anatomic relation to the aorta, lie the *celiac plexus* and the *ganglia of the autonomic nervous system*. The renal blood vessels, anterior to the renal pelvis, run medially and anteriorly from the hilus of each kidney. Consequently, each kidney is rotated so that the medial surface faces slightly anteriorly and the lateral surface somewhat posteriorly.

A *suprarenal gland* and its blood vessels lie in a layer of connective tissue close to the superior and medial aspect of each kidney. Since each suprarenal gland has

its own fascial support, it does not descend in conjunction with the kidney.

Anterior Relations

The principal anterior relationship of the kidneys is the peritoneum and those organs which, during fetal development, have come to lie in close apposition to the posterior wall of the abdominal cavity and are thus retroperitoneal. On the right, the *hepatic flexure of the colon* and the *duodenum,* and on the left, the *tail of the pancreas* and *splenic flexure of the colon* have become adherent to the respective kidneys and have lost their serosa. The areas of the kidneys in direct contact with these organs, without peritoneal covering, are thus called "bare areas."

The anterior aspect of the left kidney is covered by peritoneum superolaterally. This area assists in forming the *perisplenic peritoneal space* or *left renal fossa.* Peri-

toneum also covers the superior medial surface of the left kidney as a part of the stomach bed, and this area forms the posterior aspect of the *splenic recess of the omental bursa.* The superomedial and superolateral areas of the left kidney are separated from each other by a narrow bare area which provides attachment for the *lienorenal ligament.* Peritoneum also covers the inferior medial portion of the anterior aspect of the left kidney on which the loops of the jejunum rest.

The right kidney extends upward to the level at which the parietal peritoneum reflects onto the liver as the right *coronary ligament.* Below this point the anterior aspect of the right kidney is covered by peritoneum which forms the posterior wall of the *right subhepatic space of Morison.* As noted previously, the inferior third of the right kidney is in close apposition with the right colic flexure, without intervening serosa. Only a small portion of the inferior pole of the right kidney is

Anatomic Relations
of the Kidney

Continued

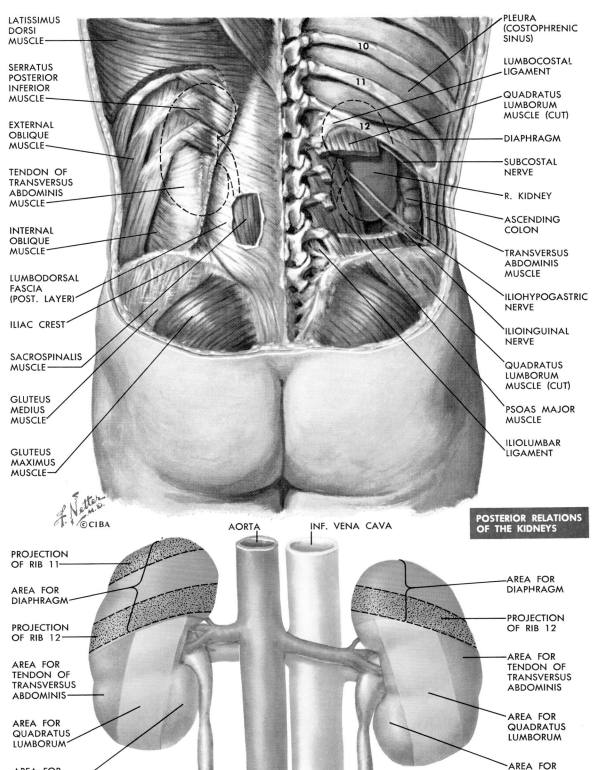

LATISSIMUS DORSI MUSCLE

SERRATUS POSTERIOR INFERIOR MUSCLE

EXTERNAL OBLIQUE MUSCLE

TENDON OF TRANSVERSUS ABDOMINIS MUSCLE

INTERNAL OBLIQUE MUSCLE

LUMBODORSAL FASCIA (POST. LAYER)

ILIAC CREST

SACROSPINALIS MUSCLE

GLUTEUS MEDIUS MUSCLE

GLUTEUS MAXIMUS MUSCLE

PLEURA (COSTOPHRENIC SINUS)

LUMBOCOSTAL LIGAMENT

QUADRATUS LUMBORUM MUSCLE (CUT)

DIAPHRAGM

SUBCOSTAL NERVE

R. KIDNEY

ASCENDING COLON

TRANSVERSUS ABDOMINIS MUSCLE

ILIOHYPOGASTRIC NERVE

ILIOINGUINAL NERVE

QUADRATUS LUMBORUM MUSCLE (CUT)

PSOAS MAJOR MUSCLE

ILIOLUMBAR LIGAMENT

POSTERIOR RELATIONS OF THE KIDNEYS

PROJECTION OF RIB 11

AREA FOR DIAPHRAGM

PROJECTION OF RIB 12

AREA FOR TENDON OF TRANSVERSUS ABDOMINIS

AREA FOR QUADRATUS LUMBORUM

AREA FOR PSOAS MAJOR

AORTA

INF. VENA CAVA

AREA FOR DIAPHRAGM

PROJECTION OF RIB 12

AREA FOR TENDON OF TRANSVERSUS ABDOMINIS

AREA FOR QUADRATUS LUMBORUM

AREA FOR PSOAS MAJOR

covered with serosa on which lie the loops of the small intestine.

Posterior Relations

Posteriorly, approximately the lower two thirds of each kidney primarily rests on the *quadratus lumborum muscle.* Medially, the *psoas muscle,* and laterally, the *aponeurosis* of the *transversus abdominis muscle* form the remainder of the kidney bed. The transverse processes of the first and second lumbar vertebrae are close to the kidney along the lateral edge of the psoas. The right kidney is crossed by the twelfth rib and the left by both the eleventh and twelfth ribs.

When viewed from the posterior aspect, three nerves lie deep to the psoas muscle and emerge from its lateral border as they descend obliquely to the inguinal region. In craniocaudal order, these nerves are the *subcostal (twelfth intercostal) nerve* near the inferior edge of the twelfth rib, and the *upper two segmental nerves of the lumbar plexus*—the *iliohypogastric* and the *ilioinguinal.*

The superior third of the left kidney, and a somewhat smaller portion of the right, are backed by the abdominal surface and lumbocostal arches (or *arcuate ligaments*) of the diaphragm. The fleshy lumbocostal portion of the diaphragm is frequently dehiscent so that the upper renal pole is separated from the rib cage only by fascia and the costophrenic sinus of the pleura, without the presence of interposed musculature.

Extraperitoneal Surgical Approach

The relations of the kidney to the more superficial structures of the back are important for the extraperitoneal approach to the organ, and therefore will be described as encountered from without inward. The procedure will vary with clinical considerations. Beneath the thick skin of the lumbar area, the *posterior layer of the aponeurotic lumbodorsal fascia* occupies a paramedian strip approximately 8 cm wide. The underlying *sacrospinalis muscle* causes this part of the fascia to bulge visibly. Laterally, the lumbodorsal fascia provides the origin for the *middle fibers of the latissimus dorsi muscle.*

The inferior and most lateral fibers of this muscle originate from the iliac crest. The lateral edge of the latissimus dorsi runs superolaterally from this origin, and together with both the almost vertical, posterior, free margin of the *external oblique muscle* and the iliac crest, forms a triangular area of variable size, called the *lumbar triangle of Petit.* The floor of this triangle is the *internal oblique* muscle whose fibers run anterosuperiorly at right angles to those of the external oblique.

When the latissimus dorsi muscle is divided and the edge of the external oblique muscle drawn anteriorly, the origin of the internal oblique muscle is seen to be from the *lateral edge of an aponeurotic sheet,* which is also the tendinous origin of the *transversus abdominis muscle.* This tendinous sheet is actually the product of fusion of all three layers of the lumbodorsal fascia. It is visible in an area bounded medially by the fascia-

covered sacrospinalis, laterally by the ascending fibers of the internal oblique muscle, and cranially by the twelfth rib. This area overlies the kidney and is called the *surgical lumbar triangle.* However, the fibers of the serratus posterior inferior muscle, attached to the twelfth rib, interfere with the triangular shape of the region.

The aponeurotic sheet in the surgical lumbar triangle must be divided, thus exposing the lateral edge of the *quadratus lumborum muscle* and the nerves derived from the twelfth thoracic and first lumbar segments. It should be noted that the inferior margin of the pleural costophrenic sinus crosses the twelfth rib approximately in the midscapular line, a relationship of significance whether or not the rib is being resected. The renal fascia, lateral to the edge of the quadratus lumborum muscle, is now exposed, except for a scanty cover of pararenal fat. □

Renal Fascia

TRANSVERSALIS FASCIA
DESCENDING COLON
PERITONEUM
LEFT KIDNEY
DUODENO-JEJUNAL FLEXURE
AORTA
PANCREAS
INF. VENA CAVA
DUODENUM
RIGHT KIDNEY
HEPATIC FLEXURE OF COLON
LIVER
EXT. AND INT. OBLIQUE MUSCLES
TRANSVERSUS ABDOMINIS TENDON
LATISSIMUS DORSI
PARARENAL (RETROPERITONEAL) FAT
PERIRENAL FAT
TRUE CAPSULE OF KIDNEY
RENAL FASCIA
PSOAS MAJOR MUSCLE AND FASCIA
SACROSPINALIS
QUADRATUS LUMBORUM
DIAPHRAGM

TRANSVERSE SECTION THROUGH 2nd LUMBAR VERTEBRA, DEMONSTRATING HORIZONTAL DISPOSITION OF RENAL FASCIA

DIAPHRAGM
DIAPHRAGMATIC FASCIA
COSTOPHRENIC SINUS
SUPRARENAL GLAND
PERIRENAL FAT
12th RIB
PARARENAL (RETRO-PERITONEAL) FAT
TRANSVERSALIS FASCIA
QUADRATUS LUMBORUM
ILIAC CREST
LUNG
LIVER
BARE AREA OF LIVER
TRUE CAPSULE OF KIDNEY
PERITONEUM
ANTERIOR AND POSTERIOR LAYERS OF RENAL FASCIA
RIGHT KIDNEY
HEPATIC FLEXURE OF COLON

SAGITTAL SECTION THROUGH R. KIDNEY AND LUMBAR REGION, DEMONSTRATING VERTICAL DISPOSITION OF RENAL FASCIA

The renal parenchyma is enclosed in a thin, fibrous, glistening membrane which represents a *true capsule.* This membrane can be stripped off easily and cleanly from the normal parenchyma. Outside this true capsule, one finds the *adipose capsule,* known as *perirenal fat.* This layer of fat varies in thickness and is traversed by sparse strands of connective tissue. Enclosing the perirenal fat is the *fibrous renal fascia of Gerota,* usually referred to as "renal fascia." This fascia separates the perirenal fat from other extraperitoneal fat found in the region of the kidney, which is called *pararenal fat.*

The fibrous renal fascia consists of a strong posterior and a more delicate anterior layer. These two layers join lateral to the kidney, and as they extend laterally blend with retroperitoneal tissues. According to Tobin, the *transversalis fascia* in this area is considered a separate structure, closely related to the parietes of the abdomen and not to the perivisceral and retroperitoneal tissues.

Anterior to the kidney, the fibrous renal fascia is thin, while near the midline it is even more elusive and fuses with the sheaths of the renal pelvis and renal blood vessels, with the sheath of the aorta, and with the sheath of the inferior vena cava.

Cranially, the renal fascia forms a fairly closed envelope for the kidney, although there is no general agreement on this point. It is agreed, however, that the fascia continues cranially, posterior to the suprarenal gland. Anterior to this gland the

fascia is thin and continuous with the connective tissue of the *diaphragmatic fascia* bilaterally, and with that of the bare area of the liver on the right.

Superior to the suprarenal gland, the anterior and posterior layers appear connected with each other, and an additional, tenuous, fascial layer separates this gland from the kidney.

Inferior to the kidneys, the compartment of the renal fascia is closed, except medially, where the ureteral sheaths descend as caudal extensions of the renal fascial apparatus. In contradiction to this description, the radiologist can perform perirenal pneumography by injecting air into the *presacral connective tissue* from the midline; the air apparently can pass, from here, freely upward between the two layers of the renal fascia (see page 99).

The results of the studies on renal fascia militate against the idea of a single "correct" version of its

anatomy. The fascia itself is tenuous and elusive, except posterolaterally, and has little similarity to the well-defined fasciae of skeletal muscles.

Moreover, one should keep in mind that connective tissue systems, such as the renal or the pelvic fasciae, lie in areas subject to heavy surgical traffic. Therefore, careful, leisurely dissection of fixed cadaver material in the laboratory cannot be compared, with assurance, to the findings in living tissues after blunt exposure on the operating table, or to the anatomical architecture revealed by frozen sections. In addition, problems of terminology, special stereotyped technics or points of view, and variations and changes because of age can contribute further to disagreement and even to outright confusion. Tobin's study of the renal fascia has gained wide acceptance, and his work has been relied upon to a considerable extent in the preceding description. □

Gross Structure of the Kidney

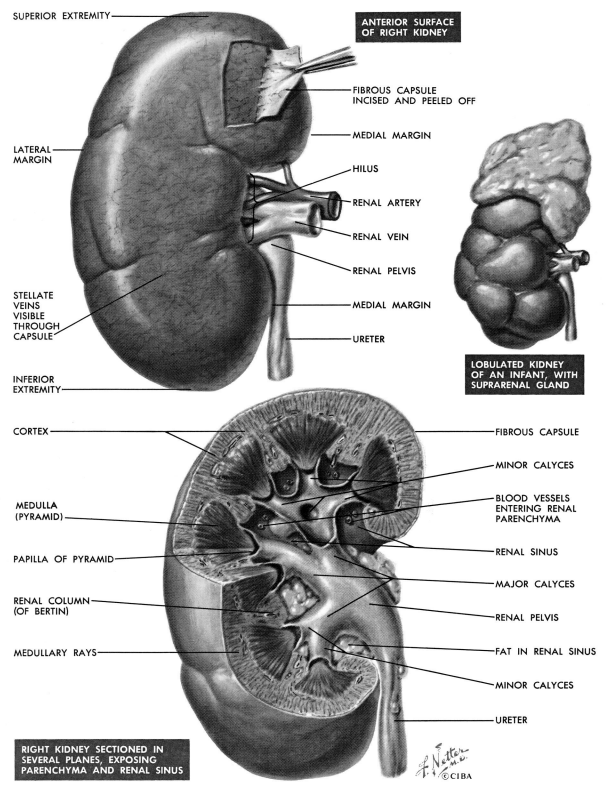

SUPERIOR EXTREMITY

ANTERIOR SURFACE OF RIGHT KIDNEY

FIBROUS CAPSULE INCISED AND PEELED OFF

MEDIAL MARGIN

HILUS

RENAL ARTERY

RENAL VEIN

RENAL PELVIS

MEDIAL MARGIN

URETER

LATERAL MARGIN

STELLATE VEINS VISIBLE THROUGH CAPSULE

INFERIOR EXTREMITY

LOBULATED KIDNEY OF AN INFANT, WITH SUPRARENAL GLAND

CORTEX

MEDULLA (PYRAMID)

PAPILLA OF PYRAMID

RENAL COLUMN (OF BERTIN)

MEDULLARY RAYS

FIBROUS CAPSULE

MINOR CALYCES

BLOOD VESSELS ENTERING RENAL PARENCHYMA

RENAL SINUS

MAJOR CALYCES

RENAL PELVIS

FAT IN RENAL SINUS

MINOR CALYCES

URETER

RIGHT KIDNEY SECTIONED IN SEVERAL PLANES, EXPOSING PARENCHYMA AND RENAL SINUS

Both the anterior and posterior surfaces of the kidney are convex, although a slight flattening of the surface may be noted posteriorly. The poles are rounded, the convex lateral edge is blunt, and the concave medial margin is deeply indented by the *hilus* which, in turn, leads into a spacious cavity, called the *renal sinus*. The renal sinus is surrounded by the kidney parenchyma and within it lie the major branches of the renal artery, the major tributaries of the renal vein, and the major and minor calyces of the collecting system. The hilus is lined by a fibrous membrane, continuous with both the true capsule and the fibrous coats of the renal vessels and collecting system. The remainder of the renal sinus is filled with adipose tissue.

The parenchyma of the kidney consists of a brownish pink *cortex* and a number of parenchymatous cones of a deeper color, called collectively the *medulla.* Each cone or *medullary pyramid* is situated with the base toward the periphery. The apex ends as a *renal papilla* toward the renal sinus.

The parenchyma served by one papilla is known as a renal lobe, and in the fetus and infant, it is outlined on the surface by a marked groove. Such a lobulated kidney *(ren lobatus)* persists in some mammalian species (ox, bear) throughout life and may occasionally be present in the human adult, although to a lesser degree. On the other hand, some species, such as the mouse and rat, possess unilobar kidneys.

The cortical areas which separate the pyramids from the surface are known as *cortical arches,* while the areas of cortex between the pyramids are called the *renal (cortical) columns of Bertin.* *

*The term "column" refers to the appearance of these cortical areas on the cut surface. As three-dimensional structures, they may be compared to the packing material in a carton of eggs, the latter being represented by the medullary pyramids whose apices stick out from the surrounding stuffing into the renal sinus.

The margins of the pyramids adjoining the renal columns are well defined, while the bases of the pyramids interdigitate with the cortex by long and delicate processes called the *medullary rays (of Ferrein).* Each medullary ray represents a *lobule,* and about 20,000 such lobules are present in each kidney.

Radial striation, apparent in each pyramid and especially well marked near the renal papilla, represents *collecting ducts.* These empty, as *papillary ducts of Bellini,* through 20 or more small pores onto the surface of the papilla *(area cribrosa).* Through these pores the urine oozes into the minor calyces.

A papilla may be connected with two and possibly more pyramids, so that the pyramids outnumber the papillae, of which there are eight to 18 in a kidney.

After leaving the papillary ducts, the urine is carried by a succession of fibromuscular tubes lined by mucous membrane. One, two, or three papillae project into

a *minor calyx.* The epithelial lining of the minor calyx is continuous with that of the mucous membrane of the papilla, and the outer fibrous coat blends with the renal capsule which lines the sinus. Two to four minor calyces join and form a *major calyx.* The resulting two or three major calyces join into the funnel-shaped *renal pelvis,* which becomes the *ureter* soon after leaving the hilus.

The muscular coat of the calyces is arranged in spirals which apparently assist in "milking" the urine out of the papillae. The mode of ramification of the major and minor calyces is variable but is nevertheless of great clinical interest.

At the hilus, the renal pelvis lies posterior to the renal vessels. It can be approached from behind with relative safety because the posterior vascular branches gain the dorsal surface of the pelvis and calyces deeper within the renal sinus. □

The Nephron

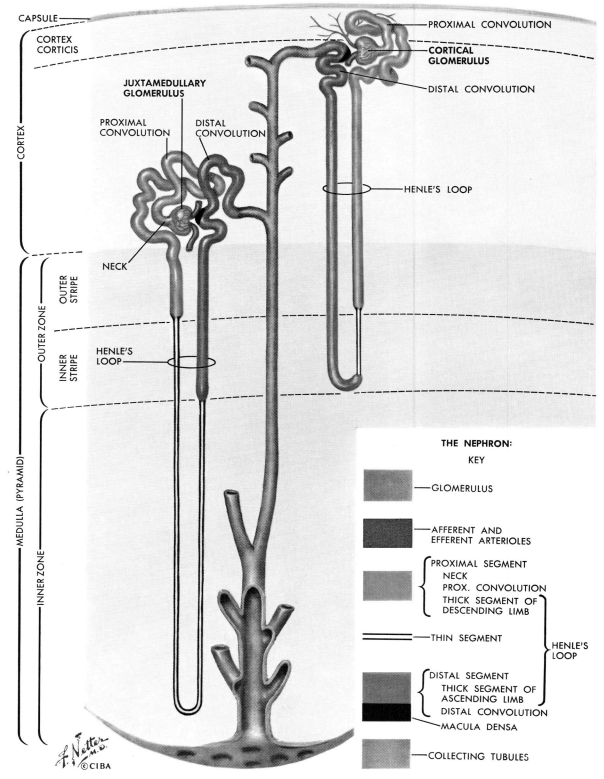

CAPSULE

CORTEX CORTICIS

CORTEX

JUXTAMEDULLARY GLOMERULUS

PROXIMAL CONVOLUTION

DISTAL CONVOLUTION

NECK

OUTER STRIPE

OUTER ZONE

INNER STRIPE

HENLE'S LOOP

MEDULLA (PYRAMID)

INNER ZONE

PROXIMAL CONVOLUTION

CORTICAL GLOMERULUS

DISTAL CONVOLUTION

HENLE'S LOOP

F. Netter M.D. ©CIBA

THE NEPHRON:

KEY

— GLOMERULUS

— AFFERENT AND EFFERENT ARTERIOLES

— PROXIMAL SEGMENT
NECK
PROX. CONVOLUTION
THICK SEGMENT OF DESCENDING LIMB

— THIN SEGMENT

HENLE'S LOOP

— DISTAL SEGMENT
THICK SEGMENT OF ASCENDING LIMB
DISTAL CONVOLUTION

— MACULA DENSA

— COLLECTING TUBULES

Each kidney is composed of between 1 million and 3 million tubular structures called *nephrons*. The relationship of each nephron to the vascular bed of the kidney is characteristic and indicates the function of the kidney, namely, regulation of the composition of the body fluids.

The nephron begins with a *renal corpuscle* (of Malpighi), a rounded body about 0.2 mm in diameter. Its bulk is formed by a skein of minute vessels, the *glomerulus*, responsible for the red color that makes the corpuscle visible to the unaided eye. The glomerulus is invaginated into the *glomerular* or *Bowman's capsule*, an epithelial sac formed by a single layer of cells. The sac receives the filtrate of the blood from the glomerular vessels.

A *vascular pole* of the corpuscle can be recognized where the *afferent arteriole* enters and an *efferent arteriole* leaves the glomerulus. The *urinary pole* is diametrically opposite the vascular pole at a site where the capsule narrows into a *tubule* which follows a typical path. The single-layered epithelium is retained, but finer histological alterations occur with great regularity along the course of all nephrons. Complex interactions between the vascular bed and the tubular epithelium account for the definitive composition of the urine, which differs profoundly from the glomerular filtrate (see pages 51–59).

The portion of the tubule adjoining the renal corpuscle is termed *proximal convoluted tubule* because it follows a very tortuous course without straying very far from its point of departure. The tubule then straightens and forms the *loop of Henle* by taking a direct course toward the center of the kidney, making a hairpin turn, and returning in a straight line to the vascular pole of its parent renal corpuscle. It now forms the *distal convoluted tubule* which becomes an *arched collecting tubule*. The nephrons join in forming *straight collecting tubules*, situated in the medullary rays of the cortex. In the inner part of the medulla, straight tubules unite to form larger ducts. By a succession of about seven such junctions, the large *papillary ducts of Bellini* are formed. These appear on the surface of the papillae.

The nephrons, while essentially similar to each other, differ in length. The shorter ones have their corpuscles in the more superficial reaches of the cortex and their loops of Henle extend only into the outer zone of the medulla. The longer nephrons begin close to the medulla as *juxtamedullary glomeruli*. Their loops extend deeply into the medulla and may almost reach the papilla.

The cortex owes its fine granular texture to the presence of glomeruli, capillary nets, and the masses of irregularly convoluted tubules. The medullary rays are macroscopically visible because they consist of parallel arrays of collecting tubules and Henle's loops. (The rays are separated from each other by cortical tissue.) The aggregate of the nephrons of one medullary ray constitutes a renal lobule.

The striated sector, near the apex of a sectioned pyramid, is called the *inner* or *papillary* zone of the medulla. The striations are caused by straight collecting ducts and vessels, which run in a radial direction through the pyramid, and by long, thin-walled loops of Henle. The *outer zone* of the medulla is characterized by the presence of thick parts of Henle's loops and the absence of very large collecting ducts. In the rat and a number of other species, this zone is further subdivided into an inner and outer stripe, but these demarcations are indistinct in man.

The anatomy and disposition of the nephrons have been investigated by various methods other than ordinary microscopy. Three-dimensional reconstructions of individual nephrons, as well as micromanipulative methods, have made it possible to observe individual nephrons *in toto*. Experimental microsurgery on parts of nephrons and electron microscopy have yielded new insights into the fine structure and the functions of the nephrons (see pages 8–13). □

Histology of Renal Corpuscle

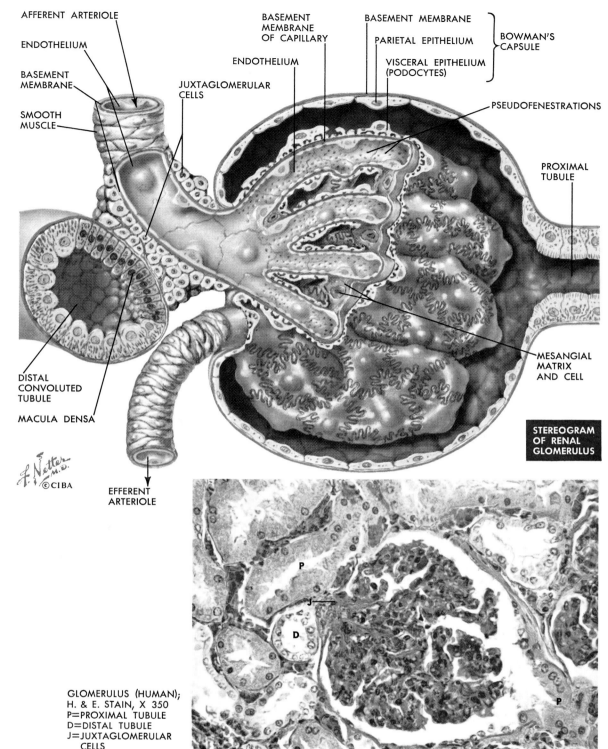

AFFERENT ARTERIOLE

ENDOTHELIUM

BASEMENT MEMBRANE

SMOOTH MUSCLE

JUXTAGLOMERULAR CELLS

BASEMENT MEMBRANE OF CAPILLARY

ENDOTHELIUM

BASEMENT MEMBRANE

PARIETAL EPITHELIUM

VISCERAL EPITHELIUM (PODOCYTES)

BOWMAN'S CAPSULE

PSEUDOFENESTRATIONS

PROXIMAL TUBULE

MESANGIAL MATRIX AND CELL

DISTAL CONVOLUTED TUBULE

MACULA DENSA

EFFERENT ARTERIOLE

STEREOGRAM OF RENAL GLOMERULUS

GLOMERULUS (HUMAN); H. & E. STAIN, X 350
P=PROXIMAL TUBULE
D=DISTAL TUBULE
J=JUXTAGLOMERULAR CELLS

The renal corpuscles are easily identifiable by the unaided eye in the routine histologic section stained with hematoxylin and eosin stain *(H. and E. Stain)*. In preparations removed at autopsy, the capillaries of the renal corpuscle, collectively called the glomerulus, appear partly filled with red blood cells, while the urinary space of Bowman's capsule is usually collapsed and difficult to see. In a normal glomerulus, neither individual cells (or cell types) nor connective tissue components, such as basement membranes and collagen, are readily distinguished. However, even a slightly diseased glomerulus will show signs of one or the other component being increased in size and number beyond normal.

The topography of individual components of the renal corpuscle has been clarified and mapped only recently. This followed the successful analysis by low magnification electron microscopy of entire corpuscles in serial sections. However, before discussing the details of the renal corpuscle, it is necessary to explain the relationship of its components.

The *afferent arteriole* contains a *tunica media* of smooth muscle cells arranged in about two layers. Near the renal corpuscle, some of the smooth muscle cells contain granules. These granules, displaying an inner crystalline structure, are probably precursors of some secretory product, generally considered to represent angiotensin, as well as erythropoietin. All smooth muscle cells are transformed into secretory cells just before the afferent arteriole disappears within the renal corpuscle.

The number of such granulated smooth muscle cells can vary greatly, and the number of granules may be dependent on the concentration of sodium in the blood plasma. However, it has been discovered that in the kidney of some rodents (rat) the *juxtaglomerular cells* of the *juxtamedullary nephrons* lack secretory granules, but the functional significance of this is not understood.

The juxtaglomerular cells of the afferent arteriole are in direct contact with the arteriolar endothelium on one side, and on the other side with the cells of the *macula densa*. This latter structure is the distal convoluted tubule contacting its own renal corpuscle (see page 6). Renal physiologists today interpret this relationship to be of great functional significance (see page 49).

Once inside the renal corpuscle, the afferent arteriole sheds its juxtaglomerular cells. It then gives rise to three to six capillary branches which, in turn, divide into smaller capillaries, the *glomerulus* or the *rete mirabile* of the renal corpuscle. Microdissections have demonstrated that the human glomerulus contains *capillary lobules*, the number determined by the initial large capillary branches. Eventually, the capillaries assemble to form an *efferent arteriole* which has only one layer of smooth muscle cells, devoid of secretory granules.

The glomerular capillaries anastomose freely. The anastomoses are usually rather narrow capillary channels, which initially led some investigators to conclude that they were too small to allow passage of erythrocytes, and that the plasma only "skimmed" through these structures.

During their course through the renal corpuscle, the capillaries are covered on at least three sides by the *visceral epithelial cells*, also called *podocytes* or *visceral cells* of the capsule of Bowman. By a special arrangement, extremely difficult to understand, the fourth side of the *main branches* of the *capillary* usually faces the central part of the glomerulus, the *glomerular stalk*. Here the deep cell or *mesangial cell* is located. The small branches of the capillaries, particularly in the periphery of each capillary lobule, are surrounded on all sides by the podocytes, as can be seen in some of the capillaries.

In order to understand the fine details that underlie some of the functions of the renal glomerular capillaries, it is necessary to discuss more thoroughly the electron microscopy of the glomerulus. □

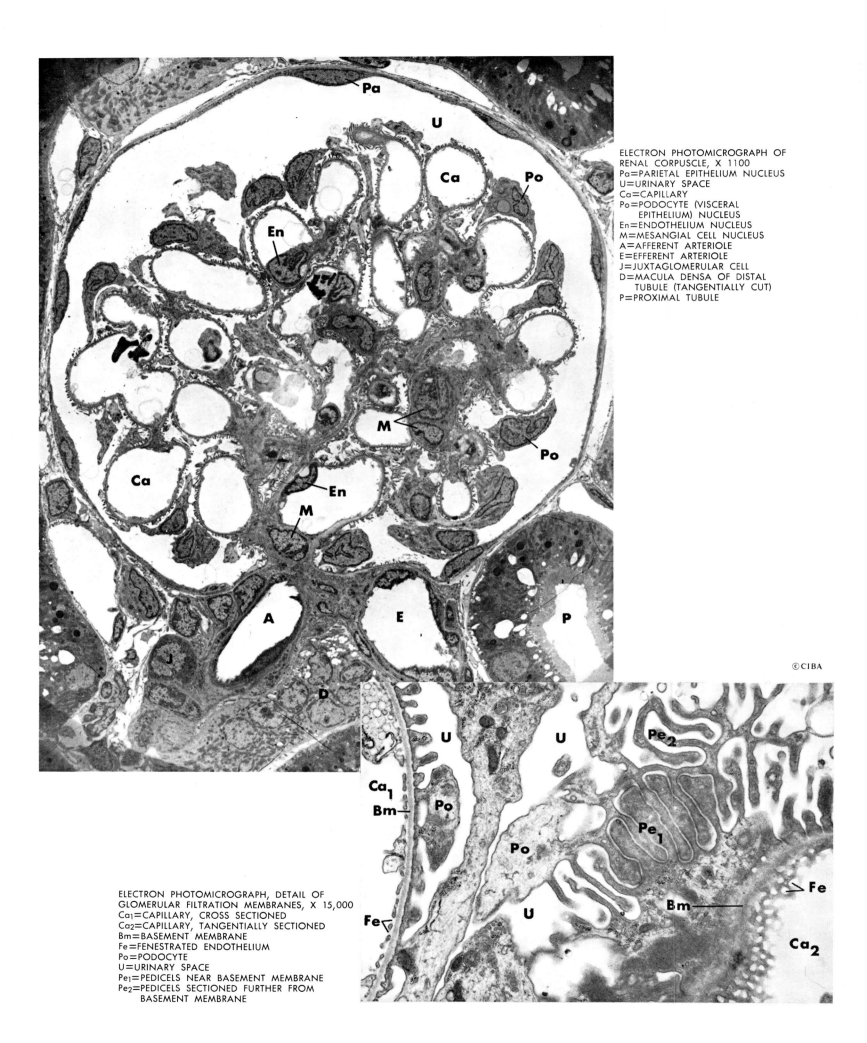

ELECTRON PHOTOMICROGRAPH OF
RENAL CORPUSCLE, X 1100
Pa=PARIETAL EPITHELIUM NUCLEUS
U=URINARY SPACE
Ca=CAPILLARY
Po=PODOCYTE (VISCERAL
    EPITHELIUM) NUCLEUS
En=ENDOTHELIUM NUCLEUS
M=MESANGIAL CELL NUCLEUS
A=AFFERENT ARTERIOLE
E=EFFERENT ARTERIOLE
J=JUXTAGLOMERULAR CELL
D=MACULA DENSA OF DISTAL
    TUBULE (TANGENTIALLY CUT)
P=PROXIMAL TUBULE

©CIBA

ELECTRON PHOTOMICROGRAPH, DETAIL OF
GLOMERULAR FILTRATION MEMBRANES, X 15,000
Ca$_1$=CAPILLARY, CROSS SECTIONED
Ca$_2$=CAPILLARY, TANGENTIALLY SECTIONED
Bm=BASEMENT MEMBRANE
Fe=FENESTRATED ENDOTHELIUM
Po=PODOCYTE
U=URINARY SPACE
Pe$_1$=PEDICELS NEAR BASEMENT MEMBRANE
Pe$_2$=PEDICELS SECTIONED FURTHER FROM
    BASEMENT MEMBRANE

Fine Structure of Renal Corpuscle

The glomerular capillaries are lined by an *attenuated endothelium*, containing regularly spaced *fenestrations* with an average diameter of 700 Å. Most of these fenestrations are open, but a large number, called *pseudofenestrations,* are closed by a thin diaphragm containing a central knob. The nucleus of the endothelial cell is usually located in that part of the capillary wall facing the central part of the glomerulus, the glomerular stalk.

This attenuated layer of *endothelial cells* comprises the *first component* of the capillary wall. The *central or second component* is a continuous *basement membrane,* probably formed by endothelial and epithelial cells (podocytes). Covering the outside of the capillary, the *podocytes* represent the *third component.*

The podocytes are highly specialized. Their cytoplasm is elaborately drawn out to form *pedicels,* or *foot processes,* which attach to the surface of the basement membrane and, at the same time, interdigitate with similar pedicels from other podocytes. The interdigitation is very close near the basement membrane *(Pe₁, see facing page)* where the bases of the pedicels flatten out slightly. This is in contrast to levels slightly away from the basement membrane *(Pe₂, see facing page).* A thin membrane, or *connecting web,* reinforced by a *median filamentous ridge,* lies between the individual pedicels.

The micrograph of the entire glomerulus shows how the pedicels extend under the main cell mass of the podocyte, where the podocyte sits as a protective "umbrella" over the pedicels and the rest of the capillary wall.

The *central stalk* of the glomerulus is occupied by *deep mesangial cells* which have distinct relations to the branching capillaries. The mesangial cell is located mostly near that part of the capillary facing the center of the glomerulus and borders directly on the endothelial cell. Only rarely is a basement membrane interposed between the two. However, the mesangial cell is often associated with accumulations of *basement membranelike material,* referred to as *mesangial stroma* or *matrix.*

The *function* of the capillary wall, or as it is often called, the *glomerular filtration membrane,* is to allow for an ultrafiltration of the blood. In separating the formed elements of the blood and the large protein molecules from the rest of

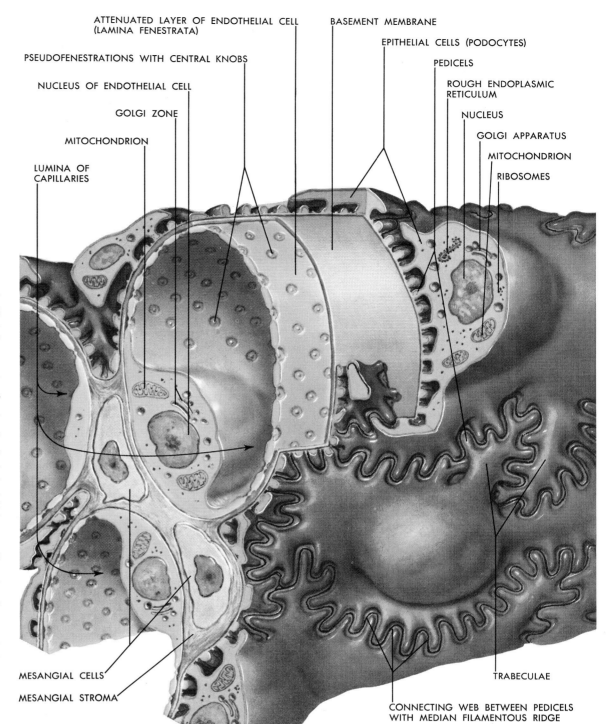

STEREOGRAM OF SEGMENT OF GLOMERULAR CAPILLARIES

the plasma, it delivers the plasma as *primary urine* to the urinary space of Bowman's capsule. The mechanism involved in this filtration process is not fully understood, since it is not known to what extent the different components of the filtration membrane actively participate in the process.

The formed elements of the blood are obviously rejected by the entire filtration membrane, while most of the large protein molecules can pass through the endothelial fenestrations but are stopped by the basement membrane. Medium-sized protein molecules penetrate the basement membrane but cannot pass through either the connecting web or the extremely small space between the pedicels, often called the slit pore. Small protein molecules (molecular weight of 70,000 and less) escape across the filtration membrane easily and most likely utilize the route between the pedicels for their crossing. The extremely long slit pore

between the pedicels therefore represents the ultimate obstacle to most molecules with a molecular weight above 70,000, and its very presence forces filtration to take place through it. Indirect evidence supporting this theory is found in the fact that when the slit pore disappears, as in certain glomerular diseases, even medium-sized and large protein molecules appear in the primary urine, probably utilizing a direct path across an impaired podocyte plasma membrane.

The mesangial cell, related to the *pericyte* of capillaries elsewhere, forms and maintains its own basement membrane or mesangial matrix. In addition, it retains the ability to form collagen which often becomes evident in the diseased glomerulus. The formation of the glomerular basement membrane is probably accomplished by both the epithelial and the endothelial cells, whereas the removal of the basement membrane is probably done by the mesangial cell. □

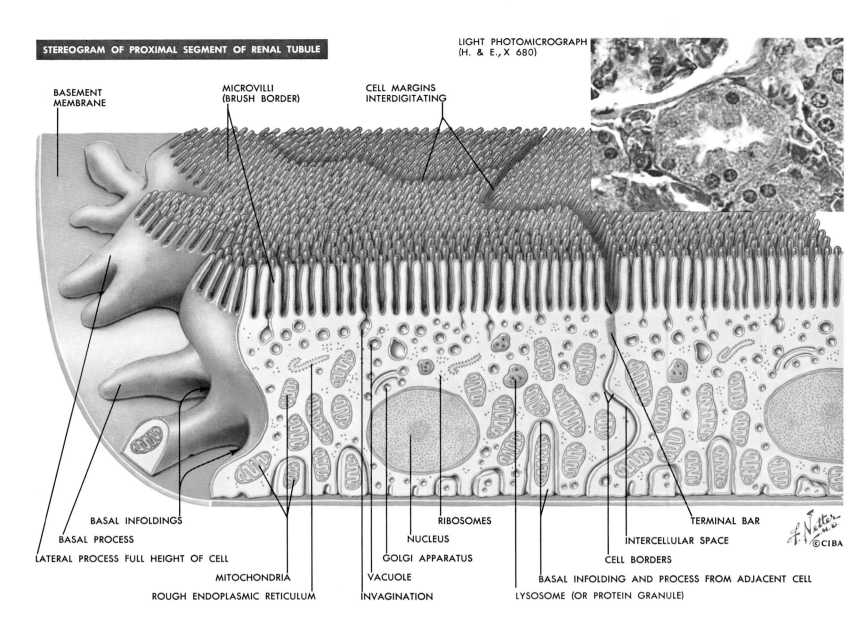

STEREOGRAM OF PROXIMAL SEGMENT OF RENAL TUBULE

LIGHT PHOTOMICROGRAPH
(H. & E., X 680)

BASEMENT
MEMBRANE

MICROVILLI
(BRUSH BORDER)

CELL MARGINS
INTERDIGITATING

BASAL INFOLDINGS

BASAL PROCESS

LATERAL PROCESS FULL HEIGHT OF CELL

MITOCHONDRIA

ROUGH ENDOPLASMIC RETICULUM

RIBOSOMES

NUCLEUS

GOLGI APPARATUS

VACUOLE

INVAGINATION

TERMINAL BAR

INTERCELLULAR SPACE

CELL BORDERS

BASAL INFOLDING AND PROCESS FROM ADJACENT CELL

LYSOSOME (OR PROTEIN GRANULE)

Proximal Segment of Renal Tubule

The proximal segment of a renal tubule is highly convoluted in its most cortical part, but as it turns toward the medulla it straightens. This straight portion is called the thick segment of the descending limb (see page 6). Both the convoluted part and the straight part are similar in structure, and there is only slight variation in the size and shape of the cells. However, numerous peritubular capillaries surround the convoluted portion.

Viewed in cross section with a light microscope, the proximal segment is round or oval, with a single layer of cells surrounding a central, irregularly shaped lumen. The cells of the tubular wall have granular cytoplasm, which with *H. and E.* stains appears strongly eosinophilic because of the large number of mitochondria. The cell margins facing the lumen have an irregular, furry, brush border. Several (four to six) nuclei may be seen in any one section, but lateral (intercellular) borders are indistinct. This apparent absence of lateral cell borders is caused by the intriguing pattern of *lateral interdigitation,* so typical of cells of both proximal and distal segments of the nephron. Primarily it is an interdigitation of the uneven *lateral portions (lateral processes)* of the cells, further elaborated

by variously shaped *basal cellular processes.* These cell processes, extending from the lateral and basal surfaces of the cell, thus become intertwined with similar processes from a neighboring cell. In the straight part of the proximal segment there are fewer lateral and basal interdigitations, but the pattern remains the same as in the convoluted portion.

The cells are held together by a junctional complex, classically referred to as the *terminal bar,* which maintains the luminal parts of the cell in close contact. One component of this complex, the *zonula occludens (tight junction),* in fact, prevents material present in the tubular lumen from escaping between the tubular cells.

The *luminal surface area* is greatly increased by the large number of *microvilli,* collectively called the brush border. The microvilli are approximately the same length throughout the proximal segment. There is, however, a tendency for the microvilli to become slightly longer in the straight part. In addition, the height of the cell decreases somewhat in this portion. Consequently, in the convoluted part of the proximal segment, the length of the microvilli is about one third the height of the rest of the cell, while in the straight portion the length of the microvilli is almost one half the cell height.

A *basal lamina* or *basement membrane* surrounds the proximal segment. It is continuous with the same structure in the capsule of Bowman. Since

there are few fibroblasts in the interstitial spaces of the cortex, the basal lamina is probably formed by epithelial cells. The thickness is about 1000 Å in the adult, but this increases with age and in reaction to different diseases.

In the living state, the proximal segment of the tubule is widely distended, and thus, the lumen is wide open and round. However, the slightest decrease in urinary filtration pressure causes a reduction in tubular diameter, and with cessation of filtration, a total collapse of the lumen. This explains the irregular lumen in histological preparations and the absence of a lumen in some of the early electron microscope preparations.

Functionally, the cells of the proximal segment are largely engaged in *reabsorbing* fluid and material from the *primary urine.* The reabsorbed substances are passed on to the interstitial spaces and to the peritubular capillaries. To a minor degree, certain substances, such as drugs or material foreign to the body, are passed across the epithelial cells in the opposite direction.

The *luminal surface,* greatly increased by the numerous *microvilli,* facilitates the reabsorption of fluid and small molecular weight substances. In turn, the *lateral* and *basal cell processes* (interdigitations) greatly increase the *basal cell surface.* They thus offer a large surface area upon or within which enzymatic reactions can take place, and across which an exchange between the cell and its extratubular environment is facilitated.

Proximal Segment of Renal Tubule
Continued

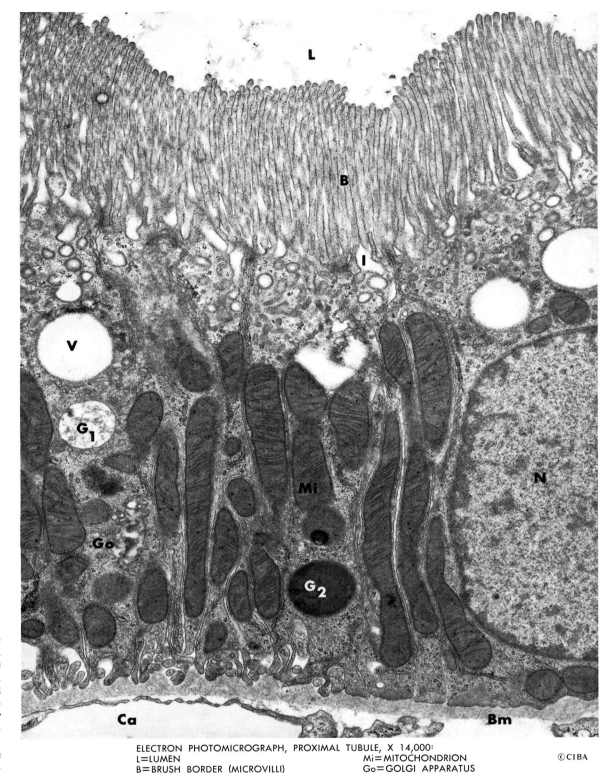

ELECTRON PHOTOMICROGRAPH, PROXIMAL TUBULE, X 14,000:
L=LUMEN
B=BRUSH BORDER (MICROVILLI)
I=INVAGINATION
V=VACUOLE
G_1, G_2=GRANULES OF VARYING DENSITY
Mi=MITOCHONDRION
Go=GOLGI APPARATUS
N=NUCLEUS
Bm=BASEMENT MEMBRANE
Ca=CAPILLARY LUMEN

©CIBA

The *microvilli* are covered by the *plasma membrane*, a *lipoprotein lamina* with a superficial *carbohydrate covering*. The transport of certain substances across this plasma membrane requires enzymatic activity, most of which is probably provided for by enzymes built into the membrane itself. Larger molecules which cannot traverse the plasma membrane are taken up near the bases of the microvilli by small *tubular invaginations* of the surface plasma membrane. This phenomenon, referred to as *micropinocytosis*, is found not only in the cells of the proximal segment of the nephron, but in many other cell types that exist throughout the mammalian body.

Following the uptake of the substance by tubular invagination, the entire structure is detached from the surface of the cell and transported to the interior of the cell. The ensuing sequence of events is not fully understood, and the following description is mostly conjectural, based on the most logical manner of interpreting some of the structures observed.

The tiny, now detached, former invaginations enlarge to form *vacuoles*, the cores of which appear empty but may contain fluid. Subsequently, the content of such vacuoles becomes denser (G_1) and finally appears solid (G_2). As such, these granules are either stored in the cell or extruded at the lumen of the tubule. There is no evidence for such extrusion at the base of the cell. Some of the dense granules may also represent *lysosomes*, which are bodies containing lytic enzymes as part of the cellular defense mechanism against foreign substances. In similarity to what

occurs in a macrophage or a leukocyte, where lysosomes are in abundance, the renal lysosomes may join with the detached *pinocytotic vacuole* to form a unit engaged in intracellular digestion of the reabsorbed substance.

Energy is required for all the activities of these cells. This is supplied by the numerous mitochondria of the cells, many of which are long and slender. The proximity of the mitochondria to the basal and lateral interdigitating cell processes with their covering plasma membrane is taken as strong evidence for the hypothesis that energy is required to complete the transport of fluid and substances which pass across the basal plasma membrane.

A *Golgi apparatus* is generally considered to be associated with secretory processes of a cell. In the prox-

imal segment, the Golgi apparatus is small. It is probably engaged only in secretory processes related to the manufacturing of substances needed for sustaining life of the cell.

The amount of *rough-surfaced endoplasmic reticulum* is small, but the number of *free ribosomes* is high, indicating that the presence of the latter is required for protein synthesis within the cell.

Little is known about which structures are involved in passing substances from the capillary, across the tubular epithelium, to the lumen of the tubule. However, there is every reason to believe that small molecules can traverse the plasma membrane in the opposite direction, and that the many vacuoles of the cell may be engaged in aiding the passage across the cell toward the lumen. □

Thin Segment of Renal Tubule

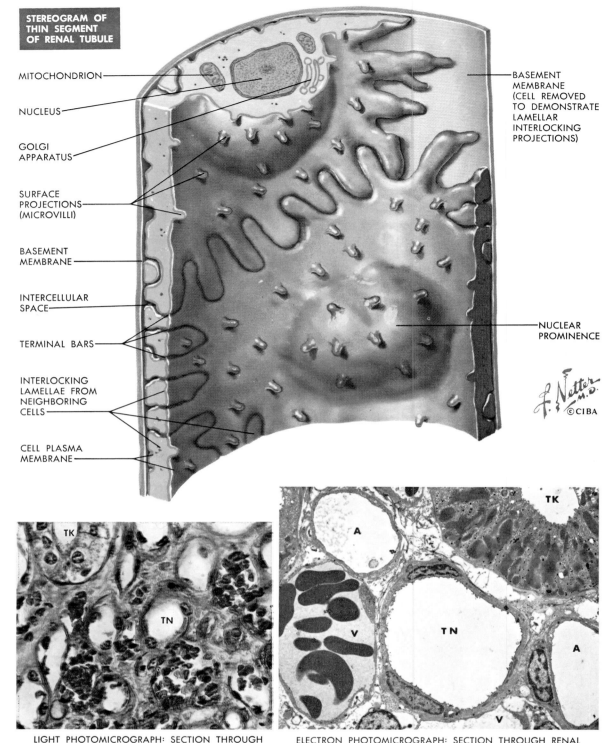

MITOCHONDRION

NUCLEUS

GOLGI APPARATUS

SURFACE PROJECTIONS (MICROVILLI)

BASEMENT MEMBRANE

INTERCELLULAR SPACE

TERMINAL BARS

INTERLOCKING LAMELLAE FROM NEIGHBORING CELLS

CELL PLASMA MEMBRANE

BASEMENT MEMBRANE (CELL REMOVED TO DEMONSTRATE LAMELLAR INTERLOCKING PROJECTIONS)

NUCLEAR PROMINENCE

The thin segment is a direct continuation of the straight descending part of the proximal segment. As indicated (see page 6), the cortical nephrons have very short thin segments, whereas juxtamedullary nephrons have long thin segments. There are probably functional differences between the two types of thin segments. However, possible structural differences have been difficult to analyze because of the problems involved in finding the segments in specimens prepared for electron microscopy. (The authors of this chapter have succeeded recently in analyzing several types of thin segments of the rat. In this species there is a clear difference at the ultrastructural level.)

The cells of the short *thin segment of a cortical nephron* are typical squamous cells. They form a rather abrupt transition from the cuboidal cells of the straight descending part of the proximal segment. The brush border is replaced by a small number of very short microvilli. The large number of mitochondria in cells of the proximal segment is reduced to a limited small number in cells of the thin segment. Attached by terminal bars, the cells generally do not show elaborate lateral interdigitations.

The long *thin segment of a juxtamedullary nephron* has two distinctly different legs. The first leg descends toward the papilla, and the second leg ascends toward the border between the cortex and the medulla. Cells of the long descending thin segment have an ultrastructural architecture similar to that characterizing the cells of the short thin segment described above. On the other hand, the cells of the long ascending thin segment have the intercellular relationship illustrated. In line with the complicated and intriguing cellular interdigitations seen in the cells of the convoluted part of the proximal segment, the cells of the thin ascending long segment show a similar topography. Only here, the cells are flattened, allowing for more pronounced intercellular cytoplasmic interlocking. Terminal bars, with tight junctions near the luminal surface, secure the entire system.

To reconcile the functional differences of the various parts of the thin segments

LIGHT PHOTOMICROGRAPH: SECTION THROUGH RENAL MEDULLA (H. & E. STAIN, X 680); TN=THIN SEGMENT OF HENLE'S LOOP TK=THICK SEGMENT OF HENLE'S LOOP

ELECTRON PHOTOMICROGRAPH: SECTION THROUGH RENAL MEDULLA (X 4000); TK=THICK SEGMENT OF HENLE'S LOOP; TN=THIN SEGMENT OF HENLE'S LOOP; A=ARTERIOLA RECTA; V=VENULA RECTA

with the ultrastructure, one must take into account other tubular structures accompanying the thin segments. In this respect, there is no special arrangement known to exist in relation to the short thin segment. However, the long thin segment is accompanied by straight vascular channels, and the entire tubular complex represents the structural basis for the countercurrent multiplier system, discussed in detail later (see pages 52–55).

The vascular channels accompanying the thin segments are derived from the efferent arterioles of the juxtamedullary nephrons. These channels are represented by the *arteriolar vasa recta* leading the blood flow down to the papilla, and by the *venular vasa recta* directing the blood back to the juxtamedullary region (see page 19).

The electron micrograph shows the general topography of a cross section of the anatomical members

of the countercurrent multiplier. The arterial vessels have a continuous, nonfenestrated endothelium, whereas the venous vessels have a thin and fenestrated endothelium. As depicted, the thin segment is a descending leg, since it shows a limited degree of interdigitations. A very important part of the countercurrent system is the thick ascending limb of the distal segment, also shown. Its structure will be discussed subsequently.

It has been suggested that the thin segmental cells are freely permeable to water. However, one must first consider the large number of cellular interdigitations, cellular junctions, and cell membranes present in one type of thin segment, versus the relative paucity of these ultrastructural characteristics in the other type. One may then assume that thin segments with numerous cell junctions are more permeable than those with few interdigitations and few cell junctions. □

Distal Segment of Renal Tubule

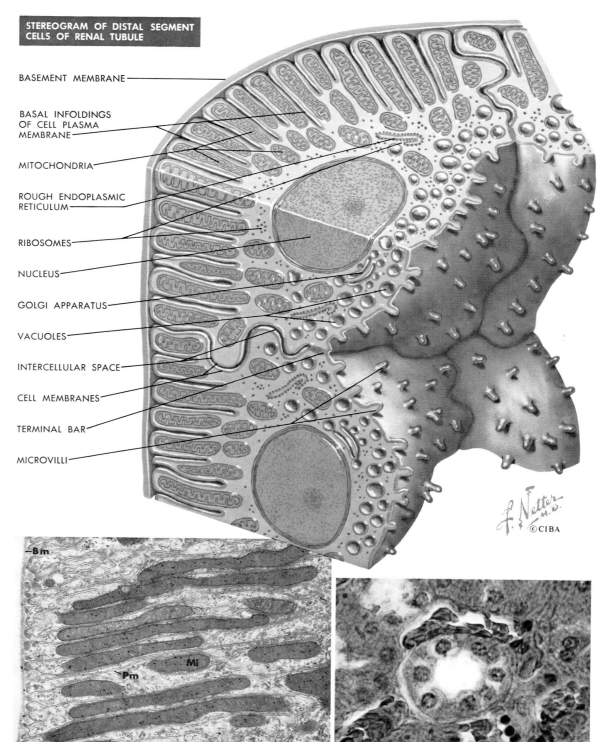

STEREOGRAM OF DISTAL SEGMENT CELLS OF RENAL TUBULE

BASEMENT MEMBRANE

BASAL INFOLDINGS OF CELL PLASMA MEMBRANE

MITOCHONDRIA

ROUGH ENDOPLASMIC RETICULUM

RIBOSOMES

NUCLEUS

GOLGI APPARATUS

VACUOLES

INTERCELLULAR SPACE

CELL MEMBRANES

TERMINAL BAR

MICROVILLI

ELECTRON PHOTOMICROGRAPH OF BASAL PORTION OF DISTAL SEGMENT CELL, X 20,000; Bm=BASEMENT MEMBRANE; Pm=PLASMA MEMBRANE (OF BASAL AND INFOLDING); Mi=MITOCHONDRION

LIGHT PHOTOMICROGRAPH, H. & E., X 680

The distal segment of the nephron is generally divided into two parts. The first part is called the *thick ascending limb* of Henle's loop, and the second part is the *distal convoluted tubule*. The *macula densa* is part of the distal convoluted tubule. In ordinary *H. and E.* sections, the distal segment may be distinguished from the proximal segment. The distal segment, in cross section, has a larger number of nuclei; the lumen of the distal segment is wider, and the distinct brush border seen in the proximal segment is missing. Often, in the cells of the distal segment, one can also discern basal striations which are caused by the long and densely packed mitochondria.

As indicated (see page 12), the ascending thick limb of the distal segment is functionally an important member of the countercurrent multiplier system (see pages 52–55), but it is important to point out the morphological basis for this theory. The cells of the thick ascending limb are generally constructed as seen in the stereogram on this page. A few small and short microvilli exist on the luminal surface. The apical part of the cell contains a large number of small vesicles or short rod-shaped profiles, but very few of these structures, if any, are seen to be connected with the *surface plasma membrane*.

The basal surface of the cell is deeply infolded, and neighboring cells interdigitate laterally to an even greater extent than in cells of the proximal segment. The long rod-shaped mitochondria fill the basal compartments of the cell. The outer limiting membrane of each mitochondrion is in very close contact with the infolded plasma membrane. In contrast, in the apical part of the cell, the mitochondria are oval or round and not very abundant.

The function of the cell, with this kind of ultrastructural design, very likely is related to processes requiring large amounts of energy. The active transport of sodium ions from the luminal fluid and reactions related to the formation of ammonia and the acidification of the urine are functions requiring energy and large surface areas for their fulfillment.

As the distal segment leaves the medulla, the cells become lower, and the shape and number of mitochondria

change. Because of these differences, one can now classify this part as the distal convolution. Of course, in addition, this segment is convoluted in contrast to the preceding straight ascending thick limb. The ultrastructure of the cell of the distal convolution is characterized by the replacement of numerous, long rod-shaped mitochondria with a few, round or oval-shaped mitochondria. The basal mitochondrial striations of the ascending thick limb are not seen, mainly because the basal plasma membrane infoldings have been reduced in depth. In fact, the basal surface of the cell of the distal convolution often displays no invaginations of the plasma membrane. Lateral interdigitations of the cells of the distal convoluted segment are also rare. As a result, the cell borders become rather straight and, occasionally, can be seen even in routine histological preparations. Small vesicles occur sporadically in the apical cell cytoplasm, and the luminal surface is pro-

vided with occasional microvilli. The overall cytoplasmic density is pronounced in these cells, owing to the large number of free ribosomes. The functional implication of some of these ultrastructural peculiarities is not clear.

When the distal segment returns to the glomerulus of its own origin, after establishing its medullary loop of Henle, it makes a short tangential contact with the afferent arteriole just before this vessel enters the glomerular capsule. The cells of the distal segment become narrow and crowded in this region, referred to as the *macula densa* (see page 7). Mitochondria are few and small in these cells, and the basal surfaces often show shallow invaginations of the plasma membrane. The physiological significance of the relationship of the macula densa cells to the secretory granules of the afferent arteriole is discussed elsewhere in this volume (see page 49). □

Collecting Tubule

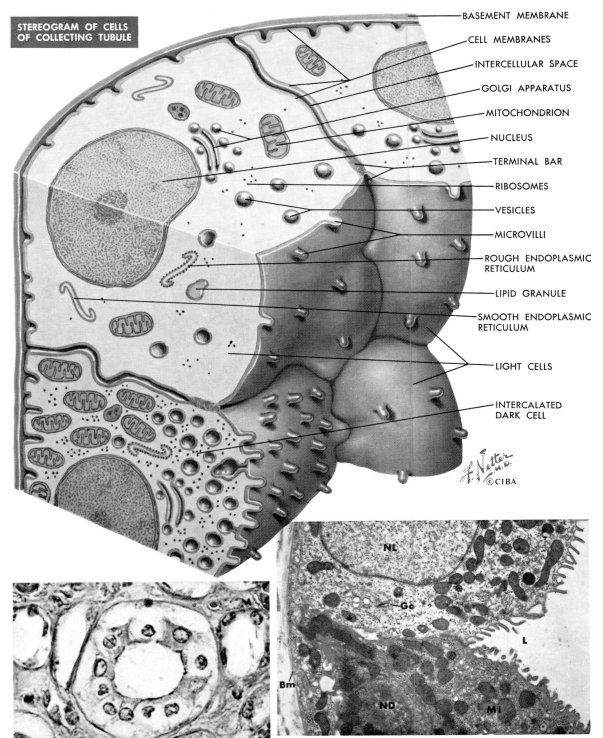

BASEMENT MEMBRANE
CELL MEMBRANES
INTERCELLULAR SPACE
GOLGI APPARATUS
MITOCHONDRION
NUCLEUS
TERMINAL BAR
RIBOSOMES
VESICLES
MICROVILLI
ROUGH ENDOPLASMIC RETICULUM
LIPID GRANULE
SMOOTH ENDOPLASMIC RETICULUM
LIGHT CELLS
INTERCALATED DARK CELL

LIGHT PHOTOMICROGRAPH OF PROXIMAL PORTION OF COLLECTING TUBULE (H. & E., X 680)

ELECTRON PHOTOMICROGRAPH: PROXIMAL PORTION OF COLLECTING TUBULE (X 10,000); NL=NUCLEUS OF LIGHT CELL; Go=GOLGI APPARATUS; L=LUMEN; Bm=BASEMENT MEMBRANE; ND=NUCLEUS OF DARK CELL; Mi=MITOCHONDRIA

Embryologically, the collecting tubules develop from the *ureteric bud* and therefore are not considered part of the nephron proper. However, the collecting tubules have several important functions as far as the composition of the urine is concerned. Therefore, they do not serve merely as urinary conduits. The collecting tubules are easy to find histologically, since their cells each have distinct and rather straight cell borders, a round central nucleus, and a light cytoplasm. In cross sections of tubules, the collecting tubule stands out with a large lumen, as opposed to the narrow lumen of the proximal segment and the medium wide lumen of the distal segment.

There are also differences between the cortical collecting tubules, the medullary collecting tubules, and the large papillary collecting tubules (ducts of Bellini). The fine structural differences are subtle, but grossly, the distinguishing feature is the height of the cells—low cuboidal in the cortex, cuboidal in the medulla, and columnar toward the tip of the papilla.

The cortical collecting tubules often have two cell types, as shown in the illustration. One type is referred to as *light cells* and the other, *dark or intercalated cells.*

The *dark cell* is quite similar in ultrastructure to the cells lining the distal convoluted tubule. It has a number of round or oval mitochondria, very few and shallow basal infoldings of the plasma membrane, and short microvilli. The number of free ribosomes is high compared to the light cells of the collecting tubule. Apical vesicles are relatively abundant. It is commonly believed that the intercalated cell is derived from the nephron proper.

The *light cell* has a scarcity of both mitochondria and ribosomes. Lipid granules occur. Often the Golgi complex is prominent, and profiles of both rough- and smooth-surfaced endoplasmic reticulum are abundant. The microvilli of the luminal border are small, but certain segments of the medullary collecting tubules may be provided with narrow ridges rather than villi. However, in a normal

section, the ridges show up as microvilli. It is only in sections tangential to the cell surface that one can see the narrow ridges forming an intricate pattern on the surface of the cell. The basal surface of the light cell is thrown into small infoldings. The lateral cell surface, particularly in the cuboidal cells of the papillary ducts of Bellini, shows small projections, shaped like microvilli.

The cells of the collecting tubules are all held together by *terminal bars* or junctional complexes at the luminal surface. However, the columnar cells of the papillary ducts may, from time to time, display *desmosomes* as an additional means of attachment. Frequently, in kidneys preserved by intravascular perfusion, the intercellular spaces of the papillary ducts are slightly distended, except in the areas of attachment. From a functional point of view, the intercellular attachment devices may be of importance, since it is

known that the antidiuretic hormone of the pituitary may influence them and open intercellular channels for transport of luminal fluid.

Finally, one must be aware of the fact that the medulla and the papilla contain a relatively large number of extracellular elements, particularly in comparison with the cortex. First, the basement membrane is continuous throughout the nephron and the collecting tubule. It terminates by fusing with the basement membrane of the epithelial cells of the renal pelvis. Second, the number of collagenous fibers increases toward the medulla and the papilla; the cells responsible for their maintenance are probably the interstitial cells, but the nature of these cells is not clear. In addition to their function as manufacturers of collagen, they may partake in urinary concentration in the papilla, in phagocytosis of materials, and in a possible contractility that affects the tubules or vessels. □

Renal Vasculature

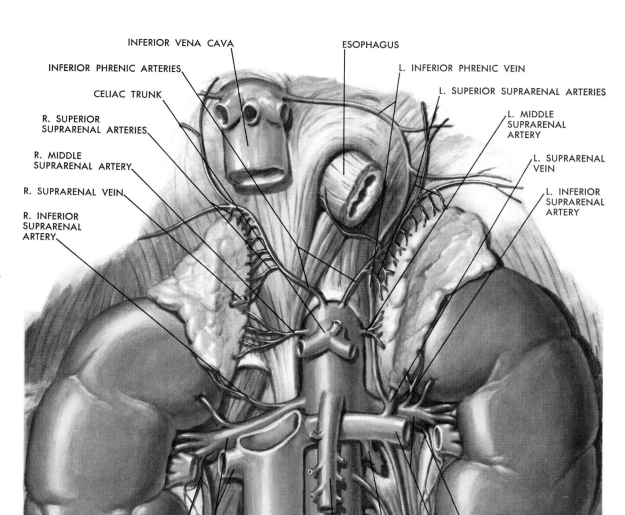

INFERIOR VENA CAVA

ESOPHAGUS

INFERIOR PHRENIC ARTERIES

CELIAC TRUNK

R. SUPERIOR SUPRARENAL ARTERIES

R. MIDDLE SUPRARENAL ARTERY

R. SUPRARENAL VEIN

R. INFERIOR SUPRARENAL ARTERY

L. INFERIOR PHRENIC VEIN

L. SUPERIOR SUPRARENAL ARTERIES

L. MIDDLE SUPRARENAL ARTERY

L. SUPRARENAL VEIN

L. INFERIOR SUPRARENAL ARTERY

URETERIC BRANCH OF L. RENAL ARTERY

L. RENAL ARTERY AND VEIN

L. TESTICULAR ARTERY AND VEIN

L. 2nd LUMBAR VEIN AND COMMUNICATION TO ASCENDING LUMBAR AND HEMIAZYGOS VEINS

URETERIC BRANCH OF R. RENAL ARTERY

R. RENAL ARTERY AND VEIN

R. TESTICULAR OR OVARIAN ARTERY AND VEIN

INFERIOR VENA CAVA

ABDOMINAL AORTA

SUPERIOR MESENTERIC ARTERY

INFERIOR MESENTERIC ARTERY

Renal Arteries

The renal arteries arise from the abdominal aorta approximately at the level of the upper margin of the second lumbar vertebra and 1 cm inferior to the origin of the superior mesenteric artery. Because the aorta is slightly to the left of the midline, the left renal artery is shorter than the right and follows a virtually horizontal course. The right renal artery arises either a little inferior to the origin of the left, or more frequently, descends obliquely to reach the kidney. During its course, the right renal artery crosses deep to the inferior vena cava and lies deep to the right renal vein, although at a somewhat more cranial level. The left renal artery is crossed, during its short course, by the left suprarenal vein. Both renal arteries are surrounded and accompanied by a dense plexus of autonomic and afferent nerves which reach the vessels by way of the celiac, superior mesenteric, and aorticorenal ganglia.

Posterior Relations. On the left, the crus, the psoas muscle, and the sympathetic trunk lie posterior to the renal artery. Also, the ascending lumbar vein (a root of the hemiazygos) lies immediately posterior to the left renal artery.

On the right side, the azygos vein, the right lumbar lymphatic trunk, and the right crus of the diaphragm lie posterior to the proximal section, and the psoas posterior to the middle section, of the artery. The right sympathetic trunk passes through or close to the crus and lies between it and the psoas.

Anterior Relations. On the left, the body of the pancreas (corpus pancreatis) lies on or slightly superior to the left renal artery, with the splenic vein between the two. Adherent to the anterior surface of the right renal artery are the duodenum and the head of the pancreas. The inferior mesenteric vein may or may not be in close relationship with the left renal vessels, depending on whether it empties into the splenic vein to the left or near the midline.

Branches. Each renal artery helps in supplying blood to the suprarenal gland on the same side by sending one or more slender inferior suprarenal arteries to that organ. (The gland receives an additional abundant supply from the middle and superior suprarenal arteries, which are variable, small, and numerous. These arteries arise from the aorta and the inferior phrenic arteries, respectively.)

Other small branches of the renal arteries arise near the hilus and ramify in the adjacent perirenal fat and renal fascia, and on the wall of the renal pelvis. One or two descend as ureteric arteries.

Numerous twigs for the true renal capsule arise from all of the branches mentioned. Near the hilus, the renal artery divides into four or five major branches which supply the parenchyma in a characteristic pattern, as described subsequently (see page 16).

Renal Veins

The veins which drain the parenchyma unite within the renal sinus and, as they leave the hilus, form the renal vein. The right renal vein occasionally assists in forming the azygos vein by means of a connecting branch. It joins the inferior vena cava after a very short course of 2 to 2.5 cm. The left renal vein is much longer than the right and empties into the vena cava at a slightly superior level. It receives the left suprarenal vein and the left testicular (or ovarian) vein, whereas the right suprarenal and gonadal veins join the inferior vena cava directly. The left renal vein connects with the hemiazygos by way of the ascending lumbar vein.

The position of the inferior vena cava to the right of the midline makes it necessary for the left renal vein to be about twice as long as the right. The positioning of the vena cava results from its development. The inferior vena cava is not derived from a midline structure but represents a chain of persisting channels that belonged to the right subcardinal and supracardinal system of veins of the embryo (see page 17 and CIBA COLLECTION, Vol. 5, pages 129–133).

The renal veins form an efficient pathway for drainage. In contrast to the arterial supply, this pathway is safeguarded by collaterals. The latter include the anastomoses between the renal and segmental veins, the veins of the azygos system, and the inferior phrenic veins. The veins of the renal fasciae connect the subcapsular intrarenal channels with those draining the adjacent body walls. *Continued on page 16*

Renal Vasculature
Continued from page 15

Segmental Branches

Just before entering the renal hilus, the renal artery divides into five *segmental arteries,* each of which is destined for one of the vascular segments of the kidney. One of these segmental arteries courses posteriorly, while the remainder lie between the veins and the renal pelvis. These segmental arteries do not anastomose with one another except by small extrarenal, capsular, and pelvic channels.

The segmental arteries eventually become *interlobar arteries* in the fat of the renal sinus, either by dividing one or more times or by continuing without dividing (see Editor's Note). The interlobar arteries enter the substance of the kidney where the cortical columns or septa of Bertin appear between the pyramids as interpapillary protrusions. Within the cortical columns, interlobar arteries lie near or alongside the pyramids and follow a gently curving course toward the cortical arches.

As each interlobar artery approaches the base of the adjacent pyramid, it divides into several (four to six) *arcuate arteries* which arch over and lie close to the convex base of the pyramid. The arcuate arteries generally do not anastomose with one another although several of them may supply the area of cortex overlying a pyramid.

The arcuate arteries give off *interlobular arteries* which lie between the medullary rays as these extend into the cortex toward the surface of the kidney. After giving off a number of interlobular arteries, some of the arcuate arteries may turn toward the surface of the kidney and terminate as interlobular arteries. Most of the interlobular arteries establish small connections with extracapsular vessels. However, the chief function of the interlobular arteries is to provide arterioles and capillaries for the renal parenchyma and especially to send afferent arterioles into the renal glomeruli. The finer details of the renal vascular bed are shown subsequently (see page 18).

Interlobular arteries may also arise directly from an interlobar artery as it passes through a cortical column. These interlobular arteries supply adjacent glomeruli in the cortical columns. In addition, *spiral arteries* arise from interlobar arteries in the cortical columns and these spiral arteries supply the neighboring portion of

Editor's Note: The terminology *interlobar artery* may be a misnomer because these arteries do not lie between two renal lobes. As Hodson has pointed out (British Journal of Urology 44:246, 1972), a renal lobe consists of a pyramid and the surrounding cortex, and the cortical columns of Bertin in actuality represent parts of two or more renal lobes. Thus, the artery lying in juxtaposition to a pyramid is *within* a renal lobe. These arteries could more properly be called *intralobar arteries.* However, because the arteries in question lie between adjacent pyramids (and the pyramids make up the bulk of a renal lobe) and also for the sake of consistency with existing nomenclature, the term *interlobar artery* will continue to be used in this volume.

It should also be mentioned that many authorities question whether a distinction between the interlobar arteries and the arcuate arteries is justified. This viewpoint is particularly cogent because the interlobar arteries follow a curving or archlike course and the arcuate arteries are merely the extension of this curve over the bases of the pyramids.

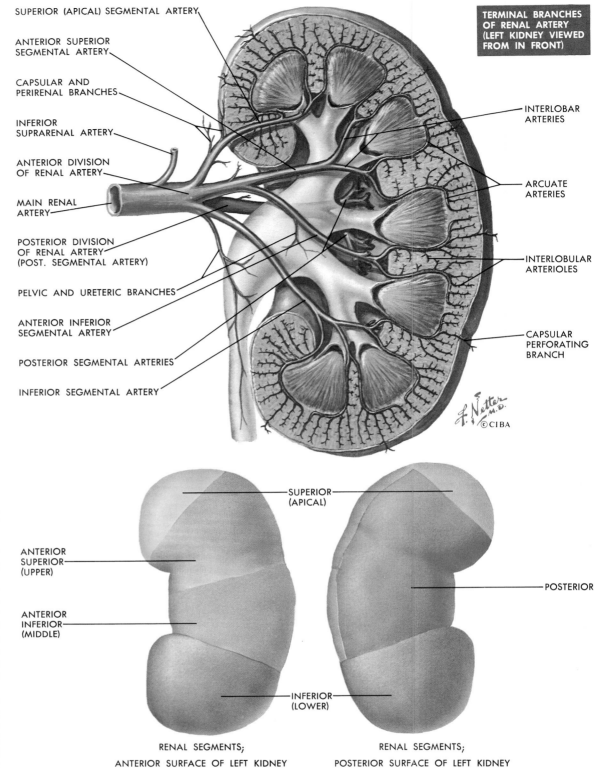

the renal pelvis and send branches into the adjacent pyramid.

The arterial supply of the kidney is vulnerable in that the renal artery itself is an end artery, solely responsible for the supply of one kidney. If accessory renal vessels do exist, each enters a certain area of the parenchyma and ramifies without forming anastomoses. Similarly, each segmental artery supplies a wedge-shaped segment of the kidney and is an end artery which seldom has precapillary anastomoses. However, when anastomoses are present, they are negligible with regard to functionally significant segant collateral circulation.

The segmental arteries of the kidney supply the organ in such a way that each renal pole receives its own artery while the anterior portion between the poles is supplied by an upper and lower segmental vessel. These two arteries also include in their territory the lateral edge of the kidney and, adjacent to

that, a strip of parenchyma on the dorsal or posterior aspect of the organ. The remainder of the posterior portion of the kidney, lying between the two poles, receives its arterial supply from the single posterior segmental branch of the renal artery.

Thus, the border between the anterior and posterior segments follows a line which closely hugs the lateral edge of the kidney on the posterior surface. This is known as the line of Brödel. No major vascular channels are likely to run beneath this line which is therefore preferred for nephrotomy incisions. The area, however, is by no means bloodless because the arterial segments are not geometrically defined and the segments interdigitate with each other by means of the smaller vessels.

Tributaries of the Renal Vein

Numerous small subcapsular veins are grouped in tiny radial arrays called *stellate veins.* These commu-

Renal Vasculature
Continued

nicate with the capsular and perirenal veins, as well as with the cortical intrinsic venous channels. The stellate veins empty into the *interlobular veins* which, in turn, drain into the *arcuate veins*. The arcuate veins empty into the *interlobar veins* following the general arterial pattern. In contrast to the arterial pattern, however, connections between intrinsic veins do exist. Eventually the veins unite into four to six trunks which converge toward the hilus and lie anterior to the arteries. Approximately 1 to 2 cm beyond the hilus, these trunks join to form the renal vein.

Embryology

Many anomalies represent persistent embryonic structures or, less frequently, occur because of delayed termination of developmental processes. The blood vessels evolve from rich and redundant embryonic plexuses. A plexus may be arranged as a net, a stepladderlike structure, or as an irregular structure similar to the skeleton of a sponge. From such a labyrinth, certain channels develop as the major vessels, while others become the capillary bed. Understanding the embryology can assist us in appreciating many seemingly odd anomalies, although we know little about the causes of the variations.

Branches of the Abdominal Aorta. During the fourth embryonic week, the two *dorsal aortas* fuse into the single abdominal aorta, and the various paired intestinal arteries fuse into unpaired, *celiac, superior,* and *inferior mesenteric arteries.* The dorsal branches of the aorta remain paired and, as *segmental arteries,* supply the central nervous system, the vertebral column, and the body wall. The latter two structures are somite derivatives.

Numerous embryonic lateral branches of the aorta are arranged in a close repeat pattern and resemble segmental vessels. However, they are unrelated to the body segments. From these arteries arise the paired lateral aortic branches to the three nephrotome derivatives—the kidneys, the suprarenal glands, and the gonads.

Anomalies of the Renal Artery

Branches of the renal artery may enter the kidney above or below the hilus. This variation is usually associated with *proximal ramification* of the renal artery. In a similar anomaly, multiple branches of the aorta persist as *supernumerary renal arteries* which arise directly from the aorta or, less frequently, from the inferior phrenic or a suprarenal artery. Almost one half the accessory renal arteries, regardless of their sources, enter the kidney at, or very close to, one of the poles. These *polar* and other *extrahilar arteries* have attracted attention because they may surprise the unwary surgeon. According to some authorities, these arteries can also cause or at least aggravate ureteric obstructions when they lie below the hilus or at the lower pole.

Anomalies of the Renal Vein

Unlike the situation in other areas of the body, anomalies of renal veins are far less common than those of the arteries. A brief summary of important developmental

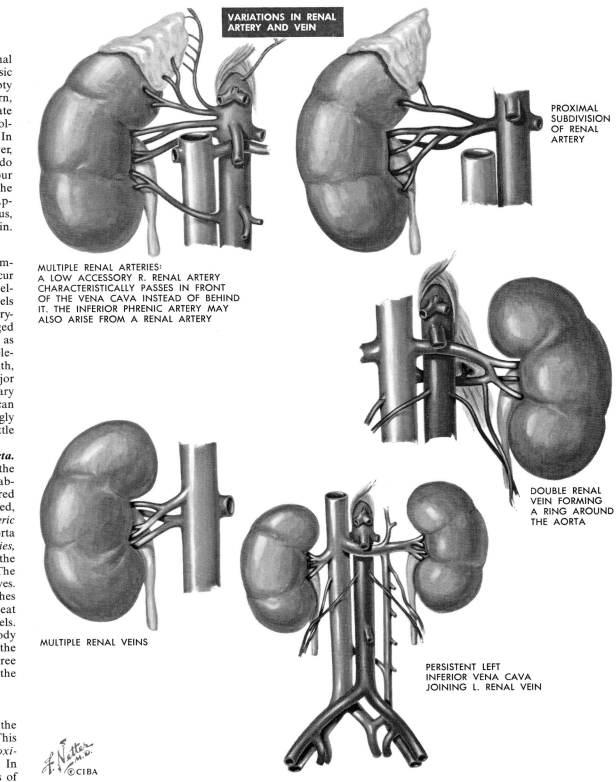

VARIATIONS IN RENAL ARTERY AND VEIN

PROXIMAL SUBDIVISION OF RENAL ARTERY

MULTIPLE RENAL ARTERIES: A LOW ACCESSORY R. RENAL ARTERY CHARACTERISTICALLY PASSES IN FRONT OF THE VENA CAVA INSTEAD OF BEHIND IT. THE INFERIOR PHRENIC ARTERY MAY ALSO ARISE FROM A RENAL ARTERY

DOUBLE RENAL VEIN FORMING A RING AROUND THE AORTA

MULTIPLE RENAL VEINS

PERSISTENT LEFT INFERIOR VENA CAVA JOINING L. RENAL VEIN

features of the veins follows (for more complete description see CIBA COLLECTION, Vol. 5, pages 129–133).

In the embryo, a plexiform collar encircles the aorta and drains the blood from the permanent kidneys. This collar connects with two sets of paired longitudinal channels, the *subcardinal* and *supracardinal veins.* Normally, only the anterior part persists and develops into the renal veins which thus lie anterior to the aorta and the renal arteries. Persistence of the whole collar on the left results in the anomalous condition of an additional renal vein which passes posterior to the aorta. If the collar persists on the right, multiple renal veins, passing both anterior and posterior to the renal pelvis, result.

The embryonic subcardinal and supracardinal veins of the left side become reduced and form discontinuous channels. The *right supracardinal vein* lies close to the posterior body wall. Caudal to the kidney, it enlarges to become the *infrarenal portion of the vena cava.* Cra-

nial to the kidney, the *right supracardinal vein* becomes the *azygos vein.*

The more ventrally placed *right subcardinal vein* forms the *suprarenal portion of the vena cava.* Thus, the inferior vena cava will be *dorsal* to a *lower polar artery* and *ventral* to the *renal* and *upper polar arteries.*

Persistence of the *left supracardinal vein,* inferior to the kidney, results in the formation of a *left inferior vena cava* which lies in a plane dorsal to the aorta. Such an anomalous inferior vena cava empties into the left renal vein. Cranial or superior to the kidney, the left supracardinal vein normally forms the *hemiazygos vein.*

Anomalies have been classified by order of frequency of occurrence by authorities such as Adachi, and with regard to the kidney, by Pick and Anson. However, even rare anomalies may be clinically significant. □

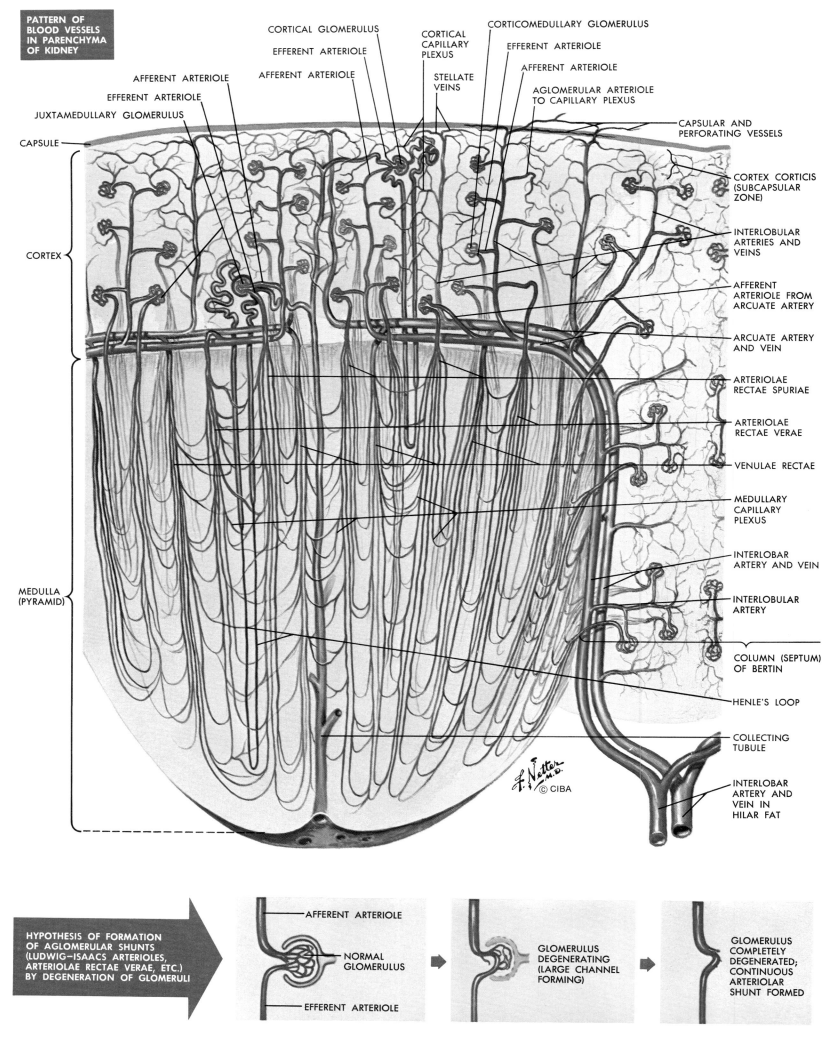

PATTERN OF BLOOD VESSELS IN PARENCHYMA OF KIDNEY

CORTICAL GLOMERULUS

EFFERENT ARTERIOLE

AFFERENT ARTERIOLE

CORTICAL CAPILLARY PLEXUS

CORTICOMEDULLARY GLOMERULUS

EFFERENT ARTERIOLE

STELLATE VEINS

AFFERENT ARTERIOLE

AGLOMERULAR ARTERIOLE TO CAPILLARY PLEXUS

AFFERENT ARTERIOLE

EFFERENT ARTERIOLE

JUXTAMEDULLARY GLOMERULUS

CAPSULE

CORTEX

MEDULLA (PYRAMID)

CAPSULAR AND PERFORATING VESSELS

CORTEX CORTICIS (SUBCAPSULAR ZONE)

INTERLOBULAR ARTERIES AND VEINS

AFFERENT ARTERIOLE FROM ARCUATE ARTERY

ARCUATE ARTERY AND VEIN

ARTERIOLAE RECTAE SPURIAE

ARTERIOLAE RECTAE VERAE

VENULAE RECTAE

MEDULLARY CAPILLARY PLEXUS

INTERLOBAR ARTERY AND VEIN

INTERLOBULAR ARTERY

COLUMN (SEPTUM) OF BERTIN

HENLE'S LOOP

COLLECTING TUBULE

INTERLOBAR ARTERY AND VEIN IN HILAR FAT

F. Netter, M.D.
© CIBA

HYPOTHESIS OF FORMATION OF AGLOMERULAR SHUNTS (LUDWIG–ISAACS ARTERIOLES, ARTERIOLAE RECTAE VERAE, ETC.) BY DEGENERATION OF GLOMERULI

AFFERENT ARTERIOLE

NORMAL GLOMERULUS

EFFERENT ARTERIOLE

GLOMERULUS DEGENERATING (LARGE CHANNEL FORMING)

GLOMERULUS COMPLETELY DEGENERATED; CONTINUOUS ARTERIOLAR SHUNT FORMED

Intrarenal Vasculature

The kidneys exert a profound regulatory influence on the composition of the blood plasma. Accordingly, the relationships between the parenchyma and the vascular bed are more specialized than in organs where tissue oxygenation is the chief function of blood vessels. Since certain aspects of renal function are incompletely understood, certain details of renal angiology are not readily explained.

It will be recalled (see page 16) that the segmental arteries divide, before entering the substance of the kidney, into *interlobar arteries* which enter the renal (cortical) columns and follow a gently curving course toward the cortical arches. Near the base of a pyramid, each interlobar artery divides into several *arcuate arteries* which lie close to the convex base of the adjacent pyramid and hence roughly parallel to the surface of the kidney. The arcuate arteries, in turn, give off the *interlobular arteries* from which the *afferent arterioles* of the glomeruli arise. Interlobular arteries also arise from the interlobar arteries as they ascend in the renal (cortical) columns. The main volume of normal circulation is routed through these lateral branches of the interlobular arteries, but a small amount of blood reaches extrarenal channels by way of the capsular anastomoses of the interlobular arteries. These capsular connections are insignificant, however, and the renal parenchyma is supplied by end arteries which have no precapillary anastomoses.

Blood Supply of Cortical Glomeruli

In the outer portion of the cortex, each afferent arteriole enters a glomerulus, divides into the glomerular capillary network, and then reunites into the efferent arteriole which leaves the glomerulus. This latter blood vessel, smaller in diameter than the afferent arteriole, then divides into a *peritubular capillary net* which still contains arterial blood.

This network supplies the tubular portion of the nephron and probably anastomoses with corresponding neighboring networks.

Venous blood from the cortical peritubular network drains into tributaries of the *interlobular veins* paralleling the arteries of the same name. In addition, blood from the *stellate veins,* which drain smaller channels of the *capsular plexus,* passes into the interlobular veins.

The interlobular veins ultimately drain into *arcuate veins* which empty into the *interlobar veins.* As in other organs, the venous channels connect with each other by anastomotic branches.

The afferent and efferent arterioles, the renal corpuscle, and the convoluted tubules of the nephron are in close anatomic relationship (see pages 6 and 7). The afferent arteriole possesses a muscular wall which is modified into an aggregate of epithelioid cells near the glomerulus. This cushion of cells is known as the *juxtaglomerular body* or *polkissen* and apparently serves secretory functions. The ascending limb of Henle's loop returns to its parent nephron, close to the juxtaglomerular body, and the distal convoluted tubule begins in this region, called the *macula densa* (see page 6).

Cortical Aglomerular Shunts

The efferent arterioles of subcapsular glomeruli send branches to the capsule as well as to the peritubular capillary networks. An additional small amount of blood (less than 10 percent) entirely bypasses the glomeruli through bypasses known as *aglomerular shunts.* These connect the arterial limb of the circulation with the capillary bed. These aglomerular shunts should be distinguished from true *arteriovenous anastomoses* which sidestep all capillary beds but which have not been observed with certainty in the renal parenchyma. (The occurrence of arteriovenous anastomoses in the renal sinus and capsule has been accepted.)

The aglomerular shunts can exist in the healthy kidney but are not common. However, their incidence is increased with age. Most of these shunts are thought to be the result of degeneration and obliteration of glomerular capillary loops, with the connection of afferent to efferent arterioles remaining pervious. These shunts have been named after their two discoverers: *arterioles of Ludwig-Isaacs.* In addition, direct connections between interlobar arteries and peritubular capillary networks have been described.

Blood Supply of Medulla

The arterial supply of the medulla is from the efferent arterioles of the *juxtamedullary glomeruli* situated in the inner one third of the cortex, particularly in the immediate vicinity of the medullary pyramids. These efferent vessels descend directly into the medulla, in contrast to the efferent arterioles of the cortical glomeruli which form peritubular capillary networks.

Between the zones of cortical glomeruli and juxtamedullary glomeruli, many renal corpuscles of the *corticomedullary* type exist. The efferent arterioles from these glomeruli supply branches for the peritubular capillary networks and also descend into the medulla.

The afferent arterioles to the juxtamedullary glomeruli may arise from interlobular arteries, or in distinction to the afferent arterioles of the cortical glomeruli, may originate directly from arcuate arteries. The efferent arterioles are at least as large as, and in some cases are larger than, these afferent vessels and descend in a radial direction into the pyramid as *vasa recta spuria.* (As will be described later, these vessels have a structure corresponding to large caliber capillaries so that the designation "arteriolae" is hardly justified.)

The vessels of the *vasa recta spuria* outnumber the thin loops of Henle around which they lie in parallel fashion. Their diameter does not appreciably change as they pursue a straight course toward the papilla, ramifying, at the same time, into several parallel vessels. At various levels, these latter vessels describe hairpin turns and return to the base of the pyramid where they empty into an *arcuate vein.* These ascending limbs of the vasa recta are wider than the descending limbs and are often referred to as *venulae rectae.*

Various interconnections exist between the ascending and descending limbs of the vasa recta as well as with neighboring arrays of straight vessels. The resulting vascular complex is called a *rete mirabile conjugatum.* This complex of retia, with paralleling loops of Henle and straight collecting tubules, forms the histological substrate for a countercurrent exchange device instrumental in the economical production of hypertonic urine (see pages 54 and 55).

Vasa Recta Vera. A distinction must be made between the *vasa recta spuria,* described above, and the so-called *vasa recta vera,* or "true" vasa recta. Insofar as the courses of the two types of vessels are concerned, there is no difference. However, the *vasa recta vera* arise directly from arcuate or interlobular arteries and not from juxtaglomerular efferent arterioles. The true vasa recta are not numerous, although there is general agreement as to their existence. Their modes of origin correspond to those of aglomerular shunts of the *Ludwig-Isaacs* type, but the degenerated glomeruli are juxtamedullary rather than cortical.

Functional Considerations. The juxtamedullary circulation of the kidney is of functional interest, although its significance for the human is insufficiently understood. In various experimental animals, renal cortical ischemia can be associated with a patent and functioning juxtamedullary circulatory bed. Anatomically, this bypass has two main characteristics. First, there is an absence of capillaries supplying the convoluted parts of the nephrons. Second, because of the large efferent arterioles, the flow of blood to the juxtamedullary glomeruli is at a filtration pressure considerably lower than that which normally prevails in the cortical glomeruli (see page 175).

Histologic Features

The larger arteries have a pronounced *elastica interna* and a well-developed media layer. The elastica interna continues, through various subdivisions, to the level of the afferent arterioles. This arrangement generally does not exist in other organs. Nerves accompany the arterial system, even to the level of the afferent and efferent arterioles. Autonomic nerve endings terminate in the connective tissue at distances of less than 0.5 micron from the medial smooth muscle cells.

The renal capillary network is characterized by *fenestrated endothelial cells.* In the glomerular capillaries these fenestrations are open to a large degree, whereas in the peritubular capillaries each is closed by a diaphragm. The endothelium of the arteriolar vasa recta is nonfenestrated, as in muscle tissue capillaries, whereas the venular vasa recta have the typical renal fenestrated endothelium of the closed variety.

Generally speaking, the veins of the renal parenchyma are thin walled. In the rat, the arcuate veins have been studied with the electron microscope. These vessels have an average inner diameter of about 200 microns. They are lined by a thin, fenestrated endothelium, a most unusual finding for a vein of this size. This ultrastructural design greatly facilitates a back diffusion of interstitial fluid and substances into the vascular lumen. The interlobular veins are also thin walled, but the renal vein is characterized by a rather heavy muscular coat, the cells of which are often arranged parallel to the long axis of the vessel. □

Urinary Bladder

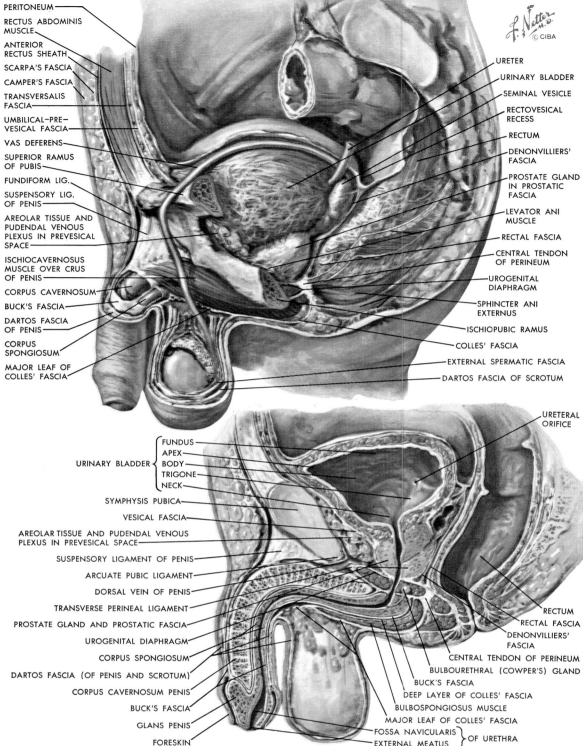

The bladder lies in the pelvis, anterior and inferior to the peritoneal cavity, and posterior to the pubic bones. In the female, it rests directly on the muscular pelvic floor, while in the male the prostate gland is attached directly to the base of the bladder and separates it from its muscular support (see CIBA COLLECTION, Vol. 2, pages 10–13, 20, 21, 92, 93, and 106, and Vol. 3/II, pages 30–34).

In the living state, the empty bladder is rarely superior to the upper edge of the pelvic bone, but as it fills with urine, it assumes an ovoid or even spherical configuration and ascends into the abdominal cavity along the anterior abdominal wall. However, when fixed *in situ,* the bladder is shaped like a round-edged tetrahedron with a superior, a posterior, and two inferior surfaces.

The *fundus* of the bladder is the large central and posterosuperior portion, while the *apex* is the anterosuperior region. Posteroinferiorly is the *body* with two *ureteral orifices.* The *urethral orifice,* in the most inferior portion, marks the *neck,* and together the three orifices mark a triangular area, the *vesical trigone.*

The base and neck of the bladder remain relatively constant in both shape and position. In the male, the internal urethral orifice lies about 1 or 2 cm superior to, and 2 cm posterior to, the inferior edge of the pubic symphysis. In the female, the position of the urethral orifice is slightly more inferior, while in the newborn, it may be situated as superior as the upper border of the pubic symphysis.

Anatomic Relations

In the female, the bladder is separated inferiorly and posteriorly from the vagina and cervix by the so-called *vesicovaginal septum* which normally consists of a small amount of areolar tissue. In the corresponding area in the male, the two *seminal vesicles* and *ampullae of the ductus deferentes* lie on each side of the midline between the bladder and the rectum. The vesicles and ductus form two sides of a small triangular area on the most inferior portion of the bladder wall. The third side of this triangle is the line of peritoneal reflection from the bladder. This area is separated from the rectum by the *rectovesical fascia of Denonvilliers.*

This rectovesical fascia becomes contin-

uous with the tough envelopes of the ampullae of the ductus deferentes and seminal vesicles. It continues posterior to the prostate as far as the perineum, and superiorly it terminates at the peritoneum of the rectovesical recess. Consequently, the fascia of Denonvilliers is also known as the *prostatoperitoneal membrane.*

The peritoneum covering the bladder is sufficiently loose to allow for distention of the organ. In the male, the peritoneum descends posteriorly between the two ductus deferentes and reflects onto the rectum, forming a cul-de-sac called the *rectovesical fossa* or *recess.* In the fetus, this is a deep excavation which dips posterior to the prostate as far as the pelvic floor. Eventually, however, the perineal section obliterates and takes part in the formation of the retroprostatic septum, or the fascia of Denonvilliers.

As the peritoneum sweeps posteriorly from the bladder to the sides of the rectum, it forms a pair of sickle-

shaped shelves called the *sacrogenital folds.* At the base of the bladder, these folds contain the terminal portions of the ureters and, in the male, the ductus deferentes. In the female, the sacrogenital folds arise from the dorsal wall of the uterine cervix.

Laterally, the walls of the bladder are covered by peritoneum to the level of the umbilical artery. Inferior to this, they are bare of serosa and are related to the sidewalls of the pelvis. The reflection of the peritoneum from the lateral wall of the bladder onto the lateral pelvic wall forms a large, shallow *paravesical fossa.* This depression reaches laterally and posteriorly to the slight fold of the ductus deferens in the male, and in the female, to the round ligament of the uterus. Superiorly, a transverse vesical fold extends across the dorsosuperior surface of the bladder, but this is effaced by distention of the organ.

Anteriorly, the apex of the empty bladder extends

Urinary Bladder

Continued

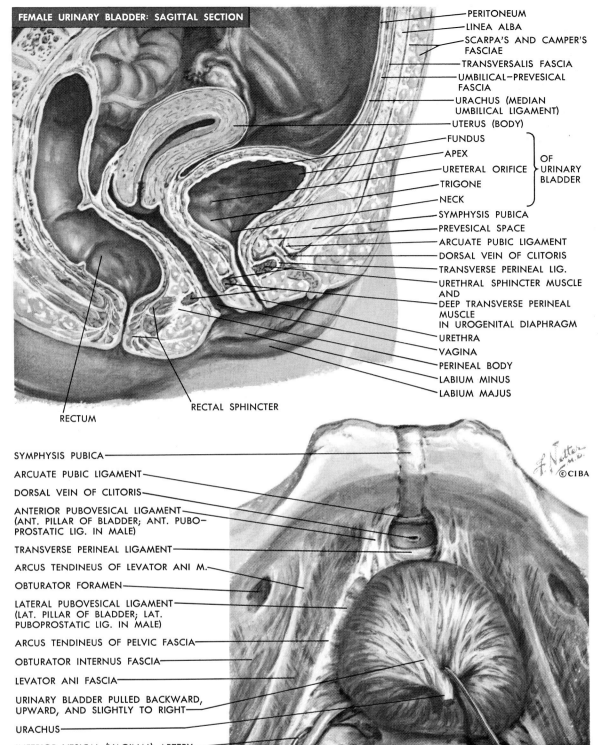

FEMALE URINARY BLADDER: SAGITTAL SECTION

PERITONEUM
LINEA ALBA
SCARPA'S AND CAMPER'S FASCIAE
TRANSVERSALIS FASCIA
UMBILICAL–PREVESICAL FASCIA
URACHUS (MEDIAN UMBILICAL LIGAMENT)
UTERUS (BODY)
FUNDUS
APEX
URETERAL ORIFICE
TRIGONE — OF URINARY BLADDER
NECK
SYMPHYSIS PUBICA
PREVESICAL SPACE
ARCUATE PUBIC LIGAMENT
DORSAL VEIN OF CLITORIS
TRANSVERSE PERINEAL LIG.
URETHRAL SPHINCTER MUSCLE AND
DEEP TRANSVERSE PERINEAL MUSCLE IN UROGENITAL DIAPHRAGM
URETHRA
VAGINA
PERINEAL BODY
LABIUM MINUS
LABIUM MAJUS

RECTUM
RECTAL SPHINCTER

SYMPHYSIS PUBICA
ARCUATE PUBIC LIGAMENT
DORSAL VEIN OF CLITORIS
ANTERIOR PUBOVESICAL LIGAMENT (ANT. PILLAR OF BLADDER; ANT. PUBO-PROSTATIC LIG. IN MALE)
TRANSVERSE PERINEAL LIGAMENT
ARCUS TENDINEUS OF LEVATOR ANI M.
OBTURATOR FORAMEN
LATERAL PUBOVESICAL LIGAMENT (LAT. PILLAR OF BLADDER; LAT. PUBOPROSTATIC LIG. IN MALE)
ARCUS TENDINEUS OF PELVIC FASCIA
OBTURATOR INTERNUS FASCIA
LEVATOR ANI FASCIA
URINARY BLADDER PULLED BACKWARD, UPWARD, AND SLIGHTLY TO RIGHT
URACHUS
INFERIOR VESICAL (VAGINAL) ARTERY
URETER

VIEWED FROM ABOVE

upward as a blunt cone. A solid slender continuation ascends in the midline of the abdominal wall as the *median umbilical ligament.* This represents a vestige of the *urachus* and rarely possesses a residual lumen. If a lumen is present, it infrequently may communicate with that of the bladder, but a urachus patent from bladder to umbilicus is most rare.

The anterior abdominal wall and the area of the pubic symphysis are separated from the bladder by the *prevesical space of Retzius.* The space contains the vesical or pudendal plexus of veins and areolar tissue. The loose areolar tissue permits the anterior peritoneal reflection to ascend as the bladder fills. Thus, the suprapubic extraperitoneal approach to the bladder is facilitated if the organ is at least partially filled.

The prevesical space is surgically most significant posterior to the lower part of the transversalis fascia and is less well defined in its cranial portion. Inferiorly, the space is bounded by the anterior ligaments of the bladder *(q.v.).* In many instances, an umbilical prevesical fascia forms a delicate layer between the two medial umbilical ligaments (obliterated umbilical arteries). This delicate layer of fascia then separates the prevesical space from the vesical fascia.

Anteriorly, the peritoneum covering the bladder reflects onto the abdominal wall and forms the paired *supravesical fossae.* These fossae flank the median umbilical fold and are bounded laterally by the folds of the obliterated umbilical arteries. Thus, if the umbilical folds are well developed, the supravesical fossae can be quite pronounced.

Ligamentous Attachments

The ligaments of the bladder and other pelvic organs are neurovasculofibrous structures which convey vessels and nerves, and often contain smooth muscle fibers. Because of the latter, terms such as "pubovesical muscle" or "pubovesical ligament" are used. In order to avoid confusion between these structures and the peritoneal folds which have similar names or locations, the neurovasculofibrous structures are called "true" ligaments, while the peritoneal folds are classified as "false" ligaments.

The inferior, anterior aspect of the bladder is connected to the pubis by a pair of ligaments which run from the vesical fascia (and the prostatic fascia) to the pelvic fascia. These ligaments clothe the anterior pelvic wall and the pelvic floor. They are called the *anterior puboprostatic ligaments* in the male, or the *anterior pubovesical ligaments* in the female. They lie close to the pelvic floor and flank the dorsal vein of the penis (or clitoris) which pierces the pelvic floor to enter the vesical venous plexus. Note that this vein passes between the *arcuate pubic ligament* (which forms the inferior margin of the pubic symphysis) and the anterior end of the urogenital diaphragm, called the *transverse perineal ligament.*

At the inferolateral border of the bladder lies the lateral ligament, or "true lateral ligament" of the bladder. In the male, it is called the *lateral puboprostatic ligament;* in the female, it is the *lateral pubovesical ligament.* It is formed by an extension of the vesical and prostatic fascial cover and encloses the inferior group of vesical arteries, the pudendal veins which drain the vesical plexus, and the autonomic nerve plexus. The terminal part of the ureter and, in the male, the ductus deferens contribute their adventitia to this ligament. Laterally, this ligament joins the pelvic fascia by attaching to the superior fascial surface of the levator ani near its origin. The linear area of attachment of the lateral puboprostatic (or pubovesical) ligament is known as the *arcus tendineus of the pelvic fascia.* (Note, however, this term is distinct from the arcus tendineus of the levator ani muscle which is the line of origin of this muscle from the obturator fascia. Both arcus tendineus, however, can be close together.)

Posteriorly, the lateral vesical ligament of the male blends with the contents of the sacrogenital (rectovesical) folds. In the female, the posterior fibers intermingle with the parametrial tissues. *Continued on page 22*

Urinary Bladder

Continued from page 21

Continued from page 21

Gross Structure

Deep to the peritoneum, a loose connective tissue layer of subserosa forms the outer or adventitial coat of the bladder wall. In areas lacking peritoneum, the thin perivesical fascia represents the outer cover. This fascia continues along the neurovascular pedicles and helps form the true vesical ligaments. In the male, strong fibrous adhesions bind the bladder to the capsule of the prostate gland.

The muscular coat (tunica muscularis) is thick and consists of three layers which are difficult to distinguish from each other.

The *outer layer* has predominantly *longitudinal muscle fibers* which are numerous in the midline region and near the neck. This layer continues into the walls of the ureters for a distance of several centimeters, to form an outer longitudinal muscular sheath. Offshoots from this layer also extend into the puboprostatic (or vesical) ligaments and the prostate gland (or the wall of the vagina). Some longitudinal muscle fibers form a hammocklike sling for the origin of the urethra.

The *middle* or *circular layer* is thin and only approximates a circular arrangement over the fundus and body. Near the neck, the fibers of this layer are more condensed and join the prostatic musculature. Some muscle bundles form a loop behind the initial portion of the urethra and so assist the longitudinal fibers in creating a sphincterlike apparatus. In the female, the circular fibers form a true ring-shaped (smooth) "sphincter vesicae" around the internal urethral orifice.

The *third layer* is usually named the *internal longitudinal*. Occasionally its sparse strands send fibers into the mucosa. However, in the region of the trigone, this layer is intimately attached to the mucosa and forms the *trigonal muscle*. In this region, the longitudinal, inner, muscular coat of each ureter also fans out into the bladder. Some of these muscle fibers run across and unite with similar strands from the opposite side, thus raising the *interureteric ridge (plica interureterica or torus uretericus)*. Other fibers spread out over the trigone itself. The sides of the trigone are outlined by yet another group of submucous fibers. These bundles, known as *Bell's muscle*, connect the ureteral muscles with the wall of the urethra, and as they converge toward the internal

urethral orifice help form a small elevation, the *uvula*. However, the high incidence of large uvulae in the bladders of aging males suggests that the underlying middle lobe of the prostate plays an equally important role in producing the uvula.

The innermost layer of the bladder is the mucosa. When the bladder is empty, the mucosa is corrugated by numerous folds, and irregular bars of hypertrophic muscles may project the mucosa, giving it a "trabeculated" appearance. However, as the bladder distends, the folds become obliterated.

The mucosal lining in the region of the trigone is anatomically and embryologically distinct from the mucosa of the remainder of the bladder. Anatomically, the trigonal mucosa is firmly attached to the muscularis so that it appears smoothly molded against the underlying musculature. Embryologically, the trigone represents a mesodermal area where the ureteric

buds arose from the mesonephric (wolffian) ducts. The remainder of the bladder, including the mucosa, was derived from the urachus which is of endodermal origin (see pages 31 – 34).

The two ureteral orifices are slitlike because of the oblique course of the ureters as they pierce the wall of the bladder in an anteromedial direction (see page 23). Each ureter is accompanied by its own longitudinal musculature throughout its course within the bladder wall. As a result, a short ridge extends laterally from the ureteral orifice.

The trigone is thought to maintain its position during expansion of the bladder. The distance between the two ureteral openings, however, may widen by 2.5 to 5 cm when the bladder is distended.

The anatomy of the urethra has been described (see CIBA COLLECTION, Vol. 2, page 20, for the male; page 106 for the female). □

FEMALE URINARY BLADDER: FRONTAL SECTION

- PERITONEUM
- FUNDUS OF BLADDER
- BODY OF BLADDER
- L. URETERAL ORIFICE
- TRIGONE OF BLADDER
- UVULA OF BLADDER
- ARCUS TENDINEUS OF LEVATOR ANI MUSCLE AT BLADDER NECK
- PARAVESICAL SPACE AND PUDENDAL VENOUS PLEXUS
- OBTURATOR INTERNUS MUSCLE
- LEVATOR ANI MUSCLE
- VESICAL FASCIA
- ARCUS TENDINEUS OF PELVIC FASCIA
- LATERAL PUBOVESICAL LIG.
- URETHRA
- INFERIOR RAMUS OF PUBIS
- URETHRAL SPHINCTER MUSCLE IN UROGENITAL DIAPHRAGM
- CRUS OF CLITORIS
- CORPUS SPONGIOSUM AND BULBOSPONGIOSUS MUSCLE
- ROUND LIG.
- VAGINA

F. Netter ©CIBA

- FUNDUS OF BLADDER
- PERITONEUM
- VAS DEFERENS
- SUP. RAMUS OF PUBIS
- R. URETERAL ORIFICE
- INTERURETERIC FOLD (BAR)
- ARCUS TENDINEUS OF LEVATOR ANI M.
- TRIGONE OF BLADDER
- PARAVESICAL SPACE AND PUDENDAL VENOUS PLEXUS
- LEVATOR ANI MUSCLE
- UVULA OF BLADDER
- PROSTATIC FASCIA
- ARCUS TENDINEUS OF PELVIC FASCIA
- LATERAL PUBOPROSTATIC LIGAMENT
- PROSTATE GLAND AND PROSTATIC URETHRA
- URETHRAL SPHINCTER M. IN UROGENITAL DIAPHRAGM
- URETHRAL BULB
- CORPUS SPONGIOSUM AND BULBOSPONGIOSUS MUSCLE
- COLLES' FASCIA

MALE URINARY BLADDER: FRONTAL SECTION

Anatomic Relations of Ureters

The ureters are a pair of mucosal-lined tubes for urine transport. Each ureter begins where the renal pelvis narrows—at, or just above, the level of the inferior pole of the kidney—and ends with insertion into the posterior bladder wall. For its entire length of 30 to 34 cm, the ureter is retroperitoneal, adhering closely to the peritoneum.

Each ureter varies in diameter from 2 to 8 mm, being small at the beginning and generally increasing in size in the lower lumbar area. As it crosses the pelvic rim, it may again decrease in diameter. However, the ureter is narrowest during its course through the bladder wall, a distance of about 12 mm.

The ureter penetrates the thick wall of the bladder, in an anteromedial direction. The orifice therefore appears as a slit in the vesical lining. The mucous membrane of the ureter is continuous with that of the bladder, and because of the oblique entrance of the ureter into the bladder, a fold of mucous membrane is formed. Formerly, this valvelike mucosal fold, together with the diagonal intramural course of the ureter and the muscular anatomy of the ureterovesical junction, was thought to prevent the reflux of urine. However, more recent clinical and experimental evidence makes the reliability of this postulate questionable.

The internal muscular layer of the ureter blends with the vesical trigonal muscle as previously described (see page 22). The superficial muscle layer of the bladder accompanies the ureter for several centimeters.

Abdominal Portion

Each ureter descends anterior to the psoas muscle and the genitofemoral nerve which it crosses. On the right, the cranial 5 to 7 cm of the ureter is covered anteriorly by the second part of the duodenum. More caudally, the right colic and ileocolic blood vessels and the root of the mesentery (containing the terminal portion of the superior mesenteric vessels) lie anteriorly.

The left ureter is crossed anteriorly by the left colic vessels and, near the rim of the true (minor) pelvis, by the sigmoid vessels. Here it is just deep to the peritoneum of the intersigmoid recess.

Near the entry into the false (major) pelvis, each ureter is crossed anteriorly, at an angle, by the gonadal (testicular or ovarian) blood vessels. The gonadal artery and vein thus enter the false pelvis slightly anterior and lateral to the ureter. As each ureter enters the true pelvis, it is anterior to the sacroiliac joint and medial to the common iliac vessels.

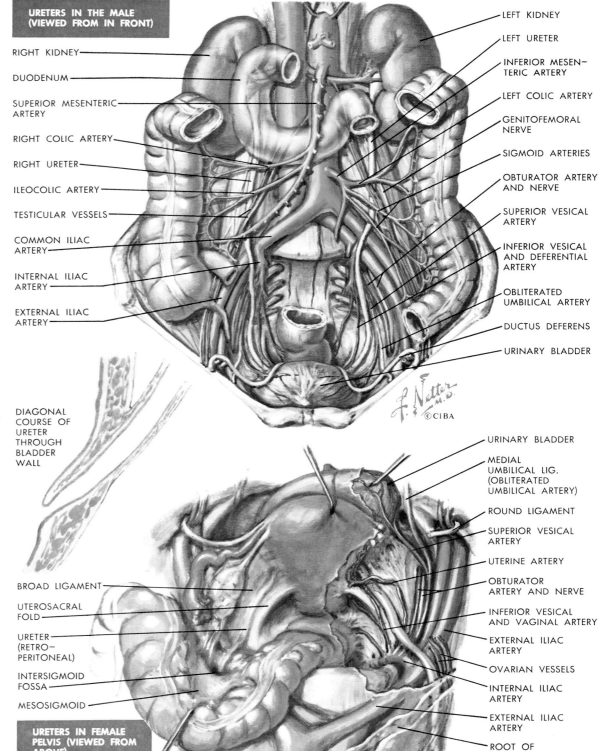

Pelvic portion

Male. The ureter descends into the true pelvis anterior to the internal iliac artery. It crosses anterior to the obturator vessels and nerve and to the superior vesical (umbilical) artery. Thus, it also lies medial to these structures. At the level of the ischial spine, the ureter turns medially and descends in the endopelvic connective tissue with branches of the hypogastric bundle of nerves (see page 27). Just before the ureter enters the bladder, it is crossed anteriorly by the ductus deferens which is on a lateral-to-medial course. At this point the ureter is superior and anterior to the top of the seminal vesicle. The ureter enters the bladder about 2.5 cm from the midline, in an anteromedial direction.

Female. The ovarian vessels are located in the suspensory (infundibulopelvic) ligament and so leave the outer wall of the pelvis and run medially. As a result, the ureter crosses these vessels posteriorly and comes to lie lateral to them. The ureter then crosses the linea terminalis and descends along the lateral pelvic wall. As in the male, it traverses the obturator artery and nerve, the superior vesical (umbilical) artery, and in addition, the uterine artery. The ureter lies closely posterior to the ovary, and as it turns medially, it is in the base of the broad ligament. About 1.5 to 2 cm lateral to the uterine cervix, the uterine artery again crosses the ureter, but this time the ureter lies posteriorly. In this region the ureter is also surrounded by a large number of veins.

In the female, the penetration of the ureter into the bladder and the associated relations are precisely the same as they are in the male, with the exception, of course, of the absence of the ductus deferens and seminal vesicle. □

Histology of Ureters and Bladder

TRANSITIONAL EPITHELIUM

TUNICA PROPRIA

LONGITUDINAL MUSCLE

CIRCULAR MUSCLE

ADVENTITIA

VEINS

ARTERIES

NERVE

Microscopically, the lower urinary tract is fairly uniform, differences being mainly macroscopic.

Adventitia. Collagenous fibroareolar tissue, with a few elastic fibers, blends with the underlying muscular coat and connects the bladder and ureter with the surrounding tissues. Blood vessels, small nerves, and tiny ganglia, singly or aggregated, lie within the adventitia (see page 28). Larger nerve strands flank the base of the bladder, but elsewhere nervous elements are sparse.

The muscle coat (tunica muscularis) is composed of two easily detectable layers in the upper part of the ureter, while in the lower portion, a third outer layer is added. The muscle bundles are sturdy and interlace freely throughout. In the bladder, however, three distinct layers are only observed in certain areas.

The inner muscular layer is composed of predominantly longitudinal fibers while the second layer consists of circular fibers. This arrangement is opposite to that which occurs in digestive organs where the circular layer is the innermost. Also, unlike the structure found in the gastrointestinal tract, the muscle layers are not separated from each other by a myenteric plexus of nerves. Instead, in the walls of the urinary passages, the delicate nerves and blood vessels course in narrow connective tissue septa among the muscles. Where a third layer of muscle is present, the fibers are longitudinal.

Mucosal Lining. From the renal cribriform area to the lower end of the bladder in the female, and into the prostatic urethra in the male, the *tunica mucosa* is covered by transitional epithelium. The calyceal epithelium may be only three cells thick, but in the ureters, this increases to four to five cells, while in the nondistended human bladder, up to eight cell layers may be identified. The superficial cells are rounded, large, and occasionally binucleated. In the deep layers, the cells are more cuboidal and usually lack the characteristic convexity of the luminal surface of superficial cells. As the bladder distends, the cells flatten but do not lose contact with their neighbors. They regroup into a squamous epithelium which may possess as few as two layers. Lymphyocytes are seen at times within the mucosa.

The *lamina propria* component of the ureteral and vesical mucosae is composed of collagenous and elastic fibers intersecting each other at various angles. Unlike other organs, no papillae are found which could project the epithelium, but blood capillaries may lie very close to, and even indent, the basal layer of epithelial cells. With a light microscope, no basement

SECTION THROUGH WALL OF URINARY BLADDER

TRANSITIONAL EPITHELIUM

TUNICA PROPRIA

MUSCLE LAYERS

ADVENTITIA (SEROSA PRESENT ONLY ON SIDES AND TOP OF BLADDER)

BLOOD VESSELS

TRANSITIONAL EPITHELIUM IN CONTRACTED STATE OF VISCUS

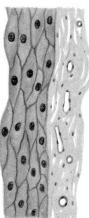

TRANSITIONAL EPITHELIUM IN DISTENDED STATE OF VISCUS

membrane can be identified between the lamina propria and the epithelium. However, a nonfibrous basement membrane of ultramicroscopic dimensions (0.1 micron) may be identified with the electron microscope.

In the ureter, the mucosa is thrown into longitudinal folds, giving it a characteristic star-shaped appearance in cross sections. Because of these longitudinal folds and the presence of well-developed longitudinal musculature, together with transitional epithelial lining, sizable calculi may distend the ureter without injury to the mucosa or wall and are passed by peristalsis. (Normally, peristaltic waves descending the ureters move only small amounts of urine which are squirted into the bladder.)

In the bladder, the folding of the mucosa is more irregular and governed in part by the underlying muscle strands. In the region of the trigone, it is, as noted

before, a tight and quite smooth mucous membrane.

At least in the human, a tunica submucosa cannot be identified in the urinary excretory structures. However, connective tissue fibers and elastic fibers abound in the lamina propria, and these become somewhat looser near the muscular layers. This feature has prompted some authors to refer to this outer zone of the propria as the submucosa. In other species, such as the rhesus monkey, a readily identified muscularis mucosa separates the tunica propria of the bladder from the submucosa.

In the mucosa of the human ureters, no glands are identified, but in the bladder, epithelial clusters of mucus-secreting cells can be found. Near the commencement of the urethra these resemble the urethral glands of Littré.

(For histology of the urethra see CIBA COLLECTION, Vol. 2, page 20, for the male; page 106 for the female.) ☐

Blood Supply of Ureters and Bladder

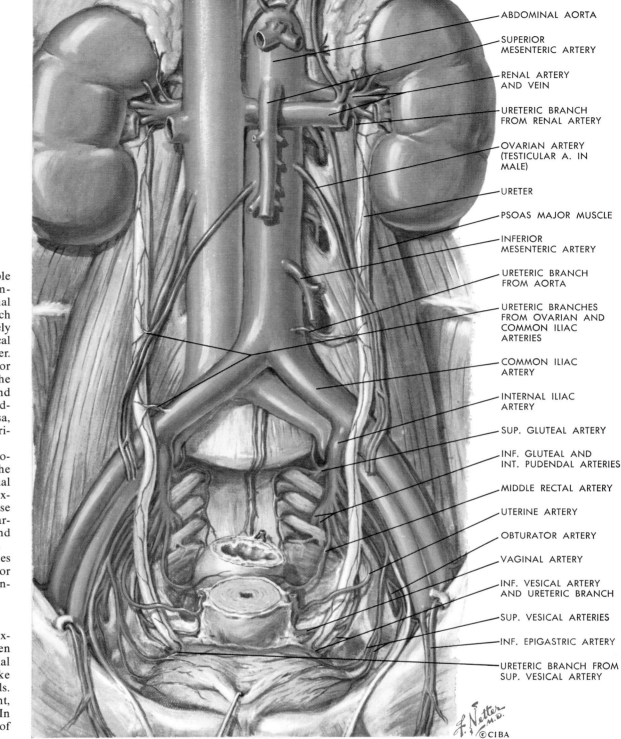

ABDOMINAL AORTA

SUPERIOR MESENTERIC ARTERY

RENAL ARTERY AND VEIN

URETERIC BRANCH FROM RENAL ARTERY

OVARIAN ARTERY (TESTICULAR A. IN MALE)

URETER

PSOAS MAJOR MUSCLE

INFERIOR MESENTERIC ARTERY

URETERIC BRANCH FROM AORTA

URETERIC BRANCHES FROM OVARIAN AND COMMON ILIAC ARTERIES

COMMON ILIAC ARTERY

INTERNAL ILIAC ARTERY

SUP. GLUTEAL ARTERY

INF. GLUTEAL AND INT. PUDENDAL ARTERIES

MIDDLE RECTAL ARTERY

UTERINE ARTERY

OBTURATOR ARTERY

VAGINAL ARTERY

INF. VESICAL ARTERY AND URETERIC BRANCH

SUP. VESICAL ARTERIES

INF. EPIGASTRIC ARTERY

URETERIC BRANCH FROM SUP. VESICAL ARTERY

F. Netter M.D.
©CIBA

Ureters

The blood supply of the ureters is variable and by no means symmetrical. Commonly, an artery stems from the renal artery, either directly or by way of a branch to the renal pelvis. Another vessel, rarely absent, arises from the inferior vesical artery near the inferior end of the ureter. Additional vessels arise from the inferior vesical, the gonadal, the common iliac, the external and internal iliac arteries, and from the aorta directly. The ureter, adherent to the posterior aspect of the serosa, also receives small twigs from minor peritoneal arteries.

The arteries form longitudinal anastomotic meshes on the outer wall of the ureter and can usually establish functional collateral circulation. However, in approximately 10 to 15 percent of cases, these collaterals fail to be efficient, and the arterial supply must be carefully noted and evaluated during operative procedures.

The ureteric veins follow the arteries and drain into the renal vein, the inferior vena cava and its tributaries, and the endopelvic venous plexus.

Urinary Bladder

The anatomy of the bladder, with the exception of its vascular supply, has been described (see pages 20–22). The arterial supply to the organ arises from the fanlike ramification of the internal iliac vessels. Since this ramification is very inconstant, the vesical arteries vary accordingly. In general, three main arteries (or groups of arteries) may be distinguished.

1. The *superior vesical artery* is the terminal branch of the *umbilical artery*. Beyond the origin of this vessel, the umbilical artery obliterates and forms the *medial umbilical ligament.** The superior vesical artery is the most constant and the most significant blood supply to the bladder. The artery may be double and it arises somewhat below the level of the pelvic brim. Its branches are tortuous, course over the superior and posterior aspects of the bladder, and anastomose with each other, with their fellows of the opposite

---

*This term for the obliterated umbilical artery was adopted by the *Nomina Anatomica* (N.A.) in 1966. The structure projects the peritoneal *medial umbilical fold.*The vestigial urachus in the midline is now named the *median umbilical ligament* (and is covered by the *median umbilical fold*). The slight ridge raised by the inferior epigastric vessels is, according to the N.A., the *lateral umbilical fold.*

---

side, and with the lower vesical arteries. Their pattern allows for changes in size of the bladder. In addition, in infants, both a small *urachal branch* to the umbilical area and anastomoses with the inferior epigastric artery may be present.

2. The *vesiculodeferential artery of the male* (or a sizable branch off a vaginal or uterine artery in the female) is usually referred to as the *inferior vesical artery*. In the male, this vessel arises most often from the *umbilical artery*, together with, or near to, the artery of the ductus deferens. The inferior vesical artery, on its way to the bladder, lies in the lateral true vesical ligament and gives off twigs to the seminal vesicle. In both male and female, it supplies the terminal portion of the ureter with an *inferior ureteric artery* and ramifies over the posterior basal part of the bladder.

3. The lower anterior and the anterior basal parts of the bladder are supplied by an artery from a prostatic

or a vaginal vessel, which in turn, arises from the internal pudendal artery. The vessel reaches the bladder via the lateral true ligament and has been more intensively studied in the male. It is sometimes called the inferior vesical artery. However, authors who use this latter term refer to the vessel described in the preceding paragraph as the middle vesical artery or vesiculodeferential artery.

The vesical veins are short and unite into a rich pudendal plexus around the base of the bladder. In the male, this plexus surrounds the prostate gland as well. It is called the *vesical* or *pudendal plexus* and has communications with the veins of the perineum and the dorsal vein of the penis (or clitoris). Multiple interconnecting channels lead from the vesical plexus into the internal iliac vein. Anastomoses with the parietal veins of the pelvis establish connections to the thigh and the buttock. □

Lymphatics of Kidneys, Ureters, and Bladder

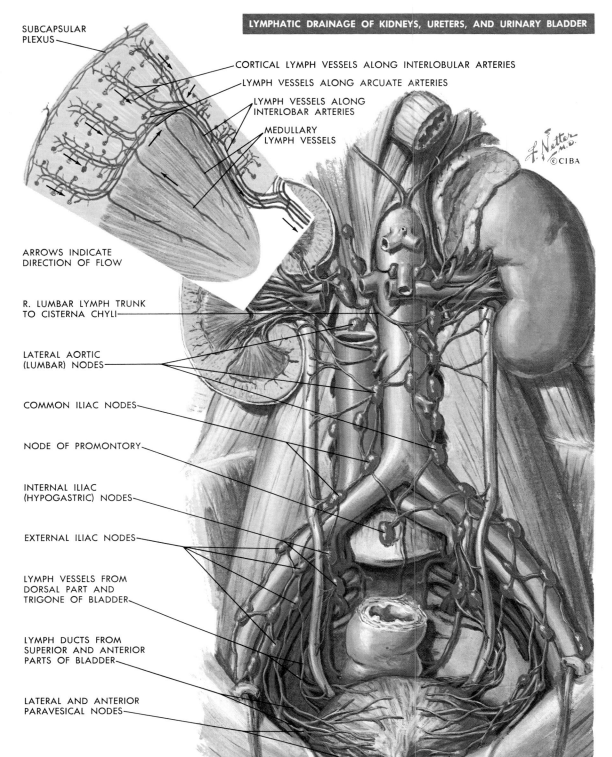

SUBCAPSULAR PLEXUS

CORTICAL LYMPH VESSELS ALONG INTERLOBULAR ARTERIES

LYMPH VESSELS ALONG ARCUATE ARTERIES

LYMPH VESSELS ALONG INTERLOBAR ARTERIES

MEDULLARY LYMPH VESSELS

ARROWS INDICATE DIRECTION OF FLOW

R. LUMBAR LYMPH TRUNK TO CISTERNA CHYLI

LATERAL AORTIC (LUMBAR) NODES

COMMON ILIAC NODES

NODE OF PROMONTORY

INTERNAL ILIAC (HYPOGASTRIC) NODES

EXTERNAL ILIAC NODES

LYMPH VESSELS FROM DORSAL PART AND TRIGONE OF BLADDER

LYMPH DUCTS FROM SUPERIOR AND ANTERIOR PARTS OF BLADDER

LATERAL AND ANTERIOR PARAVESICAL NODES

Lymph from the lower urinary tract first drains into the *submucous* network of lymph capillaries and then into an *extramuscular* plexus. This plexus, in turn, connects with vessels arising in the wall of the viscus. The plexuses are devoid of valves, unlike the vessels which drain into various groups of regional lymph nodes.

Lower Urinary Tract

Urethra. Lymph from the cavernous part of the urethra, as well as from other areas of the penis, flows to regional lymph nodes in the *deep subinguinal* group. The lymph channels from the membranous and prostatic portions of the male urethra, and the whole urethra in the female, drain into nodes situated along the internal iliac vessels—the *hypogastric nodes.*

Bladder. Drainage from the posterior wall of the urinary bladder is first to the *hypogastric nodes.* From the anterior wall of the bladder, the collecting channels enter the *external iliac nodes.* However, some vessels are interrupted by small vesical nodes of which there are anterior and lateral subgroups. The latter lie near the beginning of the obliterated umbilical artery and are regional for the apex of the bladder.

Ureter. The most inferior portion of the ureter is drained by a few lymph vessels which reach the hypogastric nodes directly or by joining the efferent vessels from the bladder. More superiorly, the channels draining the ureter enter into the *common* and *external iliac nodes,* while near the kidney, drainage is to the *aortic* and *paraaortic nodes.* Also in this region, the ureter shares regional lymph nodes with the kidney, either by direct communication or by emptying into renal lymphatic trunks.

Kidney

Beneath the surface of the kidney, a scanty *subcapsular plexus* of lymph capillaries anastomoses by means of perforating channels with the extrarenal vessels of the retroperitoneal tissues. These channels eventually drain into *superior aortic nodes.* The subcapsular plexus also communicates sparingly with lymphatics in the deeper layers of the parenchyma. Here the lymph capillaries accompany the blood vessels and are found chiefly in the connective tissue framework. Those surrounding arterioles are generally larger and more numerous than those associated with the venules.

According to most authorities, the lymphatic capillaries are in contact with the tubules in the cortex but are absent in the medullary rays and the glomeruli. However, it has been demonstrated that the glomerular capsule is surrounded by a net of lymph capillaries. Peirce considers such a relationship strictly casual and considers those lymphatics near the glomeruli as being periarterial channels.

The methods of experimentally producing stasis and congestion (Babics and Rényi-Vámos) and of observing carcinomatous permeation of the lymphatics (Rawson) bear out these statements, although some disagreements cannot be reconciled. For example, Rawson found lymph vessels ascending from the pyramidal apices through the medulla to the cortex (see insert). This finding, however, was denied by Peirce who used intravital injection methods. Attempts at direct intravascular injection of lymph channels have yielded equivocal results, and the anatomy of the intrinsic renal lymphatics, under physiologic conditions, has yet to be fully explored, particularly in man.

Accompanying the vascular tree, the large lymph vessels eventually reach the renal sinus and exit at the hilus. They are joined by vessels from the renal capsule and converge into a few valve-studded trunks which accompany the renal artery and vein. As noted previously, the first lymph nodes are the superior aortic nodes of the lumbar chain.

In summary, the lymph drainage of the lower urinary system involves the subinguinal, common, internal (hypogastric), and external iliac groups of nodes. Drainage from the upper ureter and kidney flows into the aortic and paraaortic nodes. The lymph then flows into the thoracic duct via the lumbar lymph trunk. □

Innervation of Kidneys, Ureters, and Bladder

ANTERIOR VAGAL TRUNK

POSTERIOR VAGAL TRUNK

SUPERIOR (GREATEST) THORACIC SPLANCHNIC NERVE

CELIAC PLEXUS AND GANGLIA

MIDDLE (LESSER) THORACIC SPLANCHNIC NERVE

INFERIOR (LOWEST OR LEAST) THORACIC SPLANCHNIC NERVE

AORTICORENAL GANGLION

POSTERIOR RENAL GANGLION

RENAL PLEXUS

1st LUMBAR SPLANCHNIC NERVE

RENAL AND UPPER URETERIC BRANCHES FROM INTER-MESENTERIC PLEXUS

INTERMESENTERIC (AORTIC) PLEXUS

TESTICULAR ARTERY

SYMPATHETIC TRUNK (GANGLION)

MIDDLE URETERIC NERVE

SUPERIOR HYPOGASTRIC PLEXUS

BRANCHES FROM SACRAL SYMPATHETIC TRUNK TO HYPOGASTRIC NERVE

GRAY RAMUS COMMUNICANS

HYPOGASTRIC NERVE

SACRAL PLEXUS

PUDENDAL NERVE

PELVIC SPLANCHNIC NERVES (NERVI ERIGENTES)

INFERIOR HYPOGASTRIC (PELVIC) PLEXUS WITH PERIURETERIC LOOPS AND BRANCHES TO LOWER URETER

RECTAL PLEXUS

VESICAL PLEXUS

PROSTATIC PLEXUS

Anatomical Arrangement

The kidneys are richly innervated by branches from diverse sources—the *celiac plexus*, the *thoracic* and upper *lumbar splanchnic nerves,* and the *intermesenteric (aortic)* and *superior hypogastric plexuses.* From their various origins, these renal nerves converge toward, and form an open-meshed plexus around, the renal vessels. The intrinsic renal nerves are derived from the plexus. Bilateral symmetry in the arrangement is seldom found.

The ureters, like the kidneys, are profusely innervated. Their nerve supplies originate from both abdominal and pelvic sources and are arranged in three main groups—*superior, middle,* and *inferior ureteric nerves.*

THE SUPERIOR URETERIC NERVES arise from the lower part of the homolateral renal plexus and run downward for variable distances along the upper part of the ureter. Their sympathetic fibers are derived from the same sources as those in the renal plexus (see page 28) and convey both efferent and afferent impulses. Most of the preganglionic fibers involved are believed to form synapses in ganglia in the renal plexus. Although some tiny ganglia exist upon or within the walls of the ureters, probably most of them are parasympathetic relay stations.

The parasympathetic renal branches, arising from the *superior hypogastric plexus* or the lower end of the *intermesenteric plexus* (derived ultimately from the

pelvic splanchnic nerves, see page 28), always supply one or more filaments to the upper ureter.

The superior ureteric group of nerves are usually united to the nearby gonadal nerves by delicate bundles, and both are often connected at their origins to a small ganglion or ganglia in the inferior part of the renal plexus. Together they also give off fascicles which unite with others from the lumbar splanchnic nerves and from the superior and inferior mesenteric and intermesenteric plexuses to constitute a widespread, tenuous, retroperitoneal nerve network.

THE MIDDLE URETERIC NERVES supply the intermediate part of the ureter and consist of two or more filaments from the side of the superior hypogastric plexus and from the upper end of the homolateral hypogastric nerve. They arise near, or in combination with, the middle gonadal nervelets and are associated with a small ureteric artery. (This artery arises from the

common iliac artery near its point of bifurcation, or from the external or internal iliac arteries.) The middle ureteric nerves are generally interconnected with branches supplying the ductus (vas) deferens. They sometimes communicate with iliac arterial nerves, with the lower lumbar splanchnic nerves, with rami from the upper part of the sacral sympathetic trunk, and with the genitofemoral nerve.

THE INFERIOR URETERIC NERVES supply the lower end of the ureter and are derived from the termination of the homolateral hypogastric nerve, the upper part of the inferior hypogastric plexus, or both. The nerves form one or two loops around the lowest part of the ureter. Alternately, the ureter may pass through a fenestration in the inferior hypogastric plexus. These ureteric nerves are closely associated with filaments to adjacent parts of the ductus deferens, the seminal vesicle, and the urinary bladder. *Continued on page 28*

Continued on page 28

Innervation of Kidneys, Ureters, and Bladder

Continued from page 27

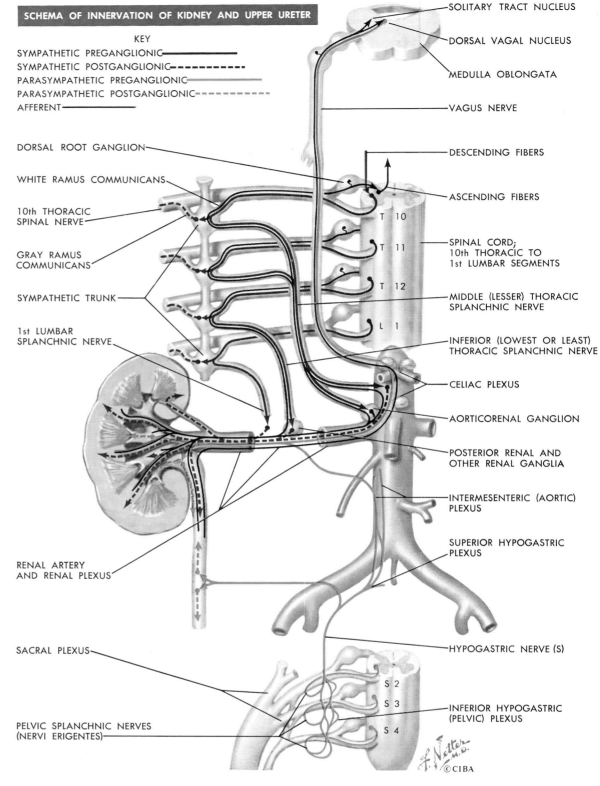

SCHEMA OF INNERVATION OF KIDNEY AND UPPER URETER

KEY

SYMPATHETIC PREGANGLIONIC ———————
SYMPATHETIC POSTGANGLIONIC – – – – – – –
PARASYMPATHETIC PREGANGLIONIC ———————
PARASYMPATHETIC POSTGANGLIONIC – – – – – – –
AFFERENT ———————

SOLITARY TRACT NUCLEUS

DORSAL VAGAL NUCLEUS

MEDULLA OBLONGATA

VAGUS NERVE

DORSAL ROOT GANGLION

WHITE RAMUS COMMUNICANS

DESCENDING FIBERS

ASCENDING FIBERS

10th THORACIC SPINAL NERVE

T 10

GRAY RAMUS COMMUNICANS

T 11

SPINAL CORD; 10th THORACIC TO 1st LUMBAR SEGMENTS

SYMPATHETIC TRUNK

T 12

MIDDLE (LESSER) THORACIC SPLANCHNIC NERVE

1st LUMBAR SPLANCHNIC NERVE

L 1

INFERIOR (LOWEST OR LEAST) THORACIC SPLANCHNIC NERVE

CELIAC PLEXUS

AORTICORENAL GANGLION

POSTERIOR RENAL AND OTHER RENAL GANGLIA

INTERMESENTERIC (AORTIC) PLEXUS

SUPERIOR HYPOGASTRIC PLEXUS

RENAL ARTERY AND RENAL PLEXUS

HYPOGASTRIC NERVE (S)

SACRAL PLEXUS

S 2

S 3

INFERIOR HYPOGASTRIC (PELVIC) PLEXUS

S 4

PELVIC SPLANCHNIC NERVES (NERVI ERIGENTES)

f. Netter m.d.
©CIBA

The urinary bladder is supplied by many nerves which arise from the anterior parts of the inferior hypogastric plexuses (sometimes termed the extrinsic vesical plexuses) and from the loops around the lower ends of the ureters.

Schema: Kidney and Upper Ureter

Sympathetic Supply. The preganglionic sympathetic nerves for the kidneys and ureters emerge from the spinal cord through the ventral nerve roots of the (tenth), eleventh, and twelfth thoracic and first lumbar spinal nerves. They then pass in white rami communicantes to adjacent ganglia in the sympathetic trunks and leave these in three or four nerves: the *middle (lesser)* and *inferior (lowest* or *least) thoracic splanchnic nerves* and the *first* (and perhaps *second*) *lumbar splanchnic nerves.*

The middle thoracic splanchnic nerve usually ends in the ipsilateral celiac or aorticorenal ganglion. The other nerves mentioned may do likewise but more often end directly in the renal plexus or in a small posterior renal ganglion lying behind the renal artery.

Most of the preganglionic fibers form synaptic relays in the celiac, aorticorenal, or posterior renal ganglia or in other, even smaller, renal ganglia incorporated at nodal points in the renal plexuses.

The postganglionic fibers form fascicles which surround and accompany the upper ureteric, pelvic, and calyceal branches,

and the segmental branches of the renal vessels *(q.v.).*

Afferent fibers from the kidney, pelvis, and upper ureter follow similar routes, but in the reverse direction. They do not form synaptic relays in peripheral ganglia, and their cell bodies are located in dorsal spinal nerve root ganglia. The central processes of these dorsal ganglion cells enter the spinal cord mainly through the dorsal nerve roots of the tenth, eleventh, and twelfth thoracic spinal nerves, and they ascend in or alongside the spinothalamic tracts and in the posterior white columns of the cord.

The parasympathetic supply is derived from two sources. One group of parasympathetic fibers is carried through the vagal contribution to the celiac plexus. Some of these vagal fibers are conveyed onward to the kidney and its vessels, through the celiac contributions, to the renal plexuses. Other parasympathetic fibers, emerging through the pelvic splanchnic nerves

(nervi erigentes), may also reach the kidney (or at least its collecting tubules), renal pelvis, and upper ureter by a more indirect route. Such an arrangement is understandable on embryologic grounds, as all the structures mentioned are derived from buds developed from the cloacal ends of the mesonephric ducts. These pelvic parasympathetic fibers (see also page 29) join the inferior hypogastric (pelvic) plexus and ascend in the hypogastric nerves to the superior hypogastric plexus *(presacral nerve).* The fibers leave the superior hypogastric plexus in fine branches which ascend retroperitoneally to enter the inferolateral parts of the homolateral renal plexus.

Intrarenal Arrangement. Within the kidney, the nerves form rich perivascular plexuses around the renal artery and its branches. The *sympathetic postganglionic* or *efferent fibers* are distributed to the vascular musculature, to the smooth muscle in the renal pelvis and

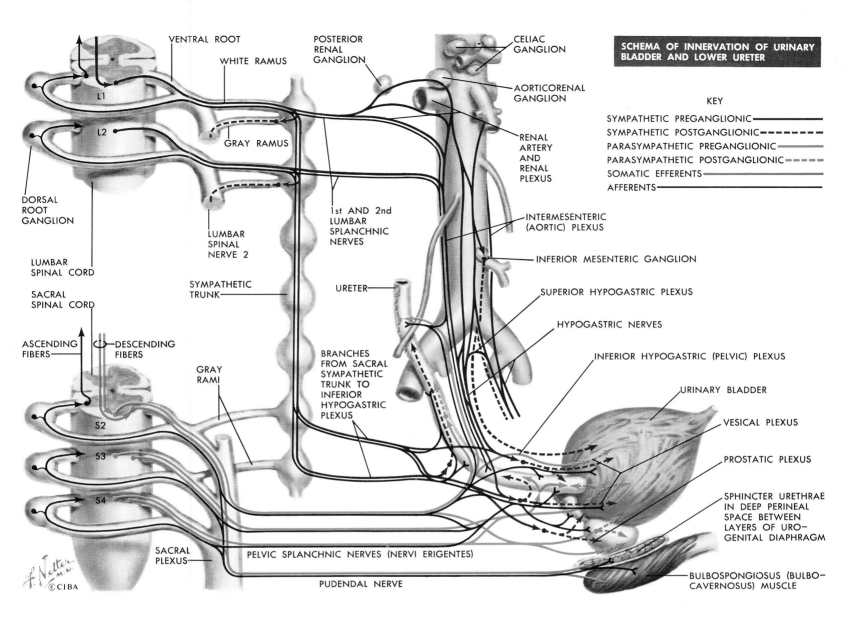

KEY

SYMPATHETIC PREGANGLIONIC————————
SYMPATHETIC POSTGANGLIONIC— — — — —
PARASYMPATHETIC PREGANGLIONIC————————
PARASYMPATHETIC POSTGANGLIONIC— — — — —
SOMATIC EFFERENTS————————
AFFERENTS————————

calyces, and probably to the renal tubules, juxtaglomerular apparatus, and glomeruli.

The *parasympathetic postganglionic fibers* supply the muscle in the upper ureter, pelvis, and calyces, but it is uncertain whether they supply the vessels and tubules.

Afferent nerve fiber terminations have been found in the adventitia of the renal vessels, near the glomeruli, and in the musculature of the pelvis. Afferent impulses from the kidney and urinary tract are also conveyed to the central nervous system through both sympathetic and parasympathetic pathways.

Schema: Bladder and Inferior Ureter

Autonomic and Afferent Supply. The sympathetic preganglionic cells concerned with vesical innervation are located in the upper two lumbar segments and perhaps also in the lowest thoracic segment of the spinal cord. The sites of synapse of the preganglionic fibers with the ganglionic neurons, where the postganglionic fibers arise, have not been determined accurately. Some writers state that the synapses occur in the inferior mesenteric ganglia, whereas others assert that the relays are in ganglia in the inferior hypogastric plexus or even in ganglia located close to, or within, the wall of the urinary bladder.

The parasympathetic preganglionic cells are located in the second to fourth sacral segments of the spinal cord. The ganglia are near, or actually within, the wall of the urinary bladder.

Afferent fibers pursue similar pathways, but in the reverse direction, so that some vesical sensory impulses enter the cord through the upper lumbar (and perhaps the last thoracic) dorsal nerve roots. Others from the neck of the bladder, and probably also from the lowest parts of the ureters, enter the cord via the pelvic splanchnic nerves and the dorsal nerve roots of the second to fourth sacral nerve segments.

Intrinsic Vesical Arrangement. The nerves enter the bladder wall mainly alongside the vessels. They divide and subdivide and are ultimately carried to all parts, forming a widespread intramural or intrinsic vesical plexus. The nerve fasciculi are most conspicuous in the trigonal and neighboring regions, becoming more scattered and attenuated toward the fundus. Many small ganglia are present on the surface or are buried within the muscular bundles, and these are also more numerous in the trigonal region.

Most of the nerve fasciculi in the urinary bladder wall contain unmyelinated or finely myelinated fibers. A small portion of larger myelinated and presumably sensory fibers are connected with complex terminal arborizations and are regarded as stretch receptors. Many other putative sensory endings have been described in the submucosa and mucous membrane.

The parasympathetic nerves may transmit many or most of the afferent fibers from the trigonal area of the urinary bladder and from the lowest parts of the ureters, including those conveying painful and thermal impulses. However, some afferents from the neck of the bladder, prostate, and prostatic urethra may reach the spinal cord via the pudendal nerves.

Functional Considerations. Sensations associated with vesical distention may be mediated through sympathetic pathways, since vague feelings of discomfort may still be experienced by patients with transverse lesions of the cord below the level of the uppermost lumbar segments. This suggests an afferent inflow from the bladder through the upper lumbar or lowest thoracic dorsal spinal nerve roots. Alternatively, such sensations may be produced by stimulation of nerve endings in the peritoneum. However, since "presacral neurectomy" (removal of the superior hypogastric plexus) alleviates discomfort in patients with painful and intractable cystitis, a portion of the vesical afferent fibers probably traverse the hypogastric nerves and superior hypogastric plexus. Afferent fibers may also travel in the perivascular plexuses of the vesical and iliac arteries and thus reach the superior hypogastric plexus. They then run in lumbar splanchnic nerves to the sympathetic trunks, pass through rami communicantes to the upper lumbar and lowest thoracic spinal nerves, and enter the cord through the dorsal roots of these nerves.

The parasympathetic supply to the bladder is actively involved in micturition and produces contraction of the walls and relaxation of the sphincteric mechanism. Most investigators associate the sympathetic supply with opposing effects, such as relaxation of the vesical walls and contraction of the sphincter. However, a minority claim that the sympathetic effects are predominantly vasomotor, and that the parasympathetic nerves are of paramount importance in controlling both the filling and emptying of the urinary bladder. □

Development of Pronephros and Mesonephros

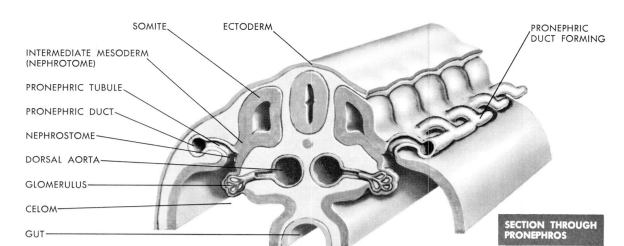

SOMITE — ECTODERM — PRONEPHRIC DUCT FORMING

INTERMEDIATE MESODERM (NEPHROTOME)

PRONEPHRIC TUBULE

PRONEPHRIC DUCT

NEPHROSTOME

DORSAL AORTA

GLOMERULUS

CELOM

GUT

SECTION THROUGH PRONEPHROS

The development of the urinary system is closely related to that of the genital system. Both are of mesodermal origin, and their excretory ducts initially enter a common cavity, the *cloaca*. The anlage of the kidney is the nephrotome which appears in the *intermediate mesoderm,* between the *somite* and the *lateral plate.* All of these structures are formed by the differentiation of the mesodermal cell. To understand the embryology of the human kidney, it is necessary to follow the phylogenetic development of the kidney, including that of the lower vertebrates, since the ontogenesis of the kidney of higher mammals recapitulates the phylogenesis.

The excretory organ which appears first in the vertebrate animals is the *pronephros.* In the majority of the adult vertebrates, it is either vestigial or completely absent, though in the lamprey, the lowest vertebrate, it functions as a permanent kidney.

In the process of development, the pronephros degenerates and is replaced by the *mesonephros* which forms caudally to it. In the higher fishes and the amphibia, the mesonephros is the final excretory organ. In the amniotes—reptiles, birds, and mammals—the mesonephros also degenerates, following the appearance of the *metanephros* still more caudally in the body. The metanephros is the permanent kidney of the amniotes, including man. Though the human kidney shows remarkable alterations in structure and location during the process of development, it is important to know that it originates in the *nephrotome* arising from the intermediate mesoderm.

In man, the nephrotome, the mother tissue of the pronephros, appears in the intermediate mesoderm at the level of the cervical and upper thoracic regions in the third fetal week. The *pronephric tubules* (seven pairs) develop in the nephrotome in the intermediate mesoderm. At the same time, the *pronephric duct* appears in the dorsal part of the nephrotome, and connects with the pronephric tubules. In man, the *pronephric tubules* rapidly degenerate without any further development, though the pronephric duct extends to the caudal part of the embryo and reaches the cloaca.

Detailed observations on the morphogenesis of the pronephros are made mainly in the lower animals, since in man, the pronephric tubules develop very poorly and degenerate before the establishment of the typical pronephros.

In the lamprey, four pairs of pronephric tubules appear in the nephrotome

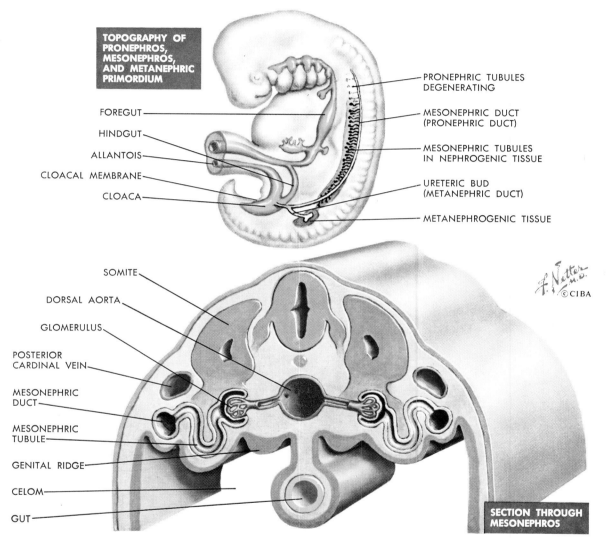

TOPOGRAPHY OF PRONEPHROS, MESONEPHROS, AND METANEPHRIC PRIMORDIUM

FOREGUT

HINDGUT

ALLANTOIS

CLOACAL MEMBRANE

CLOACA

PRONEPHRIC TUBULES DEGENERATING

MESONEPHRIC DUCT (PRONEPHRIC DUCT)

MESONEPHRIC TUBULES IN NEPHROGENIC TISSUE

URETERIC BUD (METANEPHRIC DUCT)

METANEPHROGENIC TISSUE

SOMITE

DORSAL AORTA

GLOMERULUS

POSTERIOR CARDINAL VEIN

MESONEPHRIC DUCT

MESONEPHRIC TUBULE

GENITAL RIDGE

CELOM

GUT

SECTION THROUGH MESONEPHROS

and open into the *celom* and into the cloaca. The opening into the cloaca, the *nephrostome,* is surrounded by ciliated epithelium, while the pronephric duct eventually connects with the cloaca. A branch of the *dorsal aorta* reaches beneath the lateral plate and forms a capillary glomus. Such primitive glomeruli face the celom through a thin layer of mesothelium and perform the function of a blood filter. The pronephros of the lamprey remains as the permanent kidney and functions as the excretory organ.

Though the human mesonephros is a transitory organ soon replaced by the metanephros, it attains a fairly sophisticated stage of development and acts as the excretory organ. The *mesonephric tubules* are formed in the intermediate mesoderm by the fourth fetal week. These tubules fuse with the *mesonephric duct* (wolffian duct), which is the extension of the duct of the pronephros. The successive formation of the

tubules proceeds toward the caudal part of the intermediate mesoderm. However, simultaneously, degeneration of the tubules begins in the more cranial tubules. The branched vessels from the dorsal aorta reach the blind ends of the tubules and form glomeruli. The efferent vessel from each *glomerulus* forms a capillary plexus around a tubule. Though the human mesonephros attains excretory function by the sixth fetal week, the tubules, as well as the glomeruli, begin to degenerate shortly thereafter. Some of the tubules remain and transform into the efferent ductules of the male and into the epinephron of the female. The pronephric duct in the male becomes the ductus deferens and plays a role as the sexual duct, though it vanishes entirely in the female.

Except in the lower animals such as the majority of the cyclostomes, fishes, and amphibia, the mesonephros is the transitory excretory organ. □

Development of Metanephros

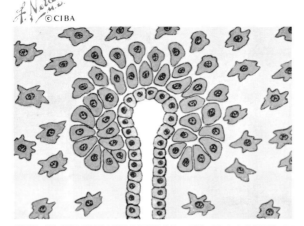

THE METANEPHRIC DUCT (URETERIC BUD) HAS GROWN OUT FROM THE MESONEPHRIC DUCT, CLOSE TO TERMINATION OF LATTER IN CLOACA, AND HAS INVADED THE METANEPHROGENIC MESODERM

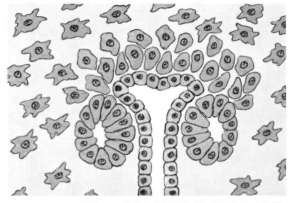

WITHIN THE METANEPHROGENIC TISSUE THE URETERIC BUD EXPANDS TO FORM A PELVIS WHICH BRANCHES INTO CALYCES, AND THESE, IN TURN, BUD INTO SUCCESSIVE GENERATIONS OF COLLECTING DUCTS

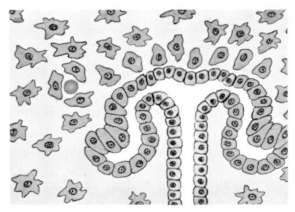

CELLS OF THE METANEPHROGENIC MESODERM AGGREGATE AROUND THE EXPANDED BLIND EXTREMITY OF EACH COLLECTING DUCT TO FORM A "METANEPHRIC CAP"

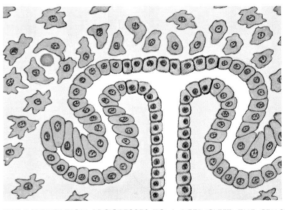

THE AMPULLAR TERMINATION OF THE COLLECTING DUCT FLATTENS AND BRANCHES; A NEST OF CELLS FORMS AND SEPARATES THE METANEPHRIC CAP ON EACH SIDE, AND ACQUIRES A LUMEN TO FORM A "METANEPHRIC VESICLE"

THE VESICLE ELONGATES AND ITS LUMEN JOINS THAT OF THE COLLECTING DUCT; AN INDENTATION APPEARS ON THE OUTER SURFACE OF THE VESICLE WHICH THUS BEGINS TO ASSUME AN "S" SHAPE

THE INDENTATION PROGRESSES TO A DEEP CLEFT; THE CELLS BORDERING THE LOWER MARGIN OF THE CLEFT BECOME TALL, WHILE THOSE ACROSS THE LUMEN FROM THEM FLATTEN

Following the regression of the mesonephros, the *metanephros* appears in the human fetus as the *permanent kidney*, possessing a highly developed excretory function. The metanephros is composed of two different systems, the *metanephric duct*, or the primitive ureter, and the *metanephrogenic tissue* from the caudal part of the intermediate mesoderm. However, both systems are of mesodermal origin. The development of the human metanephros starts with the formation of the metanephric duct. In the fourth fetal week, the duct buds from the mesonephric duct (wolffian duct) in the vicinity of the entrance of the mesonephric duct into the *cloaca*. This *ureteric bud* is a paired structure lying at the level of the fourth lumbar segment. The bud extends dorsocranially. Its end becomes enlarged to form the primitive *pelvis* which soon shows divisions into the cephalic and the caudal *primary calyces*. From each primary calyx, subdivisions occur which are called *secondary calyces*. From the tip of each secondary calyx, the *collecting ducts* generate by dichotomic *branching*. By the fifth fetal month, 10 to 12 *generations* have formed by progressive branching of the collecting duct. Also, during the development of the metanephros, the primary calyces absorb the collecting ducts of the first to fourth generations, thus enlarging the pelvis and the calyces.

In addition to the ducts, the metanephrogenic tissue contains *aggregates of mesodermal cells* which invest the tips of the terminal branches of the collecting ducts, forming *caps* which ride on the *ampullae (terminal dilations)* of the ducts.

These aggregates develop hollow vesicles *(metanephric vesicles)* around the

necks of the ampullae. The cells line the *lumina* of these vesicles in the manner of epithelial cells, forming primitive uriniferous tubules. This transformation spreads rapidly through the remaining metanephrogenic tissue in the vicinity of the ampullae. At the same time, each ampulla begins to flatten and branch. These branches, called arched collecting ducts, soon fuse with the metanephric vesicles (or primitive uriniferous tubules), forming a future passageway for urine. From each arched collecting duct, a new ampulla of the next order buds and eventually joins with another metanephric vesicle. (It is interesting to note that failure of linkage between the primitive uriniferous tubules and the collecting ducts may be the cause of polycystic kidney, see pages 226-228.)

Although the majority of the metanephrogenic cells differentiate into tubular cells, a few of them transform into the mesenchymal cells distributed in the stroma

of the metanephros. In man, formation of nephrons continues until the late stages of intrauterine life. In the tenth fetal month, the metanephrogenic tissue disappears, suggesting that the postnatal formation of nephrons does not occur.

As the differentiation of the primitive uriniferous tubule proceeds, the stroma of the metanephros becomes rich in blood vessels. The blood supply to the metanephros arises from the branches of the renal artery and so differs from the blood supply of the mesonephros which is provided by direct branches from the aorta.

Referring again to the primitive renal tubule, the cephalic part becomes *indented*, forming an *S-shaped* curve. The *indentation* or *cleft of the S* is the site of the future glomerulus.

It will be recalled that the renal glomerulus consists of four structural elements: *Continued on page 32*

Development of
Metanephros

Continued from page 31

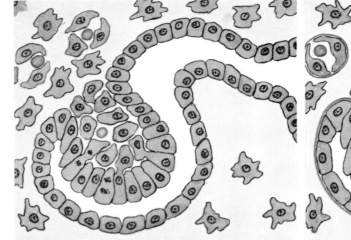

CELLS APPEAR WITHIN THE CLEFT, WHICH IS NOW SOMEWHAT BROADENED; ACCORDING TO SUZUKI AND OTHERS, THESE CELLS ORIGINATE FROM THE CELLS BORDERING THE CLEFT

BASEMENT MEMBRANE APPEARS, SEPARATING THE INTRA-CLEFTAL CELL MASS FROM THE BORDERING CELLS; THE UPPER MARGIN OF THE CLEFT PUSHES OUT TO MOVE THE CLEFT MOUTH FARTHER FROM THE TUBULE AND TO FORM A CAPSULE

THE INTRACLEFTAL CELLS DIFFERENTIATE INTO ENDOTHELIAL CELLS (YELLOW) WHICH ENCLOSE CAPILLARIES AND MESANGIAL CELLS (BLUE) THAT LIE IN THE STALKS BETWEEN THE CAPILLARIES; INDENTATIONS SEPARATE THE CAPILLARIES INTO LOBULES; THE CELLS BORDERING THE CLEFT OUTSIDE THE BASEMENT MEMBRANE BEGIN TO FORM FOOT PROCESSES, AND THE CELLS LINING THE CAPSULE FLATTEN

(a) the *epithelial cells* (parietal cell lining or Bowman's capsule, and the visceral cells or podocytes), (b) the *basement membrane,* (c) the *endothelial cells,* and (d) the *mesangium* consisting of cells and matrix (see pages 7 and 9). The development of these structural elements of the glomerulus will now be described.

Formation of Glomerulus

The formation of the renal glomerulus starts with the appearance of the mesenchymal cells in the *cleft* of the S-shaped tubule. At this early stage, the cells are few in number and are located just beneath the prospective visceral epithelium of the glomerulus *(podocytes)*. Despite the existence of the primitive blood vessels elsewhere in the myxomatous stroma, at this time there are no capillaries within the cleft. The basement membrane of the S-shaped tubule, as well as of the primitive vessels, is hardly developed. It is suggested that the mesenchymal cells in the cleft are derived from the cells of the S-shaped tubule since, at the very early stage, both cell types are similar in structure and not separated by a basement membrane.

The *basement membrane* appears as the next step of the glomerular development. A continuous layer of basement membrane is formed around the S-shaped tubule and in the cleft, clearly separating the mesenchymal cells from the tubular cells facing the cleft. The latter will differentiate into the podocytes of the glomerulus. This basement membrane is thicker than that of other parts of the S-shaped tubule, and it will form the glomerular capillary basement membrane in the future. At this stage, the mesenchymal

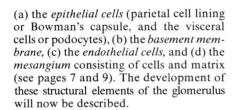

BY ACCRETION AND SUBDIVISION, THE NUMBER OF CAPILLARIES IS INCREASED; THEY COMMUNICATE WITH EACH OTHER AND WITH VESSELS IN THE SURROUNDING MESODERM; MATRIX APPEARS BETWEEN THE MESANGIAL CELLS; MUSCLE CELLS (TAN) DEVELOP AROUND THE AFFERENT AND EFFERENT VESSELS AND THE JUXTA-GLOMERULAR CELLS (PURPLE) BETWEEN THEM

cells increase in number by repeated cell division. Small spaces appear between the cells and contain red blood cells. It is not known whether these red blood cells form locally or migrate from nearby blood vessels. Some of the mesenchymal cells elongate and surround the red blood cells, thus forming the early capillary endothelium. Other mesenchymal cells give rise to the mesangial cells, though the mesangial matrix does not form until later. The layer of future podocytes gradually becomes scalloped or indented and bulges toward the lumen of the S-shaped tubule.

During the next stage, progressive organization of the glomerulus takes place. Beneath the prospective glomerular basement membrane, the mesenchymal cells are transformed into the endothelial cells, become flattened, and form junctions with other similarly flattened cells. These immature endothelial cells lack fe-

nestrae, though they are directly exposed to the blood. The majority of the mesenchymal cells still lie in the cleft, and a small amount of *mesangial matrix* appears between and around the cells. Some of these cells begin to differentiate into smooth muscle cells of the *afferent* and *efferent arterioles*. The visceral layer of the glomerular epithelium grows in complexity, and individual podocytes develop *foot processes*. In this immature glomerulus, division into lobules is not yet evident, but the arrangement of the structural elements is already established. Proceeding from Bowman's space, one encounters, in order, the epithelial cell, the basement membrane, the endothelial cell, and the mesangium. In the deep recesses between the capillaries, one finds the epithelial cell, the basement membrane, and the mesangium.

Maturation of the renal glomerulus involves various changes in its components, such as appearance of fe-

Development of Metanephros
Continued

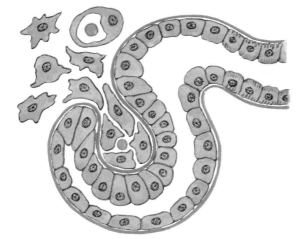

ACCORDING TO ANOTHER THEORY (JOKELAINEN), THE INTRACLEFTAL CELL MASS, FROM WHICH CAPILLARIES DEVELOP AROUND BLOOD CELLS, ARISES BY AN INGROWTH OF MESENCHYMAL CELLS

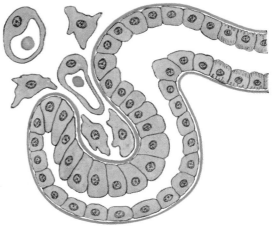

STILL OTHERS (ZAMBONI AND DE MARTINO, POTTER) BELIEVE THAT GLOMERULAR VASCULARIZATION OCCURS BY INGROWTH OF CAPILLARIES FROM THE SURROUNDING METANEPHROGENIC MESODERM

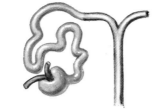

AS THE DISTAL LIMB OF THE "S"–SHAPED VESICLE DEVELOPS INTO A RENAL CORPUSCLE, THE MIDDLE AND PROXIMAL LIMBS OF THE "S" ELONGATE INTO A TUBULE CONTINUOUS WITH THE COLLECTING DUCT

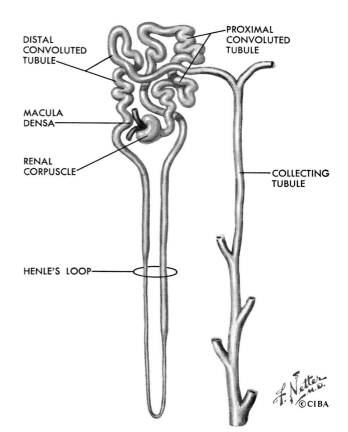

THE LOOP ELONGATES; RENAL CORPUSCLE, PROXIMAL TUBULE, HENLE'S LOOP, DISTAL TUBULE, AND MACULA DENSA OF MATURE NEPHRON ARE THUS DERIVED FROM METANEPHROGENIC MESODERM AND COLLECTING TUBULES FROM METANEPHRIC DUCT

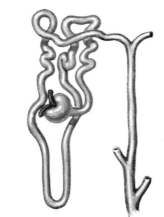

THE TUBULE LENGTHENS, COILS, AND BEGINS TO DIP DOWN TOWARD THE RENAL PELVIS, AS HENLE'S LOOP; ONE AREA OF THE TUBULE REMAINS CLOSE TO THE GLOMERULAR MOUTH, AS THE FUTURE MACULA DENSA

nestrae in the endothelium, thickening of the basement membrane, formation of trabeculae and foot processes, transformation of the mesenchymal cells into the mesangial cells, and accumulation of the mesangial matrix around the latter. During this process, some of the smooth muscle cells of the afferent arteriole develop into the *juxtaglomerular cells* containing specific granules.

From the embryological viewpoint, mesangial cells originate from the *mesenchymal cells* which appear in the *cleft* of the *S-shaped tubule*, and the mesangial cell bears an intimate relationship with the smooth muscle cell of the arterioles at the glomerular hilus. A tridimensional continuum is formed by the basement membrane system of the glomerulus, such as that of the glomerular capillary *(lamina densa)*, the mesangial matrix, and the basement membranes of the arteriole and of Bowman's capsule.

The morphogenesis of the primitive glomerular capillaries, as presented above, is not accepted by all embryologists. Some propose that the endothelial cells are derived, not from the cell mass in the cleft, but from mesenchymal cells which *grow in* from the outside. Another concept is that the *glomerular capillary* is formed *by extension* of the blood vessels already established in the vicinity of the S-shaped tubule, and that this extension is, in fact, accomplished by mitotic division of the endothelial cells and by the branching of the vessel.

After about the second fetal month, the metanephros contains glomeruli in various stages of development. It takes about 1 month from the first step of the glomerular formation to attain the comple-

tion of a fairly well differentiated glomerulus.

A new generation of uriniferous tubules and glomeruli is formed toward the outer surface of the metanephros by the eighth or ninth fetal month. Thus the kidney can be divided into zones according to the stage of glomerular development. The number of such zones is slightly greater (by one or two) than the age of the fetus expressed in months, but this formula applies only to the second half of pregnancy.

It is also believed that a certain number of glomeruli formed in the early stages of the metanephros degenerate and disappear during later stages.

Formation of the Renal Tubules

The *metanephric vesicle* (primitive uriniferous tubule), which originates from the *metanephrogenic tissue*, is the mother tissue of the entire renal tubule. It eventually differentiates into the podocytes and the capsular

cells of the glomerulus, and into the neck and convoluted and straight parts of the proximal segment, the loop of Henle, and the distal segment. However, the development of various segments does not proceed at the same pace. At the time the primitive uriniferous tubule lines up with the collecting duct and the S-shaped curve appears, the tubule is still very short. Its future segments are not yet discernible. In the course of development, the tubule becomes large and begins to coil, forming the *proximal* and *distal convolutions*. By the third fetal month, the proximal tubular cells seem to be functioning, since hyaline droplets appear in the cytoplasm. *Henle's loop* is the slowest of all segments of the tubule to develop. The loop is located initially in the vicinity of the renal glomerulus, but it eventually extends deep into the medulla, replacing, in the later stages of fetal life, the myxomatous stroma of the kidney. □

Development of Urinary Bladder

THE LOWER ENDS OF THE MESONEPHRIC DUCTS HAVE BEEN ABSORBED INTO THE CLOACA SO THAT THE METANEPHRIC DUCTS NOW OPEN DIRECTLY INTO THE CLOACA

ALLANTOIS — GENITAL TUBERCLE — CLOACA — CLOACAL MEMBRANE — MESONEPHRIC DUCT — HINDGUT — URORECTAL FOLD — METANEPHRO-GENIC TISSUE — METANEPHRIC DUCT

THE CLOACAL MEMBRANE HAS BROKEN DOWN AND THE URORECTAL SEPTUM HAS PROGRESSED CAUDALLY, DIVIDING THE CLOACA INTO THE UROGENITAL SINUS AND RECTUM; THE METANEPHROS HAS MIGRATED CRANIALLY; MESONEPHRIC AND META-NEPHRIC DUCTS HAVE SHIFTED, SO THE LATTER NOW ENTER AREA OF FUTURE URETHRA AND THE FORMER ENTER THE BLADDER

GENITAL TUBERCLE — UROGENITAL SINUS — MESONEPHRIC DUCT — METANEPHROS — MÜLLERIAN DUCTS (FUSED) — METANEPHRIC DUCT — URORECTAL FOLD — RECTUM — PERINEUM

URACHUS — BLADDER — KIDNEY — URETER — DUCTUS DEFERENS — SEMINAL VESICLE — PROSTATE — PENIS — SCROTAL SWELLING

URACHUS — UTERUS — BLADDER — VAGINA — URETHRA — CLITORIS — VESTIBULE — KIDNEY — URETER

IN MALE: MÜLLERIAN DUCTS LARGELY DEGENERATE; MESONEPHRIC DUCTS BECOME DUCTUS DEFERENS; UROGENITAL SINUS DEVELOPS INTO BLADDER AND PROSTATIC, MEMBRANOUS, AND PENILE URETHRA; PROSTATE GLAND AND SEMINAL VESICLES APPEAR

IN FEMALE: MÜLLERIAN DUCTS DEVELOP INTO UTERINE TUBES, UTERUS, AND UPPER PART OF VAGINA; MESONEPHRIC DUCTS LARGELY DEGENERATE; UROGENITAL SINUS FORMS BLADDER, URETHRA, VESTIBULE, AND LOWER PART OF VAGINA

The development of the urinary bladder and the ureter is intimately related to the structural specialization of the *cloaca.* This is the expanded blind end of the *hindgut* and is connected with the *mesonephric ducts* and the *allantoic* diverticulum (see also CIBA COLLECTION, Vol. 2, pages 2 and 3; Vol. 3/II, pages 2–7; Vol. 4, pages 113–115).

By the fourth fetal week, the *procto-deum,* the hollowed ectodermal surface located beneath the tail of the fetus, rapidly depresses toward the cloaca and comes in contact with the outer surface of the cloacal wall. The area of contact, where the ectoderm is separated by a very thin layer of tissue from the entoderm, is called the *cloacal membrane.* Simultaneously, the *urorectal fold* migrates caudally until it divides the cloaca into two parts, the posteriorly placed *rectum* and the anteriorly placed *urogenital sinus.* This series of events is called the *division of the cloaca* and is the initial step in the formation of the *bladder.*

As the development of the urogenital sinus proceeds, the ends of the *metanephric ducts (ureters)* are absorbed. Thus, the linings of four tubes, the two wolffian ducts and the two ureters, are now continuous with the mucous membrane of the sinus.

The greater part of the mucous membrane of the sinus is formed by the entodermal cells originating in the cloaca, but narrow zones where both the meso- and metanephric ducts open are occupied by the mesodermal cells derived from the intermediate mesoderm. Eventually, however, the mesodermal cells are replaced by a proliferation of entodermal cells.

With further development, the urogenital sinus differentiates into two distinct anatomical segments: (a) the *vesico-urethral canal* where the urinary bladder and the upper portion of the urethra are formed, and (b) the *definitive urogenital sinus* where the main part of the urethra is formed. The vesicourethral canal gradually enlarges, incorporating the lower allantois.

Along with the rapid development of the vesicourethral canal, both the metanephric ducts and the mesonephric ducts begin to shift. The level of the orifices of the former moves *craniolaterally* until they attain a much higher level than the orifices of the mesonephric ducts. As a result, in the later stages of development, the *metanephric ducts empty into the bladder* while the *mesonephric ducts are connected to the urethra.*

By the fourth fetal month, the vesicourethral canal assumes the characteristic shape of the adult urinary bladder, and its wall shows well-developed layers of smooth muscle cells.

Further development of the definitive urogenital sinus, comprising the pelvic and the phallic portions, follows different routes in the *male* and the *female.*

In the *male,* the pelvic portion gradually becomes a narrow tubular space forming the craniodorsally placed *prostatic urethra* and the caudoventrally placed *membranous urethra.* The phallic portion, the most caudal part of the definitive urogenital sinus, develops into the *penile urethra.*

In the *female,* the pelvic portion develops into the urethra, a part of the vestibule, and one fifth of the *vagina,* while the phallic portion also differentiates into a part of the *vestibule.*

The accessory glands derived from the urethra are different in the male and in the female. In the male, the urethra gives rise to the *prostate gland,* while in the female both urethral and paraurethral glands develop.

Eventually, the allantois is transformed into the *urachus,* the lumen of which is closed by proliferation of fibrous tissue in the late stage of intrauterine life. In postnatal life, the urachus becomes the *middle (or median) umbilical ligament.* □

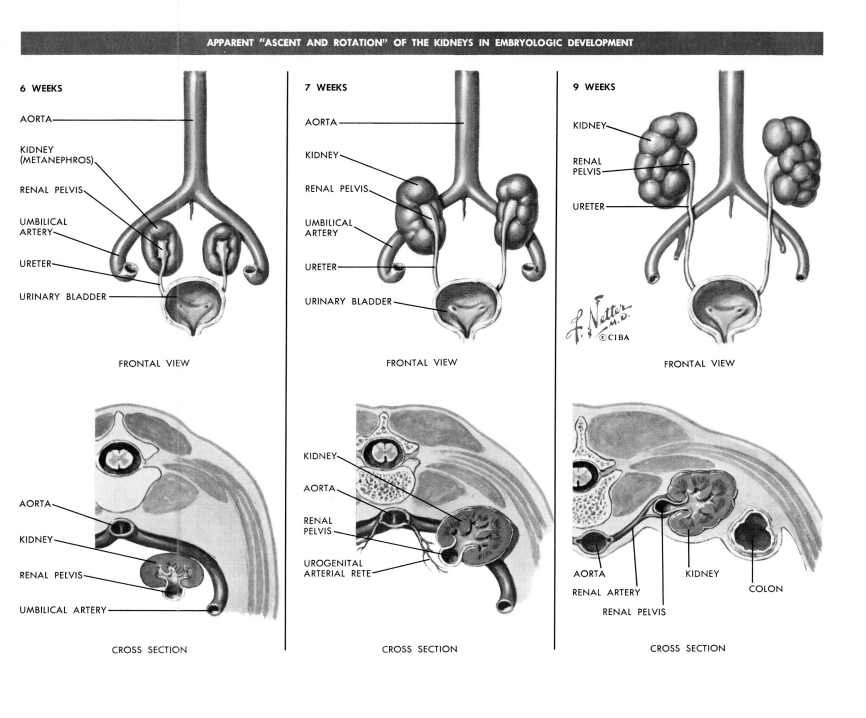

6 WEEKS

AORTA

KIDNEY (METANEPHROS)

RENAL PELVIS

UMBILICAL ARTERY

URETER

URINARY BLADDER

FRONTAL VIEW

AORTA

KIDNEY

RENAL PELVIS

UMBILICAL ARTERY

CROSS SECTION

7 WEEKS

AORTA

KIDNEY

RENAL PELVIS

UMBILICAL ARTERY

URETER

URINARY BLADDER

FRONTAL VIEW

KIDNEY

AORTA

RENAL PELVIS

UROGENITAL ARTERIAL RETE

CROSS SECTION

9 WEEKS

KIDNEY

RENAL PELVIS

URETER

FRONTAL VIEW

AORTA

RENAL ARTERY

RENAL PELVIS

KIDNEY

COLON

CROSS SECTION

Ascent and Rotation of Kidneys

The kidneys are unusual in that, unlike other organs of the body, they are ultimately located at a more cranial level than their sites of origin. This apparent cranial movement of the kidneys has been called ascent, but in reality it is a straightening of the curvature of the body which brings about this relative change in position. In addition, there is marked growth of the lumbar and sacral regions of the developing embryo, in which the ureters share, so that ultimately the kidneys lie approximately four somites superior to their origins.

The first establishment of the metanephros finds it located, in the embryo, caudal to the bifurcation of the aorta. At approximately 6 weeks, the primitive vertebral column is in the shape of an accentuated C, and the metanephros may be found at the level of somites 26 or 28, which ultimately represents the sacral region. At this time, the primitive kidney lies dorsal to the ureter and the renal pelvis. As straightening of the trunk occurs from regional differential growth, the kidneys "ascend" several somite levels.

By the end of the third month, the center of each kidney lies opposite the second or third lumbar vertebra, and at term, the apparent movement has brought the center of each kidney opposite the first lumbar vertebra.

Simultaneously, the kidneys rotate about their longitudinal axes so that the renal pelvis moves medially, and ultimately the mass of renal tissue lies lateral to the renal pelvis. The rotation, like the ascent, is more apparent than real and represents the result of differential regional growth.

As the apparent ascent and rotation occur, the kidneys come to occupy their normal retroperitoneal positions. They are subjected to compression by other viscera and assume the typical fetal lobulated appearance. Eventually the fetal lobulation is lost, and the characteristic adult shape of the kidney is assumed.

The arterial supply of the kidney arises from the mesonephric artery which, in turn, arises from the abdominal aorta and terminates in a plexus of arteries in close proximity to the renal pelvis. This plexus is called the *urogenital arterial rete*. Persistence of one branch of this plexus results in a solitary renal artery which enters and subsequently divides within the kidney. (For a discussion of renal artery anomalies see page 17). Note, however, that although kidneys in a normal position may be supplied on occasion by two or more arteries, such multiplicity of arterial supply is usually seen in ectopic kidneys.

It is obviously important to know the various anomalies of position, form, and orientation of the kidneys so that the finding of a mass in an area not normally occupied by a kidney should not exclude the possibility of this being renal tissue. If one is alerted to the possibility of anomalies of position, the occasional tragic consequences arising from surgical removal of a normally functioning organ can be avoided. This is particularly pertinent in dealing with fused pelvic kidneys or solitary ectopic kidneys (see pages 230-232). □

Section II

Renal Physiology

Frank H. Netter, M.D.

in collaboration with

Gerhard Giebisch, M.D.   *Plates 8-12, 18-21*

Albert S. Gordon, Ph.D.   *Plate 22*

Carl W. Gottschalk, M.D.   *Plates 13-17*

H. O. Heinemann, M.D.   *Plates 1-7*

Hermann Mattenheimer, M.D.   *Plates 23-24*

Introduction

The highly vascular kidneys are an integral part of the systemic circulation and receive a major portion of the cardiac output. They are intimately concerned with the regulation of the volume and composition of the extracellular fluid and the elimination of waste products.

The nephron, the basic functioning unit of the kidney, produces an essentially protein-free filtrate at the level of the glomerulus. This filtrate, by a process of selective reabsorption and secretion at various levels of the tubule, is modified to form the final urine. While glomerular filtration results solely from physical forces, the tubular functions of reabsorption and secretion involve both metabolically activated transport mechanisms and physical forces.

In adult man, the total area of the glomerular capillary membrane available for filtration is approximately 1 square meter. This membrane is normally not permeable to proteins with molecular weights in excess of 70,000; it is permeable to smaller proteins with molecular weights of 15,000 or less, while intermediate-sized molecules, between 15,000 and 70,000 molecular weight, are filtered to varying degrees.

Tubular function is complex and differs between various segments. In the proximal convoluted tubule, about 65 percent of the glomerular filtrate is selectively reabsorbed. In the ascending limb of the loop of Henle, active reabsorption of solute (mainly sodium) is preeminent. This process helps to maintain a high solute concentration in the medullary interstitial fluid, the main driving force for subsequent water reabsorption from the collecting ducts.

In the distal convoluted tubule, additional reabsorption and secretion of solutes take place, and water diffuses out of the tubule in the presence of antidiuretic hormone. Here, by subtle modification of tubular function, the "final touch" is given to the reconstitution of the extracellular fluid. At the same time, the volume as well as the composition of the remaining tubular fluid is changed.

In the collecting ducts, water conservation is one of the main features, promoted by antidiuretic hormone. This hormone facilitates back diffusion into the medullary interstitial fluid which has been made hypertonic by the active reabsorption of sodium from the ascending limb of the loop of Henle. Alternately, if antidiuretic hormone is absent, the back diffusion of water is limited. This leads to the formation of a dilute urine and elimination of excess water.

Tubular function is also intimately concerned with acid-base balance. Hydrogen ion secretion, the formation of ammonia, and the reabsorption of bicarbonate are narrowly interrelated functions which ensure stability of the extracellular fluid pH and, in the process, acidify the urine.

Finally, the kidneys also participate in extrarenal regulatory mechanisms by producing or activating components of feedback control loops. For example, renin, a proteolytic enzyme produced by the kidneys, causes the formation of angiotensin I, a polypeptide, from circulating renin substrate, an alpha-2-globulin. Similarly, erythropoiesis in bone marrow is modified by a factor which is either produced or activated by renal tissue. □

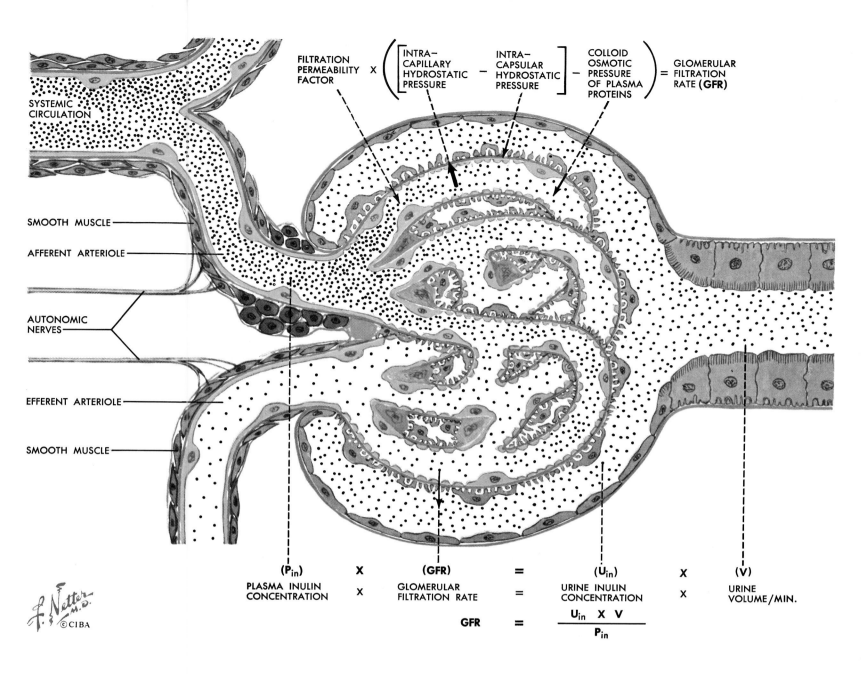

FILTRATION PERMEABILITY FACTOR X ([INTRA-CAPILLARY HYDROSTATIC PRESSURE − INTRA-CAPSULAR HYDROSTATIC PRESSURE] − COLLOID OSMOTIC PRESSURE OF PLASMA PROTEINS) = GLOMERULAR FILTRATION RATE (GFR)

| (P_{in}) | X | (GFR) | = | (U_{in}) | X | (V) |
| PLASMA INULIN CONCENTRATION | X | GLOMERULAR FILTRATION RATE | = | URINE INULIN CONCENTRATION | X | URINE VOLUME/MIN. |

$$GFR = \frac{U_{in} \times V}{P_{in}}$$

Glomerular Filtration

The basic functioning unit of the kidney is the nephron, of which there are about 2 million in man. At the level of the glomerulus, a protein-free filtrate is produced solely by physical forces.

There are several theories about filtration across the glomerular capillary membrane. According to the "pore" theory of Pappenheimer, as reviewed by Pitts, fluid passes through cylindrical channels or pores along a hydrostatic gradient. These pores are assumed to be about 75 to 100 angstroms in diameter and so would limit the passage of larger molecules.

A second theory, described by Chinard and later well reviewed by Pitts, conceives of the glomerular capillary membrane as a hydrated gel. Since the diffusion characteristics of water and other small molecules are quite similar, these substances would pass easily across the membrane. However, larger molecules would pass with difficulty, or not at all, depending on their size.

Both concepts may well be oversimplifications. Conceivably, the glomerular capillary membrane

need not be a fixed structure; pores, if present at all, need not be permanent and uniform in configuration. Aqueous channels between loosely bonded protein and lipid components of the cell membrane may exist, and these could permit the passage, by diffusion, of water and low molecular weight solutes.

The rate of glomerular filtration (GFR) is determined by the permeabilities of the capillary wall, basement membrane, and Bowman's capsule, as well as by the intracapillary hydrostatic pressure. Increased intracapsular hydrostatic pressure and increased intracapillary colloid osmotic pressure limit glomerular filtration.

Glomerular filtration is further modified by factors affecting afferent and efferent arteriolar resistance. Exercise, emotion, and change in position from supine to erect may all produce changes in vascular tone, either through direct autonomic control or through release of circulating, vasoactive catecholamines or polypeptides. Changes in vascular resistance may also alter the intrarenal distribution of blood to nephron populations with different functional characteristics, thus affecting GFR (see page 175).

The measurement of glomerular filtration can only be done indirectly, using the rate of removal from plasma to urine of a measurable substance. Any chemical compound which is freely filtered

by the glomerulus and which is not reabsorbed or secreted by the renal tubular cells is suitable. *Inulin,* a fructose polysaccharide with a molecular weight of approximately 5000, fulfills these criteria.

The blood level of inulin must be uniform during the determination of GFR. A suitable priming dose is first given, followed by a continuous infusion.

Measurement of the *concentration of inulin in plasma* (P_{in}) and in *urine* (U_{in}) and accurate determination of the *urine flow* (V) then permit calculation of *inulin clearance* (C_{in}). The clearance (C_{in}) is equal to the glomerular filtration rate (GFR). The GFR may thus be calculated according to the equation:

$$P_{in} \times GFR = U_{in} \times V$$

The equation states that the concentration of inulin in plasma, multiplied by the glomerular filtration rate, is equal to the amount of inulin appearing in the urine (product of concentration of inulin in urine and urine volume). The equation is solved for the unknown:

$$GFR = \frac{U_{in} \times V}{P_{in}}$$

The normal GFR is, on the average, 120 ml/minute and varies from moment to moment, depending on subtle hemodynamic changes. □

Clearance Principle

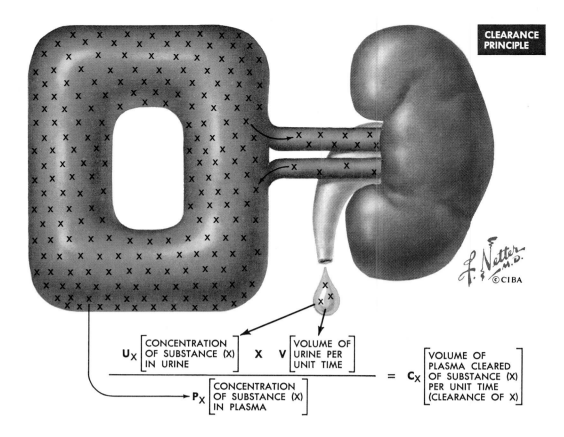

$$U_X \begin{bmatrix} \text{CONCENTRATION} \\ \text{OF SUBSTANCE (X)} \\ \text{IN URINE} \end{bmatrix} \times V \begin{bmatrix} \text{VOLUME OF} \\ \text{URINE PER} \\ \text{UNIT TIME} \end{bmatrix}$$

$$P_X \begin{bmatrix} \text{CONCENTRATION} \\ \text{OF SUBSTANCE (X)} \\ \text{IN PLASMA} \end{bmatrix} = C_X \begin{bmatrix} \text{VOLUME OF} \\ \text{PLASMA CLEARED} \\ \text{OF SUBSTANCE (X)} \\ \text{PER UNIT TIME} \\ \text{(CLEARANCE OF X)} \end{bmatrix}$$

Historically, the *clearance concept* was introduced at a time when it was thought that the sole function of the kidneys was to "clear" urea from the blood. In a broader and more modern sense, the renal clearance of any substance is the volume of plasma completely cleared of that substance per unit time (usually 1 minute). Since removal by the kidney results in the appearance of the substance in the urine, the clearance of a *substance X* (C_x), for example, can be calculated from the *concentrations of X in the urine* (U_x) and *plasma* (P_x) and the urine volume (V) according to the equation:

$$C_x = \frac{U_x \times V}{P_x}$$

Depending on how the substance is handled by the renal tubular cells, there are four possibilities:

First, a substance filtered by the glomeruli may be neither reabsorbed nor secreted by the renal tubules. The clearance rate thus *equals* the glomerular filtration rate (GFR). The polysaccharide *inulin* is such a substance and the clearance of inulin (C_{in}) equals GFR.

Second, a substance filtered by the glomeruli may also be secreted by the tubular cells, and the clearance rate then *exceeds* the GFR. *Para-aminohippurate* (PAH) is such a compound. It is so effectively excreted in one passage through the kidneys that it is used to measure renal plasma flow.

Third, a substance filtered by the glomeruli may be partly reabsorbed by the tubular cells. The clearance is *less* than the GFR, a situation shared by many substances such as *sodium, chloride,* and *calcium.*

Fourth, a substance is filtered and may be both reabsorbed and secreted. The clearance will depend upon the rates of absorption and secretion, and may be equal to, smaller than, or greater than the GFR. Uric acid is thought to be handled this way. □

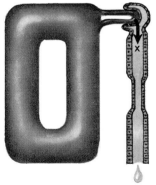

SUBSTANCE (X) FILTERED THROUGH GLOMERULI AND **NOT** REABSORBED OR SECRETED BY TUBULES (INULIN);

CLEARANCE OF X EQUALS GLOMERULAR FILTRATION RATE
$C_x = GFR$

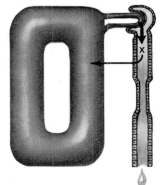

SUBSTANCE (X) FILTERED THROUGH GLOMERULI AND REABSORBED BY TUBULES;

CLEARANCE OF X EQUALS GLOMERULAR FILTRATION RATE MINUS TUBULAR REABSORPTION RATE
$C_x = GFR{-}T_x$
$C_x < C_{INULIN}$

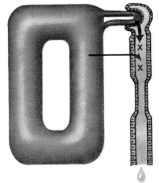

SUBSTANCE (X) FILTERED THROUGH GLOMERULI AND SECRETED BY TUBULES;

CLEARANCE OF X EQUALS GLOMERULAR FILTRATION RATE PLUS TUBULAR SECRETION RATE
$C_x = GFR + T_x$
$C_x > C_{INULIN}$

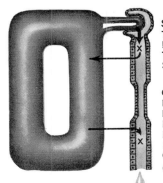

SUBSTANCE (X) FILTERED THROUGH GLOMERULI, REABSORBED BY TUBULES, AND ALSO SECRETED BY TUBULES;

CLEARANCE OF X EQUALS GLOMERULAR FILTRATION RATE MINUS NET REABSORPTION RATE OR PLUS NET SECRETION RATE
$C_x = GFR \mp T_x$
$C_x < OR > C_{INULIN}$

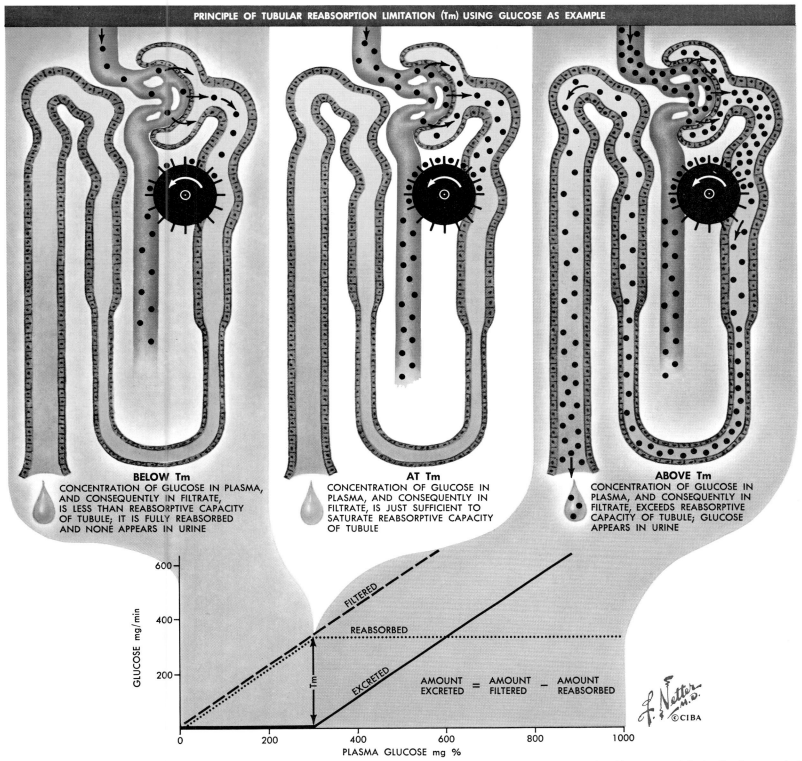

BELOW Tm
CONCENTRATION OF GLUCOSE IN PLASMA, AND CONSEQUENTLY IN FILTRATE, IS LESS THAN REABSORPTIVE CAPACITY OF TUBULE; IT IS FULLY REABSORBED AND NONE APPEARS IN URINE

AT Tm
CONCENTRATION OF GLUCOSE IN PLASMA, AND CONSEQUENTLY IN FILTRATE, IS JUST SUFFICIENT TO SATURATE REABSORPTIVE CAPACITY OF TUBULE

ABOVE Tm
CONCENTRATION OF GLUCOSE IN PLASMA, AND CONSEQUENTLY IN FILTRATE, EXCEEDS REABSORPTIVE CAPACITY OF TUBULE; GLUCOSE APPEARS IN URINE

AMOUNT EXCRETED = AMOUNT FILTERED − AMOUNT REABSORBED

Tubular Reabsorption

With the exception of proteins of large molecular weight, all constituents of the extracellular fluid are freely filtered at the glomerular level. Subsequently, selective reabsorption in the tubules helps restore essential components to the extracellular fluid. The reabsorption process may be either active or passive, the former requiring the expenditure of energy. Passive reabsorption, on the other hand, requires no energy expenditure since the substances are reabsorbed along a concentration gradient.

For various substances, active reabsorption has a limited capacity, called *tubular maximal reabsorption capacity* (Tm). For example, glucose, electrically neutral and unbound to protein, readily passes across the glomerular capillary membrane and is reabsorbed by the proximal tubular cells. Under normal conditions, virtually all filtered glu-

cose is thus eliminated from the tubular fluid. Stated another way, the capacity for tubular reabsorption of glucose exceeds the filtered load, and no glucose will be detected in the urine.

The glomerular filtration of glucose varies proportionately with the concentration of glucose in plasma. If the plasma glucose is increased above a critical level, as in disorders of carbohydrate metabolism such as diabetes mellitus, the capacity for tubular reabsorption of glucose will be exceeded, and glucose will appear in the urine. Glycosuria also may rarely be caused by a congenital defect in which the tubular cells have a limited capacity for glucose reabsorption. Glucose thus appears in the urine even though the plasma concentration of the compound is normal.

The capacity for glucose reabsorption can be assessed by increasing the plasma level of glucose, and therefore the filtered load, until glycosuria occurs. In actual practice, the plasma concentration of *glucose* (P_G), the *glomerular filtration rate* (GFR)

(determined by means of the inulin clearance), the *concentration of glucose in the urine* (U_G), and the *urine flow* (V) must all be known. The equation to calculate the *tubular maximal reabsorption capacity for glucose* (Tm_G) is:

$$U_G \times V = P_G \times GFR - Tm_G$$

This equation states that the amount of glucose appearing in the urine ($U_G \times V$) equals the filtered load of glucose ($P_G \times GFR$) minus the amount reabsorbed by the tubular cells (Tm_G). To solve the equation for the unknown Tm_G, it is rewritten:

$$Tm_G = P_G \times GFR - U_G \times V$$

or, expressed in words, the amount of glucose reabsorbed by the tubules equals the difference between the amount filtered and the amount excreted in the urine.

Tm_G, or the capacity for tubular maximal reabsorption, reflects the functional mass of proximal tubular cells. □

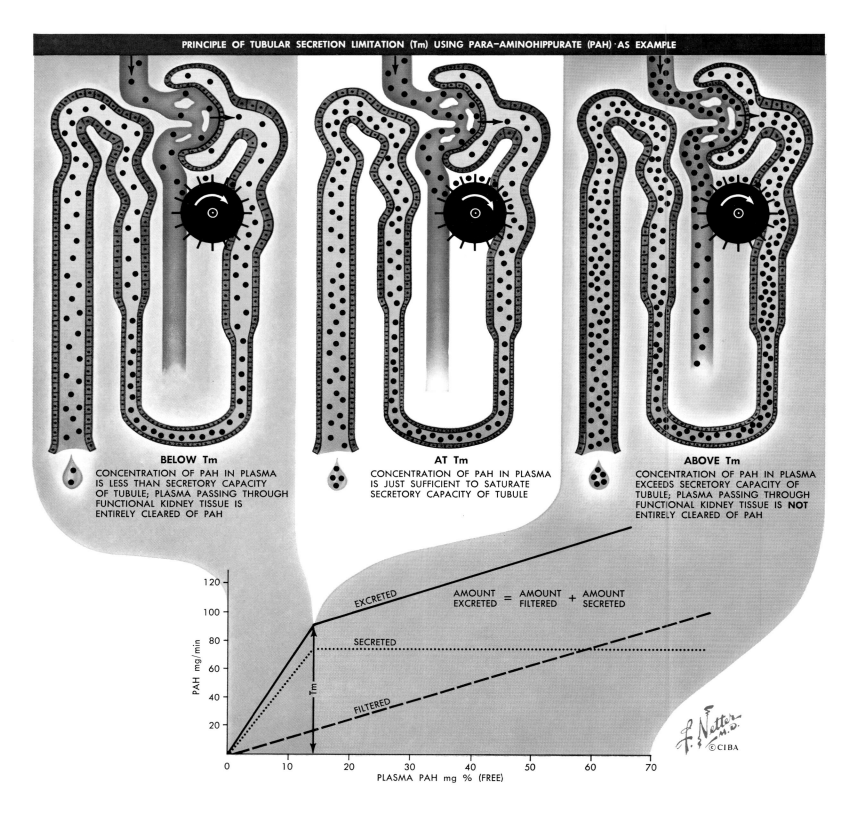

BELOW Tm
CONCENTRATION OF PAH IN PLASMA IS LESS THAN SECRETORY CAPACITY OF TUBULE; PLASMA PASSING THROUGH FUNCTIONAL KIDNEY TISSUE IS ENTIRELY CLEARED OF PAH

AT Tm
CONCENTRATION OF PAH IN PLASMA IS JUST SUFFICIENT TO SATURATE SECRETORY CAPACITY OF TUBULE

ABOVE Tm
CONCENTRATION OF PAH IN PLASMA EXCEEDS SECRETORY CAPACITY OF TUBULE; PLASMA PASSING THROUGH FUNCTIONAL KIDNEY TISSUE IS **NOT** ENTIRELY CLEARED OF PAH

$$\text{AMOUNT EXCRETED} = \text{AMOUNT FILTERED} + \text{AMOUNT SECRETED}$$

Tubular Secretion

The tubular epithelium has the capacity for secretion into the tubular lumen, in addition to its ability for reabsorption. Secretion may take place by active transport or passive diffusion along concentration gradients. The active secretory transport mechanisms also have limitations in transport capacity. Separate secretory pathways have been identified mostly for organic acids (*e.g.,* hippurate) or organic bases (*e.g.,* guanidine).

As an example, a substance like *para-aminohippurate* (PAH), which is both filtered and secreted, can be utilized to demonstrate a tubular maximum (Tm) for secretion. At low plasma concentrations, PAH is completely cleared from plasma. (Because of the rapid and effective remov-

al of PAH, its clearance is used to measure renal plasma flow, see page 43). As the concentration of PAH in plasma is increased, a level is reached at which the secretory mechanism operates at full capacity. If the plasma concentration is further increased and exceeds the secretory capacity, plasma passing through the kidney will not be completely cleared. Now renal excretion will exceed tubular secretion and be dependent on filtration.

The secretory capacity can be calculated from the filtered load and urinary excretion according to the equation:

$$U_{PAH} \times V = P_{PAH} \times GFR + Tm_{PAH}$$

This equation states that the amount of PAH appearing in the urine ($U_{PAH} \times V$) is made up of the amount filtered ($P_{PAH} \times GFR$) plus the amount

secreted by the tubules (Tm_{PAH}). By solving the equation for the unknown Tm_{PAH}, one obtains:

$$Tm_{PAH} = (U_{PAH} \times V) - (P_{PAH} \times GFR)$$

Expressed in words, the amount of PAH secreted by the tubular cells equals the difference between the amount excreted in the urine and the amount filtered by the glomeruli.

The active secretory pathway follows saturation kinetics and can be utilized by more than one compound. Simultaneous administration of two or more substances transported by this system leads to competitive inhibition. This fact has been used pharmacologically. For example, probenecid and penicillin are both secreted by tubular cells. The administration of probenecid to patients requiring penicillin delays the secretion of the antibiotic and ensures higher blood levels for a given dose. □

Renal Plasma Flow

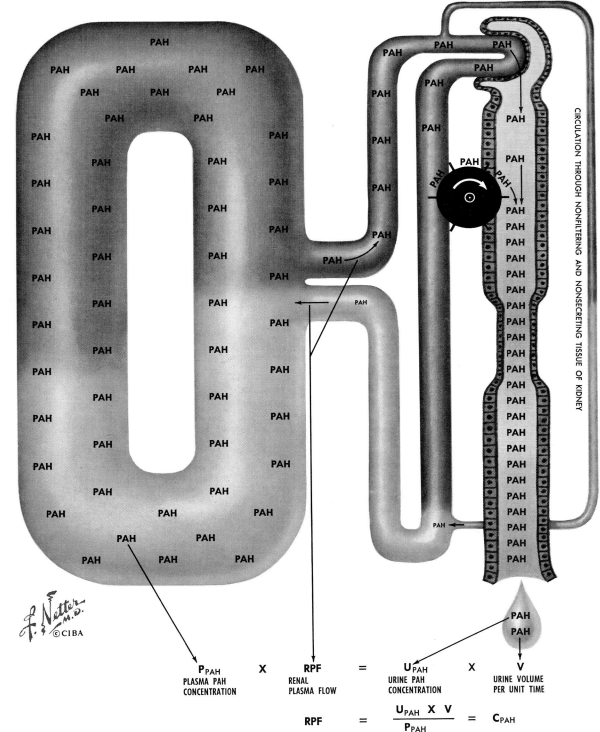

$$P_{PAH} \quad X \quad RPF \quad = \quad U_{PAH} \quad X \quad V$$

PLASMA PAH CONCENTRATION   RENAL PLASMA FLOW   URINE PAH CONCENTRATION   URINE VOLUME PER UNIT TIME

$$RPF \quad = \quad \frac{U_{PAH} \ X \ V}{P_{PAH}} \quad = \quad C_{PAH}$$

CIRCULATION THROUGH NONFILTERING AND NONSECRETING TISSUE OF KIDNEY

Substances which are effectively cleared from the plasma during a single passage through the kidney can be utilized to determine *renal plasma flow* (RPF). As noted previously (see page 42), para-aminohippurate, which is both effectively filtered at the glomerulus and secreted by the renal tubular cells, is utilized for the measurement of renal plasma flow. The procedure requires a constant plasma level which is well below the capacity of the secretory mechanism. From the *plasma concentration* (P_{PAH}) and the *rate of para-aminohippurate excretion in the urine* (U_{PAH}), the *clearance* (C_{PAH}) can be calculated:

$$C_{PAH} = \frac{U_{PAH} \times V}{P_{PAH}} = RPF$$

Renal blood flow (RBF) can be calculated from the *renal plasma flow* and the *hematocrit* (Hct), according to the equation:

$$RBF = \frac{RPF}{(1 - Hct)}$$

In actuality, the clearance of PAH only approximates the renal plasma flow, since there is always a small fraction of blood which bypasses functioning renal tissue. To emphasize this limitation, the term *"estimated renal plasma flow"* (ERPF) has been introduced.

The discrepancy between the clearance of PAH and true renal blood flow may be marked in renal disease if the intrarenal structural relationships are distorted. In this situation a larger proportion of blood bypasses functioning tissue, and the clearance of para-aminohippurate correlates poorly with the true renal blood flow.

To overcome this limitation, it is necessary to know the concentration of para-aminohippurate in the *arterial* (A_{PAH}) and *renal venous* (V_{PAH}) *blood*. The difference in arterial and venous concentrations is then used, instead of the plasma concentration, for calculation of the renal plasma flow:

$$RPF = \frac{U_{PAH} \times V}{A_{PAH} - V_{PAH}}$$

This equation is an application of the *Fick principle* (commonly used for the determination of the cardiac output, see CIBA COLLECTION, Vol. 5, page 44). According to this principle, the amount of a substance taken up or excreted by an organ is equal to the difference in concentration of that substance in arterial (A_{PAH}) and venous (V_{PAH}) blood, multiplied by the blood flow through that organ:

$$U_{PAH}V = (A_{PAH} - V_{PAH}) \, RPF$$

It is apparent that if the venous concentration approximates zero, the Fick and the clearance equations are the same. □

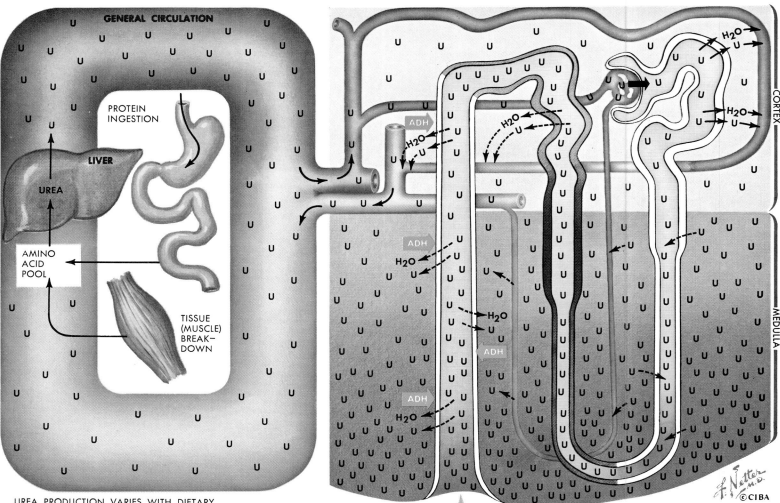

UREA PRODUCTION VARIES WITH DIETARY PROTEIN, TISSUE BREAKDOWN, AND LIVER FUNCTION (U=UREA)

IN DIURESIS (FLOW > 2 ml/min)
(SOLID ARROWS ONLY):
UREA CLEARANCE = 60% OF GFR
OR C$_{INULIN}$

IN ANTIDIURESIS (FLOW < 2 ml/min)
(SOLID ARROWS PLUS BROKEN ARROWS):
UREA CLEARANCE REDUCED

Urea Clearance

Measurement of urea excretion is of considerable historical interest since the first attempts to quantitate renal function were made with urea. Ambard and Weill (1912) in France, Addis and Watanable (1916) as well as Austin, Stillman, and Van Slyke (1921) in the United States, and Rehberg (1926) in Denmark were some of the investigators who first contributed to the development of the clearance concept.

The *clearance of urea* (C$_u$) became a standard procedure for assessment of renal function in patients. Although it continues to find use in clinical situations, the urea clearance is known to have certain limitations.

First, the rate of urea production is variable. Since urea is the end product of protein catabolism, the amount produced daily is determined by a number of factors such as dietary protein intake, endogenous protein breakdown, and the rate of conversion by the liver.

Second, renal excretion of urea is determined both by the glomerular filtration rate and varying back diffusion along the entire length of the renal tubules. The rate of back diffusion depends upon the concentration and flow rate of tubular fluid. At low flow rates, urine concentration is high; more urea diffuses back, and this limits urea excretion and reduces its clearance. At high urine flows, in excess of 2 ml/minute, the urine becomes hypotonic and back diffusion of urea is limited; the clearance is thus increased but changes little with further increments in urine volume.

Because of the flow dependency of urea clearance, the results are usually expressed in percent of an expected normal figure for any given urine flow, rather than in absolute amounts.

Urea also plays an important role in the concentrating mechanism of the kidney (see pages 56 and 58). Urea accumulates in the medullary interstitial fluid and raises the total solute content of the renal medulla. Thus urea contributes to the osmotic force which promotes water reabsorption from the collecting duct in the presence of antidiuretic hormone.

In man, the reabsorption of urea takes place by diffusion alone, although there are some nonmammalian species in which active transport of urea has been demonstrated. □

Creatinine Clearance

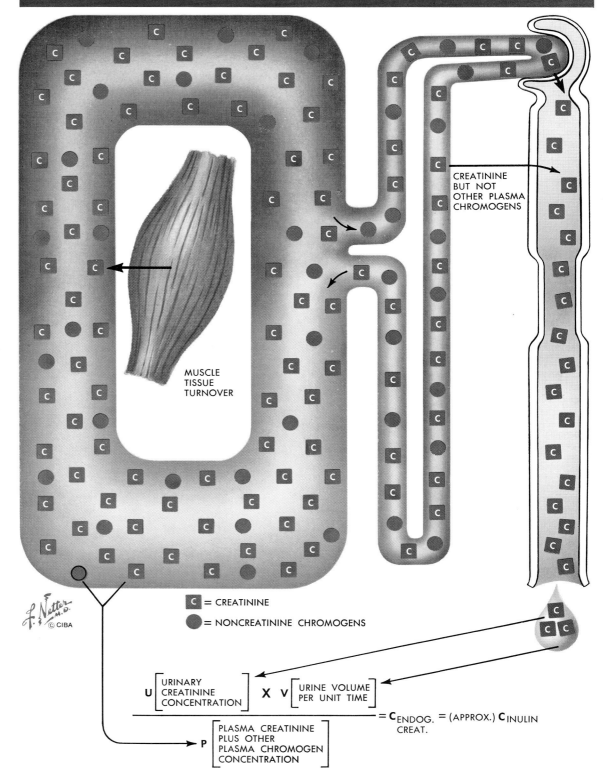

CREATININE BUT NOT OTHER PLASMA CHROMOGENS

MUSCLE TISSUE TURNOVER

C = CREATININE

● = NONCREATININE CHROMOGENS

$$\frac{U \begin{bmatrix} \text{URINARY} \\ \text{CREATININE} \\ \text{CONCENTRATION} \end{bmatrix} \times V \begin{bmatrix} \text{URINE VOLUME} \\ \text{PER UNIT TIME} \end{bmatrix}}{P \begin{bmatrix} \text{PLASMA CREATININE} \\ \text{PLUS OTHER} \\ \text{PLASMA CHROMOGEN} \\ \text{CONCENTRATION} \end{bmatrix}} = C_{ENDOG.\ CREAT.} = (APPROX.)\ C_{INULIN}$$

In the day-to-day care of patients with renal disease, it is impractical to measure the glomerular filtration rate (GFR) by means of inulin clearance (C_{in}). Instead, the *clearance of endogenous creatinine* (C_{cr}) can be employed to obtain an approximate value for glomerular filtration rate.

Creatinine originates from creatine and phosphocreatine, both largely present in skeletal muscle. Normally, the muscle mass and creatine turnover are relatively constant. This is reflected in the stable serum concentration and renal excretion rate of creatinine. Furthermore, unlike urea, creatinine excretion is not dependent upon urine volume or dietary protein intake. The stability of endogenous creatinine production makes its clearance, with few exceptions, useful for estimation of glomerular filtration rate.

However, two inherent errors in the determination of the endogenous creatinine clearance should be recognized.

First, the chemical methods employed for the determination of creatinine are all based on the so-called Jaffé reaction which detects chromogens other than creatinine. These noncreatinine chromogens are not filterable and do not appear in the urine. *Second,* creatinine enters the tubular fluid mainly by glomerular filtration, but a small fraction is also secreted by tubular cells. The errors induced by the combined effects of the factitiously high serum creatinine concentration (because of the detection of noncreatinine chromogens) and the fraction entering tubular fluid by secretion fortuitously offset each other in the calculation of the creatinine clearance.

More precise determination of glomerular filtration rate with endogenous creatinine can be obtained by using one of several available modifications of the original Folin-Wu technic which does not record noncreatinine chromogens.

In renal disease where glomerular filtration is reduced, the serum creatinine concentration rises. This is, in addition to the calculated clearance, a useful indicator for assessing the severity of impaired renal function.

In diseases where the skeletal muscle mass is reduced, the endogenous creatine pool is diminished, and thus the serum concentration and renal excretion rate of creatinine are low. In this setting, the serum creatinine concentration does not rise appropriately with impairment of renal function, and only calculation of the clearance will bring out the reduction in glomerular filtration rate. □

Sodium, Chloride, and Potassium Transport

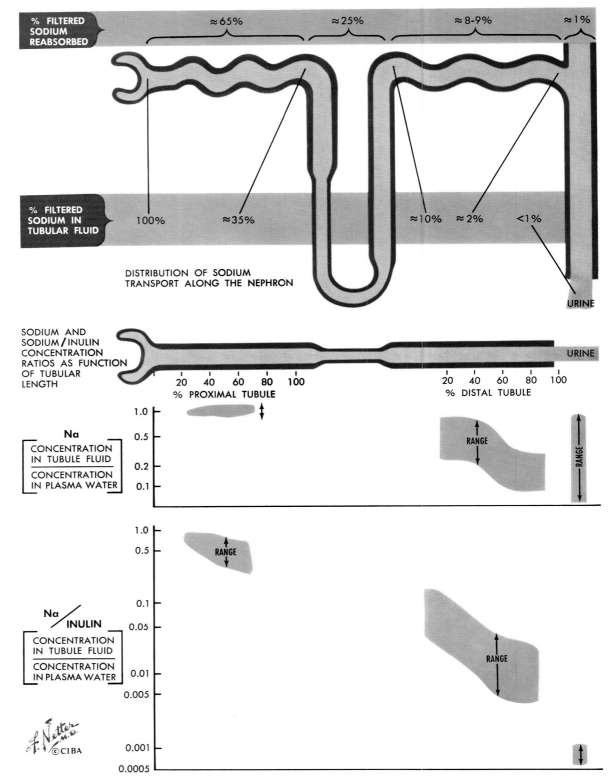

% FILTERED SODIUM REABSORBED ≈65% ≈25% ≈8-9% ≈1%

% FILTERED SODIUM IN TUBULAR FLUID 100% ≈35% ≈10% ≈2% <1%

DISTRIBUTION OF SODIUM TRANSPORT ALONG THE NEPHRON

URINE

SODIUM AND SODIUM/INULIN CONCENTRATION RATIOS AS FUNCTION OF TUBULAR LENGTH

URINE

20 40 60 80 100 % PROXIMAL TUBULE

20 40 60 80 100 % DISTAL TUBULE

Na
CONCENTRATION IN TUBULE FLUID / CONCENTRATION IN PLASMA WATER

1.0 0.5 0.2 0.1

RANGE RANGE

Na / INULIN
CONCENTRATION IN TUBULE FLUID / CONCENTRATION IN PLASMA WATER

1.0 0.5 0.1 0.05 0.01 0.005 0.001 0.0005

RANGE RANGE

Sodium Reabsorption

Reabsorption Profile Along Nephron. Renal tubular sodium (Na) reabsorption is responsible for the recovery of more than 99 percent of the glomerular filtrate from the tubular lumen. The *first stage* of tubular sodium reabsorption occurs in the *proximal tubule.* Evidence obtained by micropuncture technics and analysis of tubular fluid for inulin (a marker for transepithelial water movement), sodium, and chloride has firmly established the distribution of reabsorption along the nephron. In the mammalian nephron, under nondiuretic conditions, approximately *two thirds* of the filtered water and sodium are reabsorbed by the end of the *proximal convolution.* By the time tubular fluid has emerged from *Henle's loop,* another *25 percent* of the filtered sodium has been reabsorbed, and at this point only about 10 percent of this ion remains within the tubule. Most of the sodium load entering the distal tubule is reabsorbed there. The magnitude of the sodium transport process along the collecting ducts is small and rarely amounts to more than one percent of filtered load of this substance.

The described distribution of sodium transport along the nephron may be changed by a variety of maneuvers. Either the administration of osmotic diuretics, such as mannitol, or intravenous infusion of saline to expand extracellular volume, dramatically reduces proximal tubular sodium reabsorption. Accordingly, a disproportionately larger fraction of filtered sodium and water enters the loop of Henle and the distal nephron. However, whenever sodium reabsorption in the proximal tubule is reduced, the epithelium of the distal tubule and of Henle's loop is able to increase sodium reabsorption, a point of great functional significance. Thus, urinary loss of sodium is effectively reduced. In other words, sodium and fluid loss resulting from diminished reabsorption in the proximal tubule is greatly curtailed by the adaptive, load-dependent enhancement of sodium reabsorption along both the loop of Henle and the distal tubule.

Tubule/Plasma Concentration Ratios. It is well established that proximal tubular fluid remains isosmotic to plasma under a variety of experimental conditions. Since, under normal conditions, sodium salts represent the bulk of osmotically active material in extracellular fluid, no difference in *transepithelial* sodium concentration is established across the proximal tubular epithelium. In contrast, the sodium concentration in early distal tubular fluid is significantly less than that in plasma. Since there is no evidence that the tubular fluid is diluted by the entry of water along the loop of Henle, the significant reduction in early distal tubular sodium concentration indicates excess reabsorption of sodium relative to reabsorption of water along Henle's loop. It is this portion of the tubular sodium reabsorption process which plays a key role in the elaboration of an osmotically concentrated urine.

Intraluminal sodium concentrations further decline along the distal tubule to values as low as 10 mEq/l by the end of this segment, and additional reduction may variably occur along the collecting ducts. However, this ability of the distal nephron (the distal tubule and the collecting ducts) to lower the intratubular sodium concentration is compromised if mineralocorticoids are lacking, or if certain diuretics and cardiac glycosides are given.

Measuring the progression of Na/Inulin concentration ratios along the nephron permits a quantitative assessment of the fraction of filtered sodium which is reabsorbed as the tubular fluid passes along the proximal and distal tubule. It is apparent that a large fraction of the filtered sodium load is reabsorbed along the proximal tubule without the establishment of a transepithelial sodium concentration gradient, whereas, along the distal tubular and collecting duct epithelium, the reabsorption of a much smaller fraction of the filtered sodium load is associated with the generation of steep transepithelial concentration gradients.

Sodium, Chloride, and Potassium Transport
Continued

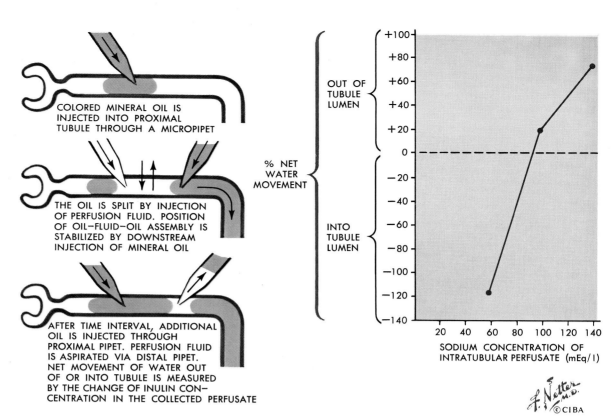

COLORED MINERAL OIL IS INJECTED INTO PROXIMAL TUBULE THROUGH A MICROPIPET

THE OIL IS SPLIT BY INJECTION OF PERFUSION FLUID. POSITION OF OIL–FLUID–OIL ASSEMBLY IS STABILIZED BY DOWNSTREAM INJECTION OF MINERAL OIL

AFTER TIME INTERVAL, ADDITIONAL OIL IS INJECTED THROUGH PROXIMAL PIPET. PERFUSION FLUID IS ASPIRATED VIA DISTAL PIPET. NET MOVEMENT OF WATER OUT OF OR INTO TUBULE IS MEASURED BY THE CHANGE OF INULIN CONCENTRATION IN THE COLLECTED PERFUSATE

% NET WATER MOVEMENT — OUT OF TUBULE LUMEN / INTO TUBULE LUMEN

SODIUM CONCENTRATION OF INTRATUBULAR PERFUSATE (mEq/l)

Mechanisms of Sodium and Water Reabsorption

Any ion movement that takes place *against a concentration gradient* is *active* and requires expenditure of energy. Sodium reabsorption, along both the distal tubule and the collecting ducts, is obviously active since it involves net movement of sodium against a concentration gradient ($U_{Na} < P_{Na}$) as well as against an electrical potential (lumen electrically negative with respect to the peritubular fluid).

Experimental Evidence of Active Transport. The nature of proximal tubular sodium transport, however, is less apparent. Extensive water and sodium reabsorption proceeds without the establishment of significant concentration differences and against, at best, very small electrical forces. However, two types of pertinent experiments, one of which uses microperfusion technics, unequivocally show that active transport participates in proximal tubular sodium reabsorption. These experiments also demonstrate that water reabsorption from the proximal tubule is dependent on both the intratubular sodium concentration and the magnitude of tubular sodium reabsorption.

The main supportive evidence is obtained from the first type of experiment. This consists of stationary perfusion of proximal tubules with solutions of different sodium concentrations containing inulin as a marker for transepithelial water movement and made isotonic by mannitol. If water reabsorption is measured by the extent to which inulin is concentrated in the collected perfusate, it is evident that sodium and water reabsorption can take place against a significant concentration gradient. This observation supports the thesis of active sodium transport in the proximal tubule. Also, this perfusion experiment clearly shows that water leaves the proximal tubular lumen in proportion to the amount of sodium reabsorbed, since the higher the concentration of sodium in the perfusate injected into the tubule, the more sodium reabsorbed, and hence the greater percentage

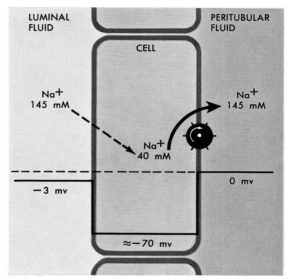

SODIUM IONS ENTER TUBULE CELL BY MOVING ACROSS LUMINAL CELL MEMBRANE, A DIRECTION FAVORED BY ELECTRICAL POTENTIAL AND CONCENTRATION GRADIENTS, BUT ARE ACTIVELY TRANSPORTED OUT OF THE CELL AT THE PERITUBULAR CELL MEMBRANE AGAINST BOTH ELECTRICAL POTENTIAL AND CONCENTRATION GRADIENTS

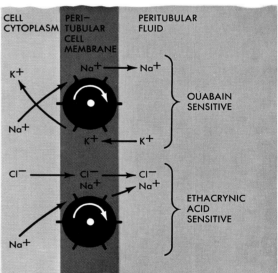

TWO TYPES OF SODIUM PUMP OPERATE AT THE PERITUBULAR CELL MEMBRANE: ONE OF THESE EXTRUDES SODIUM IONS IN EXCHANGE FOR POTASSIUM IONS; THIS MECHANISM MAY BE BLOCKED BY CARDIAC GLYCOSIDES (OUABAIN). IN THE OTHER TYPE, NO POTASSIUM EXCHANGE TAKES PLACE, BUT CHLORIDE MOVES PASSIVELY WITH THE SODIUM TO MAINTAIN ELECTRICAL NEUTRALITY; THIS MECHANISM MAY BE BLOCKED BY ETHACRYNIC ACID

of net water movement out of the tubule lumen (see graph in illustration). Thus, there is an obligatory coupling between active sodium movement and osmotically induced, passive water transfer.

Essentially similar conclusions can be reached in a second type of experiment, *in vivo,* in which the relationship between net sodium and water movement in the proximal tubule is examined during infusion of a poorly reabsorbable solute. The infusion of mannitol reduces proximal tubular water reabsorption in proportion to the decline in tubular sodium concentration. The latter falls because mannitol is retained within the lumen. Simultaneously, the sodium concentration in the reabsorbed fluid, normally osmotically equal to tubular fluid, is now raised to a level higher than that in the tubular fluid. Thus, sodium transport can occur against a sodium concentration gradient and must be an active process.

Electrical Potentials. Renal tubule cells are similar to other epithelial cells in that they are electrically asymmetrical. A stable *electrical potential* exists between the cell interior and the surrounding extracellular fluid, with the cell interior invariably negative with respect to both the tubular and peritubular fluid. This potential is in the order of a few millivolts across the proximal tubular epithelium, while a larger potential is maintained across the distal tubular epithelium, particularly in the second half of this segment.

Sodium Transport. In the proximal tubule, the concentration of sodium in the cells is lower than that in both the tubular fluid and the peritubular fluid. The same relationship probably exists in the distal tubule. Thus, sodium ions move down both an electrical potential and a concentration gradient at the luminal cell boundary but must be actively transported by a metabolically fueled *Continued on page 48*

Sodium, Chloride, and Potassium Transport

Continued from page 47

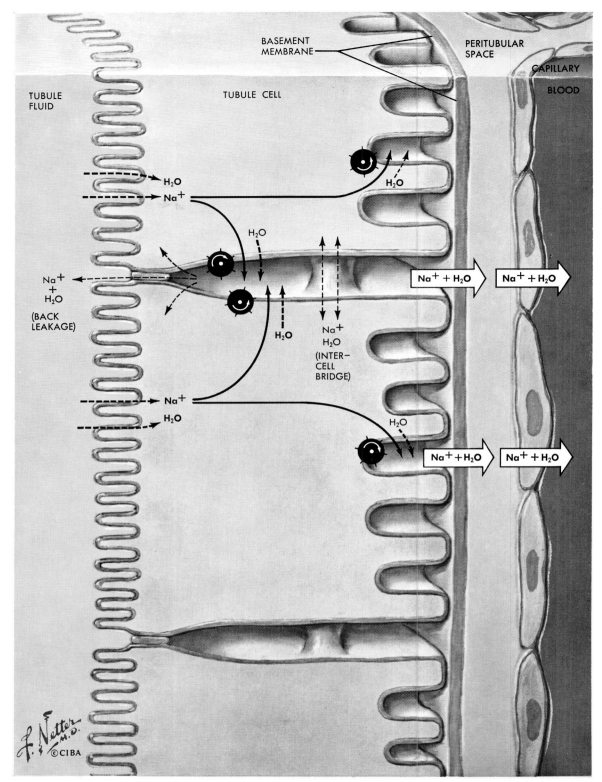

pump across the peritubular cell membrane.

Recent evidence has shown that at least two types of sodium pump operate at the peritubular cell membrane. One type extrudes sodium ions in direct exchange for potassium ions. Such a sodium-potassium exchange pump is an integral part of many body cells, and the rate of transport is sensitive to changes in the sodium and potassium concentrations in the cellular and extracellular environments. A low extracellular potassium concentration suppresses sodium extrusion from the cell interior, whereas a low intracellular sodium concentration lowers potassium uptake. In addition, these exchange pumps may be blocked by cardiac glycosides. This type of ion pumping, in addition to actively transporting sodium, helps maintain a high intracellular potassium concentration.

A second type of sodium pump moves this ion across the peritubular cell membrane without a direct exchange for potassium ion. In order to maintain electroneutrality, the transport of sodium is intimately coupled to the passive transepithelial movement of chloride ion. This type of sodium pump is insensitive to variations in extracellular potassium concentration but is sensitive to the blocking action of the diuretic, ethacrynic acid.

Chloride Reabsorption

The chloride ion concentration in the proximal tubular fluid is often significantly higher than that in the plasma, in contrast to the situation with sodium ion. The extent of the relative increase of proximal tubular chloride concentration depends on the degree of proximal tubular acidification. Hydrogen ion secretion in the proximal tubule leads to the decomposition of a large fraction of the filtered bicarbonate load. Because of the isotonic nature of proximal tubular fluid, this fall in bicarbonate concentration is regularly associated with a compensatory increase in intratubular chloride concentration to levels exceeding those in plasma. Reduction of proximal tubular acidification, on the other hand, prevents such a compensatory increase in the tubular chloride concentration.

Along the distal tubule and the collecting duct, the concentration profile of chloride follows that of sodium. An exception occurs with the administration of poorly permeant anions such as sulfate or ferrocyanide. These anions replace chloride in the tubular fluid and lead to the disappearance of all but a small fraction of the filtered chloride from the distal tubular fluid and the final urine.

Little is known about the cellular mechanism of chloride transport. It is likely that *proximal tubular chloride reabsorption* is *passive* and takes place along a small but finite electrical potential and concentration gradient favoring chloride extrusion from the tubular lumen. This occurs because the proximal tubular lumen is electrically negative with respect to the peritubular fluid, and the chloride concentration in the proximal tubular fluid is higher than in plasma. Presently, it is not clear whether the magnitude of the electrical potential across the cells of the distal tubule can account for passive transepithelial chloride reabsorption. Some studies suggest the existence of active distal tubular chloride reabsorption. Such a mechanism would have to reside within the collecting duct epithelium, since here the transepithelial concentration differences greatly exceed those which could be achieved by the relatively small electrical potential.

Routes of Sodium and Water Transport

Evidence derived mainly from work on frog skin and fish and rabbit gallbladder, but applicable to the renal tubule, shows that special *extracellular transport paths* participate in tubular sodium and water reabsorption. These paths are also the sites of action of some of the factors that are known to modulate tubular sodium and fluid transport.

Many epithelial systems, including the proximal tubular epithelium, are characterized by a *fluid space* existing *between* adjacent tubule cells. This *intraepithelial, extracellular fluid compartment* is closed off toward the tubular lumen but is open toward the peritubular space as far as the basement membrane. Sodium ions are almost certainly pumped from the cell interior into this fluid compartment, and the concentration of sodium at this site is believed to exceed that in the lumen.

Sodium, Chloride, and Potassium Transport

Continued

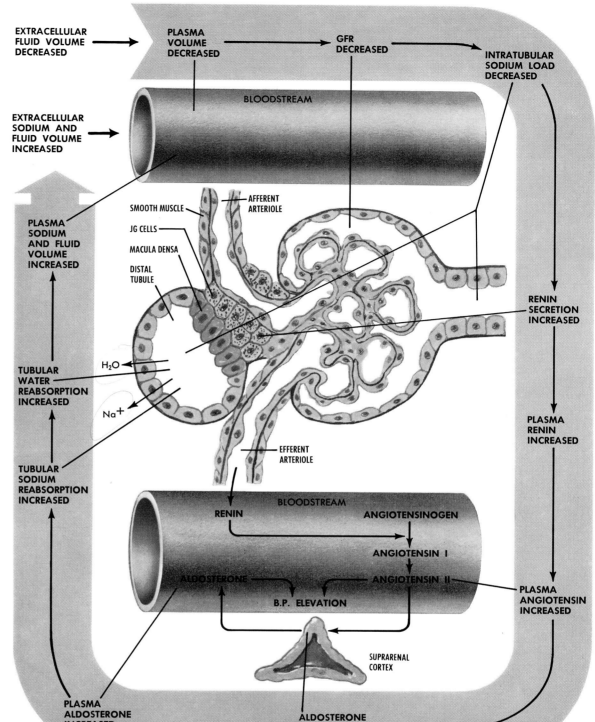

The accumulation of sodium ions within this specialized extracellular fluid compartment also affects, by local osmosis, the passive outflow of water from the tubular lumen.

A *hydrostatic pressure gradient,* between the basement membrane of the epithelium and the peritubular fluid beyond the basement membrane, is thus generated by this local fluid accumulation in the intercellular compartment. This hydrostatic pressure is responsible for the removal of fluid from the interspace compartment, through the basement membrane, into the peritubular space. The reabsorbate is ultimately moved from the interstitium into the capillary lumen by the net force of hydrostatic and oncotic pressure gradients across the capillary wall.

The fact that the terminal step of proximal tubular sodium reabsorption involves peritubular physical factors explains observations that the rate of proximal tubular sodium reabsorption is subject to modification by changes in the peritubular oncotic and hydrostatic pressures. Of particular importance are adjustments of proximal tubular sodium reabsorption in response to changes in filtered sodium load. Thus, an increase in filtration rate (GFR) is associated with both increased filtration fraction and increased peritubular oncotic pressure. The latter favors enhanced reabsorption of fluid into the peritubular capillaries. As a result, net sodium transport across the proximal tubular epithelium increases with the increase in GFR. As a consequence of this regulatory adjustment, the extracellular sodium and fluid content is maintained despite large fluctuations in the filtered sodium load.

Frequently, the rate of transepithelial sodium transfer is regulated by primary adjustments in the efficiency of moving the reabsorbate from the extracellular fluid pool, between the epithelial cells, to the capillary bed. The mechanism of this adjustment probably involves variations in the extent to which sodium leaks back into the tubule in response to changes in the hydrostatic pressure within the intercellular interspaces of the proximal tubular epithelium.

Recent data also indicate that neighboring renal tubular cells are linked to each other by low resistance bridges, permitting fairly free exchange of water and electrolytes between epithelial cells of the nephron.

Renin-Angiotensin System

Two points of view have recently emerged about the role of the *renin-angiotensin* system in the regulation of the renal tubular sodium transport. Both theories involve the *macula densa,* that area of the distal tubule where specialized cells contact the afferent arteriole of the glomerulus from which the particular tubule originated. The presence of renin in the macula densa has been established by histochemical means (see pages 6, 7, and 13).

According to one hypothesis, the rate of renin secretion depends on the distal tubular sodium load. A fall in GFR results in a concomitant reduction of distal tubular sodium delivery, and this, in turn, produces an increase in the release of renin from the specialized cells which line the arterioles of the glomerulus. Renin accelerates the conversion of angiotensinogen to angiotensin. The latter not only increases arterial blood pressure but also powerfully stimulates aldosterone secretion. Elevated aldosterone levels stimulate sodium reabsorption most effectively at the level of the distal tubule and the collecting ducts. Thus, the effect of the various mechanisms is a restoration and maintenance of a normal extracellular sodium and fluid-volume compartment by an increase in tubular sodium reabsorption, secondary to sustained aldosterone secretion.

A somewhat different view is taken by those investigators who believe that a variation in the distal tubular sodium load modifies the rate of filtrate formation by appropriate resistance changes in the glomerular arterioles. This hypothesis holds that an increase in distal tubular sodium load, resulting from a high GFR, activates a feedback system involving increased renin secretion which, in turn, lowers single-nephron GFR and thus curtails sodium loss. In this control system, the primary site of action of renin is not the suprarenal cortex through the angiotensin mechanism, but rather the intrarenal vascular system, particularly the afferent arterioles of the glomerular circulation. *Continued on page 50*

Sodium, Chloride, and Potassium Transport

Continued from page 49

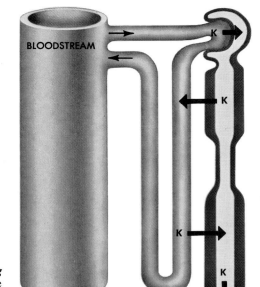

THE MAJOR PORTION OF FILTERED POTASSIUM IS REABSORBED IN THE PROXIMAL TUBULE. MOST OF THE POTASSIUM WHICH APPEARS IN THE URINE IS SECRETED IN THE DISTAL TUBULE

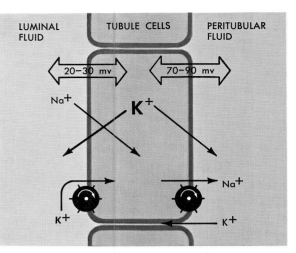

THE DISTAL TUBULE CELL MAINTAINS A HIGH INTRA-CELLULAR POTASSIUM CONCENTRATION BY VIRTUE OF THE Na^+–K^+ EXCHANGE MECHANISM: NET POTASSIUM EXCRETION IS DETERMINED BY (1) THE RATE OF ACTIVE UPTAKE ACROSS THE PERITUBULAR CELL MEMBRANE AND (2) THE DIFFERENCE BETWEEN PASSIVE MOVEMENT INTO LUMEN DOWN AN ELECTRO-CHEMICAL–POTENTIAL GRADIENT AND ACTIVE REAB-SORPTION ACROSS THE LUMINAL CELL MEMBRANE

Potassium Reabsorption and Secretion

Reabsorption and Secretion Profile Along Nephron. Although a large fraction of the filtered potassium is reabsorbed along the proximal tubule and the loop of Henle, the *highly variable secretory* activity of the *distal tubular epithelium* ultimately determines the *rate* of urinary *potassium excretion.* Accordingly, the distal tubule is the main tubular site for the translation of metabolic needs into changes in the rate of urinary potassium excretion.

In the experimental, potassium-conserving kidney (animals on low potassium diet), the concentration of potassium in the proximal tubular lumen is the same as, or slightly below, plasma levels. In the distal tubule, the concentration of potassium rises only moderately. Net potassium secretion is absent along the distal nephron, and fluid reabsorption can be shown to account fully for the observed increase in potassium concentration. In contrast, if potassium excretion is stimulated (high potassium diet), the concentration of potassium rises steeply along the distal tubule, and net addition of potassium to the tubular fluid, *i.e.,* net secretion, can easily be demonstrated.

The direction and magnitude of the tubular net movement of potassium can be assessed by following the K/Inulin concentration ratios along the nephron. Net reabsorption along the proximal tubule takes place independent of whether urinary potassium excretion is low or high. In contrast, along the distal tubule, potassium reabsorption is present in the state of experimental potassium deficiency, while massive net addition to the distal tubular fluid is responsible for the augmentation of urinary potassium excretion when potassium intake is high.

Conclusions from Experimental Evidence. Several aspects of distal tubular potassium secretion have recently become known. The main conclusions from a combination of approaches are: (1) The secretory tubule cell maintains a high intracellular potassium concentration by virtue of K-Na exchange across the peritubular cell membrane. The rate of peritubular potassium uptake is subject to regulatory modifications of potassium secretion. (2) The electrical potential across the luminal cell membrane of the secretory tubule cell is lower than the potential across the peritubular cell membrane. The luminal cell membrane is also a site of active potassium reabsorption. The intraluminal potassium concentration is deter-

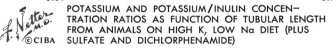

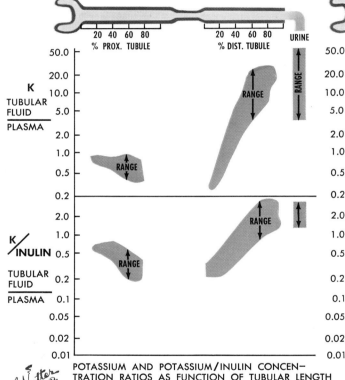

POTASSIUM AND POTASSIUM/INULIN CONCENTRATION RATIOS AS FUNCTION OF TUBULAR LENGTH FROM ANIMALS ON HIGH K, LOW Na DIET (PLUS SULFATE AND DICHLORPHENAMIDE)

POTASSIUM AND POTASSIUM/INULIN CONCENTRATION RATIOS AS FUNCTION OF TUBULAR LENGTH FROM ANIMALS ON LOW K DIET

mined by both the magnitude of the passive potassium leak from the cell potassium pool into the lumen and the rate at which potassium is pumped back from the lumen into the cell. This balance is normally in favor of net potassium secretion, but during severe potassium depletion, reversal of the direction of net potassium movement is possible. (3) It is unlikely that the secretory movement of potassium is directly linked, via a common carrier mechanism, to either sodium reabsorption or hydrogen ion secretion.

Regulating Factors. Several important factors regulate distal tubular potassium secretion. (1) A prolonged, high potassium intake sensitizes the distal tubules to exogenous potassium loads and results in a disproportionately strong stimulation of potassium secretion. (2) As a result of changes in distal cell pH, alkalosis stimulates, and acidosis depresses, potassium secretion. (3) Alterations in the level of suprarenal mineralocorti-

coids, such as aldosterone, change the potassium-secreting capacity, but the cellular mechanism of aldosterone action is unknown. (4) Poorly permeant anions make the distal tubule more electrically negative than the peritubular fluid and so promote potassium secretion. (5) High distal tubular flow rate increases potassium secretion, while a drastic reduction of distal tubular flow rate (low GFR) curtails renal potassium excretion; changes in the distal tubular sodium load are closely related to these processes.

Several diuretics (see pages 253–256) promote urinary potassium loss by increasing distal tubular flow rate and sodium delivery (furosemide, ethacrynic acid), by alkalizing distal tubular fluid (carbonic anhydrase inhibitors such as acetazolamide), or by blocking tubular potassium reabsorption (ouabain). Amiloride, a mild diuretic in promoting sodium and water loss, specifically blocks distal tubular potassium secretion. □

Urine Concentration and Dilution

ADH IS PRODUCED IN SUPRAOPTIC NUCLEI OF HYPOTHALAMUS AND DESCENDS ALONG NERVE FIBERS TO NEUROHYPOPHYSIS WHERE IT IS STORED FOR SUBSEQUENT RELEASE

BLOOD OSMOLALITY AND VOLUME MODIFIED BY FLUID INTAKE (ORAL OR PARENTERAL); WATER AND ELECTROLYTE EXCHANGE WITH TISSUES, NORMAL OR PATHOLOGIC (EDEMA); LOSS VIA GUT (VOMITING, DIARRHEA); LOSS INTO BODY CAVITIES (ASCITES, EFFUSION) OR LOSS EXTERNALLY (HEMORRHAGE, SWEAT)

ADH RELEASE IS INCREASED BY HIGH BLOOD OSMOLALITY AFFECTING HYPOTHALAMIC OSMORECEPTORS AND BY LOW BLOOD VOLUME AFFECTING THORACIC AND CAROTID VOLUME RECEPTORS. LOW OSMOLALITY AND HIGH BLOOD VOLUME INHIBIT ADH RELEASE

IN PRESENCE OF ADH, BLOOD FLOW TO RENAL MEDULLA IS DIMINISHED, THUS AUGMENTING HYPERTONICITY OF MEDULLARY INTERSTITIUM BY MINIMIZING DEPLETION OF SOLUTES VIA BLOODSTREAM

ADH CAUSES WALLS OF COLLECTING DUCTS TO BECOME MORE PERMEABLE TO WATER AND THUS PERMITS OSMOLAR EQUILIBRATION AND ABSORPTION OF WATER INTO THE HYPERTONIC INTERSTITIUM. A SMALL VOLUME OF HIGHLY CONCENTRATED URINE IS EXCRETED. IN SOME SPECIES ADH ALSO INCREASES WATER PERMEABILITY OF THE DISTAL CONVOLUTION

H_2O

As previously described (see pages 38 and 46), approximately two thirds of the filtered water and solute are reabsorbed by the end of the proximal convoluted tubule in the cortex. The proportion of water and solute reabsorbed is such that the proximal tubular fluid is isosmotic to plasma. Additional water and solute are reabsorbed in the loop of Henle in the medulla; the fluid in the early distal tubule is hyposmotic to plasma, and this indicates that there is an excess reabsorption of solute, particularly sodium, in proportion to water. As a result, the interstitial tissues of the medulla are hypertonic. These processes, occurring in the loop of Henle, are essential to the production of an osmotically concentrated urine and result from the operation of the countercurrent mechanism. This will subsequently be described in detail.

Antidiuretic Hormone

The antidiuretic hormone (ADH) has been described previously (see CIBA COLLECTION, Vol. 4, page 33). Briefly, it is produced in the supraoptic nuclei of the hypothalamus and descends along the nerve fibers to the neurohypophysis. Here it is stored for release as required.

Changes in blood osmolality and volume control the release of ADH. For instance, increased osmolality and/or decreased volume may be caused by factors such as fluid loss from vomiting, diarrhea, hemorrhage, burns, and perspiration, or by displacement of fluid as in ascites and thoracic effusion. Such increased osmolality promotes the release of ADH, which in turn, results in the ultimate conservation of fluid through excretion of an osmotically concentrated urine. Conversely, low osmolality and/or volume expansion, as from increased water intake, inhibits release of ADH, and the final urine is thus osmotically dilute.

ADH indirectly augments the key events which occur in the loop of Henle, apparently by two interrelated mechanisms. (1) The flow of blood through the vasa recta of the medulla is diminished in the presence of ADH; the reduced flow minimizes solute depletion from the interstitium which thus becomes more hypertonic. (2) ADH increases the permeability of the collecting ducts to water. Osmolar equilibration of the fluid in the collecting ducts with the hypertonic interstitium results in an osmotically concentrated urine. These steps will be subsequently described in detail (see pages 56 and 58), but first it is important to understand the countercurrent mechanism.

Countercurrent Mechanism

The *countercurrent mechanism* actually involves two basic processes, *countercurrent multiplication* in the loops of Henle and *countercurrent exchange* in the medullary blood vessels, the *vasa recta*.

In the countercurrent multiplier system, osmotic gradients are generated by active transport of sodium chloride out of the relatively water-impermeable ascending limb of the loop of Henle. In contrast, the countercurrent exchange system is a passive diffusional process in which the osmotic gradients are maintained by minimizing loss of solute from the interstitium into the blood flowing through the vasa recta of the medulla.

To understand the countercurrent mechanism, it is important to realize that all *water movement* is *passive* and *secondary to solute movement;* active transport of water as part of the process of urine concentration is not postulated. In addition, since the gradients are produced along the long axes of the straight medullary structures (whose lengths are measured in centimeters), there is no location in the kidney where large osmotic gradients must be produced and maintained by an epithelium one cell thick. *Continued on page 52*

Continued on page 52

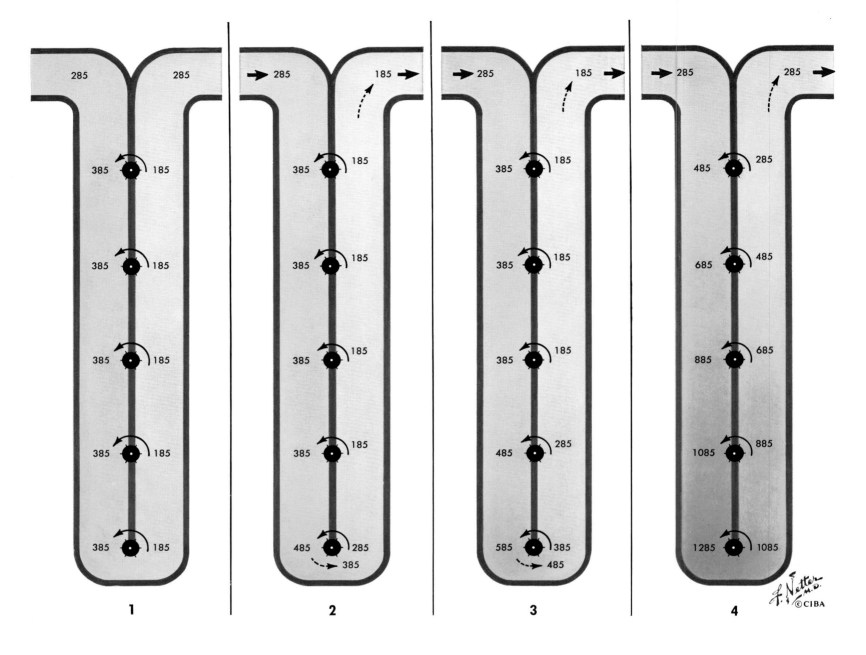

Urine Concentration and Dilution

Continued from page 51

Countercurrent Multiplication. The complicated events occurring in the kidney can best be understood by first considering a simple model, the hairpin-shaped countercurrent multiplier system (Panel 1). The dividing membrane between the two tubes is impermeable to water but does have the ability to actively transport solute from the ascending limb to the descending limb. The tube is filled with an aqueous solution of 285 milliosmoles, the approximate osmolality of the fluid entering the loop of Henle in the human kidney.

Assuming at first that there is no movement of fluid in the tube, an osmotic gradient nevertheless will be developed and maintained across the dividing membrane because solute is *actively transported* from the ascending (right) limb to the

descending (left) limb. As shown in Panel 1, a transmembrane concentration difference of 200 milliosmoles can thus be created.

In Panel 2, the fluid is moving through the tube from left to right; as fluid from the descending limb rounds the bend, the osmotic *gradient* between the two limbs is lowered, and solute from the high concentration area, the descending limb, enters the low concentration area, the ascending limb. Immediately, the membrane attempts to maintain the osmotic gradient of 200 milliosmoles, and additional solute is actively pumped from the ascending limb to the descending limb. The net effect then has been to increase the concentration at the bend in both the descending limb and the ascending limb.

As the process continues (Panel 3), the osmolality in the descending limb increases as it nears the bend. Meanwhile, fluid of higher osmolality than previously (385) is rising in the ascending limb. Solute is continuously actively pumped across the membrane and further increases the

osmolality of the fluid in the descending limb. Thus, the concentrations of solute in both limbs increase continuously, while the gradient between the two limbs is actively maintained. At this stage, the fluid leaving the system has a lower osmolality (185) than that entering (285), and a certain amount of solute is being retained in the system.

At steady state (Panel 4), the concentration in the descending limb increases progressively toward the bend, and in the ascending limb, decreases progressively away from the bend. However, the fluid leaving the system has the same osmolality as that entering the system. No *additional* solute is retained by the system, and the overall effect has been to maintain high *longitudinal* gradients while the transmembrane gradient is of a comparatively low order.

In a model more closely resembling the loop of Henle (Panel 5), the limbs of the model are separated by an interstitium. The walls of the descending limb are *freely permeable* to both water and solute. As previously described, the walls of

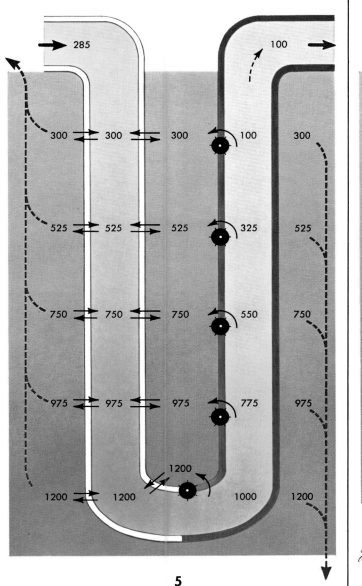

5

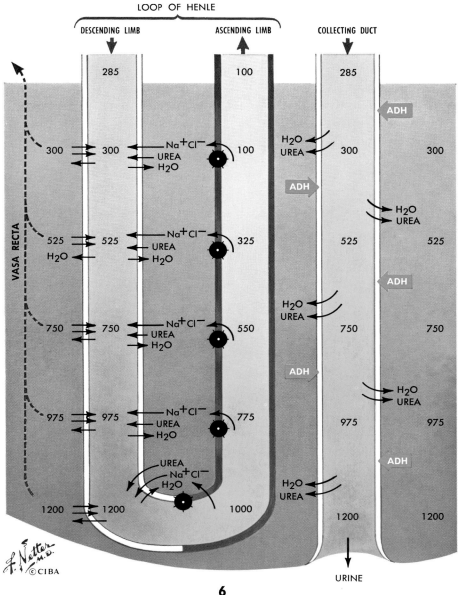

6

the ascending limb are *impermeable* to water and solute, but solute is *actively pumped* from the ascending limb into the interstitium. Since the membrane of the descending limb is permeable, solute freely diffuses into, and water out of, the descending limb. The fluid in the loop thus equilibrates osmotically with the interstitial fluid. The solute is eventually recirculated to the ascending limb.

The overall effect of this model, at steady state, would be the same as that of the previous model except for the effects of the interstitium. Some of the solute inevitably drains from the interstitium so that, if the pumping mechanism continues to maintain the transmembrane osmotic gradient, the fluid leaving the system will be hyposmotic to that entering the system. In addition, because of the drainage from the interstitium, the osmolality of the fluid in it (and consequently the osmolality of the fluid in the limbs) will not be as high as obtained in the originally described model.

In the kidney, a hairpin-shaped countercurrent multiplier is formed by the loop of Henle, as

described (Panel 6). Sodium is actively transported from the ascending limb into the interstitium, and since the epithelium of the ascending limb is almost completely impermeable to water, the tubular fluid becomes increasingly dilute as it flows up the ascending limb. When the fluid enters the distal convolution, it is hyposmotic compared to arterial plasma. The sodium pumped out of the ascending limb makes the medullary interstitium hypertonic. Since the epithelial wall of the descending limb is permeable to solutes and water, the fluid in the descending limb equilibrates osmotically with the interstitium by solute diffusing into the lumen of the descending limb and water diffusing out of the lumen into the interstitium.

In the presence of ADH, the epithelium of the collecting duct is permeable to water, and water thus passes from the lumen of the collecting duct into the interstitium. The net effect is to establish osmotic equilibrium between the interstitium and the fluid in the collecting duct. As a result, the

final urine is osmotically concentrated. Thus, the loops of Henle make a countercurrent multiplier system which is responsible for creating a high osmolality in the renal papilla and, in the presence of ADH, creates a hypertonic final urine.

Urea plays a role in the mammalian kidney in establishing a high osmolar gradient in the interstitium. In the presence of ADH, urea leaves the collecting ducts with the water which diffuses out, and it accumulates in the medullary interstitium. Here the urea attains a high concentration, and some of it passes into the descending limb of Henle's loop to be recirculated, via the ascending limb and distal convoluted tubule, to the collecting duct.

In the arrangement as described so far, there is a tendency for water to accumulate in the interstitium as it leaves the descending limb and the collecting duct. This accumulation of water would impair the countercurrent multiplier system were it not for the vasa recta which remove water and solute from the interstitium. *Continued on page 54*

Continued on page 54

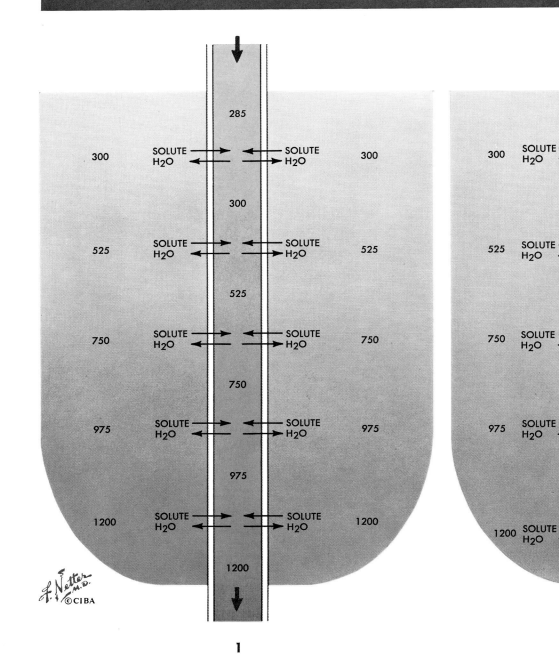

1   2

Urine Concentration
and Dilution

Continued from page 53

Countercurrent Diffusion (Exchange). If blood vessels were to pass straight through the interstitium as in the model (Panel 1), the blood would become osmotically concentrated by a loss of water and a gain of solute; thus the medulla would be depleted of its high solute content. Instead, if the

blood vessels were to turn back upon themselves as in the model (Panel 2), a *countercurrent exchanger* would be in operation. By passive diffusion, which is characteristic of countercurrent exchange, the blood tends to equilibrate osmotically with medullary interstitial fluid; as the blood flows through the descending limb into the medulla, the solute diffuses in and water diffuses out—the opposite of the events which occur in the ascending limb. Thus, the loops of the vasa recta

form a countercurrent exchange system which minimizes the loss of solute from the interstitium.

The countercurrent multiplier system, as represented by the loops of Henle, and the countercurrent exchange system, as represented by the vasa recta, are shown diagrammatically in Panel 3 as they are thought to interact. In this model, the loop of Henle creates a high osmolality in the interstitium, but the fluid leaving the medulla in the ascending limbs is hyposmotic to that entering

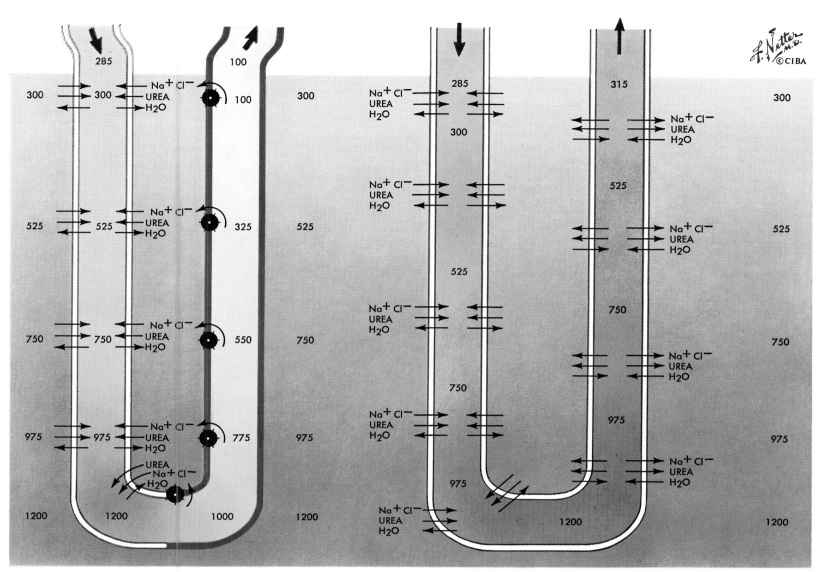

LOOP OF HENLE
(COUNTERCURRENT MULTIPLIER SYSTEM)

VASA RECTA
(COUNTERCURRENT EXCHANGE SYSTEM)

3

through the descending limbs. The vasa recta, acting as the countercurrent exchange system, minimize the dissipation of the high osmolality of the renal papilla which has been created by the loops of Henle. Movement of solutes and water across the walls of the vasa recta is by diffusion, and fluid in the descending limbs (arteriolae rectae) tends to equilibrate osmotically with the interstitium. Thus, sodium, chloride, and urea enter the descending blood vessels as they pass through the progressively higher osmolality of the interstitium, and water leaves the vessels. In the ascending limbs (venulae rectae), the opposite events take place, and sodium, chloride, and urea diffuse into the interstitium while water is reabsorbed into the blood vessels. However, the blood leaving the medulla is not completely equilibrated and thus is presumed to be hyperosmotic, to some unknown extent, to that entering.

In summary, the anatomical configuration of the vasa recta minimizes, but does not prevent, solute loss from the medulla via the blood supply. Consequently, the osmolality of the medulla will vary *inversely* with the rate of blood flow through the vasa recta. Fortunately, both the blood flow rate per gram of medullary tissue and the linear velocity of blood flow in medullary tissue are quite low. Thus, efficient operation of the countercurrent exchange system, in order to maintain medullary hyperosmolality, is assured. *Continued on page 56*

Urine Concentration and Dilution

Continued from page 55

Concentrating Kidney

Theoretical considerations indicate that solute transport against a total solute concentration gradient, with restricted water movement, must occur from a tubular structure in those portions of the kidney which have an increasing interstitial osmotic gradient. It is generally agreed that the thick ascending limb of the loop of Henle, situated in the outer medulla, functions as described previously in the explanation of the countercurrent mechanism. Although there is no general agreement as to the mechanism by which osmotic gradients in the inner medulla are produced, the evidence favors the concept that the thin ascending limb of the loop of Henle functions in a similar fashion to that of the thick portion. For instance, species-to-species variation in urine-concentrating ability generally correlates well with the relative thicknesses of the cortex and medulla; the major increases in osmolality occur in the inner medulla where both limbs of Henle's loop have thin segments. In fact, only nephrons which have thin, as well as thick, ascending limbs are sufficiently long to dip into the inner medulla.

The percent of nephrons with long loops is a species variant. In dogs and cats, all nephrons have long loops; in humans, probably only one in eight nephrons has a loop of Henle which dips into the inner medulla. In man, such nephrons originate from juxtamedullary glomeruli. The remainder of the nephrons in the human kidney arise from glomeruli located more superficially in the cortex, and the loops of Henle generally turn at the boundary between the inner and outer zones of the medulla. At this point, the thin descending limb is transformed into the thick ascending limb. As noted previously, the maximum concentration of fluid at the bend of the loop is a function of the location of the bend within the medulla. Thus, only a small fraction of the fluid flowing through the loops of Henle in man becomes as concentrated as the final urine.

Diagrammatically depicted is a long loop of Henle representing the countercurrent multiplier system, a single arteriola recta and venula recta of the vasa recta functioning as a countercurrent exchange system, and a collecting duct.

The interstitial tissues of the cortex and the glomerular filtrate are isosmotic to plasma. The tubular fluid entering the descending limb of the loop of Henle is also isosmotic to plasma. In the steady state, as depicted, the tubular fluid becomes progressively concentrated toward the bend, while in the ascending limb it becomes less concentrated as it moves toward the cortex; in the distal tubule the fluid is hypotonic as it reenters the cortex. (Note that the figures given are exemplary rather than specific.)

Under the influence of ADH, blood flow through the vasa recta is decreased, and osmotic equilibration of blood in the vasa recta with medullary interstitial fluid is enhanced. However, solute is lost from the system via the vasa recta, and the blood leaving the medulla in the venulae rectae is thus slightly hypertonic.

The epithelium of the collecting ducts is freely permeable to water in the presence of ADH and permits osmotic equilibration between the tubular fluid and the interstitial fluid. In the cortical reaches of the kidney, the fluid in the collecting tubules becomes isotonic since it equilibrates with the surrounding interstitium. Water and solutes which enter the interstitium of the cortex are carried away by the peritubular capillaries and thus do not interfere with the concentrating operations of the kidney.

As the fluid moves through the medullary portions of the collecting tubules, there is equilibration with the surrounding interstitium which is progressively hypertonic toward the innermost zone. This equilibration occurs because of the diffusion of water from the tubular lumen into the interstitium. Active transport of sodium also occurs from the tubular fluid; this may take place in exchange for potassium, hydrogen, and ammonium, or be associated with anion reabsorption.

The withdrawal of water from the collecting tubules leads to high concentrations of urea in the collecting tubule fluid. A gradient which thus favors diffusion of urea from the collecting ducts into the interstitium is established. The urea subsequently diffuses from the interstitium into the descending limb of the loop of Henle. This urea is thus recirculated through the ascending limb and distal convolutions to the collecting ducts and contributes to the high urea content of the medulla in the concentrating kidney.

In the presence of ADH, the amount of water removed from the collecting ducts is limited only by the volume flow of fluid through them and not by their osmotic permeability. Thus, when only a small volume of tubular fluid is presented to the medullary collecting ducts, as in the case of hydropenia, only a little water is present to diffuse across their walls. *Continued on page 58*

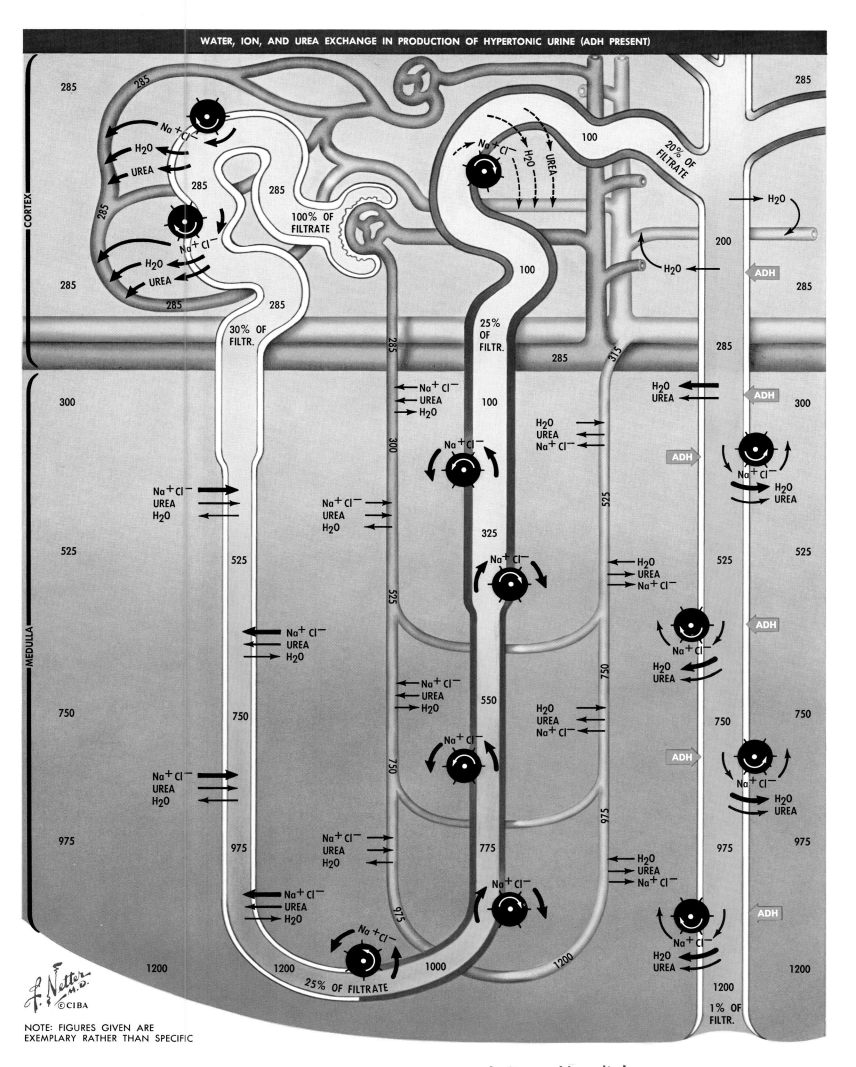

NOTE: FIGURES GIVEN ARE
EXEMPLARY RATHER THAN SPECIFIC

14031

Urine Concentration and Dilution

Continued from page 56

Diluting Kidneys

When ADH is absent, the interstitial osmolality of the medulla is lower than in the presence of ADH. However, the exact mechanism which produces this change is not well understood.

The fluid entering the distal convoluted tubule from the ascending limb of the loop of Henle is hypotonic, just as it is in the presence of ADH. The fluid remains hypotonic throughout the distal convolution and the entire length of the collecting tubule because of this low permeability to water in the absence of ADH. Some reabsorption of both solute and water continues from these structures, but the net effect is the production of a hypotonic urine.

In addition, in the diluting kidney very little urea diffuses from the collecting tubules into the interstitium. One obvious reason is that the urea concentration in the collecting tubule is decreased, and therefore a large gradient promoting diffusion is not established. In addition, however, the permeability of the collecting tubule epithelium to urea is probably less in the absence of ADH. Consequently, high medullary concentrations of urea are not seen in the diluting kidney. Parenthetically, it will be recalled that renal excretion of urea is partially dependent on urine flow rates, in either the presence or absence of ADH (see page 44).

In addition to the changes described, the blood flow to the inner medulla is greater in the absence of ADH; this presumably leads to additional loss of solute and helps account for the decreased osmolality of the medullary interstitium. However, it is not clear whether the increase in blood flow is secondary to a direct vasoactive effect of ADH.

Alternatively, the increased blood flow could result from an indirect effect of ADH. In the presence of high medullary osmolality, there is an increased tendency for diffusion of water across the "tops" of the vascular loops. Since the osmotic gradient in the medulla is lower in the absence of ADH, there would be less "short-circuiting" and thus increased flow to the inner medulla.

The lower medullary osmolality observed in water diuresis, as compared to antidiuresis, is caused to a great extent by the fact that the amount of water removed from the collecting ducts is greater during water diuresis than during antidiuresis. Although this fact appears paradoxical in view of the lower permeability to water of the collecting duct epithelium in the absence of ADH, it results from the greater delivery of tubular fluid to the collecting ducts during water diuresis. In the absence of ADH, diffusional water loss from the collecting ducts is limited only by the permeability of the epithelium. In the presence of ADH, it is limited by the rate of urine flow. □

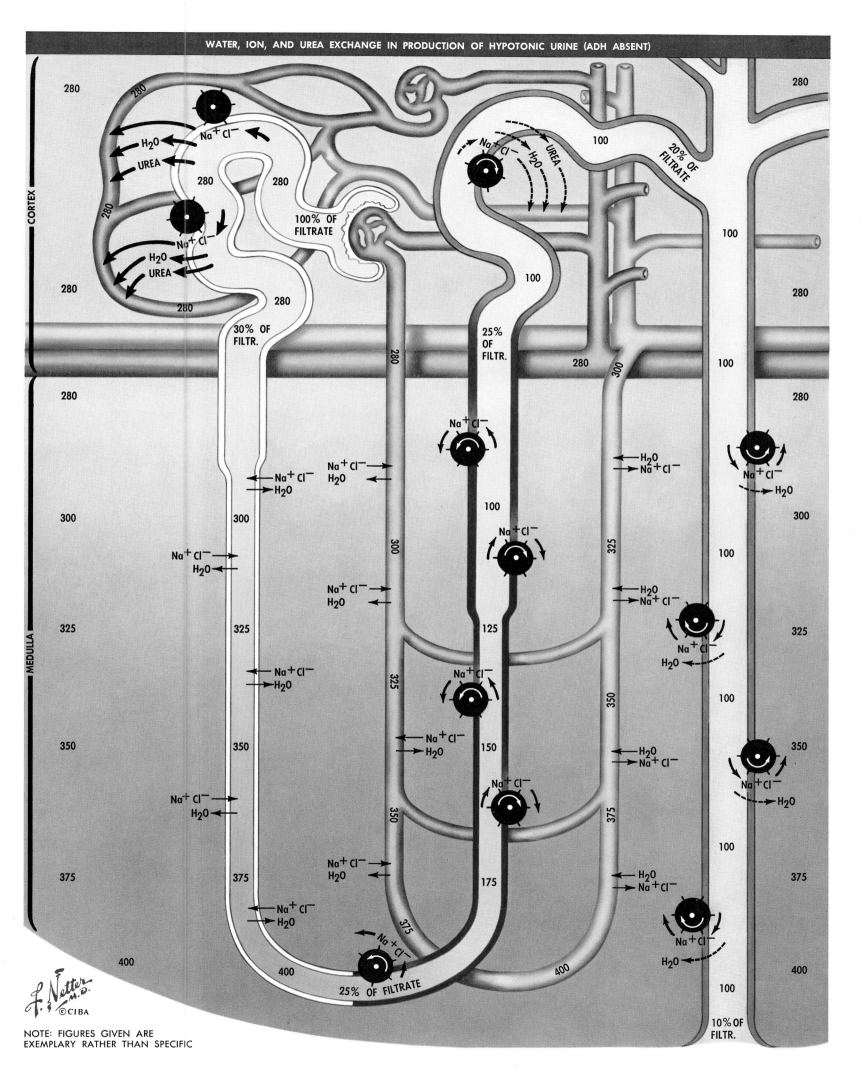

NOTE: FIGURES GIVEN ARE
EXEMPLARY RATHER THAN SPECIFIC

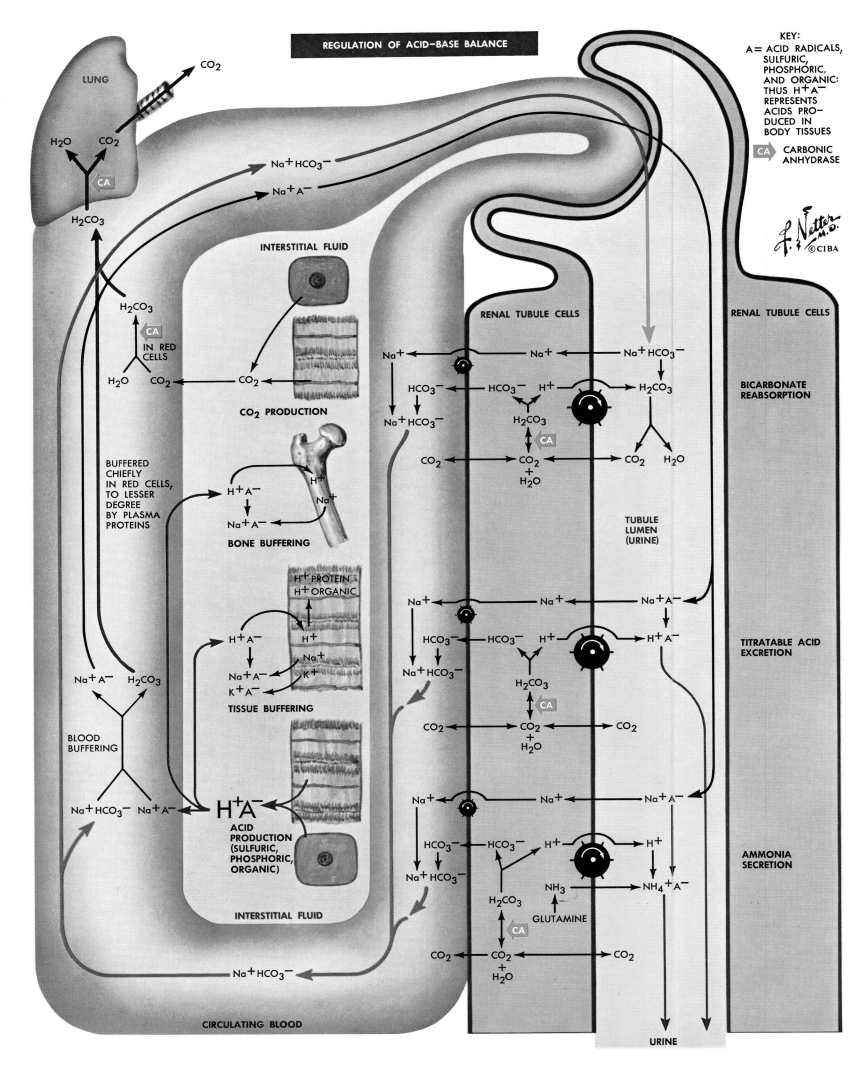

REGULATION OF ACID–BASE BALANCE

LUNG

CO_2

H_2O CO_2

CA

H_2CO_3

$Na^+HCO_3^-$

Na^+A^-

H_2CO_3

CA

IN RED CELLS

H_2O CO_2 CO_2

INTERSTITIAL FLUID

CO_2 PRODUCTION

BUFFERED CHIEFLY IN RED CELLS, TO LESSER DEGREE BY PLASMA PROTEINS

H^+A^- H^+

Na^+

Na^+A^-

BONE BUFFERING

H^+ PROTEIN
H^+ ORGANIC

H^+A^- H^+

Na^+A^- Na^+
K^+A^- K^+

TISSUE BUFFERING

Na^+A^- H_2CO_3

BLOOD BUFFERING

$Na^+HCO_3^-$ Na^+A^-

H^+A^-

ACID PRODUCTION (SULFURIC, PHOSPHORIC, ORGANIC)

INTERSTITIAL FLUID

$Na^+HCO_3^-$

CIRCULATING BLOOD

RENAL TUBULE CELLS

Na^+ Na^+ $Na^+HCO_3^-$

HCO_3^- HCO_3^- H^+ H_2CO_3

$Na^+HCO_3^-$

H_2CO_3

CA

CO_2 CO_2 CO_2 H_2O
$+$
H_2O

Na^+ Na^+ Na^+A^-

HCO_3^- HCO_3^- H^+ H^+A^-

$Na^+HCO_3^-$

H_2CO_3

CA

CO_2 CO_2 CO_2
$+$
H_2O

Na^+ Na^+ Na^+A^-

HCO_3^- HCO_3^- H^+ H^+

NH_3 $NH_4^+A^-$

H_2CO_3 GLUTAMINE

CA

CO_2 CO_2 CO_2
$+$
H_2O

TUBULE LUMEN (URINE)

RENAL TUBULE CELLS

BICARBONATE REABSORPTION

TITRATABLE ACID EXCRETION

AMMONIA SECRETION

URINE

Acid-Base Regulation

The stability of the hydrogen ion concentration in the body's fluid compartments is maintained through the operation of a number of specific biological buffering mechanisms. Without these, the body fluids would become increasingly acidified by the continuous formation of strong acids, mainly phosphoric and sulfuric, derived from the metabolism of phospholipids and proteins. The normal acid-ash diet thus constitutes a continuous threat to the maintenance of the pH of the extracellular fluid within the narrow limits of 7.34 to 7.45. On the other hand, a number of effective mechanisms also protect against the danger of inordinate alkalinization of the body fluids.

Three systems operate to safeguard the maintenance of an appropriate pH in the body fluids. The quickest to respond to an acid or base invasion are the *chemical buffers in body fluids and tissues*. These neutralize acids or bases which either are produced within the tissues or are extraneously derived. A second line of defense is the *respiratory system*. The lungs are the main route of elimination of carbon dioxide, which is another major acid end product of metabolism. Respiratory control of pCO$_2$ (see Editor's Note, below) is also of prime importance in setting the ratio of bicarbonate to carbonic acid, one of the most decisive factors

Editor's Note: The term pCO$_2$ is used here to mean the partial pressure of carbon dioxide. It should be distinguished from P used elsewhere in this book to mean plasma concentration, *e.g.*, P$_{in}$ or P$_{urea}$. The term pH stands for the negative logarithm of the hydrogen ion concentration (or the logarithm of the reciprocal of the hydrogen ion concentration). Similarly K, the dissociation constant, is expressed as pK, its negative logarithm.

determining extracellular pH. The third and most sluggish line of defense, but ultimately no less important in the overall defense of a normal pH, is the *renal elimination of nonvolatile acids and bases*. The kidney is responsible for excess acid and base excretion, as well as for maintaining the extracellular level of bicarbonate ions. It thereby assists in a major way in maintaining both the body buffer stores and the optimum body fluid reaction.

Chemical Buffering

If acid of either endogenous or exogenous origin is added to the extracellular fluid, it is first buffered by the circulating plasma proteins. The second buffering system involves extracellular bicarbonate and leads to a dramatic fall in the bicarbonate concentration. Penetration of the acid into cells calls into play the third reaction, the exchange of extracellular chloride for intracellular bicarbonate. The last, but no less important, operation is buffering of extracellular acid by exchange of intracellular potassium and sodium for extracellular hydrogen ions. In this reaction, intracellular proteins and phosphates participate in the buffering of hydrogen ions entering the cell. A fraction of the sodium-hydrogen exchange also involves sodium stores in bone, particularly when acidosis is of a chronic nature.

The result of these interactions between extracellular hydrogen and both cell and bone cations is an increased buffering capacity of the body at the expense of an increased hydrogen ion concentration within structures outside the readily diffusible extracellular fluid. These ion exchange processes between extracellular fluid and intracellular buffer stores, and mainly involving sodium, potassium, and hydrogen ions, are also involved in the buffering in *metabolic alkalosis* as well as in acid-base disturbances of respiratory origin.

Role of the Respiratory System

The bicarbonate/carbonic acid buffer system is physiologically unique in that the concentration of each of the two components is under separate physiologic control: the bicarbonate concentration is regulated by the kidney, the carbonic acid concentration (pCO$_2$) by the respiratory system. Within the multibuffer systems of the body fluids, the concentrations of these two compounds maintain the pH according to the Henderson-Hasselbalch equation: pH = pK + log bicarbonate/carbonic acid.

The respiratory system (the lungs and those parts of the central nervous system which are uniquely sensitive to changes in extracellular pCO$_2$) is responsible for the effective elimination of metabolically generated carbon dioxide. This large acid load corresponds, in the normal adult, to about 13,000 mEq of carbonic acid per day. Were it not for such "blowing off" of CO$_2$ (H$_2$CO$_3$ $\rightleftharpoons$ H$_2$O + CO$_2$), a severe *respiratory acidosis* would develop. An increase in pCO$_2$ thus stimulates respiration while a decrease depresses pulmonary ventilation. These rapid responses to changes in blood gas tension are effectively mediated by a respiratory control system involving the medullary section of the brain stem (chemosensitive receptors) and those parts of the neuromuscular apparatus which serve external ventilation.

The effective maintenance of a normal pCO$_2$ (40 mm Hg) and the stimulating effect upon respiration of low body fluid pH also aid in the compensation of metabolic acid-base disorders. Thus, pCO$_2$ is initially increased as the interaction of strong acids with extracellular bicarbonate leads to the release of CO$_2$:

$$NaHCO_3 + HCl \rightleftharpoons NaCl + H_2CO_3 \text{ (and)}$$
$$H_2CO_3 \rightleftharpoons H_2O + CO_2$$

Both the subsequent elimination of the extra CO$_2$ as well as the stabilization of pCO$_2$ at subnormal values (respiration is stimulated by a low pH) partly compensate the acidosis. This eventual lowering of pCO$_2$ is then a physiologic adjustment returning the bicarbonate/carbonic acid ratio toward normal.

Renal Factors

The renal tubules are endowed with the capacity to secrete hydrogen ions into the tubular lumen. This process is fundamental to the three renal operations which play key roles in the defense of a normal body pH: bicarbonate reabsorption, titratable acid excretion, and ammonia secretion (see pages 63 and 64).

In both the excretion of titratable acid and the secretion of ammonia, the process of hydrogen ion secretion results in a net excretion of acid. This is on the order of 50 to 70 mEq/day in man. In contrast, the process of bicarbonate reabsorption, although dependent on hydrogen ion secretion, does not affect net acid-base balance; hydrogen ions are neither lost from, nor added to, the body fluids. However, reabsorption of bicarbonate, aided by the enzyme *carbonic anhydrase* (CA), results in the recovery of over 99 percent of the filtered bicarbonate, thus preserving this important buffer.

The extent to which tubular hydrogen ion secretion is involved in bicarbonate reabsorption, titratable acid excretion, or ammonium secretion is determined by the bicarbonate and non-bicarbonate buffer concentration profiles along the nephron and the general acid-base status of the organism (see page 64).

Tubular bicarbonate reabsorption is also dependent upon the pCO$_2$ of arterial blood. An increase in arterial pCO$_2$ enhances bicarbonate reabsorption, while a fall in pCO$_2$ reduces reabsorption. Such alterations in pCO$_2$ presumably affect the renal transport of bicarbonate via changes in intracellular hydrogen ion concentration. It is virtually certain that an increase in pCO$_2$ of extracellular fluid is associated with a proportional increase in pCO$_2$ within tubule cells. This, in turn, would accelerate the formation of carbonic acid and so augment the intracellular hydrogen ion supply for bicarbonate reabsorption. Conversely, a fall in extracellular pCO$_2$ would reduce renal tubular bicarbonate reabsorption.

These adjustments to changes in arterial pCO$_2$ are important for renal compensation in both primary respiratory acidosis and alkalosis. With retention of CO$_2$, as in respiratory acidosis, the extracellular bicarbonate concentration increases and hence tends to compensate the acidosis. The rise in bicarbonate concentration in respiratory acidosis is initially accomplished to a considerable extent by extrarenal mechanisms (sodium-hydrogen and potassium-hydrogen exchanges between extracellular and intracellular fluids). However, this change in extracellular bicarbonate concentration can only be sustained by appropriate increments in renal bicarbonate reabsorption.

In *respiratory alkalosis*, particularly of a chronic nature, the plasma concentration of bicarbonate decreases as a consequence of diminished reabsorption. Although compensation is not perfect, stabilization of the plasma bicarbonate level at subnormal levels aids in the restoration of a less-distorted bicarbonate/carbonic acid ratio.

Bicarbonate reabsorption is also sensitive to changes in the body stores of potassium. Potassium depletion accelerates hydrogen ion secretion while potassium excess decreases hydrogen ion secretion and bicarbonate reabsorption. Although the underlying mechanisms of these adjustments are not clear, it is probable that they are mediated by changes which occur in the intracellular hydrogen ion concentration. *Continued on page 62*

Acid-Base Regulation

Continued from page 61

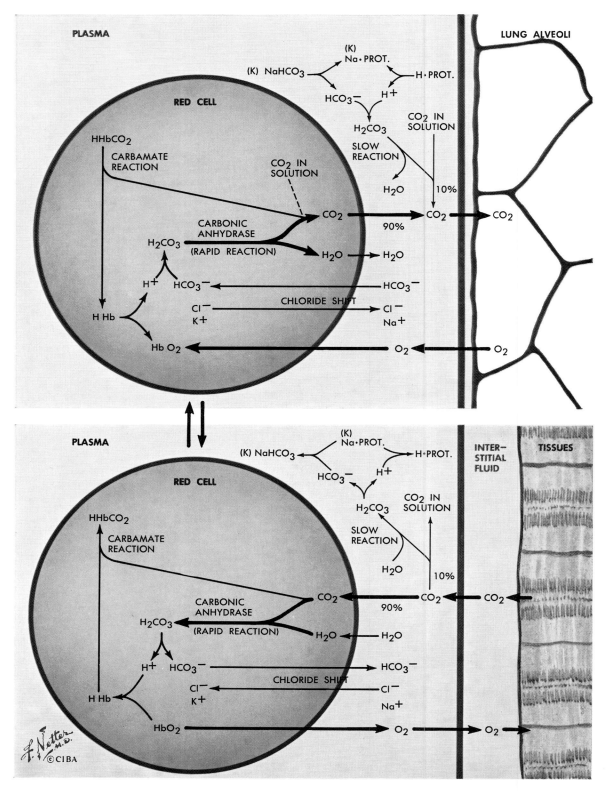

Carbon Dioxide Transport and Buffering

Hemoglobin plays a key role in the blood transport of oxygen and carbon dioxide. Within peripheral capillaries, deoxygenation of hemoglobin (relatively low pO_2) coincides with the release of metabolically generated carbon dioxide from tissues. Accordingly, the pCO_2 of plasma and red cells is elevated. About 10 percent of CO_2 is normally buffered in plasma either by conversion to bicarbonate or by combining with proteins. The remainder moves along a diffusion gradient into erythrocytes. Of the carbon dioxide entering the red cells, somewhat less than one third combines directly with hemoglobin (HHb)* to form carbaminohemoglobin (HHbCO$_2$). The remaining two thirds is buffered by hemoglobin via a number of specific and enzyme-dependent reactions. The following two reactions are involved:

$$CO_2 + H_2O \overset{CA}{\rightleftharpoons} HCO_3^- + H^+ \text{ (and)}$$
$$Hb + H^+ + HCO_3^- \rightleftharpoons HHb + HCO_3^-$$

The first reaction is greatly accelerated by the enzyme carbonic anhydrase (CA). This enzyme is found in high concentrations within erythrocytes but is absent from plasma. Its main function is to catalyze the sequence of reactions involved in the buffering of carbonic acid, within the short time that venous blood remains in the tissue capillaries.

The degree of oxygenation also determines the efficiency of the buffering capacity of the hemoglobin-oxyhemoglobin system. Reduced hemoglobin (HHb) is a weaker acid than oxyhemoglobin (HHbO$_2$). Hence, exposure of oxyhemoglobin to an environment with a relatively low pO_2, as in the peripheral tissues, initiates the release of oxygen, the partial conversion of oxy- into reduced hemoglobin, and an ensuing increase in buffer capacity.

Uptake of hydrogen ions by hemoglobin (and the subsequent accelerated formation of bicarbonate) results in the generation of a concentration gradient for bicarbonate ions from red cells to plasma. Owing to the inherently low cation permeability of the erythrocyte membrane, bicarbonate egress can occur only if enough chloride ions enter the cells in exchange for bicarbonate ions. This *chlo-*
*See Glossary

ride shift is made possible by the high chloride permeability of red cells and is essential for the maintenance of electroneutrality within the cell compartment of erythrocytes.

Changes occurring in the pulmonary capillaries are the reverse of those in tissue capillaries. Exposure of hemoglobin to the gas tensions of the alveolar air (relatively high pO_2, low pCO_2) promotes diffusion of CO_2 from erythrocytes and plasma toward the alveolar gas compartment. Concomitantly, oxygen diffuses into erythrocytes, converting hemoglobin into oxyhemoglobin, the more acidic form of the hemoglobin molecule. Via formation of carbonic acid, carbon dioxide is released and diffuses out of the red cell. The direction of the chloride shift is reversed as bicarbonate enters the cell to buffer the hydrogen ions released by the more acidic oxyhemoglobin. The carbamate reaction,*
$RNCOO^- + H^+ \rightleftharpoons RNH + CO_2$, is also shifted to the

right since oxygenation of hemoglobin reduces its ability to bind carbon dioxide.

Theoretical Concepts of Bicarbonate Reabsorption

Hydrogen ion secretion represents the basic mechanism underlying bicarbonate reabsorption as well as titratable acid excretion and ammonium secretion (see pages 61 and 64). Previously, this concept was based on indirect evidence, but recently, direct experimental confirmation of this thesis has been obtained.

In principle, however, two hypotheses can account for bicarbonate reabsorption: (1) hydrogen ion secretion, *i.e.,* operationally linked sodium-hydrogen exchange, or (2) direct reabsorption of bicarbonate ions from the lumen into the peritubular fluid without intervention of intermediate reactions. Obviously, the consequences of these two mechanisms upon intratubular pH are different and should be examined in detail.

Acid-Base Regulation

Continued

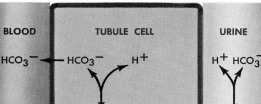

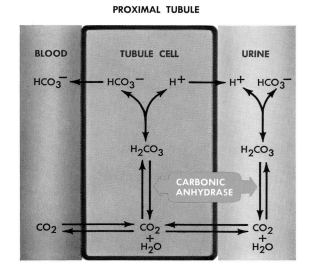

H⁺ SECRETION

HCO₃⁻ REABSORPTION

PROPOSED MECHANISMS OF PROXIMAL AND DISTAL TUBULAR URINARY ACIDIFICATION

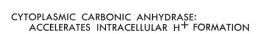

PROXIMAL TUBULE

DISTAL TUBULE

CYTOPLASMIC CARBONIC ANHYDRASE:
ACCELERATES INTRACELLULAR H⁺ FORMATION

LUMINAL MEMBRANE CARBONIC ANHYDRASE:
CATALYZES H_2CO_3 BREAKDOWN AND PREVENTS
GENERATION OF STEEP pH GRADIENTS

CYTOPLASMIC CARBONIC ANHYDRASE:
ACCELERATES INTRACELLULAR H⁺ FORMATION

LUMINAL MEMBRANE CARBONIC ANHYDRASE
ABSENT

According to hypothesis 1, secretion of hydrogen ions and the subsequent reaction with filtered bicarbonate result in the formation of carbonic acid. Since the uncatalyzed dehydration of carbonic acid to carbon dioxide and water is inherently slow, excess carbonic acid would then accumulate and lower the luminal pH below that predicted for complete equilibrium. In addition, the rate of hydrogen ion secretion necessary to accomplish the high rate of bicarbonate reabsorption dictated by the large filtration rate would further serve to lower luminal pH.

From the known rate of the uncatalyzed reaction and the known kinetics of tubular bicarbonate reabsorption, a "disequilibrium pH" can be calculated. In the rat proximal tubule, this is in the order of 0.4 to 0.8 pH unit.

In hypothesis 2, neither the generation of excess carbonic acid nor the presence of an acid "disequilibrium pH" would be expected, since carbonic acid is not formed during the transport process.

Direct measurement *in situ* of the intratubular pH, using either glass or antimony pH-sensitive microelectrodes, helps to distinguish between the two mechanisms, and also provides information about proximal and distal tubular acidification. In the proximal tubule, a significant "disequilibrium pH" is initially absent and only appears after the administration of a potent carbonic anhydrase inhibitor. Thus, it appears that carbonic anhydrase is normally in functional contact with luminal fluid and effectively prevents, by catalytic acceleration of carbonic acid breakdown, the accumulation of excess carbonic acid.

Accordingly, carbonic anhydrase plays a dual role in proximal tubular epithelium. It ensures an adequate hydrogen ion supply for the pumping mechanism at the luminal membrane, and it prevents excess accumulation of carbonic acid within the proximal tubular lumen. By this latter luminal action, carbonic anhydrase greatly reduces the hydrogen ion gradient against which transport must proceed. The presence of a significant "disequilibrium pH" at the proximal tubular level after administration of a carbonic anhydrase inhibitor indicates that hydrogen ion secre-

tion does indeed participate importantly in tubular bicarbonate reabsorption.

In the distal tubule the situation is different. At this tubular level a significant "disequilibrium pH" is normally present, and this can be obliterated with infusion of carbonic anhydrase. These observations prove that hydrogen ion secretion is directly involved in distal tubular bicarbonate reabsorption. In addition, the evidence stresses an important difference between proximal and distal tubular mechanisms for hydrogen ion secretion: *in the distal tubule, carbonic anhydrase apparently does not have access to luminal fluid and thus cannot prevent accumulation of excess carbonic acid.* Consequently, secretion of hydrogen ions has to proceed against relatively large concentration gradients.

Two factors determine the magnitude of the "disequilibrium pH": the rate of hydrogen ion secretion and the tubular bicarbonate load. If these parameters

increase, accentuation of "disequilibrium pH" conditions may be expected.

Secretion of Hydrogen Ions

The pH profile along the nephron determines the fraction of total hydrogen ion secretion utilized in bicarbonate reabsorption, titratable acid excretion, or ammonium secretion. Recent studies on the single-nephron level have not supported the previously held concept that only the distal tubular epithelium has the ability to establish significant hydrogen ion concentration gradients between tubular lumen and plasma. Rather, there is now general agreement that in the mammalian nephron the filtrate becomes acidified along the entire nephron.

Assuming no major differences in pCO_2 between tubular fluid and plasma, the pH changes along the proximal tubule indicate that, at the *Continued on page 64*

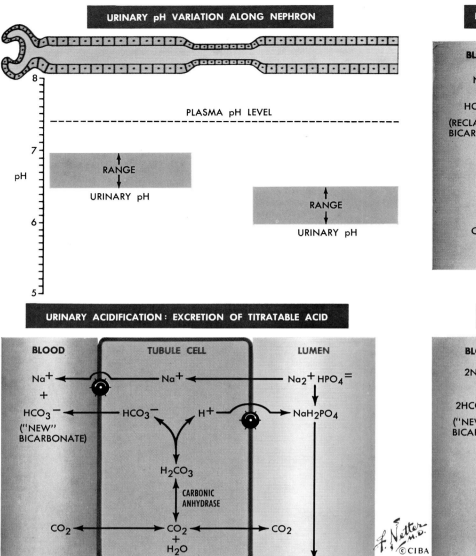

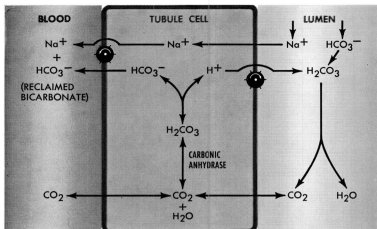

URINARY ACIDIFICATION: EXCRETION OF TITRATABLE ACID

URINARY ACIDIFICATION: SECRETION OF AMMONIUM

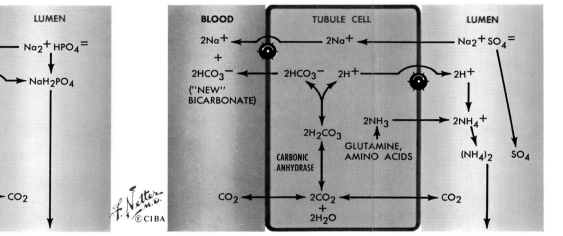

Acid-Base Regulation

Continued from page 63

end of the proximal convoluted segment, the luminal bicarbonate concentration has dropped to about one half or one third of its original level in the glomerular filtrate. With adjustments made for the simultaneous decrease in volume of the glomerular filtrate by reabsorption of water in the proximal tubule, it is calculated that 80 to 90 percent of the filtered bicarbonate is reabsorbed along the proximal tubule.

Final acidification of the urine takes place in the collecting ducts, where maximal hydrogen ion gradients are established. The limiting gradient against which hydrogen ions can be pumped is of the order of 1000:1, corresponding to urine pH values of about 4.0 to 4.5.

Bicarbonate Reabsorption

At normal or elevated plasma bicarbonate levels, tubular hydrogen ion secretion mainly promotes bicarbonate reabsorption, and little is used for the excretion of titratable acid or ammonium. Tubular bicarbonate reabsorption is virtually complete at plasma concentrations below normal, so that body stores are maintained at optimal levels. If the plasma bicarbonate concentration is above the normal "threshold," bicarbonate appears in the urine. Hence, the excess is effectively excreted and the plasma level will again approach the normal range of 25 to 27 mEq/l.

Carbonic anhydrase inhibitors significantly depress tubular bicarbonate reabsorption, thereby increasing bicarbonate excretion. Thus, carbonic anhydrase appears to play a key role in the reabsorptive transport mechanism. Its participation in accelerating the generation of intracellular hydrogen ions and its role in the luminal cell membrane of proximal tubule cells in reducing the transmembrane hydrogen ion concentration gradient have already been discussed (see page 63).

Excretion of Titratable Acid

The exchange of hydrogen for sodium may also involve nonbicarbonate buffers, of which phosphate buffers are of greatest significance. Net hydrogen ion secretion converts the filtered dibasic phosphate to the acid monobasic form and thus effects net acid excretion.

Factors determining the rate of titratable acid formation are the rate of buffer excretion and the acid-base balance of the organism. Increased quantities of titratable acid formation will thus result from either an absolute increase in the tubular buffer load or a relative increase because of lowered bicarbonate load, as in metabolic acidosis. The pK′ of the buffer is another factor governing acid formation. The transtubular concentration gradient, against which hydrogen ions may be pumped, is limited so that a buffer with a relatively high pK′, such as phosphate (pK′:6.8), is most effective. Thus, more hydrogen ions can be buffered by phosphate than by buffers with a lower pK′, such as creatinine (pK′:4.97) or para-aminohippurate (pK′:3.83).

As noted above, in the healthy individual titratable acid is mainly monobasic phosphate, and its availability is limited by the rate of glomerular filtration of phosphate buffers. If acidosis is prolonged, additional phosphate may be mobilized from stores in bone. However, in diabetic acidosis, β-hydroxybutyrate constitutes an additional and highly important source of buffer and greatly aids in the excretion of titratable acid.

Ammonia Secretion

Ammonia is a buffer synthesized by the renal tubules, mainly from amide and amino nitrogens of glutamine (see pages 66 and 67). Under conditions of low urinary buffer excretion, the free base NH_3 is formed in increasing amounts in renal cortical tissue. This highly diffusible, free base NH_3 penetrates the luminal cell membrane and is converted, in acid tubular fluid, into the relatively poorly permeant ammonium ion (NH_4^+). This secretory mechanism is one of "diffusion trapping." The free base NH_3 is trapped in tubular fluid by conversion into ammonium ions which do not diffuse back into cells to any appreciable degree. Thus, energy is utilized directly, not in the transfer of NH_3 from cell to tubular lumen, but only in the synthesis of ammonia and the generation of the hydrogen ion gradient.

Ammonia is secreted in both the proximal and distal tubules of mammalian kidneys, but recent evidence indicates that most of the urinary ammonia is derived from proximal ammonia secretion. Ammonia secretion in normal man shows the phenomenon of adaptation; secretion increase is manifold in severe chronic acidosis. On the other hand, in renal failure with acidosis, ammonia secretion fails to rise sufficiently to prevent a severe cation loss. □

Renal Erythropoietic Function

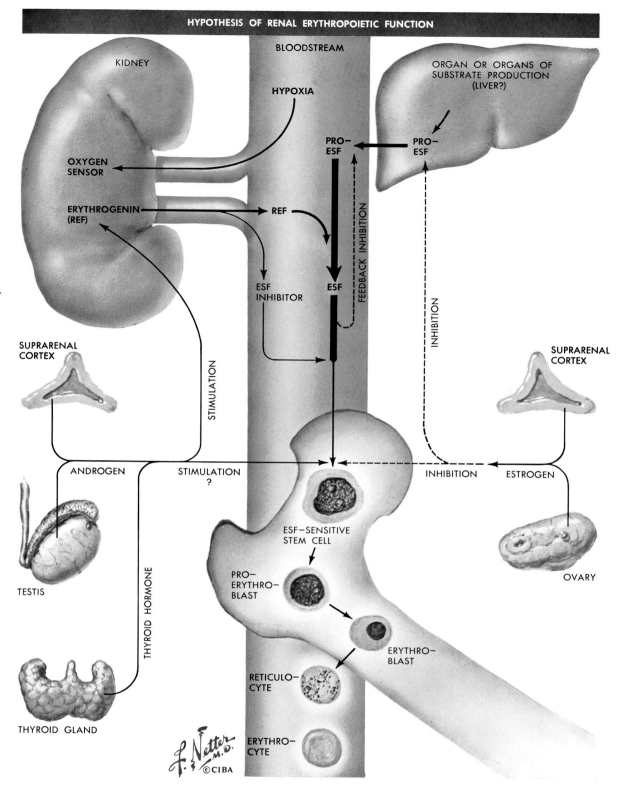

Clinical observations provide evidence of a role of the kidney in erythropoiesis. For instance, moderate to severe anemia often accompanies chronic renal insufficiency, while, conversely, erythrocytosis may be associated with renal tumors. Experimental data corroborate the clinical observations, and the kidney is now acknowledged to be the chief site of either the production or the activation of a circulating *erythropoiesis-stimulating factor* (ESF *or erythropoietin*). This substance has been identified as a glycoprotein with a molecular weight of 45,800.

Experimentally, animals with bilateral nephrectomies exhibit diminished capacities to produce ESF in response to a variety of hypoxic stimuli. However, it must not be assumed that this post-nephrectomy depression in ESF production results from uremia or the accumulation of other unexcreted wastes. Bilateral ureteral ligation in rats, which produces uremia equivalent to that seen following renal ablation, does not appreciably reduce the capacity to produce ESF.

Current Concepts. Two main concepts for the renal production of ESF have been suggested. One view is that the kidney elaborates a *precursor of* ESF which, upon combining with a serum protein, yields the functional ESF. On the other hand, there is growing evidence for the second concept that the kidney produces an enzymatic factor, *renal erythropoietic factor* (REF or *erythrogenin*), which converts a precursor (proESF or *erythropoietinogen*) in plasma to ESF. The distribution of erythrogenin observed in the kidney suggests that it is tubular in origin.

It appears that the concentration of erythrogenin (REF) in the kidney is controlled by the availability of oxygen to this organ. Thus, hypoxia is the fundamental erythrocytogenic stimulus which triggers the renal production and release of REF. This substance then reacts with a substrate in plasma, proESF, to produce circulating ESF.

This system of erythrogenin, plasma proESF, and ESF superficially resembles the renin-angiotensinogen-angiotensin mechanism. However, there is no relationship between the two systems since neither renin nor angiotensin stimulates erythropoiesis in test animals. Moreover, neither erythrogenin nor ESF exerts vasopressor effects in either mice or rats.

Feedback mechanisms operate in the production and/or activities of the plasma substrate, renal erythrogenin, and ESF. For instance, administration of exogenous ESF, by suppressing plasma proESF, inhibits the expected rise in endogenous ESF which accompanies exposure to hypoxia. Thus, ESF functions as a negative feedback on its own production. Also, another regulatory mechanism is suggested by the existence of an ESF inhibitor in kidney tissue.

As noted previously, the oxygen supply to the kidney provides additional control of the concentration of REF. Renal levels of erythrogenin increase when the oxygen supply of the kidney is reduced and decrease when more oxygen is available as, for example, after transfusion of red cells in the experimental animal.

Role of Other Hormones. Hormones of various glands affect metabolic processes and would also be expected to influence red cell formation. Indeed, androgenic and thyroid hormones stimulate erythropoiesis, and this action is mediated, at least in part, through increased elaboration of ESF. This in turn is probably secondary to augmented production of erythrogenin. On the other hand, the depression in erythropoiesis caused by estrogens results from both an inhibitory effect on the plasma substrate for erythrogenin and a decreased response of the blood-forming tissues to ESF. Thus, it appears that the hormones which influence the rate of erythropoiesis do so, in part, by affecting ESF levels, most likely by changing the production of either erythrogenin or the plasma substrate. Alternately, both erythrogenin and the plasma substrate could be affected. There are also indications that certain types of erythropoietic dyscrasias in both man and animals may be attributed to alterations in the amounts and activities of the three components of the ESF biogenesis system. □

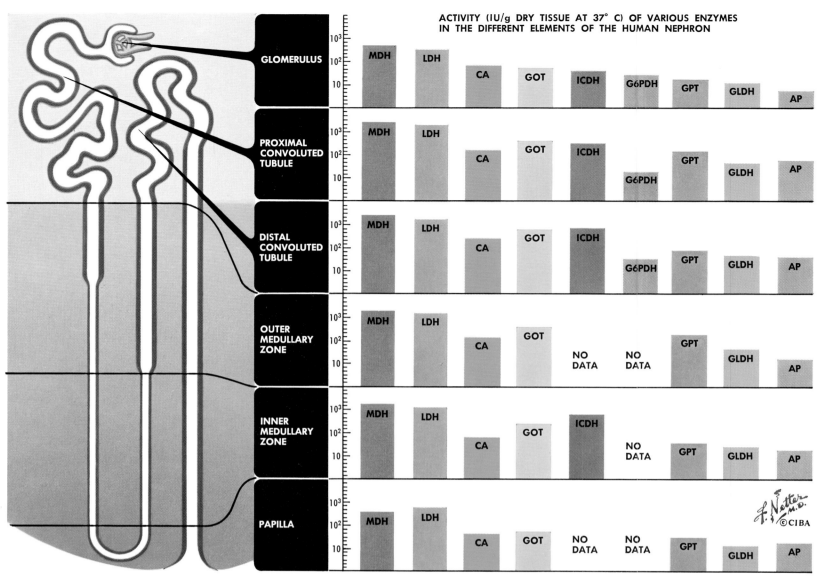

ACTIVITY (IU/g DRY TISSUE AT 37° C) OF VARIOUS ENZYMES IN THE DIFFERENT ELEMENTS OF THE HUMAN NEPHRON

Enzymology of the Nephron

Enzymes catalyze many of the cellular mechanisms responsible for the physiologic processes of tubular reabsorption and secretion. Accordingly, knowledge of the quantitative distribution patterns of enzymes in the various anatomic and functional parts of the nephron appears essential to comprehend fully renal function, particularly urine formation. Moreover, it is possible that the renal enzymes which may appear in the urine or blood can provide important diagnostic information about early damage to specific structures of the nephron.

The complexity of the kidney, however, restricts the value of classic quantitative methods of enzyme assay using tissue homogenates or slices, so that newer methodology is necessary. The development of an exact dissection technic, together with precise micro- and ultramicrochemical analyses, thus made a quantitative enzyme study possible.

The enzyme activities in the human nephron, as determined to date, are highest in the proximal and distal convoluted tubules, with one exception: the activity of *glucose-6-phosphate dehydrogenase* (G-6-PDH) is slightly higher in the glomeruli than in the distal convoluted tubules.

It has not yet been possible to dissect, routinely, single collecting ducts or Henle's loops because of difficulty in recognizing them with certainty in unstained, frozen, dried sections. However, information representative of cross sections through these segments of the nephron can be obtained from the data on the outer and inner zones of the medulla and on the papilla. In addition, since the activity of the glutaminases is rapidly destroyed and not detectable in frozen dried sections, measurements were made from fresh homogenates from the cortex, medulla, and papilla.

Role of Enzymes in Production and Excretion of Ammonia and Hydrogen Ions

Formation of Ammonia. Plasma glutamine is the major precursor of urinary ammonia and contributes both the amide and the amino nitrogen to the formation of ammonia. *Glutaminase I,* activated by phosphate, splits glutamine to ammonia (NH_3) and glutamate. *Glutaminase II,* activated by pyruvate, or another 2-oxo-acid, hydrolyzes the amide bond after the amino group has been transferred to the 2-oxo-acid. If the receiving acid is 2-oxo-glutarate, glutamate is formed. This glutamate, together with that generated by glutaminase I, can be deaminated by *glutamate dehydrogenase* (GLDH).

The site of ammonia excretion varies with the species. In the rat, information obtained by micropuncture of the nephron indicates that all parts of the nephron contribute to urinary ammonia excretion. The pattern of glutaminase distribution in homogenates from separate zones of the rat kidney is consistent with this observation. However, nothing is known about the site of ammonia excretion in the human nephron, although the high glutaminase activity in the cortex and the relatively low activity in the medulla and papilla suggest that most of the ammonia may be added to the urine in the cortical convoluted tubules. One can calculate that the ratio of the combined activities of the glutaminases in total cortex to the combined activities in total medulla and papilla is ~9 in man, ~7 in the dog, and only ~2 in the rat, thus supporting the concept that the medulla and papilla contribute comparatively little to ammonia production in both man and dog (see page 64).

Hydrogen ion excretion must accompany ammonia excretion in order to form nondiffusible ammonium (NH_4^+) and thus prevent back diffusion of ammonia (NH_3). Since *carbonic anhydrase* (CA) catalyzes the reversible reaction:

$$CO_2 + H_2O \rightleftharpoons H_2CO_3 \rightleftharpoons H^+ + HCO_3^-$$

it is the key enzyme in the excretion of both hydrogen ion (H^+) and ammonium ion (NH_4^+).

Carbonic anhydrase is also a key enzyme in the reabsorption of filtered bicarbonate. Located in the cytoplasm of probably all tubular cells, the enzyme generates H^+ intracellularly. This ion is then excreted into the tubular fluid in exchange for sodium ion of dissolved sodium bicarbonate ($NaHCO_3$). Carbonic acid (H_2CO_3) is thus formed. Dehydration of the acid by contact with carbonic anhydrase, thought to be present also in the luminal membrane of the proximal tubular cells, leads to the reabsorption of CO_2 (see page 64).

In the rat nephron, data obtained by micropuncture indicate that the pH in the tubular fluid decreases slightly in the more distal segments of the proximal convolutions, with an additional slight decrease in the distal convoluted tubules. The greatest fall in pH, however, is found in the collecting ducts. In the human nephron, the data on the quantitative distribution of CA suggest that both the mechanism and the site of bicarbonate reabsorption, as well as hydrogen ion excretion, are similar to those of the rat.

The precise role of the other enzymes in the excretion and reabsorption processes remains unknown. However, *glutamate oxaloacetate transaminase* (GOT) and *glutamate pyruvate transaminase* (GPT) probably contribute to ammonia production via the GLDH reaction described previously.

Renal Tubular Dysfunction

Renal Tubular Acidosis and Lowe's Syndrome. The capacity of the kidney to produce an acid urine and to excrete ammonia is impaired in patients with renal tubular acidosis and in patients with Lowe's syndrome (oculocerebrorenal disease). Since the activities of CA, the glutaminases, and GLDH were found to be normal in the kidneys of patients suffering from these diseases, the impaired hydrogen ion and ammonia excretion are not caused by a deficiency of these enzymes. However, the possibility cannot be excluded that the enzyme activity is in some way inhibited *in vivo* (see page 248).

Hypokalemic Nephropathy. The activity of *lactate dehydrogenase* (LDH) was increased twofold in the proximal tubules of five patients with hypokalemic nephropathy (see page 178). One explanation is that observed morphologic changes in the mitochondria of cells of the proximal tubules might have been associated with decreased *oxidative phosphorylation,* an aerobic process involving the citric acid cycle and the cytochrome electron transport chain. One can then speculate that an alternate source of *adenosine triphosphate* (ATP) synthesis was necessary, and the glycolytic anaerobic pathway became the predominant system. An important sequence in this pathway requires the use of *nicotinamide adenine dinucleotide* (NAD) as a coenzyme essential for the generation of phosphate bonds of high energy.

The first step in the sequence of reactions in which two molecules of ATP are generated for each three-carbon fragment of glucose requires NAD:

$$\text{glyceraldehyde-3-phosphate} + P_i + NAD^+$$
$$\rightleftharpoons \text{1,3-diphosphoglycerate} + NADH + H^+$$

In the second step, 1,3-diphosphoglycerate is enzymatically dephosphorylated:

$$\text{1,3-diphosphoglycerate} + ADP$$
$$\rightleftharpoons \text{3-phosphoglycerate} + ATP$$

The availability of NAD is thus critical for the continued operation of the glycolytic pathway. The depletion of NAD is prevented by the reduction of pyruvate to lactate, a reaction catalyzed by LDH, which regenerates NAD:

$$\text{pyruvate} + NADH + H^+ \xrightleftharpoons{LDH}$$
$$\text{lactate} + NAD^+$$

Glycolysis can thus proceed under anaerobic conditions, and this may account for the observed increase in LDH activity.

Renal Transplantation

In patients with long-surviving renal homografts and progressively decreasing glomerular filtration, the activity of G-6-PDH (*hexose monophosphate shunt*), measured in the glomeruli and proximal convoluted tubules, was found to be decreased in response to the progressive ischemia. In the same patients, the activities of *isocitrate dehydrogenase* (ICDH), also measured in the glomeruli and proximal convoluted tubules, and *succinate de-*

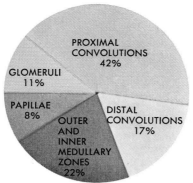

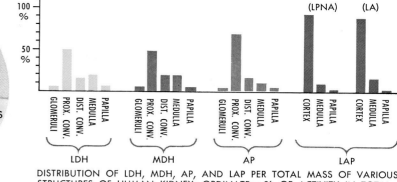

RELATIVE MASS OF THE VARIOUS STRUCTURES AND ZONES OF THE HUMAN KIDNEY

DISTRIBUTION OF LDH, MDH, AP, AND LAP PER TOTAL MASS OF VARIOUS STRUCTURES OF HUMAN KIDNEY: ORDINATE = % OF ACTIVITY IN TOTAL KIDNEY MASS. SUBSTRATES FOR LAP: LPNA = LEUCINE–p–NITROANILIDE; LA = LEUCINAMIDE. TOTAL ACTIVITIES IN BOTH KIDNEYS (300 g) IN μ MOLE/MIN, LDH = 81000 (37°C); MDH = 89000 (37°C); AP = 3600 (37°C); LAP (LPNA) = 1800 (25°C); LAP (LA) = 4100 (25°C)

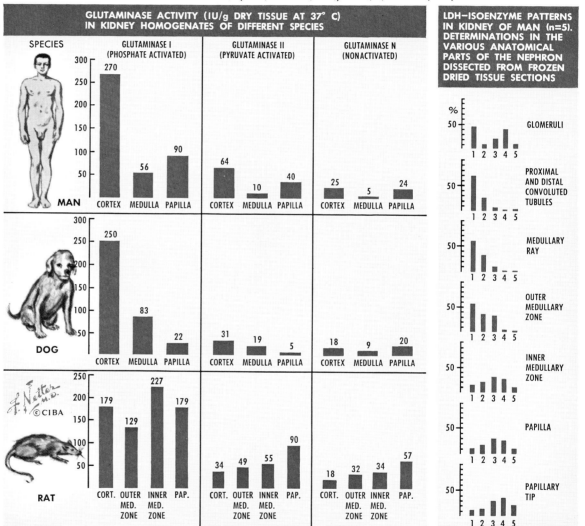

hydrogenase, demonstrated histochemically, were greatly reduced. Only the activity of LDH remained unchanged. A similar pattern, using a larger spectrum of enzymes, was observed in cats during the early rejection phase of homotransplanted kidneys. In these animals, the activities of enzymes of glycolysis and the hexose monophosphate shunt remained unchanged or were increased, while the activities of those enzymes of fatty acid oxidation, the citrate cycle, and amino acid metabolism were decreased.

Kidney as a Source of Enzymes in Urine and Serum

Renal tissue is the main source of those enzymes in the urine with a molecular weight of >70,000 and which therefore are excluded from significant filtration in the glomeruli. The high activity of most enzymes in the proximal and distal tubular cells and the substantial mass of the convoluted tubules indicate that renal enzymes found in the urine are derived mainly from cortex, at least under physiologic conditions. In fact, the LDH-isoenzyme pattern in normal urine, which predominantly contains LDH-1, closely resembles the isoenzyme pattern in the convoluted tubules.

It is not known, however, how much the kidney contributes to the normal enzyme levels of the serum. Since the organ is relatively small, and some renal enzymes are constantly excreted into the urine, the amounts of enzymes released into the bloodstream are probably small. Unlike the situation existing in patients with diseases of the liver, heart, and other organs, diagnostic enzymology of the serum in kidney diseases has not gained importance. Renal infarction appears to be the only condition in which kidney enzymes are released into the blood in measurable amounts, and the LDH-isoenzyme pattern observed suggests that the enzymes originate mainly in the renal cortex. □

Section III

Diagnostic Technics

Frank H. Netter, M.D.

in collaboration with

Richard E. Buenger, M.D. and Suresh K. Patel, M.D.   *Plates 18-31*

Robert M. Kark, M.D., F.R.C.P.   *Plates 1-15, 36-37*

J. U. Schlegel, M.D.   *Plates 32-35*

Howard G. Worthen, M.D., Ph.D.   *Plates 16-17*

Collection of Urine Specimens

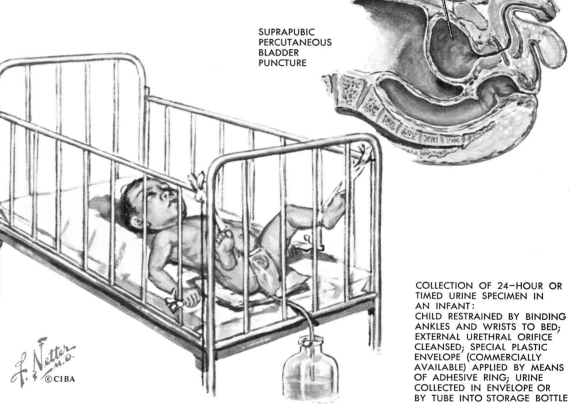

COLLECTION OF CLEAN VOIDED SPECIMENS

FEMALE: PATIENT SQUATS OVER BEDPAN OR TOILET; LABIA SEPARATED, URETHRAL MEATUS AND VESTIBULE SWABBED GENTLY FROM BEFORE BACKWARD BY PATIENT OR ATTENDANT, 5 TIMES WITH BENZALKONIUM CHLORIDE AND 3 TIMES WITH STERILE WATER; PATIENT VOIDS INTO PAN OR TOILET AND MIDSTREAM IS CAUGHT IN STERILE CONTAINER

MALE: FORESKIN DRAWN BACK; MEATUS AND GLANS CLEANSED WITH BENZALKONIUM CHLORIDE AND STERILE WATER; PATIENT VOIDS INTO STERILE CONTAINER

SUPRAPUBIC PERCUTANEOUS BLADDER PUNCTURE

COLLECTION OF 24−HOUR OR TIMED URINE SPECIMEN IN AN INFANT: CHILD RESTRAINED BY BINDING ANKLES AND WRISTS TO BED; EXTERNAL URETHRAL ORIFICE CLEANSED; SPECIAL PLASTIC ENVELOPE (COMMERCIALLY AVAILABLE) APPLIED BY MEANS OF ADHESIVE RING; URINE COLLECTED IN ENVELOPE OR BY TUBE INTO STORAGE BOTTLE

For urine examinations, including bacteriologic cultures, clean-voided specimens should be collected in sterile receptacles. The first morning specimen, which is concentrated, is best for examination. The urine should be examined within 30 minutes after collection, but if this is not possible, half the specimen should be refrigerated for bacteriologic examination and chemical analysis, and the other half treated with a commercially available preservative tablet. This tablet makes the urine both acid and highly osmotic and preserves casts and cells.

For bacteriologic studies of urine from the bladder and upper urinary tract, the specimen must be free of contaminating bacteria from the urethra, external genitalia, and perineum (see page 81). The technic used to obtain clean urine differs among men, women, and infants.

Voided Urine. In men, the glans penis is carefully cleansed with soap, water, and wet sponges. During forceful urination the stream is caught consecutively in three clear, sterile, disposable plastic cups, each of which is immediately capped with a tight-fitting lid and labeled.

The first specimen contains urine from the anterior urethra and appendages, such as the prostate. It should be cultured if urethritis or prostatitis is suspected (see CIBA COLLECTION, Vol. 2, pages 37 and 49). The second, or midstream, specimen contains urine from the bladder and is used for bacteriologic examination and sensitivity studies whether or not it is normal in appearance (see page 81). The third specimen is said to consist of urine from the upper urinary tract. This concept is erroneous. Nevertheless, this specimen can be used for urinalysis as can the midstream specimen.

In women, additional care is required. Collection can be made on the toilet, over a washbowl, or on a special urologic examining table. Detailed instructions, printed on a card and given to the patient, have proved helpful. As in men, the first specimen is from the anterior urethra. It should be cultured if "honeymoon" urethritis or other lower urinary tract diseases are suspected, whereas the midstream specimen is routinely cultured, and the third specimen is used for urinalysis (see CIBA COLLECTION, Vol. 2, page 131).

In infants or very young children, a sterile, plastic, urine-collecting bag can be used. It is put on after the genitalia have been properly cleansed and is held in place by a tight-fitting diaper or plastic device. The bag must be removed as soon as the infant voids. If no urine appears in 45 minutes, the entire procedure must be repeated with a new bag.

Catheterization may lead to genitourinary tract infection and therefore is considered by many authorities to be unnecessarily dangerous. It should be done only when the patient cannot pass urine normally, and then with great care and aseptic technic.

Percutaneous Bladder Puncture. Many nephrologists, however, avoid catheterization by doing percutaneous needle puncture of the bladder. This is a safe and painless procedure which is used routinely in some hospitals to collect urine for culture. Percutaneous puncture is easy to perform in adults, but in infants it is difficult and should only be done by those who have acquired the skill by training and practice.

Visual Examination. All specimens should be visually inspected for gross abnormalities such as blood, blood clots, and threads of pus.

If the color or odor of the urine is abnormal, the cause should be sought. Various *red hues* are produced by hemoglobin, erythrocytes, porphyrins, urorosein, some foods such as beets and red candies, and drugs such as aminopyrine and phenazopyridine. In porphyrinuria the urine may turn *purple.* Melanin or homogentisic acid may make the urine *dark brown or black. Blue green* colors come from drugs like methylene blue, or from Evans blue dyes used to observe blood volume.

Urine from patients with maple-syrup disease has a characteristic, diagnostically useful odor. Similarly, the urine from ketotic patients usually has a pearlike smell. In urinary tract infections, the urine smells fishy and ammoniacal. □

Urine Examination

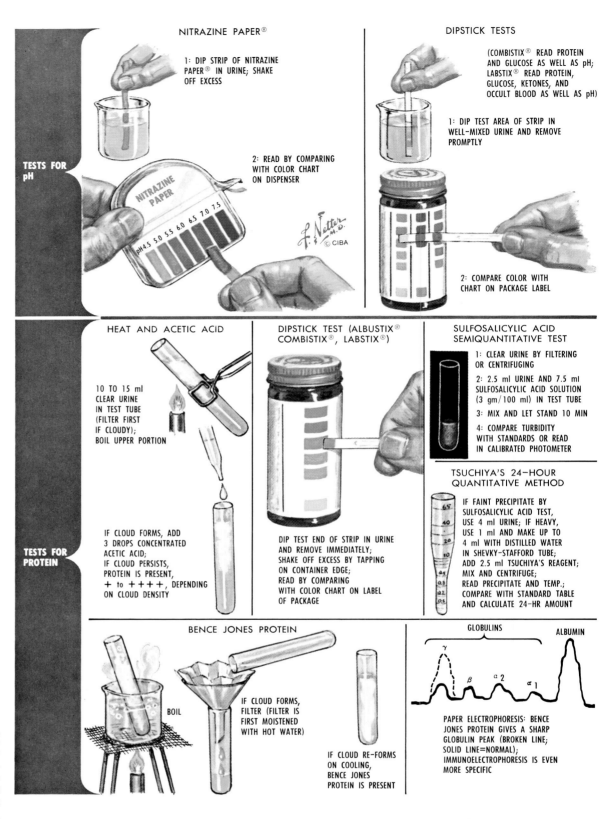

TESTS FOR pH

NITRAZINE PAPER®

1: DIP STRIP OF NITRAZINE PAPER® IN URINE; SHAKE OFF EXCESS

2: READ BY COMPARING WITH COLOR CHART ON DISPENSER

NITRAZINE PAPER

pH4.5 5.0 5.5 6.0 6.5 7.0 7.5

DIPSTICK TESTS

(COMBISTIX® READ PROTEIN AND GLUCOSE AS WELL AS pH; LABSTIX® READ PROTEIN, GLUCOSE, KETONES, AND OCCULT BLOOD AS WELL AS pH)

1: DIP TEST AREA OF STRIP IN WELL-MIXED URINE AND REMOVE PROMPTLY

2: COMPARE COLOR WITH CHART ON PACKAGE LABEL

TESTS FOR PROTEIN

HEAT AND ACETIC ACID

10 TO 15 ml CLEAR URINE IN TEST TUBE (FILTER FIRST IF CLOUDY); BOIL UPPER PORTION

IF CLOUD FORMS, ADD 3 DROPS CONCENTRATED ACETIC ACID; IF CLOUD PERSISTS, PROTEIN IS PRESENT, + to + + + +, DEPENDING ON CLOUD DENSITY

DIPSTICK TEST (ALBUSTIX® COMBISTIX®, LABSTIX®)

DIP TEST END OF STRIP IN URINE AND REMOVE IMMEDIATELY; SHAKE OFF EXCESS BY TAPPING ON CONTAINER EDGE; READ BY COMPARING WITH COLOR CHART ON LABEL OF PACKAGE

SULFOSALICYLIC ACID SEMIQUANTITATIVE TEST

1: CLEAR URINE BY FILTERING OR CENTRIFUGING

2: 2.5 ml URINE AND 7.5 ml SULFOSALICYLIC ACID SOLUTION (3 gm/100 ml) IN TEST TUBE

3: MIX AND LET STAND 10 MIN

4: COMPARE TURBIDITY WITH STANDARDS OR READ IN CALIBRATED PHOTOMETER

TSUCHIYA'S 24-HOUR QUANTITATIVE METHOD

IF FAINT PRECIPITATE BY SULFOSALICYLIC ACID TEST, USE 4 ml URINE; IF HEAVY, USE 1 ml AND MAKE UP TO 4 ml WITH DISTILLED WATER IN SHEVKY-STAFFORD TUBE; ADD 2.5 ml TSUCHIYA'S REAGENT; MIX AND CENTRIFUGE; READ PRECIPITATE AND TEMP.; COMPARE WITH STANDARD TABLE AND CALCULATE 24-HR AMOUNT

BENCE JONES PROTEIN

BOIL

IF CLOUD FORMS, FILTER (FILTER IS FIRST MOISTENED WITH HOT WATER)

IF CLOUD RE-FORMS ON COOLING, BENCE JONES PROTEIN IS PRESENT

GLOBULINS   ALBUMIN

γ   β   α 2   α 1

PAPER ELECTROPHORESIS: BENCE JONES PROTEIN GIVES A SHARP GLOBULIN PEAK (BROKEN LINE; SOLID LINE=NORMAL); IMMUNOELECTROPHORESIS IS EVEN MORE SPECIFIC

Urine pH

Healthy kidneys produce urine with pH ranging widely from 4.5 to 8, but the pooled daily specimen is usually acid (pH 6). Decreased pulmonary ventilation during sleep produces respiratory acidosis and a highly acid urine. After a meal, the urine becomes less acid (alkaline tide), and a few hours later more acid. Because of these physiologic swings and because pH may change during storage, pH should be measured only in fresh specimens.

A diet rich in animal protein, typical of the western hemisphere, results in an acid urine, while a predominantly vegetable diet results in an alkaline urine. A hot, dry climate will often yield a highly concentrated, acid urine which may be irritating when passed.

Persistently acid urine may occur in metabolic acidosis (diabetic ketosis, starvation, diarrhea), respiratory acidosis (CO_2 retention), pyrexia, tuberculosis of the kidney, methyl alcohol poisoning, and metabolic disorders (phenylketonuria, alkaptonuria).

Alkaline urines are usually found in patients with certain urinary tract infections (especially those caused by *Proteus*), respiratory alkalosis (hyperventilation), or metabolic alkalosis (overdosage of alkali, loss of gastric acid from vomiting as in pyloric stenosis or high intestinal obstruction). Alkaline urine may also occur in patients who have primary hyperaldosteronism or some forms of Cushing's disease, or who have ingested diuretics that inhibit carbonic anhydrase (particularly acetazolamide).

Urinary pH is important in three other conditions: (1) In *renal tubular acidosis* (see page 248), the pH is usually 6.5 or higher because of the inability of the tubules to conserve fixed base. (2) In *potassium depletion* (see page 178), the tubules lose the ability to produce urine more acid than pH 6.5, with a resultant loss of the nocturnal acid tide. (3) In *Fanconi syndrome* (see page 247), ammonium excretion is defective,

potassium depletion is common, and the pH of urine varies within a narrow range, usually weakly acid or alkaline.

In the management of certain clinical conditions, urinary pH should be kept persistently high or low by various diets or drugs. *Alkaline urine* is desirable: (1) in the treatment of patients with urinary calculi (see page 200) which develop in acid urine (calcium oxalate, uric acid, and cystine stones) and (2) during therapy with sulfonamides or streptomycin. An *acid urine* is necessary: (1) for the treatment of patients with stones which arise in alkaline urine (calcium phosphate or carbonate stones and magnesium ammonium phosphate calculi), (2) in the treatment of urinary tract infections and persistent bacteriuria, especially those resulting from urea-splitting organisms, and (3) during methenamine therapy. For such regimens to be effective, urinary pH must be tested frequently by the properly instructed

Urine Examination

Continued

Healthy adults normally excrete small amounts of protein (less than 250 mg/day), consisting of albumin, globulin, and 20 or so other proteins from the plasma. Other sources of protein found in the urine are the lower genitourinary tract, including the seminal fluid. *Tamm-Horsfall* mucoprotein is secreted by the distal tubule and, as will be discussed later (see page 76), is a major constituent of the matrix of urinary casts.

Detection of Protein. Despite the growing sophistication of tests for proteinuria, the clinician must keep constantly in mind that all currently used methods, both sophisticated and simple, have inherent limitations. Thus the finding of a 1 +, 2 +, or 3 + proteinuria on routine examination is only a signal for further investigation. In other words, a single finding of proteinuria—regardless of how much—does not point to a specific disorder or diagnosis.

None of the three commonly used tests for proteinuria (dipstick, heat and acetic acid, and sulfosalicylic acid) is entirely satisfactory. Because it is easy to use and generally accurate, the *dipstick* is most frequently employed. Interpretation may be difficult. For example, a positive "trace" reading, indicating 30 mg protein/100 ml urine, is an accurate result. However, if a "trace response" were found in a concentrated, early morning, but randomly obtained urine specimen, the indicated amount of protein excretion would probably be within normal limits, less than 150 to 200 mg protein/24 hours. On the other hand, if the urine tested were very dilute (specific gravity 1.008), a "trace response" might in fact indicate excessive protein excretion.

The dipstick may give false-positive results with highly buffered urines, particularly those which are highly alkaline. Also, this test does not always detect *Bence Jones protein,* and therefore some laboratories routinely test for protein with either the salfosalicylic acid test or the heat and acetic acid test.

Either the heat and acetic acid test or the sulfosalicylic acid test may give false-positive reactions when urine contains X-ray contrast media, tolbutamide metabolites, penicillin in large amounts, or para-aminosalicylic acid. The sulfosalicylic acid test may also give a false-positive reaction when sulfisoxazole metabolites are present, and both this test and the heat and acetic acid test may give false-negative results in highly buffered alkaline urine.

Electrophoresis can help identify serum proteins found in the urine. For instance, it can distinguish "glomerular" proteinuria (over 70 percent of the protein is albumin), "tubular" proteinuria (low molecular weight proteinuria), and the protein spike seen in the urine of some patients who have myeloma.

Significant Proteinuria. If protein in excess of the normal daily excretion is discovered, it is important to determine whether such proteinuria is *transient or fixed and reproducible.* The latter may be either *orthostatic* or *persistent.*

Transient proteinuria may occur with acute febrile disorders, in abdominal crises, and in association with heart disease, severe anemia, thyroid disorders, and central nervous system lesions. In these conditions, proteinuria is minimal, and renal function tests, examination of the urinary sediment, and intravenous pyelography show no abnormality. The proteinuria disappears as soon as the underlying illness has run its course or has been therapeutically controlled.

Orthostatic or postural proteinuria is common in children, adolescents, and young adults. Urine collected in the recumbent position (*e.g.,* immediately after a night's sleep) contains either no protein or normal amounts of protein, while that collected when the individual is erect and moving about contains large amounts of protein. A finding of orthostatic proteinuria in a young person usually indicates a benign situation, but in the older patient, such a finding often indicates serious parenchymal changes.

Persistent proteinuria is associated with primary renal disorders and systemic disorders producing renal vascular or parenchymal changes. Heavy proteinuria may be considered as greater than 0.3 gm/kg of body weight/24 hours and usually raises the suspicion of the presence of the nephrotic syndrome (see pages 123-127). Less protein may indicate chronic renal medullary syndrome (see pages 77-78) or other disorders.

Bence Jones Proteinuria. Up to 80 percent of patients with myeloma (see page 180) may have proteinuria. Approximately 40 percent have heavy proteinuria, and a few may develop the nephrotic syndrome. A number of patients excrete low molecular weight Bence Jones protein, which is characteristically precipitated in weakly acid urines at 56°C and usually, but not always, redissolves on boiling. Bence Jones protein and its fragments (lambda and kappa chains and Fc piece fragments) are also found in *Waldenström's gamma globulinemia* and in the urine of other forms of monoclonal gammopathies. These conditions are most accurately detected by immunologic analysis.

Electrophoretic analysis of the urine protein is also useful to detect Bence Jones protein. However, immunoelectrophoresis is more specific, since the type of immunoglobulin in the urine of patients with myeloma is variable and depends upon the particular low molecular weight proteins circulating in the serum.

Glucose and Other Reducing Substances

In addition to glucose, there may be many reducing substances in the urine, including lactose, galactose, the pentoses, homogentisic acid, and ascorbic acid. The reagent tablet test and Benedict's test detect reducing substances in the urine and are not specific for glucose. Thus, the reagent tablet test is useful for all *initial* examinations of the urine, since it will detect uncommon diseases like fructosuria, galactosuria, pentosuria, and alkaptonuria, as well as relatively common abnormalities such as lactosuria of pregnancy and glycosuria of diabetes mellitus. Further identification of reducing substances may be made by paper chromatography.

Paper impregnated with the dye orthotolidine and the enzyme glucose oxidase turns blue (oxidized orthotolidine) in urine containing glucose but will not react with the other reducing substances. This principle is the basis for the commercially available dipsticks and testing tapes used for the detection of glucose. Such tests are particularly helpful to the diabetic patient for regular urine testing. However, false-negative glucose oxidase tests may occur when the urine contains metabolites of drugs such as L-dopa, which act directly on orthotolidine to prevent oxidation.

Glycosuria commonly occurs during intravenous glucose infusions, in diabetes mellitus, and in pregnancy. It may also be the result of excitement, brain injury, or renal tubular dysfunction, including genetic, familial, and parenchymatous kidney disorders. Glucose may also appear in the urine following anesthesia or if patients have destructive pancreatic disease. Glycosuria is a hallmark of various endocrine diseases, including pheochromocytoma, Cushing's syndrome, acromegaly, and thyrotoxicosis. It is sometimes induced by treatment with steroids, diuretics, and other drugs.

Glucose alone appears in the urine of about 25 percent of pregnant women, while lactose alone is present in almost 50 percent. Both occur together in approximately 15 percent. *Continued on page 74*

patient who is checked, from time to time, by his physician.

Measurement of pH. The use of litmus paper is too crude to be practical and has been replaced by commercially available rolls of indicator paper which has a range of pH 4.5 to 7.5, or by dipsticks which have a range of pH 5 to 9. In the laboratory situation, a pH meter may be used.

Protein

The clinical examination of every patient should include urinalysis, particularly testing for urinary protein. This should be done at each visit to the physician's office, on admission to the hospital, and at least weekly during the hospital stay. Urinalysis and testing for protein should also be done as part of routine physical examinations for college, military service, employment, and life insurance.

Urine Examination

Continued from page 73

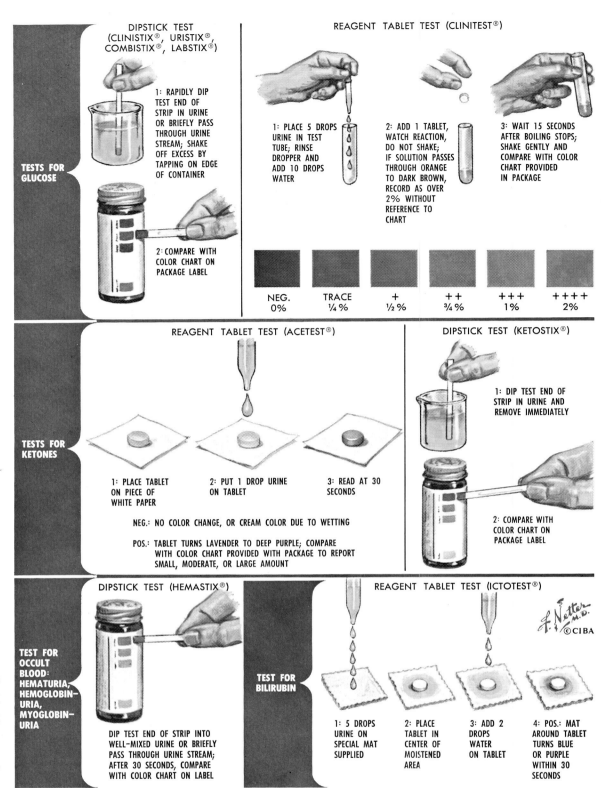

TESTS FOR GLUCOSE

DIPSTICK TEST (CLINISTIX®, URISTIX®, COMBISTIX®, LABSTIX®)

1: RAPIDLY DIP TEST END OF STRIP IN URINE OR BRIEFLY PASS THROUGH URINE STREAM; SHAKE OFF EXCESS BY TAPPING ON EDGE OF CONTAINER

2: COMPARE WITH COLOR CHART ON PACKAGE LABEL

REAGENT TABLET TEST (CLINITEST®)

1: PLACE 5 DROPS URINE IN TEST TUBE; RINSE DROPPER AND ADD 10 DROPS WATER

2: ADD 1 TABLET, WATCH REACTION, DO NOT SHAKE; IF SOLUTION PASSES THROUGH ORANGE TO DARK BROWN, RECORD AS OVER 2% WITHOUT REFERENCE TO CHART

3: WAIT 15 SECONDS AFTER BOILING STOPS; SHAKE GENTLY AND COMPARE WITH COLOR CHART PROVIDED IN PACKAGE

NEG. 0%	TRACE ¼ %	+ ½ %	++ ¾ %	+++ 1%	++++ 2%

TESTS FOR KETONES

REAGENT TABLET TEST (ACETEST®)

1: PLACE TABLET ON PIECE OF WHITE PAPER

2: PUT 1 DROP URINE ON TABLET

3: READ AT 30 SECONDS

NEG.: NO COLOR CHANGE, OR CREAM COLOR DUE TO WETTING

POS.: TABLET TURNS LAVENDER TO DEEP PURPLE; COMPARE WITH COLOR CHART PROVIDED WITH PACKAGE TO REPORT SMALL, MODERATE, OR LARGE AMOUNT

DIPSTICK TEST (KETOSTIX®)

1: DIP TEST END OF STRIP IN URINE AND REMOVE IMMEDIATELY

2: COMPARE WITH COLOR CHART ON PACKAGE LABEL

TEST FOR OCCULT BLOOD: HEMATURIA; HEMOGLOBINURIA, MYOGLOBINURIA

DIPSTICK TEST (HEMASTIX®)

DIP TEST END OF STRIP INTO WELL-MIXED URINE OR BRIEFLY PASS THROUGH URINE STREAM; AFTER 30 SECONDS, COMPARE WITH COLOR CHART ON LABEL

TEST FOR BILIRUBIN

REAGENT TABLET TEST (ICTOTEST®)

1: 5 DROPS URINE ON SPECIAL MAT SUPPLIED

2: PLACE TABLET IN CENTER OF MOISTENED AREA

3: ADD 2 DROPS WATER ON TABLET

4: POS.: MAT AROUND TABLET TURNS BLUE OR PURPLE WITHIN 30 SECONDS

After delivery, the glycosuria stops but the degree of lactosuria increases. In addition, the incidence of lactosuria is higher in the postpartum period than during pregnancy.

Ketones

Ketone bodies are present in the urine of patients suffering from uncontrolled diabetes mellitus, starvation, vomiting, and dehydration, or following anesthesia, exposure to cold, and severe exercise. Such ketones may be detected with commercially available tablet or dipstick tests. The latter is particularly useful for the diabetic patient who tests his own urine.

Parenthetically, the tablet test can also be used to measure plasma ketone levels. In fact, the estimation of the amount of *ketonemia* is a reliable indicator of the severity of diabetic ketosis and of the response to treatment. A drop of blood from a fingertip puncture is allowed to clot on the tablet for 10 minutes; the clos is then removed, and the tablet color is compared with the chart.

Mild ketonuria develops in a large number of hospitalized patients who do not have diabetes mellitus. For example, it may be observed in association with febrile diseases, dietary imbalance, starvation, cachectic conditions, digestive disturbances, eclampsia, pernicious vomiting of pregnancy, cyclic vomiting in children, and diarrhea, and following anesthesia.

Occult Blood

The dipstick test for occult blood is most reactive with free hemoglobin in urine. However, it also detects both hemoglobin in intact red blood cells and myoglobin. Thus, it is an excellent screening rest for hematuria, hemoglobinuria, and myoglobinuria. Any urine which is positive for occult blood should be examined both microscopically for red blood cells (see page 75) and spectroscopically for myoglobin and hemoglobin. As with the other dipstick tests, the occult blood test can also be used as a self-testing device by patients to follow the course of hematuria during treatment.

Bilirubin

Bilirubin appears in the urine when there is partial or complete obstruction of the intra- and extrahepatic biliary system, including the hepatocytes (see CIBA COLLECTION, Vol. 3/III, pages 47-49). Clinical jaundice appears when the plasma level of conjugated bilirubin rises because of backflow from obstruction of the hepatic ducts (as the result of stones blocking the common duct, the presence of periportal inflammation or fibrosis, swelling and necrosis of liver cells, or damage to hepatic cells). This conjugated form of bilirubin is excreted by the kidneys and can be detected in the urine by the reagent tablet test. However, if jaundice is caused by excessive hemolysis, abnormal synthesis of pigment, or when bilirubin circulates in the unconjugated form in disorders such as Gilbert's disease, the serum level of the unconjugated form of bilirubin rises. This is not excreted by the kidneys. □

Microscopic Urine Examination

Organized Urinary Sediment

The urine from healthy persons usually contains a small amount of sediment consisting of a few hyaline and granular casts, cells, and debris from the entire urinary tract. Casts are formed in the nephrons and vary in shape and appearance. Epithelial cells are shed into the urine from the nephrons, pelves, ureters, bladder, and urethra. In the male, the prostate may contribute cells and mucous threads, while in the female, the vagina and periurethral glands may supply these elements. In addition, spermatozoa may occasionally be found in the male. A few erythrocytes and leukocytes may be seen, and these are thought to enter the urine by diapedesis from any part of the tract.

Generally, in patients with renal parenchymal disease, increased numbers of cells and casts are discharged from the kidney. However, the urinary sediment may appear *normal* in some patients with advanced parenchymal disease, such as chronic renal medullary syndrome. (For a description of chronic renal medullary syndrome see pages 77-78.) In these patients, special methods and technics are necessary to detect the few abnormal casts discharged (see page 77).

Technic. Proper examination of the sediment requires a consistency in technic so that patient-to-patient and day-to-day comparisons of specimens can be made. Thus, the amount of urine centrifuged, the centrifuge speed, the kind of tube used, and the time should remain constant, *e.g.,* 15 ml at 1500 rpm for 10 minutes. After centrifuging, the tube containing the specimen is quickly inverted and the supernatant urine poured off. The tube is then placed upright and the sediment resuspended in the small amount of urine which remains. This suspension is transferred by pipet to a hemacytometer for quantitative counts. Alternately, for semi-quantitative counts, the material may be transferred by pipet or glass rod to a slide. Regardless of the method used, the whole counting chamber or slide should be examined for abnormalities.

If the standard light microscope is used for examination, the low power objective is first employed with the condenser lowered and the diaphragm closed. This produces a subdued light which assists in identifying hyaline casts and observing the matrices of other casts. In addition, since many of the formed elements are somewhat refractile and difficult to distinguish, the fine focus of the microscope should be continuously changed.

Cellular Elements. Up to five *red blood cells* per high power field may be observed in urine from healthy subjects. In febrile conditions, or after strenuous exercise, there may be a transient increase in the number of red blood cells present. If the number of red cells is increased consistently above five per high power field, or if there is gross hematuria, one may be dealing with a serious disorder and the cause must be sought. Renal parenchy-

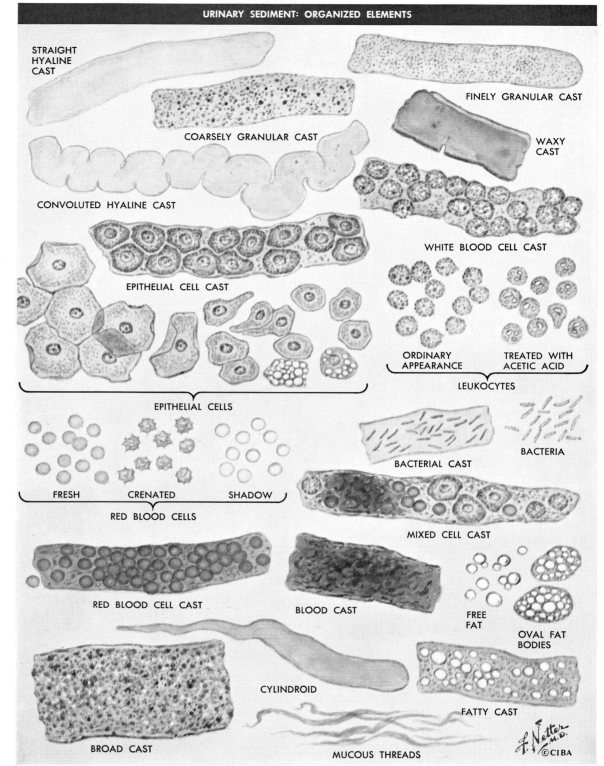

URINARY SEDIMENT: ORGANIZED ELEMENTS

STRAIGHT HYALINE CAST — FINELY GRANULAR CAST — COARSELY GRANULAR CAST — WAXY CAST — CONVOLUTED HYALINE CAST — WHITE BLOOD CELL CAST — EPITHELIAL CELL CAST — ORDINARY APPEARANCE — TREATED WITH ACETIC ACID — LEUKOCYTES — EPITHELIAL CELLS — FRESH — CRENATED — SHADOW — RED BLOOD CELLS — BACTERIAL CAST — BACTERIA — MIXED CELL CAST — RED BLOOD CELL CAST — BLOOD CAST — FREE FAT — OVAL FAT BODIES — CYLINDROID — FATTY CAST — BROAD CAST — MUCOUS THREADS

F. Netter M.D. ©CIBA

mal diseases, such as glomerulonephritis, and lesions in any part of the urinary tract (such as arteriovenous fistulae, calculi, infections, schistosomiasis, or neoplasms) should all be considered in the differential diagnosis. Diseases such as periarteritis nodosa, subacute bacterial endocarditis, scurvy, sickle cell anemia, blood dyscrasias, and malignant hypertension may also be causes of hematuria. One should not overlook the possibility of hemorrhage arising from the use of drugs, such as anticoagulants, or from various nephrotoxic agents. Renal infarction and certain congenital anomalies, such as polycystic kidneys, are also possible causes of excess red cells in the urine.

In dilute urine, red blood cells may hemolyze. Ghost forms may develop and be difficult to differentiate from yeast cells. In acute glomerulonephritis, the red blood cells may be crenated, while in lupus nephritis, helmet cells, burr cells, and red cell fragments may be

seen. In sickle cell disease, sickle cells may be found.

The presence of excessive numbers of *white blood cells* in the urine, either free or in clumps, indicates an inflammatory process. This may be an acute infection or be the result of an inflammatory disorder such as lupus nephritis (see page 141).

Bacteriologic cultures should always be made when excessive numbers of white blood cells are found (see page 81). If the urine is repeatedly sterile, one may be dealing with unusual infections, such as tuberculosis or candidiasis, and special culture media may have to be used. Alternately, the acute infection may have been adequately treated, and the presence of white cells in the urine may reflect the presence of a healing, infective, inflammatory process. For example, pus cells may appear in the urinary sediment for at least 10 days after adequate treatment and sterilization of the urine of a patient with *Continued on page 76*

Microscopic Urine Examination

Continued from page 75

acute pyelonephritis caused by *E. coli*.

Pyuria in association with sterile urine may reflect the presence of one of the collagen disorders, chronic renal medullary syndrome, or that peculiar disorder, rapidly contracting kidneys with sterile pyuria.

At times, it is very difficult to distinguish white blood cells from small epithelial cells. An excess of the latter in the urine may simulate pyuria. White blood cells and epithelial cells can clearly be distinguished from each other by the Prescott-Brodie stain which colors white cells purplish black but does not stain epithelial cells. Formerly, acetic acid, or methylene blue, or the Sternheimer stain was used to assist in making a distinction between the two types of cells.

Casts. All casts arise in the kidney. They consist of a mucoprotein matrix, the Tamm-Horsfall mucoprotein, in which cells or debris are embedded and in which a variety of serum and renal proteins may be absorbed. The Tamm-Horsfall mucoprotein is secreted by the cells of the distal convolutions of the tubules. As it passes down the tubules, it dehydrates, precipitates, and conglutinates and so forms the hyaline cast. If tubular cell debris is caught up in, and molded into, the hyaline matrix

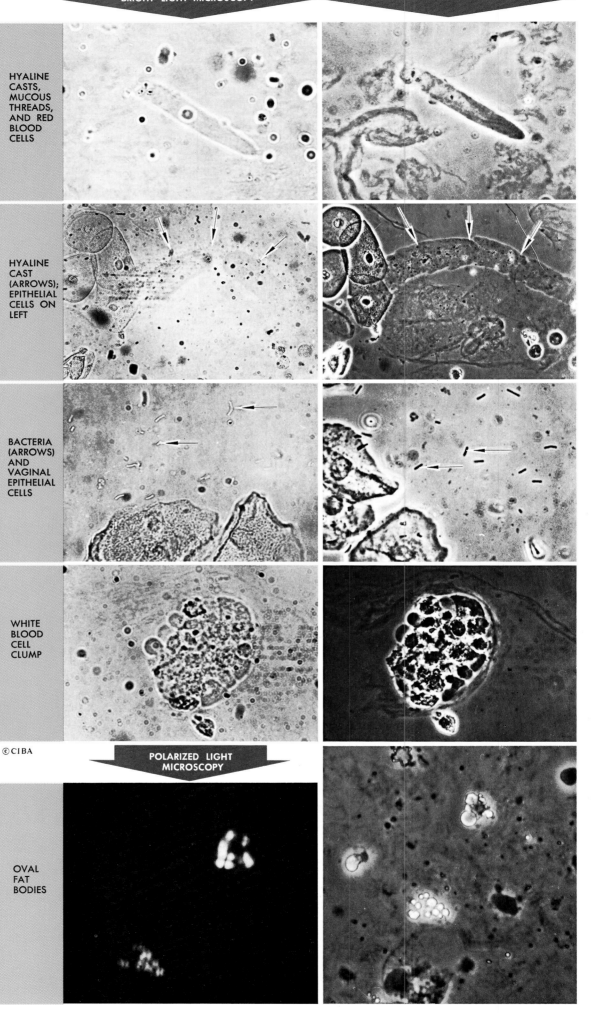

BRIGHT LIGHT MICROSCOPY

PHASE CONTRAST MICROSCOPY

HYALINE CASTS, MUCOUS THREADS, AND RED BLOOD CELLS

HYALINE CAST (ARROWS); EPITHELIAL CELLS ON LEFT

BACTERIA (ARROWS) AND VAGINAL EPITHELIAL CELLS

WHITE BLOOD CELL CLUMP

© CIBA

POLARIZED LIGHT MICROSCOPY

OVAL FAT BODIES

Microscopic Urine Examination

Continued

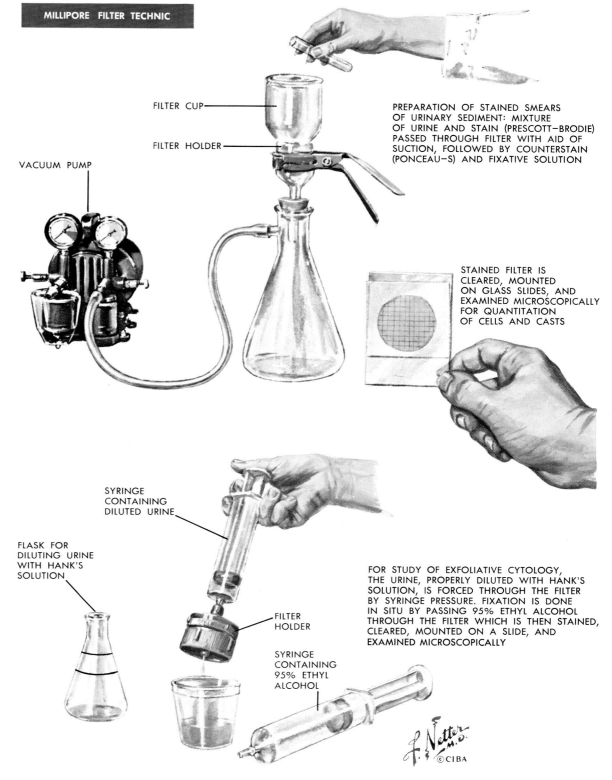

FILTER CUP

FILTER HOLDER

VACUUM PUMP

PREPARATION OF STAINED SMEARS OF URINARY SEDIMENT: MIXTURE OF URINE AND STAIN (PRESCOTT—BRODIE) PASSED THROUGH FILTER WITH AID OF SUCTION, FOLLOWED BY COUNTERSTAIN (PONCEAU—S) AND FIXATIVE SOLUTION

STAINED FILTER IS CLEARED, MOUNTED ON GLASS SLIDES, AND EXAMINED MICROSCOPICALLY FOR QUANTITATION OF CELLS AND CASTS

SYRINGE CONTAINING DILUTED URINE

FLASK FOR DILUTING URINE WITH HANK'S SOLUTION

FILTER HOLDER

SYRINGE CONTAINING 95% ETHYL ALCOHOL

FOR STUDY OF EXFOLIATIVE CYTOLOGY, THE URINE, PROPERLY DILUTED WITH HANK'S SOLUTION, IS FORCED THROUGH THE FILTER BY SYRINGE PRESSURE. FIXATION IS DONE IN SITU BY PASSING 95% ETHYL ALCOHOL THROUGH THE FILTER WHICH IS THEN STAINED, CLEARED, MOUNTED ON A SLIDE, AND EXAMINED MICROSCOPICALLY

during passage down the nephron, granular casts (fine or coarse) are formed. When cells are molded into the Tamm-Horsfall mucoprotein, red cell, white cell, epithelial cell, or mixed cell casts may be formed. Waxy casts are thought to indicate stasis in nephrons. All casts, excluding hyaline and granular but including the broad casts formed in the collecting ducts, indicate renal disease. Broad casts indicate chronic renal failure.

Fatty Substances. Fatty casts, oval fat bodies, and free fat are excreted by patients who have the nephrotic syndrome (see page 123) and occasionally by patients with diabetes mellitus (see page 149). The fatty casts and oval fat bodies contain cholesterol esters and take on a Maltese-cross appearance when viewed in polarized light.

Phase Microscopy

The optical characteristics of the bright light microscope produce a well-known lack of precision in recognizing the elements of the urinary sediment; many casts are never seen, and many cells and casts are misidentified. However, phase microscopes, now available for routine use, provide a new order of precision in the identification of cells, casts, and other

material in the urinary sediment. These instruments are relatively inexpensive, save time, and are easy to use.

Most standard microscopes may be converted to phase microscopes by use of phase contrast accessories. As noted, such instruments are accurate and simple to operate, and phase microscopy should be used for the routine study of urinary sediment in both the physician's office and the hospital laboratory.

It is possible to visualize transparent objects, without loss of definition, with phase contrast microscopy. Not only are casts clearly visible, but there is maximum definition of other elements of the sediment.

The differences between bright light microscopy and phase contrast microscopy are readily apparent in the illustration. With phase microscopy one can also distinguish fragmented particulate debris from bacteria, yeast cells from red blood cells, and small epithelial

cells from polymorphonuclear leukocytes. In addition, oval fat bodies and oval fat casts are usually visible as glittering, rounded dots reflecting light. One does not normally need polarized light to recognize them.

For instance, one can see that epithelial cells have a smooth outline as compared with leukocytes; the cytoplasm is dark whereas that of the leukocyte is mottled; and the nucleus is central with a very well marked central nucleolus, while the leukocyte nucleus is lobed. These distinctions are virtually impossible to see with bright light microscopy.

Millipore Filter Technic

In the past, a wide variety of disorders which involve the renal medulla and papilla have been classified under the term "chronic pyelonephritis." This assortment of diseases comprises the *chronic renal medullary syndrome* and includes the various Continued on page 78

Microscopic Urine Examination

Continued from page 77

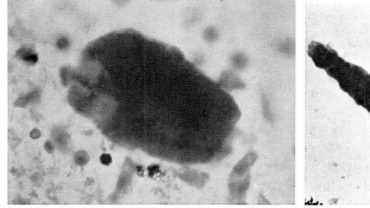

HYALINE CAST

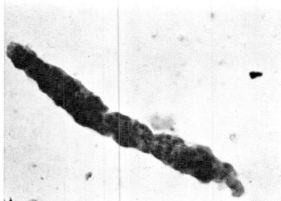

GRANULAR CAST

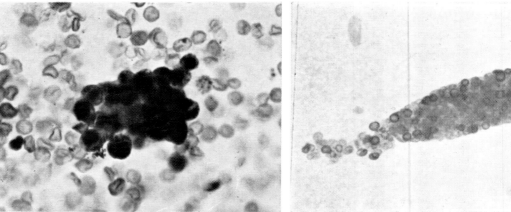

WHITE BLOOD CELL CAST; RED BLOOD CELLS IN BACKGROUND

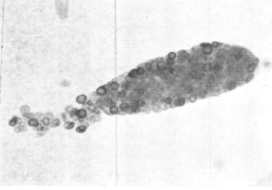

RED BLOOD CELL CAST

©CIBA

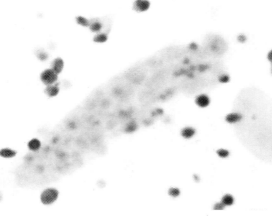

EPITHELIAL CELL CAST; WHITE CELLS (BLACK) IN BACKGROUND

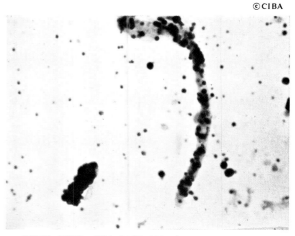

LONG MIXED CELL CAST AND SMALL WHITE CELL CAST (BLACK)

forms of renal ischemia (either with or without hypertension, see pages 153–158, and CIBA COLLECTION, Vol. 5, page 228), analgesic abuse (see page 169), interstitial nephritis (secondary to either drug reactions and sensitivity, or infectious and immunologic reactions, see page 144), chronic granulomatous disorders (such as sarcoidosis and tuberculosis, see page 196), renal fibrosis from chronic potassium deficiency (see page 178), Balkan nephritis (see page 145), parasitic disorders (such as bilharziasis), sickle cell disease, gouty infiltration, and chronic bacterial pyelonephritis (see page 191).

These diseases are slowly progressive and very often are extremely difficult to diagnose until patients suddenly develop symptoms of chronic renal failure. Even when parenchymatous involvement is severe, the urinary findings may be minimal. The specific gravity is somewhat reduced, but there is a paucity of cells and casts. In fact, hyaline and granular casts may be completely absent, in contrast to the situation with the urine of healthy persons in which small numbers of hyaline and granular casts are usually found. Occasionally, there may be increased numbers of leukocytes in the urine but usually without the presence of bacteria.

In this situation, if one of the diseases of the chronic renal medullary syndrome is suspected, one could examine numerous specimens of urine in an attempt to find a single abnormal cast, such as a white cell cast, which would indicate an inflammatory process. One could then confirm the diagnosis with a renal biopsy (see page 107).

Fortunately, a newer technic involving the use of Millipore filters has largely overcome the problem and allows an accurate count of the total number of casts passed per unit of time. Parenthetically, the Addis count was originally developed to obtain such an accurate count, per unit of time, of the various cells and casts in the urine; however, it is not satisfactory since many cells and casts are destroyed while others are not well displayed.

Technic for Urinary Sediment. The patient's urine is collected (see page 71) for a fixed period of time,

usually 30 minutes to an hour, and immediately transported to the laboratory. The volume is measured, and a 10 ml aliquot is mixed with 10 drops of prefiltered Prescott-Brodie stain. The colored urine is poured into the filter cup of the Millipore holder which is attached, using a rubber cork, to a vacuum flask and vacuum pump. The contents of the filter cup are cleared by vacuum into the flask; the pump is shut off to leave the filter moist. Normal saline is next added to the cup and filtered. Then 5 ml of prefiltered Ponceau-S stain is added to the cup and allowed to remain on the filter for 5 minutes. The pump is now turned on, and the stain is filtered until the filter is just moist. Thereafter, 95 percent alcohol and a mixture of 50 percent absolute isopropanol and 50 percent xylol are successively added and filtered. Finally, xylol alone is added and is allowed to remain in contact with the filter for 5 minutes before being filtered. The Millipore

Microscopic Urine Examination

Continued

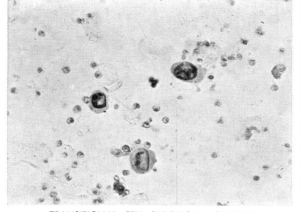

TRANSITIONAL CELL CARCINOMA OF RENAL PELVIS (PAPANICOLAOU STAIN)

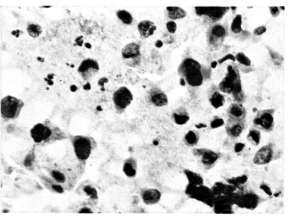

TRANSITIONAL CELL CARCINOMA OF URINARY BLADDER (PAPANICOLAOU STAIN)

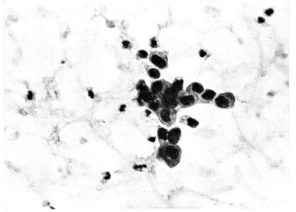

TRANSITIONAL CELL CARCINOMA OF URINARY BLADDER (PAPANICOLAOU STAIN)

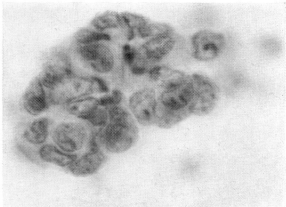

METASTATIC MELANOMA OF KIDNEY (PAPANICOLAOU STAIN)

MEASLES GIANT CELL (PAPANICOLAOU STAIN)

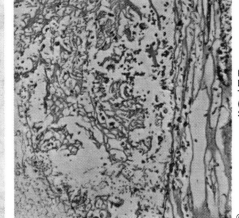

PAPILLARY NECROSIS TISSUE (H. AND E. STAIN)

©CIBA

filter is removed, trimmed, and mounted on a slide under a coverslip. It is ready for examination under both low and high power. The slide can also be filed indefinitely for future reference.

Red blood cells, white blood cells, and epithelial cells are on the filter, whereas bacteria and small amorphous crystals either pass through the filter or are trapped within its matrix. The filter is not dissolved but is cleared and rendered transparent. The different types of casts can be clearly distinguished and are counted, providing both total and differential cast counts.

Hyaline casts and the matrix of other casts stain *clear pink* (Ponceau-S stain), while *white blood cells,* if present on the membrane, are stained *black* (Prescott-Brodie stain). However, if the white blood cells are within the casts, they are seen as rows of black blobs surrounded by a pink matrix. *Red blood cells* within red cell casts appear as rows of round red-rimmed dots buried in a pink matrix. *Epithelial cells* in casts usually are seen as deep pink rectangular (or round) rows of cells in a light pink matrix. The *granular cast* is obvious as a series of round dark pink granules within the light pink matrix. *Mixed casts,* consisting of red cells, white cells, and epithelial cells, can be readily

identified, the differently colored cells embedded within the light pink matrix.

Technic for Neoplastic Cells in Urine. Neoplasms in the kidneys, renal pelves, ureters, and bladder, whether primary or metastatic, shed cells into the urine providing there is a connection with the urinary conduit. Detection of these cells in the urinary sediment would thus permit diagnosis of such neoplasms early in development. In addition, the effects of treatment can be followed by repeated study of the cells in the urinary sediment. (One exception, however, is *hypernephroma* which does not involve the tubular lumen early in development. Early detection of this tumor is thus not possible by examination of the urine.)

In the past it has been difficult to recognize malignancy of the kidney, ureter, or bladder by examination of the urine. For instance, the old method of blocking the 24-hour sediment in paraffin, staining with Papani-

colaou's stain, and examining sections was unsatisfactory; the cells were distorted and difficult to classify.

At present, the *method of Frost,* or suitable modifications, should be employed.

As illustrated in Plate 6 (see page 77), the urine is collected directly into alcohol and Hank's solution, and, since the morphology of the cells is better the sooner they are fixed, the specimen is *immediately* passed through a Millipore filter, in a portable filter holder, by gentle pressure, using a syringe. (Note that the pore size of the Millipore filter used for exfoliative cytology is smaller than that of the filter used for collection of urinary casts.) This portion of the procedure can be done at the bedside or in the physician's office and has the added advantage of reducing to a minimum the number of cells lost.

The cells on the surface of the filter are next fixed with a syringe of alcohol. Staining *Continued on page 80*

Microscopic Urine Examination

Continued from page 79

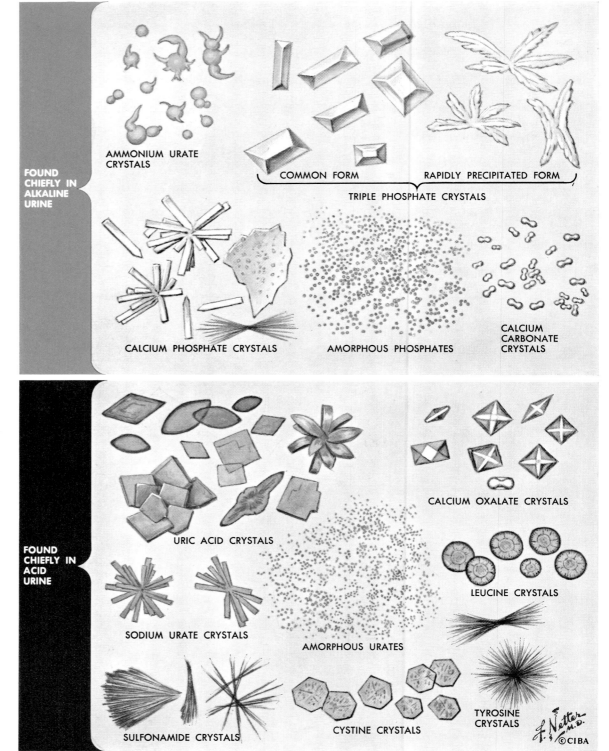

is accomplished by passing all the Papanicolaou solutions through the filter. The filter is *not* dipped in the staining jars.

This modification improves on the Frost method by greatly increasing the yield of cancer cells (up to fivefold) and by improving the morphology. It eliminates cell deterioration, cell loss, and the danger of false-positive preparations caused by cell transfer.

A number of abnormal cells are illustrated, as found in urinary sediments using the Millipore filter technic. Both false-negative and false-positive interpretations can occur, but their incidence can be minimized if the cytologist is well trained. When abnormal cells are found, the study should be repeated to be certain of the nature of the cells and also to try to determine their origin. Further investigation, including radiologic studies, such as renal angiograms, will be necessary to pinpoint the exact location of the suspected lesion.

The described method also permits identification, at times, of cells containing *inclusion bodies,* the result of viral infections. In the case of measles, for instance, the characteristic cell may often be found in the urine even before the appearance of Koplik's spots in the mouth.

Crystals in the Urine

The urine contains crystals and amorphous compounds, which together represent both the end products of tissue metabolism (urates, carbonates, and ammonium) and the excesses of consumed nutrients (calcium, phosphorus, and amino acids). These substances combine to form characteristic crystals which abound in the urine and which often interfere with both examination of the sediment and chemical analysis.

In the past, the presence of crystals and amorphous compounds was given more emphasis in diagnosis and was used to formulate regimens of treatment. Now, there is little significance assigned to the presence of many substances, while the finding of others suggests disease. For instance, it is recognized that excessive leucine or tyrosine crystals are present in urine from patients with *rapidly progressing hepatic disintegration,*

such as occurs in acute yellow atrophy. Also, the characteristic hexagonal crystals of cystine may appear in the urine of patients with *cystinuria,* whether or not the patients have renal calculi. However, the presence of other crystals or of amorphous salts is not considered to have any particular clinical meaning at the present time.

Certain crystals are found in alkaline urine, while others are seen in acid urine.

In *alkaline urine* the following crystals (with their somewhat colorful nicknames) may be found: ammonium urate ("thorn apples"); triple (ammonium and magnesium) phosphate ("coffin lids"); calcium carbonate ("dumbbells"); calcium phosphate (amorphous or wedge shaped). In *acid urine* these crystals occur: uric acid (red rhombic prisms); sodium urate (amorphous brown clumps, or needles, or fan-shaped clusters); calcium oxalate ("envelopes"). □

Bacteriologic Examination of Urine

Freshly passed, centrifuged urine can be examined with phase microscopy (see page 76) and, if bacteria are detected, a useful estimation of their number made. If two or more organisms are seen with phase microscopy, or 20 with bright light examination, in each of nine high power fields, the presumptive diagnosis of significant bacteriuria is justified, and cultures and sensitivity tests must be prepared.

If the physician deems it necessary, treatment may be started immediately without waiting for the results of the culture which must be done. The patient's response to treatment can also be assessed by frequent reexamination of the urine with phase microscopy while awaiting culture reports. If treatment is successful, viable organisms will disappear from the urinary tract within 24 to 48 hours and will not be seen on subsequent microscopic examinations.

Methodology

Urine specimens must be cultured within 15 minutes of collection or immediately refrigerated for later culture. Urine can be stored for as long as 48 hours at 4°C without significant growth of bacteria. The urine may be cultured on an agar pour plate, and at 24 or 48 hours, bacterial numbers are estimated by colony count.

Streak Plates. The urine is inoculated on the surface of a nutrient plate, using a calibrated platinum loop which delivers 0.001 ml of urine. Instead of a nutrient plate, a blood agar plate may be used to give a total bacterial count, and highly selective media, such as eosin methylene blue (EMB) may be used to detect gram negative organisms.

Technically, streaks are made in the center of each plate. The inoculum is then worked to the periphery four times, using a large loop, properly flamed. The plates are incubated at 37° for 24 hours.

Counts of 100 or more colonies (*i.e.,* more than 10^5 or 100,000 organisms per milliliter of urine) are significant. If a single, properly obtained, urine sample is used, the distinction between pathogenic bacteria and contaminant bacteria can be made correctly in eight out of 10 cases, *i.e.,* with a confidence limit of 80 percent. If, however, two separate urine samples are collected for culture, the confidence limit increases to 95 percent.

Contamination should be suspected if replicate cultures, or cultures made at different times, do not agree in either number or type of organisms. If two or more organisms are isolated in large numbers, or if organisms such as diphtheroids, staphylococci, or microaerophilic streptococci are predominant, contamination is likely.

Escherichia coli is the causative organism in nearly all urinary tract infections. However, in complicated cases, one or more species of *Proteus, Klebsiella, Aerobacter, Pseudomonas,* or, rarely, *Staphylococcus aureus* or certain other organisms are likely to be encountered. If symptoms and signs continue unabated and if cultures are sterile, the infection may be caused by *Mycobacterium* tubercu-

losis or anaerobic organisms which must be cultured by special technics.

The dipslide method is exceedingly simple and accurate. A microscopic slide is coated on one side with a few drops of nutrient agar and on the other side with a selective agar, such as EMB or MacConkey's, and kept in a sterile plastic vial until used. The slide is dipped in urine, allowed to drain, and returned to the plastic tube to incubate. The density of colony growth after suitable incubation is compared to a printed standard.

The method has been carefully evaluated by Cohen and Kass. Correlation with pour plates is virtually 100 percent, with no false negatives. These dipslides are now available commercially, and one can clearly distinguish between significant (10^5 or more) and insignificant (less than 10^5) bacteriuria in asymptomatic patients.

The direct sensitivity test is extremely helpful in rapidly assessing a choice of antimicrobial agents. A sterile cotton swab is dipped in urine and streaked over the surface of the nutrient agar plate. Sensitivity discs are added, and the plate is incubated overnight. It is ready for reading the next morning.

Since *gonorrhea* has become so widespread in recent years, a comment on detection is appropriate. Culture of the urine has no value, but in the male, the urethral discharge obtained following prostatic massage should be cultured. In the female, cultures should be obtained from the urethra and cervix, and in both the male and female, from the anus as well. Gonorrhea is covered more completely in CIBA COLLECTION, Volume 2.

In summary, the physician can make a presumptive diagnosis with the microscope, do a confirmatory quantitative culture, and have sensitivity information the next morning to guide his treatment. □

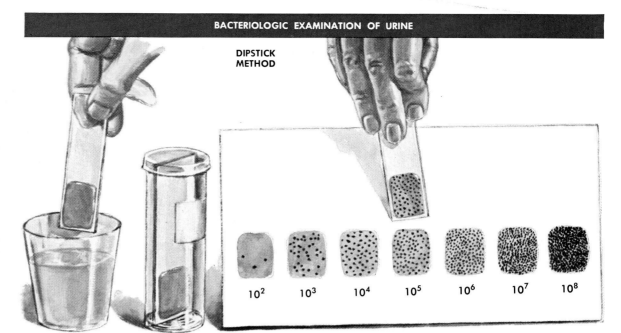

DIPSTICK METHOD

10^2 10^3 10^4 10^5 10^6 10^7 10^8

SPECIAL URINE CULTURE PLATE DIPPED INTO CLEAN VOIDED URINE FRESHLY COLLECTED IN STERILE CONTAINER, AND SHAKEN FREE OF EXCESS

PLATE PLACED IN SPECIAL TUBE AND INCUBATED AT 37° C FOR 24 HOURS

RESULTS READ BY COMPARING DENSITY OF COLONIES ON THE PLATE TO THE CHART. THE CHART REPRESENTS DENSITY OF BACTERIAL COLONIES FROM 10^2 TO 10^8/ml OF URINE. SIGNIFICANT BACTERIURIA IS 10^5 COLONIES/ml, OR HIGHER. ONE SIDE OF THE PLATE CARRIES NUTRIENT AGAR ON WHICH MOST PATHOGENS AND CONTAMINATING ORGANISMS GROW; THE OTHER SIDE CARRIES EOSIN METHYLENE BLUE (EMB) AGAR ON WHICH ONLY GRAM NEGATIVE BACTERIA GROW

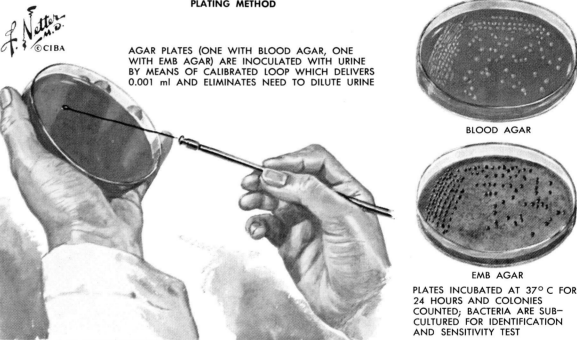

PLATING METHOD

AGAR PLATES (ONE WITH BLOOD AGAR, ONE WITH EMB AGAR) ARE INOCULATED WITH URINE BY MEANS OF CALIBRATED LOOP WHICH DELIVERS 0.001 ml AND ELIMINATES NEED TO DILUTE URINE

BLOOD AGAR

EMB AGAR

PLATES INCUBATED AT 37° C FOR 24 HOURS AND COLONIES COUNTED; BACTERIA ARE SUB-CULTURED FOR IDENTIFICATION AND SENSITIVITY TEST

Tests of Concentration and Dilution

The concentrations of all solids in the urine are determined by instruments which measure *specific gravity, refractive index,* or *osmolality.* The clinical hydrometer, which is notoriously inaccurate, measures specific gravity; the osmometer (which is accurate but expensive) determines osmolality by measuring freezing point depression; the total solids meter provides an accurate, rapid, and simple measurement of the total solids in a drop of urine (or serum). The total solids meter is a clinical refractometer and is calibrated to display results as either the specific gravity or the refractive index.

In a patient eating a normal diet, inability to concentrate or dilute the urine may point to renal structural damage *(q.v.).* A *highly concentrated urine* implies dehydration or the abnormal presence of solutes in the urine such as glucose or organic iodide compounds (after an intravenous pyelogram).

Dilute urine is found in patients who: are compulsive water drinkers, have diabetes insipidus, have ingested diuretic drugs, or have renal disease. The ability to concentrate urine maximally is lost early in patients with chronic renal medullary syndrome, and eventually only a dilute urine of fixed specific gravity of 1.010 is excreted (hyposthenuria).

Concentration Test

Most persons usually pass an early morning urine with specific gravity greater than 1.020. If routine, repeated testing indicates that a patient does not concentrate the morning urine, an overnight concentration test should be done. The patient should produce a urine of specific gravity of 1.026 when dehydrated. If not, antidiuretic hormone can be given and the urine retested hourly. However, water deprivation and the use of antidiuretic hormone depend on the clinical state of the patient.

Maximum concentration of urine may not be achieved if the patient has been on a low protein or salt-restricted diet or has had a high fluid intake prior to the test. The test should not be run if the patient is having a spontaneous or drug-induced diuresis.

The clinical value of the concentration test lies in its ability to detect early disturbances of renal function, as in patients with *asymptomatic bacteriuria of pregnancy.* (The test usually returns to normal after appropriate antibiotic therapy.) The test also may be abnormal in diabetes insipidus before other tests are. It is also useful in the assessment of patients with suspected *intrinsic tubular defects, renal parenchymal disorders of the medulla, hypercalcemia,* and *potassium deficiency.* However, the concentration test is of little value, and in fact is dangerous, if patients have chronic renal failure.

Newer Tests. Determination of the *osmolar clearance* and the *urine-to-serum*

osmolar ratio is gradually replacing the specific-gravity concentration tests. Simultaneous measurements of serum osmolality (normally 290 mOsm/1) and urine osmolality (800 to 1400 mOsm/kg water) are made. For instance, in acute renal failure of parenchymatous origin (see page 111), the urine osmolality tends to be low, whereas in the prerenal type of failure it is high. Moreover, if in acutely oliguric patients the ratio of urine osmolality to serum osmolality is less than 1.35, renal failure from parenchymatous causes is the most likely diagnosis.

Patients with malignant tumors, diseases involving the central nervous system, and diseases of the lung may present with very low serum sodium levels. These patients excrete sodium despite severe hyposmolality of the serum, and the urine osmolality is greater than that appropriate for the concomitant tonicity of the plasma. When the patients are studied, there is no

evidence of constricted fluid volume, and there is normal renal and suprarenal function. These findings of hyposmotic serum levels and normal or hyperosmotic urine levels are typical of the syndrome of inappropriate secretion of antidiuretic substances.

Dilution Test

The *dilution test* was commonly used in the past to detect chronic renal disease. If the kidneys have lost the ability to concentrate and dilute, the urine is excreted with a specific gravity fixed at about 1.010, even when the dilution test is performed. The test also indicates an inability to dilute urine, as in Addison's disease, in salt-losing nephritis, and in other disorders in which there is an imbalance or deficiency of one or more electrolytes. Now, many simpler, faster, more accurate procedures detect these abnormalities so that the dilution test is used infrequently. □

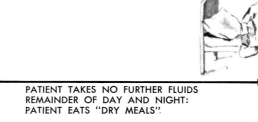

TOTAL SOLIDS METER READS SPECIFIC GRAVITY AS WELL AS TOTAL SOLIDS

OSMOMETER READS OSMOLALITY OF URINE OR SERUM BY FREEZING POINT DEPRESSION

URINOMETER READS SPECIFIC GRAVITY

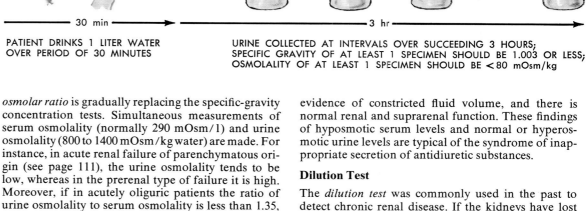

CONCENTRATION TEST — SHOULD NOT BE DONE IF PATIENT IS HAVING DIURESIS DUE TO DIURETICS OR SPONTANEOUSLY

PATIENT EATS NORMAL BREAKFAST (PT. SHOULD HAVE BEEN ON NORMAL DIET AND NORMAL FLUID INTAKE PREVIOUSLY, AND OFF DIURETICS)

PATIENT TAKES NO FURTHER FLUIDS REMAINDER OF DAY AND NIGHT: PATIENT EATS "DRY MEALS".

FIRST URINE, ON AWAKENING NEXT MORNING, DISCARDED

NEXT VOIDED URINE SHOULD HAVE SP. GR. OF 1.026 OR HIGHER; OSMOLALITY OF 800 mOsm/kg OR HIGHER

DILUTION TEST — SHOULD NOT BE DONE IN PRESENCE OF AZOTEMIA OR ELECTROLYTE IMBALANCE OR DEFICIENCY

← 30 min → ← 3 hr →

PATIENT DRINKS 1 LITER WATER OVER PERIOD OF 30 MINUTES

URINE COLLECTED AT INTERVALS OVER SUCCEEDING 3 HOURS; SPECIFIC GRAVITY OF AT LEAST 1 SPECIMEN SHOULD BE 1.003 OR LESS; OSMOLALITY OF AT LEAST 1 SPECIMEN SHOULD BE < 80 mOsm/kg

Clearance Tests

BLOOD SAMPLE TAKEN

←——————— 24 HOURS ———————→

PATIENT VOIDS ON ARISING (7 A.M.); URINE DISCARDED

URINE COLLECTED FOR 24 HOURS, INCLUDING SPECIMEN ON ARISING FOLLOWING MORNING (7 A.M.)

Renal clearance (see page 40) can be measured most accurately with inulin, but the technic is too complex for routine clinical use. However, the endogenous creatinine clearance test is extremely useful for studying patients with renal dysfunction and for following their progress. The creatinine clearance has virtually supplanted the urea clearance tests for reasons described both elsewhere (see pages 44 and 45) and below.

The serum creatinine levels depend virtually on the integrity of the nephrons, while the blood urea level can and does change rapidly in response to diet, changes in hepatic function, the presence of blood in the gut, and as a result of catabolic processes. Moreover, unlike urea, creatinine is not freely reabsorbed by the tubules, and its excretion is not related directly to urine flow. However, one must bear in mind that urea is more easily and accurately measured in the laboratory and that, at low levels of renal clearance, urea clearance values are more accurate than creatinine clearance.

Both creatinine and urea clearance require an accurately timed period of urine collection (usually 2 hours). To ensure a good urine flow, a good fluid consumption precedes the test. Creatinine clearances are also done with 12- or 24-hour collections of urine.

Accurate collection of urine is crucial, particularly with the 2-hour test, and patients should be instructed to strain hard to squeeze the last drops of urine out of the bladder at the time of final voiding. The tests are not valid in patients with large residual urine volumes, but catheterization of the bladder for this procedure is not warranted.

mg %
1.6
1.4
1.2
1.0
0.8
0.6
0.4
0.2

NORMAL RANGE OF PLASMA TRUE CREATININE

$$C_{CREAT.} = \frac{U \times V}{P}$$

$C_{CREAT.}$ = CLEARANCE OF CREATININE
U = CONCENTRATION OF CREATININE IN URINE, mg/100 ml
V = VOLUME OF URINE, ml/min
P = CONCENTRATION OF CREATININE IN PLASMA, mg/100 ml
NORMAL $C_{CREAT.}$ = 80 to 110 ml/min/1.73 m^2

BLOOD SAMPLE TAKEN ABOUT MIDPOINT OF TEST PERIOD

PATIENT DRINKS 2 GLASSES OF WATER, SHORTLY BEFORE TEST, TO ENSURE ADEQUATE URINE FLOW

PT. VOIDS COMPLETELY; URINE DISCARDED

URINE COMPLETELY COLLECTED OVER APPROXIMATELY 2 HOURS, ACCURATELY TIMED IN MINUTES

mg %
30
20
10

NORMAL RANGE OF BLOOD UREA NITROGEN (BUN)

$$C_{UREA} = \frac{U \times V}{B}$$

U = CONCENTRATION OF UREA IN URINE, mg/100 ml
V = VOLUME OF URINE, ml/min
B = CONCENTRATION OF UREA IN BLOOD, mg/100 ml

IF V > 2.0 ml/min (MAXIMUM CLEARANCE)
NORMAL = 64 to 99 ml/min/1.73 m^2
AVERAGE 75 ml/min/1.73 m^2

IF V < 2.0 ml/min (STANDARD CLEARANCE)
NORMAL = 40 to 60 ml/min/1.73 m^2
AVERAGE 54 ml/min/1.73 m^2

EXPRESS AS % OF NORMAL
NORMAL C_{UREA} = 75 to 120% OF MAXIMUM CLEARANCE OR OF STANDARD CLEARANCE

Creatinine Clearance

Venous blood is taken for analysis, preferably at the midpoint of the urine collection period, or, instead, at the beginning or end. The creatinine clearance can then be calculated if the concentration of creatinine in the serum, the duration of the urine collection period (in minutes), the volume of urine, and the total excretion of creatinine (in milligrams per volume of timed urine collected) are all known (see also page 45). Clearances are usually expressed as milliliters per minute per 1.73 square meters of body surface. Calculation of the excretion per 1.73 square meters body surface is not essential in adults but is absolutely necessary in infants and children.

Values between 80 and 110 ml/minute/1.73 m^2 are normal for creatinine clearance; 24-hour clearance in health tends to give results around 80 ml/minute/1.73 m^2 while 2-hour clearances show results of 110 ml or higher. When the GFR (see page 39) is about 15 ml/minute, the ratio of creatinine to inulin approaches unity; at low GFR, creatinine clearance is overestimated, and at high GFR, clearance relative to inulin is underestimated (see pages 40, 44, and 45).

Urea Clearance

The procedure for performing urea clearance is similar to, but not identical with, that for creatinine clearance.

In health, urea clearance is about 60 percent of inulin clearance. Values for maximal clearance (i.e., when urine flow during the test is greater than 2 ml/minute) are between 64 and 99 ml/minute/1.73 m^2. For standard clearances the values obtained are lower, usually 40 to 60 ml/minute/1.73 m^2, since urine flow is low and less urea is excreted.

Clinical Uses

Clearances have a wide variety of practical uses: to determine if renal function is deteriorating or improving; to select dietary levels of protein intake in chronic renal failure (e.g., 20 grams of protein per day if creatinine clearance is between 2 and 5 ml/minute and 40 gm/day if it is over 10 ml, see also page 120); to assist in diagnosis; to classify patients; to provide evidence of degree of renal dysfunction for medicolegal purposes; and for prognosis.

Clearances up to three times normal are found in pregnancy (particularly in the early part of the third trimester) and in some cases of nephrotic syndrome, particularly in patients with very low serum albumin levels and lipoid nephrosis (see page 123). □

Phenolsulfonphthalein Excretion Test

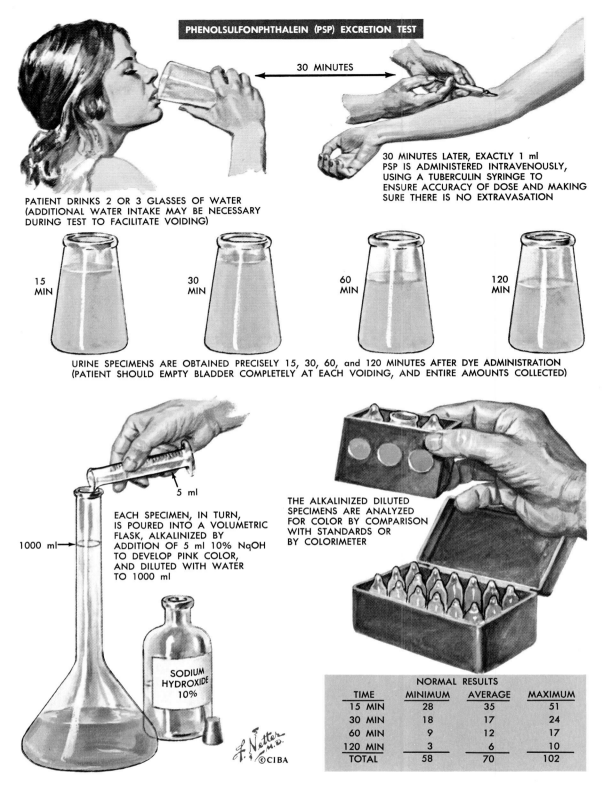

PHENOLSULFONPHTHALEIN (PSP) EXCRETION TEST

30 MINUTES

PATIENT DRINKS 2 OR 3 GLASSES OF WATER (ADDITIONAL WATER INTAKE MAY BE NECESSARY DURING TEST TO FACILITATE VOIDING)

30 MINUTES LATER, EXACTLY 1 ml PSP IS ADMINISTERED INTRAVENOUSLY, USING A TUBERCULIN SYRINGE TO ENSURE ACCURACY OF DOSE AND MAKING SURE THERE IS NO EXTRAVASATION

15 MIN   30 MIN   60 MIN   120 MIN

URINE SPECIMENS ARE OBTAINED PRECISELY 15, 30, 60, and 120 MINUTES AFTER DYE ADMINISTRATION (PATIENT SHOULD EMPTY BLADDER COMPLETELY AT EACH VOIDING, AND ENTIRE AMOUNTS COLLECTED)

5 ml

1000 ml

EACH SPECIMEN, IN TURN, IS POURED INTO A VOLUMETRIC FLASK, ALKALINIZED BY ADDITION OF 5 ml 10% NqOH TO DEVELOP PINK COLOR, AND DILUTED WITH WATER TO 1000 ml

SODIUM HYDROXIDE 10%

THE ALKALINIZED DILUTED SPECIMENS ARE ANALYZED FOR COLOR BY COMPARISON WITH STANDARDS OR BY COLORIMETER

	NORMAL RESULTS		
TIME	MINIMUM	AVERAGE	MAXIMUM
15 MIN	28	35	51
30 MIN	18	17	24
60 MIN	9	12	17
120 MIN	3	6	10
TOTAL	58	70	102

Injected phenolsulfonphthalein (PSP) is transferred from blood to urine by *active transport*. Since the dye passes from the peritubular blood vessels across the cells of the tubules into the lumina, its urinary excretion, per unit of time, depends on: (1) the integrity of the blood vessels and the rate of blood flow; (2) the integrity of tubular function; (3) a patent and normally functioning urinary conduit; (4) the presence or absence of inhibiting or competing drugs (*e.g.,* probenecid).

If there is *urinary tract obstruction* with both normal blood flow and normal nephron function, there will be delayed but complete excretion of the dye. On the other hand, if there is a normal conduit with normal blood flow and normal glomerular function but *tubular disease* (*e.g.,* Fanconi syndrome), excretion of PSP in 15 minutes will be abnormally reduced. In this situation of pure tubular disease, the creatinine clearance is normal, reflecting normal glomerular structure and normal blood flow and function. However, despite the normal peritubular blood supply, active transfer of PSP across the tubular cells is disturbed, and excretion is reduced from 25 percent in 15 minutes to about two to five percent.

Normal creatinine clearance with low PSP excretion is not a common finding because pure tubular disorders are not common. It is much more usual to find both creatinine clearance and PSP excretion low. This situation reflects *glomerular disease* or *interstitial disease* or *renal vascular disease* or *mixtures* of the three. In essence, any of the three diseases, either alone or together, can damage the peritubular blood vessels secondarily and/or disturb their flow.

It should be recalled that the peritubular arterioles arise mainly from the efferent vessels of the glomerular tufts. As Jean Oliver has shown by nephron dissection, disease of the glomerular tuft is followed first by disease of the peritubular vessels (with consequent reduction in peritubular blood flow) and ultimately by degeneration and loss of function of tubular cells. Therefore, a low PSP test, like a reduced creatinine clearance level, usually indicates *general loss of nephron function*.

The PSP test has the advantage that it can be done in a short time. However, the test suffers from the disadvantage that precise data are difficult to obtain. First, the amount injected must be *precisely* 1 ml, and second, the patient must *completely* empty the bladder *exactly* 15 minutes after

the dye has been injected intravenously.

One way of assuring a complete 15-minute urine collection is to give a patient several glasses of water to drink and then wait until he has the urge to void. At this point, exactly 1 ml PSP is injected with a tuberculin syringe. The patient continues to hold his urine for the next 15 minutes and then urinates with pressure. *All* urine is collected and measured. The total amount of PSP excreted in 15 minutes is expressed as a percentage of the amount injected.

Today, very few physicians collect the 30-, 60-, and 120-minute specimens. Although conduit obstruction would be suggested if these specimens were to contain increasing amounts of dye, obstruction is more readily and clearly studied by radiography.

Other drawbacks of the PSP test are that either excretion or chemical analysis for the dye is altered by *liver disease, low serum albumin, heart failure,* certain

drugs *(penicillin, sulfonamides, salicylates,* and *diuretics),* and even an erect position of the patient.

Currently under trial are three recent modifications intended to improve the usefulness of the PSP test. One method, which relates the intravenous dose of PSP to body surface (18 mg/m²), was reported to have good correlation between the 15-minute excretion and serum creatinine level. Another modification used a dose of PSP of 1 mg/kg body weight, and the 15-minute PSP excretion also correlated well with creatinine clearance. With a third variation, 60 mg of PSP was injected and the plasma concentration measured at 60 minutes. The result was stated to have correlated well with creatinine clearance.

It appears that one or more of these modifications, if done correctly, will be more useful clinically than the standard PSP method and may replace the creatinine clearance for follow-up assessment of the patient. □

Renal Artery Stenosis

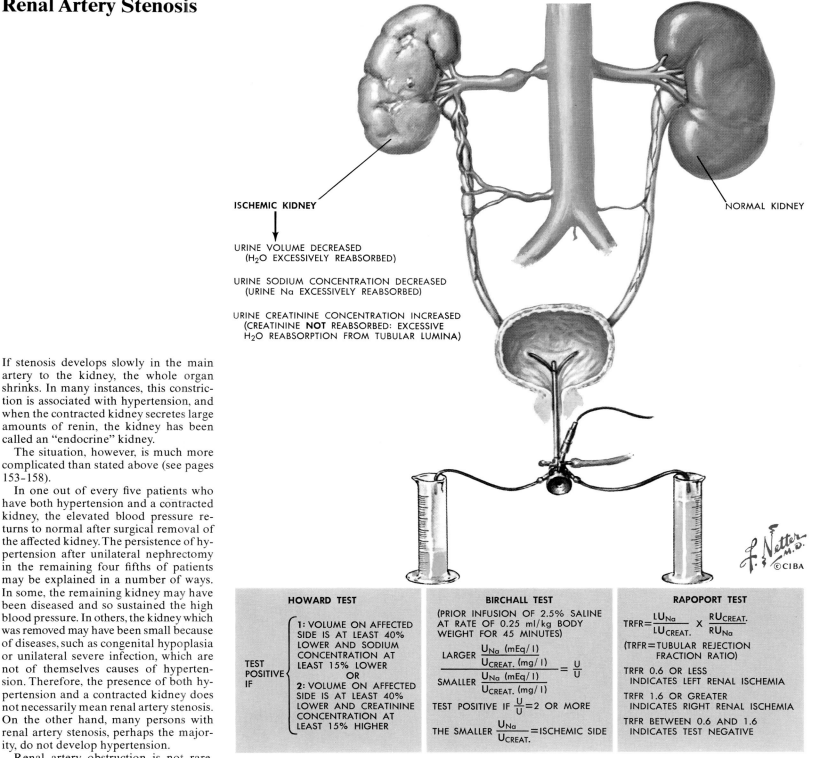

ISCHEMIC KIDNEY

NORMAL KIDNEY

URINE VOLUME DECREASED
(H_2O EXCESSIVELY REABSORBED)

URINE SODIUM CONCENTRATION DECREASED
(URINE Na EXCESSIVELY REABSORBED)

URINE CREATININE CONCENTRATION INCREASED
(CREATININE **NOT** REABSORBED: EXCESSIVE
H_2O REABSORPTION FROM TUBULAR LUMINA)

HOWARD TEST	BIRCHALL TEST	RAPOPORT TEST
TEST POSITIVE IF { **1:** VOLUME ON AFFECTED SIDE IS AT LEAST 40% LOWER AND SODIUM CONCENTRATION AT LEAST 15% LOWER OR **2:** VOLUME ON AFFECTED SIDE IS AT LEAST 40% LOWER AND CREATININE CONCENTRATION AT LEAST 15% HIGHER	(PRIOR INFUSION OF 2.5% SALINE AT RATE OF 0.25 ml/kg BODY WEIGHT FOR 45 MINUTES) LARGER $\dfrac{\dfrac{U_{Na}\ (mEq/l)}{U_{CREAT.}\ (mg/l)}}{\dfrac{U_{Na}\ (mEq/l)}{U_{CREAT.}\ (mg/l)}}$ SMALLER $= \dfrac{U}{U}$ TEST POSITIVE IF $\dfrac{U}{U}=2$ OR MORE THE SMALLER $\dfrac{U_{Na}}{U_{CREAT.}}$ = ISCHEMIC SIDE	$TRFR = \dfrac{LU_{Na}}{LU_{CREAT.}} \times \dfrac{RU_{CREAT.}}{RU_{Na}}$ (TRFR = TUBULAR REJECTION FRACTION RATIO) TRFR 0.6 OR LESS INDICATES LEFT RENAL ISCHEMIA TRFR 1.6 OR GREATER INDICATES RIGHT RENAL ISCHEMIA TRFR BETWEEN 0.6 AND 1.6 INDICATES TEST NEGATIVE

If stenosis develops slowly in the main artery to the kidney, the whole organ shrinks. In many instances, this constriction is associated with hypertension, and when the contracted kidney secretes large amounts of renin, the kidney has been called an "endocrine" kidney.

The situation, however, is much more complicated than stated above (see pages 153–158).

In one out of every five patients who have both hypertension and a contracted kidney, the elevated blood pressure returns to normal after surgical removal of the affected kidney. The persistence of hypertension after unilateral nephrectomy in the remaining four fifths of patients may be explained in a number of ways. In some, the remaining kidney may have been diseased and so sustained the high blood pressure. In others, the kidney which was removed may have been small because of diseases, such as congenital hypoplasia or unilateral severe infection, which are not of themselves causes of hypertension. Therefore, the presence of both hypertension and a contracted kidney does not necessarily mean renal artery stenosis. On the other hand, many persons with renal artery stenosis, perhaps the majority, do not develop hypertension.

Renal artery obstruction is not rare, particularly in people over the age of 50. In these patients, renal artery blood flow may be compromised by arteriosclerosis at the origin of one or both main renal arteries or by atheromatous plaques in the renal arteries (see also CIBA COLLECTION, Vol. 5, page 228). Such renal artery lesions are often incidentally discovered in patients with normal blood pressure who have angiography done to assess the status of limb or abdominal blood vessels.

In summary, it is not known why some patients with renal artery stenosis develop hypertension and others do not. Previously, it was thought that the "tightness" (or degree) of stenosis was a factor, but measurements of pressure across stenotic renal arteries have not confirmed this concept.

In younger patients, particularly women under the age of 40, fibromuscular disorders of the renal vessels (see also CIBA COLLECTION, Vol. 5, page 228) may be responsible for the obstruction with decreased blood flow and pulse pressure to the kidney. In these patients, soft systolic bruits may be heard with a stethoscope on the upper lateral abdominal wall or on the back near the articulations of the eleventh and twelfth ribs with the vertebrae. However, systolic abdominal bruits are more frequently found with increasing patient age, presumably because atheromatous lesions in the large intraabdominal arteries cause turbulence in blood flow.

These common obstructive lesions of the renal vasculature can usually be very well delineated by angiography, particularly selective examination of the renal arteries. However, as discussed, renal artery stenosis is not invariably the cause of any coexisting hypertension, and it is important to assess the clinical significance of the vascular lesion before surgery.

Physiologic Responses to Ischemia

The two well-known physiologic responses to renal artery stenosis are *disturbance of water reabsorption* in the ischemic kidney and the release of *renin*. Studies on dogs have indicated that clipping one renal artery produces increased reabsorption of water from the respective kidney. Thus, there is less volume of urine formed, per unit of time, by the ischemic kidney as compared to the normal organ. The increased reabsorption of sodium and water from the ischemic nephrons is not associated with an increased reabsorption of creatinine.

Howard found that the ischemic kidneys of patients with renal artery stenosis behave similarly to the experimental ischemic kidneys of dogs. He devised a test, which bears his name, for differential assessment of renal function in patients with *Continued on page 86*

Renal Artery Stenosis

Continued from page 85

Continued from page 85

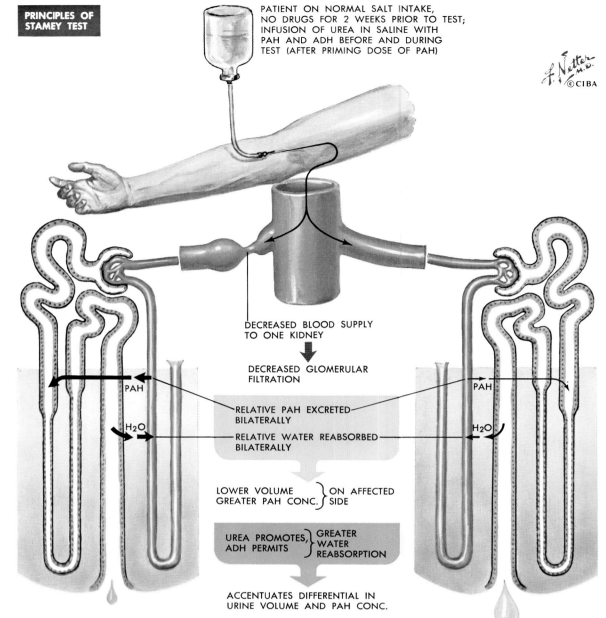

PATIENT ON NORMAL SALT INTAKE, NO DRUGS FOR 2 WEEKS PRIOR TO TEST; INFUSION OF UREA IN SALINE WITH PAH AND ADH BEFORE AND DURING TEST (AFTER PRIMING DOSE OF PAH)

DECREASED BLOOD SUPPLY TO ONE KIDNEY

DECREASED GLOMERULAR FILTRATION

PAH

H₂O

RELATIVE PAH EXCRETED BILATERALLY

RELATIVE WATER REABSORBED BILATERALLY

LOWER VOLUME GREATER PAH CONC. } ON AFFECTED SIDE

UREA PROMOTES, ADH PERMITS } GREATER WATER REABSORPTION

ACCENTUATES DIFFERENTIAL IN URINE VOLUME AND PAH CONC.

INTERPRETATION OF STAMEY TEST

POSITIVE TEST { 3:1, OR GREATER, DIFFERENTIAL IN URINE VOLUME (AFFECTED SIDE LOWER) AND 100%, OR GREATER, DIFFERENTIAL IN PAH CONCENTRATION (AFFECTED SIDE HIGHER)

A 2:1 DIFFERENTIAL IN URINE VOLUME AND LESS THAN 100% DIFFERENTIAL IN PAH CONCENTRATION ARE COMPATIBLE WITH:
A. ESSENTIAL HYPERTENSION WITH DISPARITY IN NEPHROSCLEROSIS BETWEEN THE KIDNEYS
B. LESION IN BRANCH OR IN ACCESSORY RENAL ARTERY ON ONE SIDE
C. BILATERAL RENAL ARTERY STENOSIS WITH DISPARITY IN DEGREE

renal artery stenosis and hypertension. Ureteral catheters are inserted bilaterally, and urine is collected from each kidney. (The test is sometimes called the "split-function test.") During 20 minutes of collection, a smaller volume of urine is obtained from the ischemic kidney as compared to the normal side. Also, the creatinine concentration on the ischemic side is increased and sodium concentration decreased. Howard set arbitrary limits for the test; patients with *positive* test results were considered candidates for either removal of the ischemic kidney or arterial reconstruction, sometimes with a bypass prosthesis from the aorta to the renal artery beyond the site of obstruction.

Both *Birchall* and *Rapoport* modified the technic of Howard's method and have analyzed the data differently in attempts to refine the selection process.

Stamey Test

Stamey refined Howard's method in order to select for operation hypertensive patients with stenosis of a *branch* of a renal artery, or of an *accessory* renal artery, as well as those patients with unilateral or bilateral *main renal artery* obstruction. The refinement is based on two observations. First, during an intravenous pyelogram in patients with unilateral renal artery stenosis, the contrast medium is more concentrated in the pelvis and ureter of the affected side. Second, in dogs with experimentally induced unilateral renal ischemia, para-aminohippurate (PAH), which is related chemically to radiologic contrast material and which is secreted by the renal tubules (see pages 42 and 43), is also concentrated on the stenotic side.

The normal kidney can be physiologically stimulated to produce an excellent flow of dilute urine per unit of time. Stamey found that an infusion of urea and ADH in saline produced this anticipated response in the normal kidney and, importantly, enhanced the reabsorption of water by the ischemic kidney. Thus, if PAH is simultaneously administered, it will appear in increased concentration in urine from the ischemic kidney.

The recommended procedure in hypertensive patients, in order to accentuate differences in PAH concentration and urine volume, is to discontinue all drugs,

including diuretics and saluretics, 2 weeks prior to the test and to *restore body sodium* to normal by a normal salt intake. At the time of the test, *saline* is infused to provide diuresis on the normal side. *ADH* is added in physiologic amounts to ensure maximum stimulus to concentration on the affected side, while *urea* is used to accentuate the countercurrent concentration mechanism on the affected side and to act as an osmotic diuretic on the normal side (see also pages 51-59).

Stamey defined a *positive* test result as a 3:1 or greater differential in urine volume (affected side lower) together with a 100 percent or greater differential in PAH concentration (affected side higher). This indicates *significant renal artery stenosis,* while a 2:1 differential in volume and less than 100 percent differential in PAH concentration are compatible with either a *branch (or accessory) renal artery stenosis* or *disparate bilateral nephrosclerosis* and *essential hypertension.*

Incidentally, at present the most reliable screening test for renal artery stenosis in hypertensive patients is a properly interpreted *timed nephrogram* (see page 95). Stenosis is probable if radiographic dye excretion is concentrated in the pelvis and ureter of the affected side, particularly if the appearance of the contrast material on that side is delayed.

Since the recent development of *radioimmune assays of renin in blood,* the differential clearance methods have become less popular in the accurate diagnosis of hypertension. Renin assays are done on blood taken from peripheral veins and preferably from both renal veins. It is important to note, however, that measurement of renin is fraught with difficulties. Since its production varies with position, the time of day, aldosterone activity, levels of sodium in the body, and the sodium intake and output, rigid controls must be maintained when blood is collected for renin assays. □

Acid-Loading Tests

Acid-loading tests provide a quantitative assessment of the ability of patients who are suspected of having renal tubular acidosis (see page 248), but who do not exhibit spontaneous acidosis, to excrete administered hydrogen ions. The tests are also used to evaluate distal tubular function in patients having other forms of renal disease.

Tests designed to measure the maximum acid-excreting capacity of the kidney have been in use for many years. However, free hydrogen ion excretion, as measured by urinary pH, accounts for only a minute fraction of the acid excreted by the kidney. Actually, most hydrogen ion is excreted either in combination with buffer anions which are so poorly dissociated as to keep the concentration of free hydrogen ion at a low level, or in combination with ammonia to form ammonium ion which neutralizes the anions of strong acids (chloride, sulfate). The hydrogen ions in these strong acids dissociate completely and would thus produce excessively high hydrogen ion concentration were they to be excreted free rather than combined with ammonium.

The drop in urine pH and the increase in urinary titratable acidity occur rapidly after the acid load has been administered. However, the excretion of ammonium ion usually requires 4 to 5 days, following induction of acidosis, to reach its maximum. For this reason, acid-loading tests have traditionally been carried out for a 5-day period to produce the maximum stimulus for the secretion of ammonia. Nevertheless, Wrong and Davis, and subsequently other workers, have found that a shorter acid-loading test produces sufficient stimulus to the acidification mechanisms of the kidney for separation of normal individuals from those having reduced acid-excreting capabilities. The 5-day test is still used for patients in whom measurement of maximum ammonia-secreting ability is desirable.

The short and long tests are performed in nearly the same way. *Titratable acidity, pH,* and *ammonia content* are measured on control urines and urines collected during the administration of ammonium chloride. For the long test, urines generally are collected under oil with toluene or thymol added as a preservative. For the short acid-loading test, pH is measured immediately and the urine kept from exposure to air until the ammonia and titratable acidity have been measured. If studies cannot be made rapidly, urine should be collected under oil with thymol or toluene, as in the long acid-loading test.

With both tests, the larger the dose of ammonium chloride used, the greater the likelihood that the urine will be adequately acidified. However, recent data suggest that once the serum bicarbonate has been depressed below the bicarbonate threshold, the response cannot be augmented by more acidifying salt or further depression of bicarbonate.

The *maximal hydrogen ion excretion* is determined by adding the titratable acid

SHORT ACID-LOADING TEST

| 2 CONTROL COLLECTIONS OF 1 HOUR EACH: pH, NH₄⁺, AND TITR. ACID DETERMINED | ←— 1 HOUR —→ 75 mEq/m² (2 TO 3 mEq/kg) NH₄ Cl P.O. IN DIVIDED DOSES (0.5 TO 1.0 g GELATIN CAPSULES) OVER 1 HOUR, PLUS 1 LITER WATER | ←——— 5 HOURS ———→ URINE MAY BE COLLECTED AT HOURLY INTERVALS FOR 8 HOURS, BUT CHANGES ARE MAXIMAL AND RELATIVELY CONSTANT AFTER 5 HOURS, SO A SINGLE COLLECTION AT THAT TIME SUFFICES | URINE COLLECTION: pH, NH₄⁺, AND TITR. ACID DETERMINED |

LONG (3-DAY) ACID TEST

←— 24 hr —→ ←— 24 hr —→ | 100 mEq/m² NH₄ Cl P.O. IN DIVIDED DOSES ←— 24 hr —→ | 100 mEq/m² NH₄ Cl P.O. IN DIVIDED DOSES ←— 24 hr —→ | 100 mEq/m² NH₄ Cl P.O. IN DIVIDED DOSES ←— 24 hr —→

2 DAYS OF CONTROL COLLECTIONS: pH, NH₄⁺, AND TITR. ACID DETERMINED

URINARY pH DETERMINED DAILY; AMMONIUM AND TITR. ACID ON 3rd DAY

MAXIMAL H⁺ SECRETION

$$H^+ = TITRATABLE\ ACID + NH_4^+ - HCO_3^-\ (ALL\ IN\ \mu Eq/min)$$

H⁺ ION CLEARANCE INDEX

$$H^+\ CLEARANCE\ INDEX = \frac{MAX.\ H^+\ SECRETION}{H^+\ CONCENTRATION\ IN\ PLASMA} = \frac{U_{H^+} \times V}{P_{H^+}}$$

OR

$$H^+\ CLEARANCE\ INDEX = \frac{MAX.\ H^+\ SECRETION}{1/TOTAL\ PLASMA\ CO_2} = \frac{U_{H^+} \times V}{1/Total\ P_{CO_2}}$$

TmHCO₃⁻

BICARBONATE INFUSED TO RAISE SERUM LEVEL WELL ABOVE THRESHOLD

$$Tm_{HCO_3^-} = (PLASMA_{HCO_3^-} \times GFR) - (URINE_{HCO_3^-} \times URINE\ VOL.)$$

NORMAL AND ABNORMAL FINDINGS IN INDUCED OR SPONTANEOUS ACIDOSIS

	NORMAL	PROX. TUBULAR ACIDOSIS	DIST. TUB. ACIDOSIS	INCOMPLETE R. T. A.
pH	4.5 TO 5.31	GREATER THAN 5.0	6.5 TO 7.5	6 TO 7
TITRATABLE ACIDITY μEq/min/1.73 m²	20 TO 50	LOW: ABOVE HCO₃⁻ THRESHOLD NORMAL: BELOW THRESHOLD	LOW	LOW
AMMONIUM μEq/min/1.73 m²	35 TO 100	LOW: ABOVE HCO₃⁻ THRESHOLD NORMAL: BELOW THRESHOLD	LOW	LOW
BICARBONATE	ABSENT	PRESENT: ABOVE THRESHOLD ABSENT: BELOW THRESHOLD	PRESENT	UNKNOWN
MAXIMUM TOTAL H⁺ EXCRETION μEq/min/1.73 m²	60 TO 135	LOW: ABOVE HCO₃⁻ THRESHOLD NORMAL: BELOW THRESHOLD	LOW	LOW
H⁺ CLEARANCE INDEX	1.5 TO 3.0	NORMAL OR LOW	LOW	LOW
BICARBONATE THRESHOLD mM/liter	INFANTS, 21.4 to 24 ADULTS, 24 to 28	LOW	NORMAL	UNKNOWN
TmHCO₃⁻	2.5 TO 2.8 mM/ 100 ml GFR	LOW	NORMAL	UNKNOWN

and ammonia excreted and subtracting the bicarbonate excreted (all in $\mu Eq/min$). Since bicarbonate is normally absent from the urine during induced acidosis, this total is usually simply the sum of titratable acid plus ammonia. The hydrogen ion clearance index, developed by Elkington *et al.,* is simply the total hydrogen excretion divided by the plasma hydrogen ion concentration. This index is nearly equal to the hydrogen excretion divided by the reciprocal of the plasma bicarbonate, which is usually expressed more simply as the hydrogen excretion multiplied by the serum or plasma bicarbonate. The index is useful at serum bicarbonate values from normal down to the bicarbonate threshold, with a rough correlation between the ability to excrete acid and the index. However, at serum bicarbonate levels below the threshold, total hydrogen excretion plateaus and the index continues to fall. Thus, the hydrogen ion clearance index is usually not

calculated if the bicarbonate is less than 20 mM/liter. Instead, total hydrogen excretion more accurately reflects acidifying ability.

Bicarbonate threshold is usually determined at the same time as the other studies, by measurement of serum and urine bicarbonate during the induction of acidosis. The serum level at which bicarbonate disappears from the urine is considered the threshold.

The *bicarbonate Tm* (Tm_{HCO_3}) has also been used to characterize the tubular mechanism responsible for renal tubular acidosis. However, recent studies suggest that the bicarbonate Tm performed by the usual technic is not a valid measure of bicarbonate reabsorptive capacity since the process of raising the serum bicarbonate also expands plasma volume. The expansion in turn depresses bicarbonate reabsorption. Therefore, bicarbonate Tm does not appear useful in the evaluation of patients with renal tubular acidosis. □

Cystometry

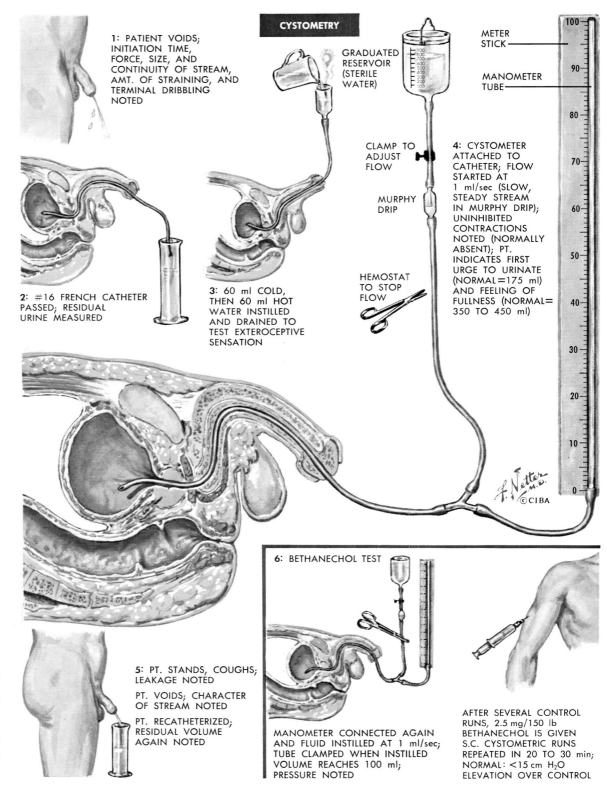

1: PATIENT VOIDS; INITIATION TIME, FORCE, SIZE, AND CONTINUITY OF STREAM, AMT. OF STRAINING, AND TERMINAL DRIBBLING NOTED

GRADUATED RESERVOIR (STERILE WATER)

METER STICK

MANOMETER TUBE

CLAMP TO ADJUST FLOW

MURPHY DRIP

HEMOSTAT TO STOP FLOW

4: CYSTOMETER ATTACHED TO CATHETER; FLOW STARTED AT 1 ml/sec (SLOW, STEADY STREAM IN MURPHY DRIP); UNINHIBITED CONTRACTIONS NOTED (NORMALLY ABSENT); PT. INDICATES FIRST URGE TO URINATE (NORMAL=175 ml) AND FEELING OF FULLNESS (NORMAL= 350 TO 450 ml)

2: #16 FRENCH CATHETER PASSED; RESIDUAL URINE MEASURED

3: 60 ml COLD, THEN 60 ml HOT WATER INSTILLED AND DRAINED TO TEST EXTEROCEPTIVE SENSATION

6: BETHANECHOL TEST

5: PT. STANDS, COUGHS; LEAKAGE NOTED

PT. VOIDS; CHARACTER OF STREAM NOTED

PT. RECATHETERIZED; RESIDUAL VOLUME AGAIN NOTED

MANOMETER CONNECTED AGAIN AND FLUID INSTILLED AT 1 ml/sec; TUBE CLAMPED WHEN INSTILLED VOLUME REACHES 100 ml; PRESSURE NOTED

AFTER SEVERAL CONTROL RUNS, 2.5 mg/150 lb BETHANECHOL IS GIVEN S.C. CYSTOMETRIC RUNS REPEATED IN 20 TO 30 min; NORMAL: <15 cm H₂O ELEVATION OVER CONTROL

Cystometry is a useful procedure in the functional evaluation of micturition. In particular, it is helpful in deciding whether disorders of micturition are caused by neurologic disease or are secondary to obstruction. The cystometric study also proves useful in distinguishing various types of neurogenic bladder which may require, and respond to, different forms of therapy.

However, cystometry must be used in conjunction with other studies—*e.g.*, intravenous pyelography (see page 91), voiding cystourethrography (see page 97), cystoscopy, and urethral calibration—to obtain accurate interpretations, since on occasion, cystometric findings resulting from obstructive lesions will simulate those resulting from neurologic disorders.

Apparatus used for cystometry varies from the relatively simple, illustrated setup to complex, electronically monitored measuring equipment. The procedures pictured, which show cystometry combined with other ancillary steps, provide most of the information required to evaluate a patient.

Technic. Observation of the patient's voiding furnishes useful information on the time and amount of effort required to initiate urination, the character of the stream, and terminal dribbling. Immediately after voiding, the patient is catheterized and the volume of any residual urine measured. With the catheter left in place, exteroceptive sensation is tested by instilling cold water followed by warm water.

Next, the manometric apparatus is connected to the catheter, and the bladder is filled gradually to determine pressures and volumes at which the initial urge to void occurs and at which the bladder feels full. These pressures and volumes are plotted to form the *cystometrogram*.

With the bladder still full, the catheter is removed and the patient asked to cough to determine stress incontinence. Then the voiding pattern is reobserved. Next, the catheter is reinserted to measure residual urine. With the catheter in place, the bethanechol test can be performed to determine the patient's reaction to parasympathetic stimulation. First, 100 ml of water is instilled into the bladder and the pressure measured. This is repeated for several control periods. Then the patient receives 2.5 mg of bethanechol/150 pounds body weight. After 20 to 30 minutes, cystometric measurements are again made.

In the normal person, pressure after instillation of 100 ml of water will increase following bethanechol to a maximum of 15 cm of water greater than the control. The response to bethanechol is positive (*i.e.*, pressure rises more than 15 cm of water over the control) among patients who exhibit the uninhibited type neurogenic bladder and the reflex type neurogenic bladder. As a general rule, a positive bethanechol test occurs in patients who exhibit lesions of the lower segmental reflex arc in which the ganglionic synapse and neuromuscular junctions become supersensitive to bethanechol. □

Radiography

Throughout most of the nineteenth century, physicians could directly visualize the urinary tract in the living patient only at surgery. However, in 1879 Nitze introduced the first practical lighted instrument for cystoscopy. The discovery of roentgen rays in 1895 permitted additional major advances in the diagnosis of renal pathology, and within a year, Guyon used X-rays to detect urinary calculi. By the end of another decade, Voelcker and Von Lichtenberg had developed a technic for retrograde pyelography.

In 1923, Rowntree and his colleagues at the Mayo Clinic developed technics to visualize the urinary tract using intravenous and oral administration of large amounts of a solution of sodium iodide. However, the method proved impractical. Visualization of the renal pelvis was too poor for exact interpretation, and untoward reactions resulted from absorption of large amounts of iodine. By 1928, Roseno had succeeded in improving visualization using a combination of urea with sodium iodide. Unfortunately, this combination proved too toxic for use. One year later, Swick solved both problems, and the first satisfactory excretory method became available. He used a compound, readily soluble in water, called Iopax in the United States and Uroselectan in Europe. It was relatively nontoxic and was excreted by normal kidneys in a concentration of approximately five percent.

Many other contrast media have been developed during the past four decades, but all those currently in use are basically substituted triiodobenzoic acid derivatives first introduced in 1950.

Plain Film Radiography

The simplest form of radiographic examination of the urinary system is the plain film of the abdomen, also called the KUB (kidney, ureter, bladder) or scout film. As such, it should precede all other radiographic procedures including tomography, pyelography, retroperitoneal pneumography, and angiography (q.v.).

The plain film of the abdomen is taken with the patient supine and includes the renal, ureteral, and bladder areas. The shadow created by the kidney is influenced by the thickness of the fatty capsule as well as by the mass of the kidney itself. If the fatty capsule is thin, as in infants, elderly patients, and lean individuals, definition of the kidneys may be improved by taking oblique views.

Kidney Size. In adults, the kidneys usually measure about 11 to 12 cm long by 5 cm wide and vary little with change in body size or physique. A difference in length of 1.5 cm or more is significant.

A unilateral small organ suggests ischemia (see page 157), chronic pyelonephritis (see page 191), or hypoplasia (see page 224). Progressive decrease in size over a period of months suggests continuing vascular insufficiency. Unilateral enlargement suggests new growth (see pages 205-207), compensatory hyperplasia, or hydronephrosis (see page 186). An irregularly enlarged kidney suggests tumor, cyst (see page 227), or abscess (see page 195); if accompanied by calcification, tumor is more likely.

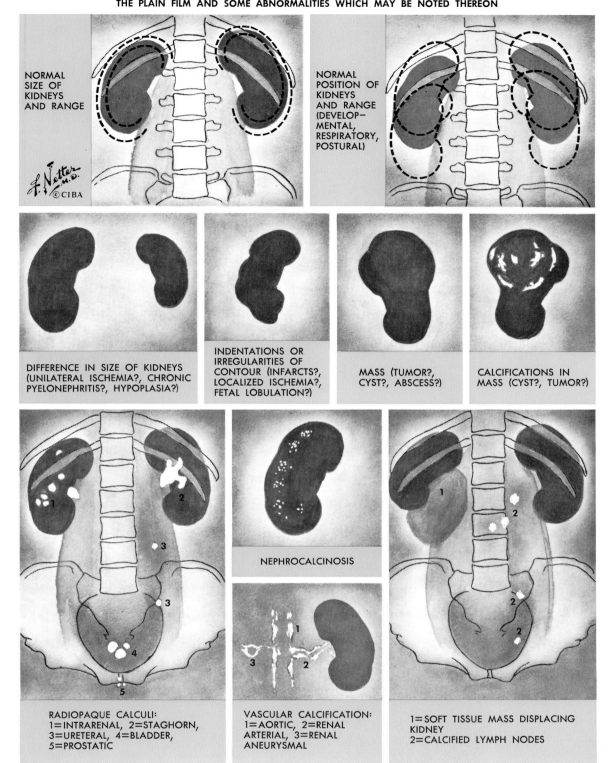

Kidney Shape. An irregularly shaped kidney, if unilateral, suggests an infarct, focal pyelonephritis, or localized ischemia. On the other hand, the uniformly ischemic kidney is regular in outline in contrast to the multipitted kidney of unilateral chronic pyelonephritis. Bilateral irregularity would lead one to suspect a congenital or hereditary disorder such as fetal lobulation or bilateral chronic pyelonephritis.

The position of the kidney in the normal supine adult is from just above the body of the twelfth thoracic vertebra to about the midpoint of the third lumbar vertebra on the left. The right kidney usually sits about 1.5 cm below the left. In the young child (until some time between the ages of 5 and 13 years) both organs are lower than in the adult. The medial borders of the kidneys lie about 5 cm from the midline in the male but are nearer the midline in the female.

Although ventrodorsal and mediolateral mobility is small, craniocaudal movement is appreciable. If the patient is in a head down position, the kidney may move cranially so that the superior pole of the left kidney reaches the tenth intercostal space, whereas that of the right kidney reaches the eleventh intercostal space. With deep inspiration, or in the upright position, the left kidney may descend to a point where the inferior pole is just above the interiliac line; the inferior pole of the right kidney may reach or even descend below this line.

Displacement of the kidney, particularly if unilateral, may be caused by a soft tissue mass such as a tumor in nearby organs or tissues.

Calcification should be looked for. If noted, oblique views must be taken to determine whether such calcification lies within the kidney or is located in nearby tissues. Calcification in lymph nodes may be mistaken for renal or ureteral calculi (see pages 200-202). □

Tomography

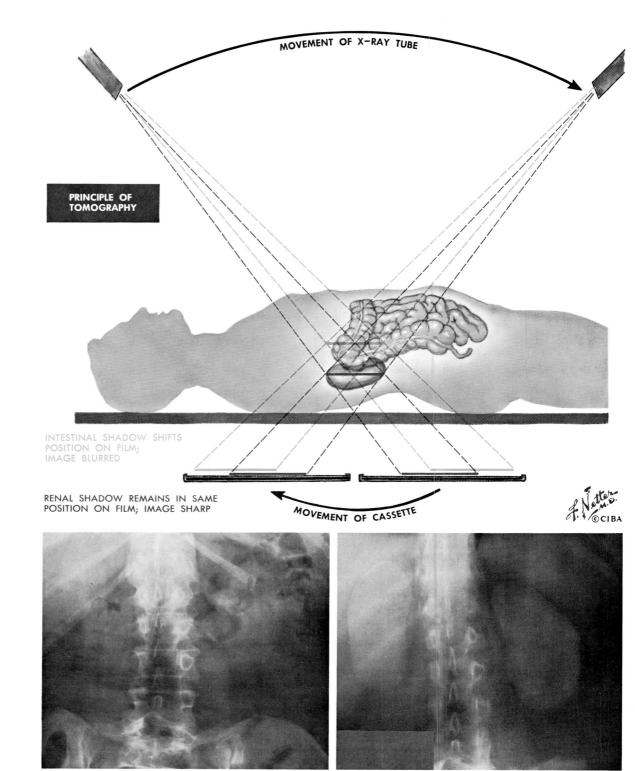

PRINCIPLE OF TOMOGRAPHY

MOVEMENT OF X-RAY TUBE

INTESTINAL SHADOW SHIFTS POSITION ON FILM; IMAGE BLURRED

RENAL SHADOW REMAINS IN SAME POSITION ON FILM; IMAGE SHARP

MOVEMENT OF CASSETTE

PLAIN X-RAY: SHADOW OF KIDNEY OBSCURED BY OVERLYING GAS IN BOWEL

TOMOGRAM: SHADOW OF KIDNEY IN PLANE OF FULCRUM WELL DEFINED, BUT BOWEL SHADOW BLURRED BY MOVEMENT

Tomography is also known as body section radiography, laminography, and planigraphy. In 1922, Bocage invented a device to radiograph a desired level of the body while blurring structures in front of and behind this level.

Principle. The tube and film move during exposure so that the roentgenographic shadow of a selected plane in the body remains stationary. The shadows of all other planes are in motion during exposure. Therefore, they are blurred to varying degrees. The image of the stationary plane remains in focus because that plane is at the level of the axis of rotation of the X-ray tube and film carrier.

Technic. In practice, the X-ray tube and film carrier are connected by a metal rod. The axis of rotation, or fulcrum, of the rod is adjustable for various heights above a tabletop and corresponds to that plane

of the body which will be in focus. Of course, both the connecting rod and fulcrum mechanisms are outside the path of the X-ray pattern.

The simplest pattern of motion of the tube and film carrier is rectilinear, the tube and film carrier moving in opposite directions. Since structural lines which lie parallel to the direction of motion are not blurred, the tomography plate is streaky. This streakiness is minimized if pluridirectional motion is utilized whereby the tube and carrier describe a circular, spiral, or hypocycloid path.

Multitomography, a modification of linear tomography, provides a series of body section plates with a single excursion of the tube, using a special "book" cassette. In this cassette, each film is placed between a pair of intensifying screens, and each such sandwich is separated from the next by a radiolucent spacer. The thicknesses of these spacers correspond to the desired

distances between tomographic body section plates.

Because of the absorption of the X-rays by the layers within the cassette, the speeds of the intensifying screens must be graduated, with the slower screens at the top and the faster ones at the bottom. As a result, exposure of the patient to radiation is about equal to that required for a similar number of individual tomograms. However, image definition is poorer than with conventional tomograms. Nevertheless, the chief advantage of multitomography is the timesaving achieved.

Indications. In the diagnosis of renal disorders, tomography is used primarily to blur shadows of overlying gas and feces in the intestinal tract as well as shadows of other abdominal viscera. Therefore, when patients have poorly cleansed colons, tomography of the kidneys is useful in association with retroperitoneal pneumography and nephrography (see pages 98 and 99). □

Intravenous Pyelography (Excretory Urography)

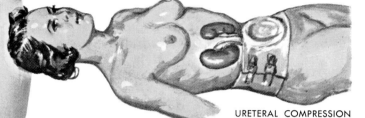

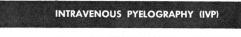

INTRAVENOUS PYELOGRAPHY (IVP)

30 ml CONTRAST MATERIAL INJECTED INTRAVENOUSLY IN 2 TO 3 MINUTE PERIOD; CONTRAST MATERIAL CIRCULATES VIA BLOOD-STREAM AND HEART TO KIDNEYS WHERE IT IS EXCRETED, OPACIFYING THE COLLECTING SYSTEM;
FILMS TAKEN AT 5, 10, AND 15 MINUTES WITH PATIENT IN SUPINE POSITION; OBLIQUE AND PRONE FILMS ALSO TAKEN;
FINALLY CONED—DOWN FILMS OF BLADDER ARE MADE BEFORE AND AFTER VOIDING

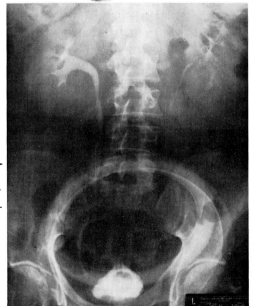

URETERAL COMPRESSION

← INTRAVENOUS PYELOGRAM

→ SAME CASE WITH URETERAL COMPRESSION; BETTER VISUAL—IZATION OF DISTENDED COLLECTING SYSTEM WITH PARTIAL BLOCK OF RIGHT URETER NEAR PELVIC BRIM

The purpose of intravenous pyelography is to visualize the renal parenchyma, as well as the calyces, pelves, ureters, and urinary bladder, by injection of a contrast medium which is excreted principally through the kidneys.

Contrast media in use today are triiodobenzoic acid derivatives excreted either through the kidney or via the liver through the bile. Those eliminated in the urine usually have completely substituted benzene rings and are not appreciably bound to serum proteins at physiologic pH. They are cleared from the plasma almost exclusively by glomerular filtration. Contrast media excreted through the bile generally have high molecular weights, incompletely substituted rings, and are bound strongly to serum albumin at physiologic pH.

The preparations currently used for excretory urography are sodium salts, methylglucamine salts, or a combination of both. As a general rule, sodium salts are less viscous, whereas glucamine reduces toxicity, avoids high sodium ion concentration, and lessens tissue irritability. The adult dose, usually 50 ml, varies somewhat with the particular preparation. Larger doses may be required on occasion, particularly in obese patients. In infants and children, dosage is calculated for the age or weight of the patient according to the manufacturer's instructions. If intravenous injection is not possible, certain preparations can safely be administered by the intramuscular route.

Preparation of the patient is important to obtain optimal visualization. Castor oil or another suitable laxative should be given on the evening before the study to remove gas and fecal material from the colon. In adults and older children, mild dehydration can be achieved by omitting fluids for 12 to 15 hours before examination. This helps minimize the diuretic action of the contrast medium and increases the concentration of the medium in the urine. However, dehydration is not recommended for infants and young children. In these patients, a carbonated beverage is given at the time of the study to distend the stomach with gas; this will displace the bowel enough to allow visualization of the renal shadows through the gas-filled stomach.

Precautions. Prior to injection of the contrast medium, it would be wise to question the patient concerning a history of allergy, including asthma and a sensitivity to iodine, since allergic reactions to the medium can occur. Although results are not always reliable, a test of 0.5 to 1 ml of contrast medium may be injected intravenously prior to the regular dose in an effort to ascertain if a patient is allergic to the material. The limitations of this test lie in the fact that a reaction to the test dose may in itself be severe or may be delayed sufficienctly to give a false-negative reaction.

Although idiosyncrasy to iodine is not an absolute contraindication, extreme caution is advised. Caution is also advised with patients who have severe cardiovascular disease. If, in spite of adequate precautions, allergic or other reactions occur, it is essential that provision for intensive treatment be available. The room in which the examination is performed must be equipped to handle any emergency that may arise.

Contrast media have also been shown to promote the phenomenon of sickling, in individuals who are homozygous for sickle cell disease, when the material is injected intravenously or intraarterially.

A definite risk exists in the performance of excretory urography in patients who are *Continued on page 92*

Intravenous Pyelography
(Excretory Urography)

Continued from page 91

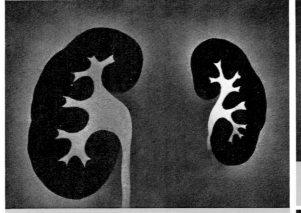

SMALL ATROPHIC KIDNEY DUE TO UNILATERAL RENAL ISCHEMIA: INCREASED OPACITY AND INCOMPLETE DISTENTION OF PELVIS OF ISCHEMIC KIDNEY

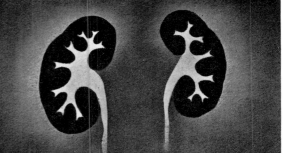

BILATERALLY SHRUNKEN KIDNEYS, WITH RELATIVELY THIN CORTEX, WHICH MAY APPEAR IN LATE CHRONIC GLOMERULONEPHRITIS OR IN NEPHROSCLEROSIS

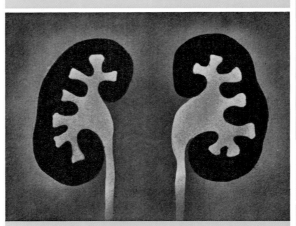

MILD CLUBBING OF CALYCES WHICH MAY BE SEEN IN EARLY CHRONIC PYELONEPHRITIS

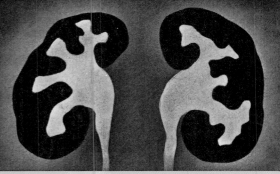

GREAT IRREGULARITY AND CLUBBING OF CALYCES, WITH LOSS OF PARENCHYMAL SUBSTANCE AND INDENTATIONS OF RENAL CONTOUR, WHICH MAY BE FOUND IN ADVANCED CHRONIC PYELONEPHRITIS. PAPILLARY NECROSIS—LOWER POLE L. KIDNEY

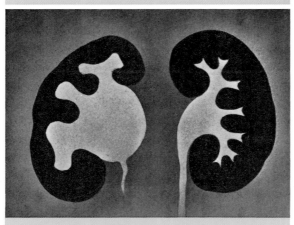

CHRONIC OBSTRUCTION OF URETEROPELVIC JUNCTION WITH DILATATION OF PELVIS (RIGHT)

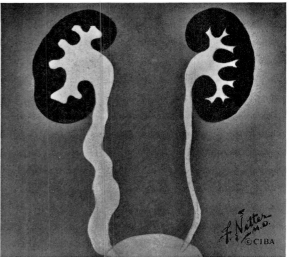

LOW OBSTRUCTION WITH GREAT DILATATION OF URETER (MAY ALSO OCCUR BILATERALLY); DILATATION ALSO MAY BE DUE TO URETERAL REFLUX

known to have multiple myeloma. Partial dehydration is not recommended as this may predispose to precipitation of myeloma protein in the kidney tubules.

Since water-soluble contrast media cause a marked elevation of the protein-bound iodine level, thyroid function studies should be performed in advance of radiographic studies if clinically indicated.

Technic. Immediately before the contrast medium is injected, the patient should be instructed to empty the bladder. Otherwise, collection of the medium into a bladder already partially filled with urine may produce a cystogram of sufficient size and density to obscure the lower portions of either ureter. The dilution effect may also make interpretation of the bladder outline difficult, and small tumors of the bladder may be missed.

After the plain film of the abdomen has been checked for adequate preparation of the patient and for any abnormalities, 50 ml of the contrast medium is injected intravenously in 2 to 3 minutes. Films are exposed (with the patient in a supine position) 5, 10, and 15 minutes after injection. In addition, one oblique projection of each kidney and one prone film are obtained. Subsequently, coned-down films of the bladder, both before and after voiding, are taken.

The technic of *ureteral compression* is often employed during the early part of the procedure. With the patient supine, the lower abdomen is compressed by an inflated rubber bag, thus partially occluding the ureters at the level of the pelvic brim. Such compression causes the contrast medium to remain proximal to the pelvic brim, resulting in better filling and opacification of the renal calyces and pelves. Unfortunately, this procedure may cause the patient some discomfort and does not always give the desired result. Instead, the patient may also be put in a moderate, recumbent, head down position to help prevent overly rapid emptying of the renal pelves.

In the supine position, the superior pole of each kidney is situated more dorsally than the inferior pole, and the medial border more ventrally than the lateral. Therefore, filling of the inferior calyces, the pelves, and upper ureters is aided by turning the patient to the prone position.

Pre- and postvoiding films of the bladder help assess the amount of residual urine and detect the presence of small tumors (see page 209) and diverticula (see page 218).

Delayed films, up to 7 hours, are obtained when indicated, *e.g.,* in patients with acute ureteral obstruction (see page 183).

Reactions to Contrast Media. Faulty technic may cause hematomas and ecchymoses (because of extravasation from the vein) and pyrogenic reactions. Cardiovascular effects include vasodilatation with flushing, mild hypotension, and (rarely) vein cramp or thrombophlebitis. More serious reactions include rare cases of cardiac arrhythmias, shock, and cardiac arrest.

Allergic manifestations are nasal and conjunctival symptoms, dermal reactions such as urticaria, and rarely, anaphylactic reactions which may be fatal. Severe allergic reactions may also cause asthma and/or laryngeal edema with manifested dyspnea, cyanosis, and perhaps pulmonary edema.

The nervous system symptoms which may occur are restlessness, confusion, and convulsions. Other possible reactions include nausea, vomiting, excessive saliva-

Intravenous Pyelography (Excretory Urography)

Continued

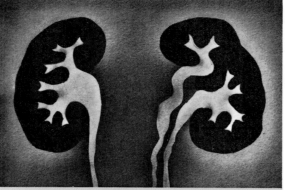

DOUBLE URETER (LEFT); EXTRINSIC VASCULAR IMPRESSIONS ON L. UPPER URETER

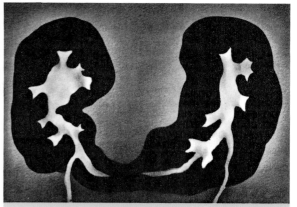

HORSESHOE KIDNEY

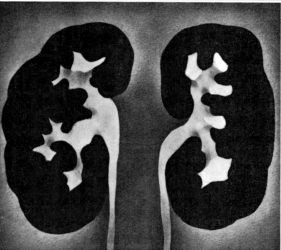

POLYCYSTIC KIDNEYS

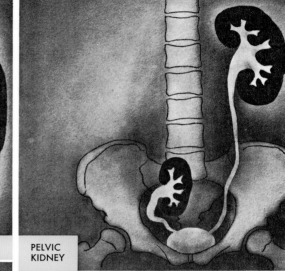

PELVIC KIDNEY

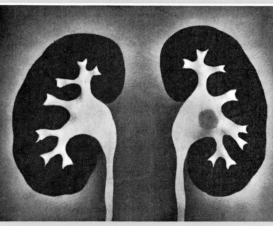

RADIOLUCENT STONE APPEARS AS FILLING DEFECT IN RENAL PELVIS (LEFT)

RADIOPAQUE SHADOW (STONE) CONFIRMED AS BEING WITHIN URETER

tion, headache, and dizziness.

Infrequently, "iodism" (salivary gland swelling) from organic compounds appears the second day after exposure and subsides by the sixth day. The incidence of fatal reactions from contrast media is about seven or eight per 1 million examinations.

Indications and Advantages. The chief advantage of excretory urography is the visualization of the urinary tract without the need for cystoscopic examination. In renal tuberculosis (see page 196) particularly, excretory urography eliminates the danger of disseminating the infection which could occur if retrograde pyelography (see page 96) were employed. Ureteral anomalies (see pages 234-237), such as duplication, and injury to the urinary tract from accidents or surgical procedures (see pages 213-217) can be well demonstrated by IVP. This examination is especially useful in children, and when catherization of the ureters is either impossible or not practical because of the risk of causing excessive trauma. Such a risk exists if there is marked enlargement of the prostate gland (see CIBA COLLECTION, Vol. 2, pages 51-53), if large tumors of the bladder involve the ureteral orifices (see page 209), and after implantation of the ureters into the bowel.

The excretory urogram is also valuable as a rough test of renal function. In general, prompt visualization of good intensity denotes good renal function. However, the reverse is not true because absence of visualization does not necessarily indicate absence of function (*e.g.*, temporary obstruction of the ureter by a calculus, see page 202).

Interpretation. Correct interpretation of the IVP depends upon adequate observation of the size, shape, number, and position of the calyces, their relationship to the soft tissue shadow of the kidney parenchyma, the size, shape, and position of the renal pelvis and ureter, and a comparison of one side with the other. For instance, as illustrated, an increased concentration of the contrast medium associated with incomplete distention of the renal pelvis and a small renal tissue shadow may be associated with an atrophic kidney, such as caused by ischemia (see page 156-157).

Certain technical factors may interfere with the visualization of the urinary tract, the most important being inadequate preparation of the patient and injection of too little contrast medium.

Inadequate visualization may also result from a number of pathologic conditions. For instance, unilateral inhibition of secretion of urine may occur if there are ureteral calculi on that side. Also, obstruction of the ureter, such as occurs with hydronephrosis (see page 186) or neoplasm of the kidney, ureter, or bladder (see pages 205-212), may prevent adequate outline of the urinary tract. Renal atrophy, diffuse unilateral pyelonephritis (see page 191), congenital hypoplasia (see page 224), renal agenesis (see page 223), renal tumor, and renal tuberculosis (see page 196) may all be associated with poor visualization.

If the blood urea nitrogen (BUN) is above 75 mg percent, there may be inadequate secretion of a normal dose of contrast medium. In such patients, the drip infusion technic should be used (*q.v.*). Peristalsis may cause fragmentary visualization of any portion of the renal pelvis or ureters.

Notching of the pelvis and upper ureter strongly suggests the presence of a blocked renal artery. Other causes of notching are varicose Continued on page 94

Intravenous Pyelography
(Excretory Urography)

Continued from page 93

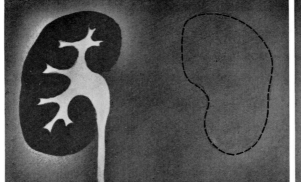

COMPLETE NONFUNCTION OF ONE KIDNEY: MAY BE DUE TO COMPLETE OBSTRUCTION, EXTENSIVE UNILATERAL RENAL DISEASE SUCH AS MARKED ISCHEMIA, EXTENSIVE INFARCTION, OR CONGENITAL ABSENCE

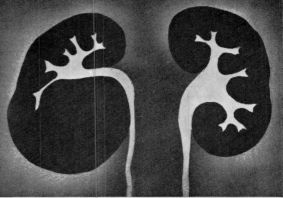

SPACE–OCCUPYING LESION (TUMOR OR CYST), DISTORTING PELVIS AND CALYCES OF ONE KIDNEY

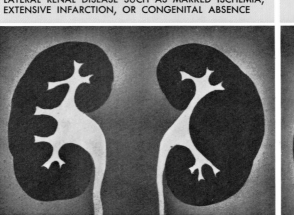

DEEP–SEATED TUMOR OR CYST, DISPLACING THE CENTRAL CALYCES BUT CAUSING LITTLE DEFORMITY OF RENAL CONTOUR; UPPER AND LOWER CALYCES APPEAR STRETCHED AROUND LESION

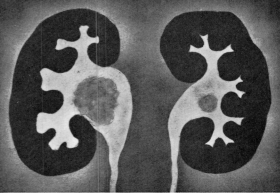

FILLING DEFECTS CAUSED BY PAPILLOMATOUS TUMOR OF RIGHT RENAL PELVIS AND RADIOLUCENT STONE IN LEFT RENAL PELVIS

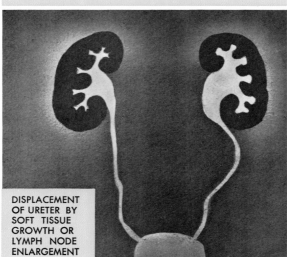

DISPLACEMENT OF URETER BY SOFT TISSUE GROWTH OR LYMPH NODE ENLARGEMENT

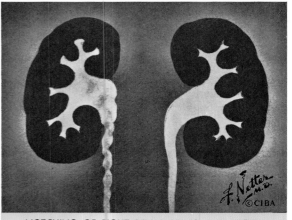

NOTCHING OF RIGHT RENAL PELVIS AND URETER BY VARICOSITIES SUGGESTIVE OF RENAL VEIN THROMBOSIS OR RENAL ARTERY STENOSIS

ureteral veins, arteriovenous fistula, and enlarged lymph nodes. Unilateral absence of excretion of the contrast medium in association with normal retrograde pyelography is practically pathognomonic of blockage of the main renal artery.

Drip-Infusion Pyelography

This method of excretory urography requires rapid intravenous infusion of a large volume of diluted contrast medium. It was described by Schencker, and by Harris and Harris in 1964. The technic has been employed widely since then and has proved to be a safe and efficient method for obtaining a clear demonstration of the renal collecting systems. Complications and contraindications are the same as for conventional IVP.

The prime advantages of drip-infusion pyelography are improved overall concentration of contrast medium, a denser nephrogram, and avoidance of prior dehydration. However, preliminary dehydration further improves the opacification of the urinary tract. The technic is considerably more costly than routine IVP. The recommended dose of the contrast medium is 1 ml/pound of body weight diluted with an equal amount of sterile water for injection or with 5 percent glucose in water. Prediluted solutions are also available commercially in 300-cc bottles; the recommended dose is 2 ml/pound of body weight. The diluted solution is administered by intravenous drip over a period of 8 to 10 minutes. Films are taken during and after infusion as necessary.

Indications. These are numerous and include:

1. Clarification of a poor or equivocal IVP—drip IVP offers a valid alternative to retrograde pyelography.

2. Demonstration of ureters—drip IVP is particularly suitable for "emergency" investigation of patients having ureteric colic, with or without evidence of a calculus on the plain film. It is also useful in demonstrating ureteric stenosis or fistula, periureteric fibrosis, possible involvement of the ureter in pelvic malignancy, and in the investigation of retroperitoneal tumor.

3. BUN levels between 40 and 120 mg percent—drip-infusion pyelography is the method of choice in the presence of impaired renal function and may afford the only prospect of opacifying the renal tract other than by retrograde pyelography. No significant alterations of BUN have been reported in such patients following drip IVP.

4. Nonopacification of one kidney by IVP—drip IVP may often demonstrate hydronephrotic, pyelonephritic, or hypoplastic kidneys.

5. Renal cyst vs. tumor—when combined with tomography, drip IVP sometimes permits differentiation of renal cysts from tumors.

6. Hematuria—the improved overall opacification can be very valuable in demonstrating small lesions of the pelvicalyceal system or of the ureters.

7. Renal trauma—since abdominal compression is contraindicated and preparation of the patient is generally poor, drip IVP is more valuable than conventional IVP.

8. In children—drip IVP eliminates the need for energetic preparation, prior dehydration, and abdominal compression. However, because of the practical problems involved, drip IVP should be performed in children only when otherwise indicated.

9. Miscellaneous indications—drip IVP can be employed following renal transplantation and following ileal-bladder and other diversionary operations. □

Timed Intravenous Pyelography

1–MINUTE FILM: CONTRAST MATERIAL IN CAPILLARIES AND TUBULES DELINEATES RENAL CONTOURS AND DIMENSIONS (NEPHROGRAPHIC PHASE)

3– AND 5–MINUTE FILMS: CONTRAST MATERIAL IN RENAL CALYCES AND PELVIS (PYELOGRAPHIC PHASE)

NORMAL KIDNEY

NORMAL BLOOD FLOW TO GLOMERULI; GOOD FILTRATION RATE AND URINE FLOW THROUGH TUBULES; WATER NORMALLY REABSORBED FROM TUBULES RESULTS IN SOME CONCENTRATION OF CONTRAST MATERIAL AND MODERATE OPACIFICATION

ISCHEMIC KIDNEY

IMPAIRED BLOOD FLOW TO GLOMERULI DECREASES GLOMERULAR FILTRATION; URINE FLOW THROUGH TUBULES IS SLOWED, RESULTING IN GREATER REABSORPTION OF WATER AND GREATER CONCENTRATION OF CONTRAST MATERIAL

NORMAL RENAL SIZE AND CONTOUR; CALYCES FAIRLY WELL FILLED; MODERATE OPACIFICATION

KIDNEY SMALL; OPACIFICATION USUALLY INCREASED; IRREGULAR FILLING DUE TO DECREASED VOLUME (SPIDERING); PYELOGRAM DELAYED (IN SEVERE ISCHEMIA, OPACIFICATION MAY BE DIMINISHED OR VERY POOR, DUE TO IMPAIRED EXCRETION)

Information obtained from differential studies of kidney function using bilateral ureteral catheterization (see pages 85 and 86) has shown physiological abnormalities upon which are based an understanding of the radiographic findings in the timed pyelogram. This is an important procedure in the diagnosis of renovascular hypertension (see pages 156-157).

If a kidney exhibits decreased blood flow, there is resultant diminished glomerular filtration rate and, more specifically, increased water and sodium reabsorption by the tubules. Those components of the glomerular filtrate which do not undergo tubular reabsorption (including organic iodides used in radiography) are thus excreted in increased concentrations in the urine of the ischemic kidney.

Technic. Timed pyelography requires the same preparation as routine intravenous pyelography (see page 91). A plain film of the abdomen is taken, followed by rapid injection of contrast material. Exposures are made at 1, 3, and 5 minutes and at conventional times. The 1-minute film represents the *nephrographic phase* from which the renal dimensions and contours may be evaluated. The 3- and 5-minute films should show satisfactory simultaneous filling of the major and minor calyces and the renal pelvis.

Several modifications of the technic may be utilized:

1. In the so-called minute-sequence pyelogram, exposures are made at 30 seconds, 1, 2, 3, 4, and 5 minutes, with subsequent films at conventional times.

2. Different nephropacification may be obtained by routine or laminographic films of the kidneys taken 15 seconds after rapid injection of about 50 ml of contrast material. This may improve opacification and assist in the evaluation of kidney size, contour, and parenchymal density.

3. Mild to moderate hydration by ingestion of water immediately preceding or following the injection of contrast material has been proposed to emphasize any different diuretic responses of the two kidneys which may exist. Under these circumstances, the normal kidney would show poor opacification because of diuresis, whereas excretion of the contrast material by the ischemic kidney would be in greater concentration and result in greater opacification.

4. Severe diuresis may be attempted using urea washout. Following preliminary dehydration and rapid intravenous injection of contrast material, early exposures are made. If bilateral visualization of the kidneys is noted, 500 ml of eight percent urea solution is rapidly injected intravenously and exposures are made at intervals of 3 to 5 minutes. A normal kidney will respond with diuresis and "washout" of the pyelogram, but an ischemic kidney will maintain its opacity. However, this modification of the test should not be performed on patients with elevated blood urea nitrogen levels or in congestive heart failure.

Interpretations. The appearances of an ischemic kidney on plain film have been discussed previously (see page 89); also a number of findings to be expected on intravenous pyelogram if ischemia exists have been discussed on pages 92 and 93. In addition, however, the nephrographic phase (1-minute film) may show a diminished intensity on the affected side if ischemia is present. The 3- and 5-minute films (pyelographic phase) may show delay in opacification of the calyces. Also, the calyces may appear "spidered" because incomplete distention results from decreased urine flow.

In moderate degrees of renovascular disease, decreased glomerular filtration is compensated for by increased tubular reabsorption of water. Consequently, there is hyperconcentration of the contrast material. However, in severe degrees of renovascular disease so little contrast material is filtered by glomeruli that the pyelogram appears hypoconcentrated. In these patients other signs of severe renal disease will be apparent clinically. □

Retrograde Pyelography

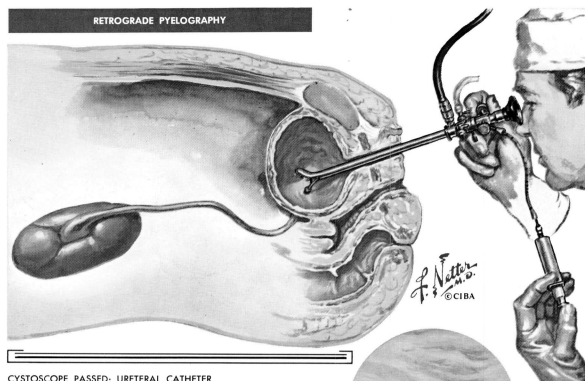

CYSTOSCOPE PASSED; URETERAL CATHETER
INTRODUCED THROUGH SCOPE AND GUIDED TO
URETERAL ORIFICE; IF CONE–TIPPED CATHETER
IS USED, IT IS SIMPLY IMPACTED IN THE ORIFICE,
BUT, IF PLAIN–TIPPED CATHETER IS EMPLOYED, IT
IS PASSED UP THE URETER FOR VARIABLE DISTANCE;
5 ml CONTRAST MEDIUM IS THEN INJECTED VIA
CATHETER TO OPACIFY THE COLLECTING SYSTEM,
AND PICTURES ARE TAKEN

CYSTOSCOPIC
VIEW

Retrograde pyelography is performed by introducing a contrast medium into the renal collecting system through a ureteral catheter. It is complementary to intravenous pyelography (see page 91) and offers several advantages. The degree of visualization is not influenced by impaired renal function, and in most patients, the dense concentration of contrast material outlines the calyces, pelvis, and ureters on one film. Furthermore, retrograde pyelography is an effective method for determining moderate degrees of stasis within the pelvis and ureters when complemented by delayed films.

Indications. Usually retrograde pyelography is used to confirm findings obtained with intravenous pyelography or to clarify the situation if the intravenous pyelogram is either unsatisfactory or inconclusive. If hematuria is present, the side from which bleeding arises can sometimes be determined at cystoscopy (see also page 73).

Contraindications and Disadvantages. Cystoscopic examination and catheterization of the ureters carry risk of infection. Retrograde pyelography can produce oliguria or anuria and is thus inadvisable in patients who already have renal damage from diseases such as pyelonephritis (see page 191), glomerulonephritis (see pages 131–139), and arteriolar nephrosclerosis (see page 153). Also, since severe reactions to contrast material can occur (see pages 91 and 92), the contrast material should not be routinely injected beyond an obstructing lesion.

Technic. Preparation of the patient is the same as for intravenous pyelography, except that dehydration is not necessary. Following preliminary cystoscopy under local anesthesia, catheters are introduced into the ureters with extreme care. (If the ureter is traumatized during manipulation, it becomes spastic and subsequent ureterograms will suggest abnormality.) After the tip of the catheter is advanced well into the renal pelvis, a plain film of the abdomen is exposed.

Ureteral catheters are either radiopaque or nonopaque, the former being

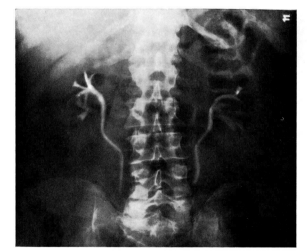

IVP: DISTORTION OF COLLECTING SYSTEM ON
LEFT, WITH INCOMPLETE VISUALIZATION OF LOWER
CALYCES; FURTHER STUDY INDICATED

RETROGRADE PYELOGRAM OF SAME CASE REVEALS
NORMAL COLLECTING SYSTEM

more frequently used because they aid in localization of shadows over the ureteral area on a plain film. Blunt-tipped (cone-tipped) catheters are less likely to traumatize and irritate the ureter. However, point-tipped (plain-tipped) catheters are easier to introduce into small ureteral orifices and are more readily passed beyond an obstruction.

The two principal methods for introducing contrast media are by gravity and syringe. The gravity method offers less danger of overdistending the pelvis and calyces, with subsequent extravasation.

A number of contrast materials are available: (1) a 12 percent solution of sodium iodide or bromide, which, although it provides excellent roentgenologic contrast, does irritate the mucosal lining of the urinary tract and occasionally produces severe reactions; (2) a 30 percent solution of sodium orthoiodohippurate in thimerosal and water; and (3) a 20 to 30 percent

solution of any of the contrast media used for intravenous pyelography.

Normally, 5 to 10 ml of contrast medium will provide a satisfactory pyelogram. However, a sense of fullness or pain in the patient's renal region indicates that the injection should be terminated.

Films are exposed with the patient in the supine and oblique positions and are developed immediately. If indicated, additional films can then be taken. A final exposure is made while simultaneously withdrawing the catheters and injecting contrast medium. In suspected urinary stasis, a delayed film is taken after the patient has been upright and moving about to determine if the contrast medium is retained in the pelvis and calyces. Though retained contrast medium indicates a delay in emptying time, it must be remembered that stasis may be secondary to spasm of the ureter produced by irritation from the catheter. □

Cystourethrography

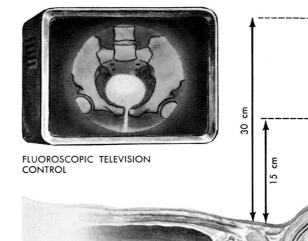

FLUOROSCOPIC TELEVISION CONTROL

CYSTOURETHROGRAPHY

CONTRAST MEDIUM INTRO- DUCED INTO BLADDER BY GRAVITY WITH FLUID LEVEL IN CONTAINER 15 cm ABOVE PUBIS. WHEN FLOW STOPS, CATHETER IS CLAMPED AND FILMS TAKEN. CONTAINER IS THEN RAISED TO 30 cm, ADDITIONAL FLUID ADDED TO CAPACITY, AND PICTURES AGAIN TAKEN

CATHETER REMOVED, PATIENT PLACED IN OBLIQUE POSITION AND INSTRUCTED TO VOID. X-RAYS TAKEN AS PATIENT VOIDS. WITH THIS TECHNIC, REFLUX MAY BE NOTED AS OCCURRING AT LOW PRESSURE, AT HIGH PRESSURE, OR ONLY AS BLADDER CONTRACTS, AND OTHER ABNORMALITIES OF BLADDER OR URETHRA MAY BE VISUALIZED

Cystourethrography is the roentgenologic study of the bladder and urethra. *Cystography* is indicated when a filling defect within the bladder is suspected, *e.g.,* calculus (see page 203) or tumor (see pages 209-211), or for demonstration of vesicoureteral reflux, bladder diverticula, and bladder fistulas (see page 218) or placenta previa (see CIBA COLLECTION, Vol. 2, page 222). Urethrography is indicated in suspected cases of urethral stricture, valves, diverticula, calculi, or fistulas (see CIBA COLLECTION, Vol. 2). However, if there is acute infection or acute traumatic injury of the urethra, the procedures are contraindicated.

Cineroentgenography is widely used in cystourethrography and has proven very valuable for demonstrating fleeting vesicoureteral reflux and for delineation of the bladder neck. It also reveals the importance of performing the examination under fluoroscopic control.

Because of inherent poor detail with cine films, a new method has been devised that uses fluoroscopy and multiple photo-timed spot films. According to some authors, the spot-film method is as good as the cine method for demonstrating ureteral reflux and is superior for demonstrating pathologic anatomy. Both methods have gained wide acceptance.

Technic. Fluoroscopy should be available for the examination. Since active co-operation is very desirable, the patient receives no premedication. With the patient in a supine position, a catheter is passed under aseptic conditions. Alternatively, a percutaneous suprapubic puncture of the bladder may be used (see page 71), particularly if bacteriuria is suspected and urine samples are to be collected.

The bladder may be filled with contrast medium either by injection or by gravity. If injection is used, the criteria for ade-

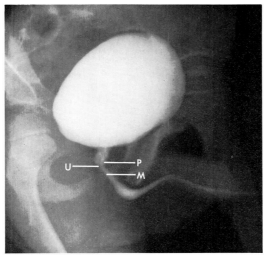

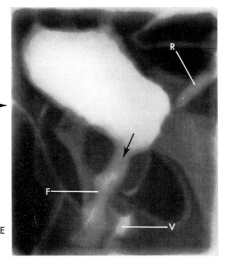

NORMAL MALE VOIDING CYSTO- URETHROGRAM:
P = PROSTATIC URETHRA
U = UTRICLE
M = MEMBRANOUS URETHRA

FEMALE VOIDING CYSTOURETHRO- GRAM:
R = URETERAL REFLUX
F = NARROWING BY PELVIC FLOOR
V = REFLUX INTO VAGINA (NORMAL)
ARROW = TRIGONE DESCENT IN VOIDING

quate filling are the fluoroscopic appearance of the bladder, discomfort of the patient, and the presence of either reflux or spontaneous voiding around the catheter. The gravity method carries the advantage of gradual distension of the bladder.

Among the most commonly employed contrast media are five to 10 percent sodium iodide, and 12 percent sodium orthoiodohippurate, or diatrizoate sodium, or meglumine diatrizoate.

After adequate distension of the bladder is obtained, spot films are exposed in supine, oblique, and lateral projections. With the patient in the right posterior oblique position, the catheter is removed. When the patient begins to void, multiple spot films are taken that include the bladder as well as the urethra. (If the cine method is used, both filling and emptying of the bladder and urethra are recorded.)

Good *cystograms* often can be obtained following

conventional excretory urography if the kidneys are functioning well and sufficient time is allowed for the bladder to be adequately distended with the contrast-medium. Semivoided cystograms help in the detection of small polypoid tumors of the bladder which may be obscured by a bladder fully distended with contrast medium.

Air-filled cystograms are of value in demonstrating small filling defects within the urinary bladder. However, the possible danger of air embolism should be kept in mind.

For *retrograde urethrography* in males, a cannula having a cone-shaped rubber mouthpiece is inserted into the external urethral orifice and secured to the penis by a specially designed clamp. Either water-soluble or viscous contrast medium (20 to 30 ml) is injected manually with a slow steady pressure, and radiographs are exposed. □

Nephrotomography

Basically, nephrotomography is a form of excretory urography which is combined with body section radiography for filming the kidney during the period of parenchymal opacification (*the nephrographic phase*, see page 95). By a nicety of timing, one can obtain roentgenographic delineation, not only of the renal parenchyma (in both the arterial and nephrographic phases), but also of the renal pelvis and calyces, and often of the abdominal aorta and the main renal arteries as well. However, the opacification of the aorta and the renal arteries is very poor and does not compare with the excellent detail obtained with renal arteriography. The tomograms permit unobstructed visualization of multiple planes through the opacified kidney.

Nephrotomography is particularly helpful when unsatisfactory results are obtained with intravenous or retrograde pyelography. It is also helpful to distinguish cysts (see page 227) from neoplasms (see pages 205-207) of the kidney. Essentially, the contraindications are the same as for intravenous pyelography. Complications are usually minor and transient and include nausea and vomiting, urticaria, and pain and burning at the site of injection.

Unsatisfactory results with the procedure usually stem from poor demonstration of the small renal vessels or inadequate opacification of the kidneys.

Technic. An understanding of the principles involved can best be appreciated from a review of the procedure:

1. Plain films of the renal area provide a check on radiologic technic, positioning, and tomographic levels.

2. Arm-to-tongue circulation time, determined by injection of sodium dehydrocholate through a 12-gauge angiographic needle, gives a close approximation of the arm-to-kidney circulation time. The needle is left in place.

3. A loading dose of 50 percent diatrizoate injected intravenously intensifies the nephrographic effect and opacifies the renal collecting system.

4. Immediately, 50 ml of 90 percent sodium and meglumine diatrizoates is injected as rapidly as possible, preferably within 2 to 3 seconds. Rapid injection ensures that a high concentration of contrast medium is presented to the kidney.

5. A film exposed at the predetermined arm-to-kidney circulation time demonstrates the renal arteries.

6. Immediately, tomograms at levels 1 cm apart demonstrate the entire thickness of the opacified kidney.

A simplified technic, utilizing drip-infusion pyelography and tomography, was introduced in 1965 and has become very popular at most institutions. □

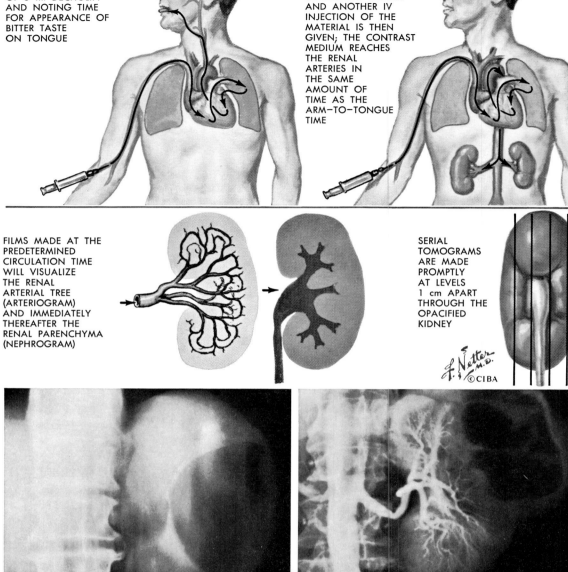

ARM-TO-TONGUE CIRCULATION TIME DETERMINED BY INTRAVENOUS INJECTION OF 5 ml DECHOLIN® AND NOTING TIME FOR APPEARANCE OF BITTER TASTE ON TONGUE

A LOADING DOSE OF CONTRAST MATERIAL IS GIVEN INTRAVENOUSLY TO OPACIFY THE COLLECTING SYSTEM AND ANOTHER IV INJECTION OF THE MATERIAL IS THEN GIVEN; THE CONTRAST MEDIUM REACHES THE RENAL ARTERIES IN THE SAME AMOUNT OF TIME AS THE ARM-TO-TONGUE TIME

FILMS MADE AT THE PREDETERMINED CIRCULATION TIME WILL VISUALIZE THE RENAL ARTERIAL TREE (ARTERIOGRAM) AND IMMEDIATELY THEREAFTER THE RENAL PARENCHYMA (NEPHROGRAM)

SERIAL TOMOGRAMS ARE MADE PROMPTLY AT LEVELS 1 cm APART THROUGH THE OPACIFIED KIDNEY

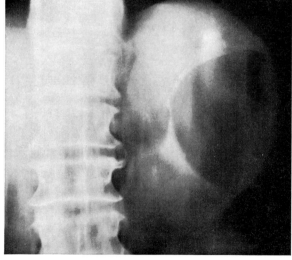

NEPHROTOMOGRAM: LARGE HOMOGENEOUSLY RADIOLUCENT MASS WITH THIN SMOOTH MARGINS IN SUPEROLATERAL ASPECT OF L. KIDNEY (RENAL CYST)

L. RENAL ARTERIOGRAM: THE INTRARENAL ARTERIES ARE DISPLACED MEDIALLY AND DOWNWARD BY A RADIOLUCENT MASS, CONFIRMING DIAGNOSIS OF RENAL CYST ON NEPHROTOMOGRAPHY

Renal Cysts vs. Neoplasm

	Arteriographic Phase	
	Cyst	**Neoplasm**
Vessels	None in mass	Tumor type in mass
Opacification	None of mass	Irregular ("puddling") in mass
	Nephrographic Phase	
Density	Radiolucent	Variable; may contain irregular radiolucent areas
Consistency	Homogenous	Irregular
Wall	Thin and well defined	Thick and irregular
Interface with normal tissue	Sharp demarcation	Poorly defined

Retroperitoneal Pneumography

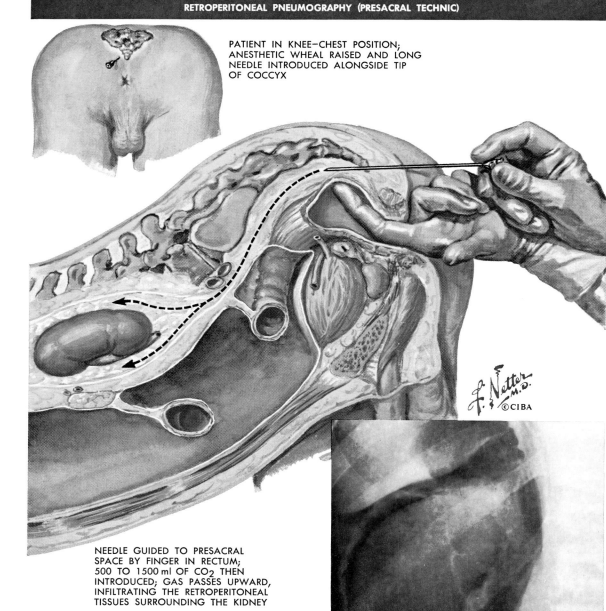

PATIENT IN KNEE–CHEST POSITION;
ANESTHETIC WHEAL RAISED AND LONG
NEEDLE INTRODUCED ALONGSIDE TIP
OF COCCYX

NEEDLE GUIDED TO PRESACRAL
SPACE BY FINGER IN RECTUM;
500 TO 1500 ml OF CO₂ THEN
INTRODUCED; GAS PASSES UPWARD,
INFILTRATING THE RETROPERITONEAL
TISSUES SURROUNDING THE KIDNEY

RETROPERITONEAL PNEUMOGRAM:
EXCELLENT DELINEATION OF
RENAL CONTOUR BY GAS IN
SURROUNDING TISSUES

When it becomes difficult to demonstrate the kidneys and suprarenal glands by plain roentgenography, gas may be injected into the retroperitoneal space to increase the contrast between these organs and the surrounding tissues.

Indications for retroperitoneal pneumography are suspected suprarenal lesions, renal tumors or hyperplasia, perirenal lesions, cysts or tumors, and other retroperitoneal masses.

Apart from its value as a diagnostic procedure with a high level of accuracy, retroperitoneal pneumography offers the advantages of safety (with very few complications) and little patient discomfort.

The *direct flank technic* was introduced in 1921 by Carelli, who injected carbon dioxide around the kidney *(perirenal insufflation)*. In 1935 Cahill simplified the technic by using air instead of carbon dioxide. However, this modification did not become popular because of deaths that occurred from air embolism.

Retroperitoneal gas insufflation utilizing the *presacral approach* was introduced by Rivas in 1950. The procedure is quite safe and has largely superseded the direct flank technic.

Anatomically, the kidneys, suprarenal glands, and retroperitoneal organs are embedded in more or less fatty connective tissue, continuous with connective tissue in other regions, including pelvic connective tissue. This retroperitoneal connective tissue is voluminous in the paravertebral areas of the lumbar region and contains the kidneys and suprarenal glands within the renal fascia. Although this fascia surrounds the kidneys and suprarenal glands, it is more or less wide open caudally (see page 4). Gas injected retrorectally can pass superiorly through the connective tissue interstices into the retroperitoneal space and, via the caudal opening, enter the renal fascia and surround the kidney and suprarenal gland.

Technic. The patient is prepared with purgatives and an enema. Carbon dioxide, oxygen, nitrous oxide, or helium may be used as the gaseous medium. Carbon dioxide is the most commonly employed medium,

being highly soluble in blood (20 times more soluble than oxygen) and thus entailing little risk of gas embolism.

With the patient in the knee-chest position, the skin just lateral to the coccyx is anesthetized and an ordinary lumbar puncture needle is introduced. The tip of the needle is directed medially and cranially toward the sacrum. Penetration of the rectum can be avoided by palpation with a finger in the rectum. If aspiration produces no blood, sterile carbon dioxide is injected. Image amplification and tomography may be used to advantage following gas insufflation.

Some of the hazards of retroperitoneal gas insufflation are gas embolism, bleeding and hematoma formation, infection, and emphysema of the scrotum, mediastinum, and neck. The procedure is contraindicated in patients whose general condition is poor or when infection is present at the site of injection. □

Aortorenal Angiography

In 1929 the feasibility of catheter angiography was first demonstrated by Forssmann. In the same year dos Santos introduced aortography and visceral arteriography by means of translumbar percutaneous needle puncture. However, neither technic received wide application at the time because of the highly toxic contrast media available.

Abdominal aortography using a catheter inserted through a surgically exposed femoral artery was reported by Farinas in 1941. Ten years later Peirce devised the percutaneous approach, inserting a catheter through a needle introduced into the femoral artery. Seldinger further revolutionized abdominal aortography in 1953 with his percutaneous transfemoral approach.

The term *renal angiography* implies visualization of the whole arterial tree, the capillaries, and the venous drainage. *Renal arteriography* implies visualization of only the arteries. Both can be performed either as aortorenal angiography (injection of the contrast medium into the abdominal aorta) or as selective angiography (injection of the medium directly into the renal artery orifice).

Indications and Advantages

Aortorenal angiography is indicated in patients suspected of having aneurysm, arteriovenous fistula, other vascular malformations, or renovascular hypertension. It is used to evaluate patients who have obstruction of the renal collecting systems (see page 183) and certain architectural or positional anomalies (see pages 231-232) such as horseshoe kidney (in order to visualize the precise vascular supply prior to surgery). The examination is helpful in differentiating renal cysts from malignant tumors (see page 98), in defining or excluding suspected renal or suprarenal masses, in visualizing the extent of vascular and parenchymal damage in patients who have suffered renal trauma (see pages 213-214), and in demonstrating renal vein thrombosis (see page 173) when there is complete occlusion of the inferior vena cava.

The procedure is particularly important in the study of patients suspected of having renal vascular disease and renovascular hypertension (see page 156). In these diseases, detection of intraaortic plaques in the region of the ostia and of plaques lying in the ostia or proximal centimeter of the renal arteries is highly important. Equally important is visualization of aberrant renal arteries (see page 17).

Selective renal angiography offers the additional advantages of detailed visualization of the renal vessels and vascular architecture, without superimposition of other visceral arteries which often are unavoidably opacified by aortorenal angiography.

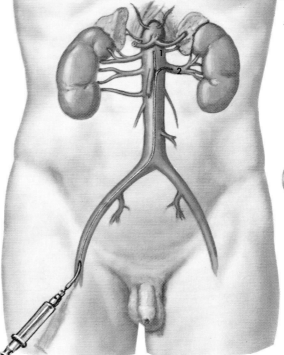

CATHETER INTRODUCED VIA FEMORAL ARTERY TO DESIRED LEVEL OF AORTA, AND CONTRAST MEDIUM INJECTED WHICH THEN FLOWS INTO NORMAL AND ACCESSORY RENAL ARTERIES AND POSSIBLY ALSO INTO OTHER AORTIC BRANCHES (AORTORENAL ANGIOGRAPHY, 1); OR CATHETER MAY BE MADE TO ENTER RENAL ARTERIES FOR DIRECT INJECTION (SELECTIVE RENAL ANGIOGRAPHY, 2)

SELDINGER TECHNIC FOR CATHETERIZATION OF FEMORAL ARTERY

1: NEEDLE INTRODUCED INTO ARTERY

2: GUIDE WIRE PASSED THROUGH NEEDLE

3: NEEDLE WITHDRAWN

4: CATHETER INTRODUCED OVER WIRE

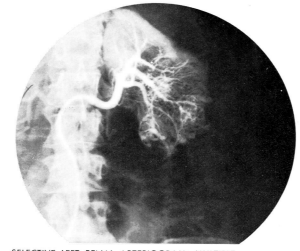

SELECTIVE LEFT RENAL ARTERIOGRAM: MULTIPLE TUMOR VESSELS IN LOWER POLE OF LEFT KIDNEY SUGGESTIVE OF HIGHLY VASCULAR TUMOR (HYPER-NEPHROMA)

AORTORENAL ANGIOGRAM: BEADED APPEARANCE OF LEFT RENAL ARTERY IS EVIDENCE OF FIBROMUSCULAR HYPERPLASIA; ANEURYSM AT BIFURCATION OF RIGHT RENAL ARTERY

Transfemoral Approach

Because the method is selective and permits injection of contrast medium into any part of the aorta or into one or both renal arteries, the percutaneous transfemoral approach is the method of choice. The Seldinger technic is simple and should be used except in patients who exhibit advanced aortoiliac atheromatous disease or extreme torsion of the iliac arteries.

Catheterization is done under local anesthesia and fluoroscopy. Once the catheter is in place, it is periodically flushed with heparinized saline to prevent clotting at the catheter tip or side hole.

As a rule, 30 to 50 ml of contrast medium is injected with a pressure injector in 1.5 to 2 seconds. For selective study, lesser amounts of contrast material (8 to 10 ml) may be used. Serial films are taken immediately after injection.

Translumbar Approach

When the transfemoral approach is contraindicated or unsuccessful, a translumbar approach may be utilized. This procedure is simple and rapid. When performed with care it is relatively safe. It is very helpful in suspected renal artery lesions but is not of much value in suspected renal parenchymal lesions. Additional disadvantages are relative nonselectivity of renal artery opacification and possible obscuration of renal arteries by simultaneous opacification of other visceral arteries.

The properly prepared and moderately sedated patient is placed in the prone position. Under local anesthesia a translumbar needle, with stylet in place, is introduced through the skin at a point just below the inferior margin of the left twelfth rib, about 8 to 10 cm lateral to the midline. The needle is advanced cranially, medially, and ventrally through the para-

Aortorenal Angiography

Continued

spinal tissues at an angle which permits entry into the aorta above the origin of the renal arteries.

When the needle comes in contact with the wall of the aorta, the pulsations of the vessel are transmitted to it. At this point, the needle is sharply advanced a short distance. If the puncture is successful, pulsatile arterial blood will flow from the needle when the stylet is removed. Flexible tubing is used as a precaution against mechanical dislodgment of the needle during injection. A test injection of 5 ml of contrast medium, observed fluoroscopically, will confirm the position of the needle tip. If a free intraluminal position has been achieved, 30 ml of contrast medium is injected manually as rapidly as possible, and serial exposures are made. (The pressure injector must not be used with metallic needles because of the possibility of laceration of the aorta. Teflon sleeve needles with guide wires are available for such purposes.)

Alternate Approaches. Other technics of renal angiography that may be employed, but will not be described here, are the percutaneous transbrachial or transaxillary catheterization method, the percutaneous noncatheter brachial method, and intravenous abdominal aortography. The last-mentioned technic is useful only as a screening procedure because it does not provide detailed visualization of the renal vasculature.

Complications

The various effects of contrast media have been described elsewhere (see pages 91–94). Of course, angiography should not be performed in patients sensitive to iodine. Local complications include hemorrhage and hematoma formation, and angiography should not be performed on patients with hemorrhagic tendencies. Infection, arterial thrombosis, and damage to atheromatous plaques—with subintimal dissection or possible embolization —are also possible complications.

Rarely, with the transfemoral approach, the tip of the guide wire may break off or perforate the arterial wall. There is also the possibility that a false aneurysm or arteriovenous fistula will form at the site of arterial puncture. In addition, with the translumbar approach, periaortic injection of contrast medium may occur.

Renal damage may occur and apparently is related to the amount and concentration of contrast medium reaching the renal parenchyma. Additionally, the time during which the medium is in contact with the kidneys is significant. This is known as application time and is dependent on the volume and rate of injection and the rate of renal blood flow. Clinical manifestations of renal insufficiency may appear within 3 days after angiography is performed. If renal dam-

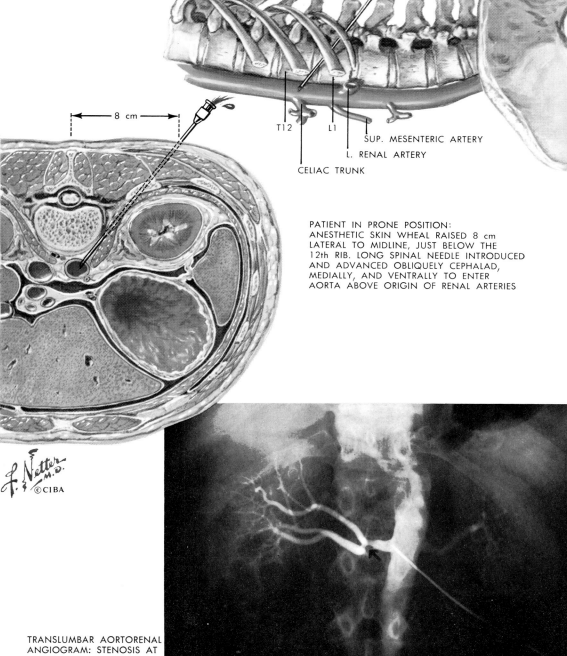

T12 L1 SUP. MESENTERIC ARTERY
L. RENAL ARTERY
CELIAC TRUNK

PATIENT IN PRONE POSITION: ANESTHETIC SKIN WHEAL RAISED 8 cm LATERAL TO MIDLINE, JUST BELOW THE 12th RIB. LONG SPINAL NEEDLE INTRODUCED AND ADVANCED OBLIQUELY CEPHALAD, MEDIALLY, AND VENTRALLY TO ENTER AORTA ABOVE ORIGIN OF RENAL ARTERIES

TRANSLUMBAR AORTORENAL ANGIOGRAM: STENOSIS AT BIFURCATION OF RIGHT RENAL ARTERY

age is severe, there is albuminuria, hematuria, oliguria, and an increase in blood urea.

In addition to the neurologic complications which may occur from intravenous use of contrast media (see pages 91 and 92), spinal cord damage is a very rare but important complication of abdominal aortography. Damage is attributable to the direct toxic action of the contrast medium on the spinal cord, the blood supply of which is through the major radicular and other arteries. (The major radicular artery arises from the left lumbar artery at the level of the second lumbar vertebra.)

Also, poor technic with the translumbar approach may place the needle within the spinal canal. Intrathecal injection would thus occur if the position of the needle were not checked.

A slight fall in blood pressure of 10 to 20 mm Hg occurs from 20 to 40 seconds after injection; blood pressure returns to the preinjection level in 1 to 2

minutes. Occasionally, more severe hypotension may occur. In patients suffering from pheochromocytoma, the contrast medium may induce hypertensive crises.

Interpretation. There are three phases of renal angiography:

1. Arterial phase, occurring during the first 3 to 4 seconds after injection and providing excellent opacification of the main renal artery and its branches.

2. Nephrographic phase, beginning 6 to 8 seconds after injection and lasting about 10 to 12 seconds; during this phase there is diffuse opacification of the capillary system, delineating clearly the extent and contour of the organ.

3. Venous phase, occurring about 15 to 20 seconds after injection; the renal vein is opacified. However, the opacification frequently is very poor because most of the contrast medium is rapidly excreted into the renal collecting system. □

Renal Cyst Puncture and Venous Studies

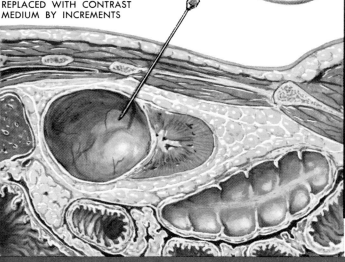

NEEDLE INTRODUCED INTO RENAL CYST; FLUID REMOVED AND REPLACED WITH CONTRAST MEDIUM BY INCREMENTS

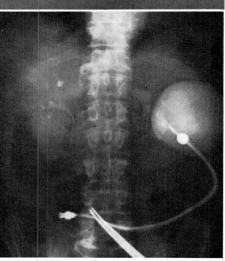

CYST OPACIFIED WITH CONTRAST MEDIUM BY DIRECT PUNCTURE

Direct puncture of a renal cyst is called for when other radiographic studies (IVP, see page 91, retrograde pyelogram, see page 96, nephrotomogram, see page 98, or angiogram, see pages 100 and 101) indicate a diagnosis of renal cyst. However, puncture should not be attempted if an abscess is suspected, if a hemorrhagic disorder is present, or in the presence of hematuria and elevated sedimentation rate, temperature, or lactic acid dehydrogenase in urine. (The latter signs favor a diagnosis of renal tumor.)

Technic. With the patient prone, the kidney is opacified with contrast material excreted into the pelvicalyceal system. Under fluoroscopic control, a 20-gauge needle is inserted into the lesion. (The needle will move with respiration when it enters the kidney.) Usually clear amber fluid will flow briskly from the needle when the cyst is entered.

The fluid is exchanged for contrast material—in increments to prevent collapse of the cyst and dislodgment of the needle. Of course, the fluid should be saved for a Papanicolaou smear (see also page 79). Carbon dioxide may also be injected to produce a double-contrast study.

After the needle is withdrawn, roentgenograms are obtained in prone, supine, upright, decubitus, and Trendelenburg positions. This technic permits evaluation of the entire wall of the cyst.

Criteria for Diagnosis of Benign Cyst. If a cyst is benign, the fluid is crystal clear, usually yellowish, and more than 15 ml should be readily aspirable; the Papanicolaou smear of the fluid should be negative; the cystic space outlined by the contrast medium should conform to either the deformity seen on IVP or the nonopaque mass seen on nephrotomograms or arteriograms; the cyst wall should be smooth, with no intraluminal masses; and the aspirated fluid should be free from fat (see also page 98).

Venous Studies

Inferior vena cavography is indicated if one suspects thrombosis of the inferior

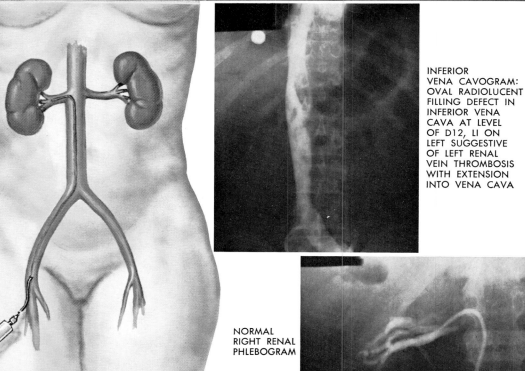

CATHETER INTRODUCED INTO FEMORAL VEIN AND PASSED UP TO RENAL VEIN; CONTRAST MATERIAL INJECTED

INFERIOR VENA CAVOGRAM: OVAL RADIOLUCENT FILLING DEFECT IN INFERIOR VENA CAVA AT LEVEL OF D12, LI ON LEFT SUGGESTIVE OF LEFT RENAL VEIN THROMBOSIS WITH EXTENSION INTO VENA CAVA

NORMAL RIGHT RENAL PHLEBOGRAM

vena cava or renal veins (see page 173). If renal vein thrombosis exists, there will be little or no streaming of unopacified renal blood to wash contrast material out of the inferior vena cava. There may also be marginal filling defects and partial or even complete caval occlusion. In other words, if the inferior vena cava is patent and contrast material is washed from it by a good stream of unopacified renal blood, main renal vein thrombosis does not exist. If the inferior vena cava is completely thrombosed, selective renal arteriography may permit adequate visualization of the renal veins.

Selective renal venography is useful in detecting small thrombi in the main renal vein or its intrarenal tributaries and in the study of the patency of splenorenal anastomoses. With cine films, renal venography also is finding use in the study of renovascular hypertension (see pages 156-157) to determine the *renal venous*

washout time. This is the total elapsed time from injection of contrast material (into the renal vein) to disappearance—normally between 1.5 and 3 seconds. Significant renal artery stenosis, with reduction in renal blood flow, usually prolongs renal washout time. However, in the absence of significant renal artery stenosis, the washout time may also be prolonged if profound arteriolar nephrosclerosis (see page 153) and a consequent diminution in renal plasma flow exist.

Technic. Both femoral veins are punctured and contrast material is simultaneously injected bilaterally. If the inferior vena cava is patent and free of thrombi, a catheter is passed into the inferior vena cava up to the level of the renal veins, which then may be catheterized selectively. Next, retrograde injection of 10 to 20 ml of contrast material is performed to opacify the renal vein and its major branches. Both studies may be performed while rapid serial exposures are made. □

Radioisotope Renography

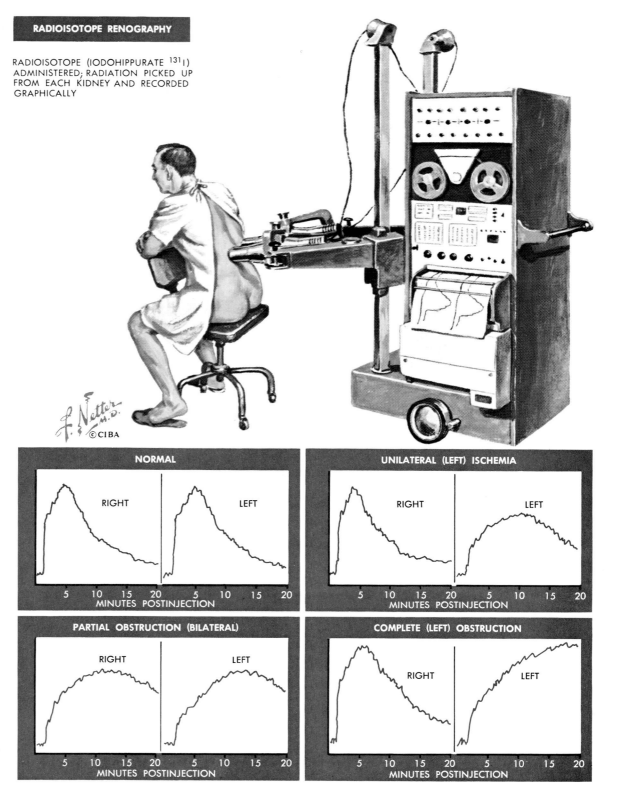

RADIOISOTOPE RENOGRAPHY

RADIOISOTOPE (IODOHIPPURATE ^{131}I) ADMINISTERED; RADIATION PICKED UP FROM EACH KIDNEY AND RECORDED GRAPHICALLY

NORMAL
RIGHT   LEFT
5 10 15 20   5 10 15 20
MINUTES POSTINJECTION

UNILATERAL (LEFT) ISCHEMIA
RIGHT   LEFT
5 10 15 20   5 10 15 20
MINUTES POSTINJECTION

PARTIAL OBSTRUCTION (BILATERAL)
RIGHT   LEFT
5 10 15 20   5 10 15 20
MINUTES POSTINJECTION

COMPLETE (LEFT) OBSTRUCTION
RIGHT   LEFT
5 10 15 20   5 10 15 20
MINUTES POSTINJECTION

The means for evaluating total kidney function by noninvasive procedures have been available to physicians for many years. However, before the post-World War II period, little information could be obtained about individual kidney function without resorting to ureteral catheterization. Such a procedure carries a certain morbidity, especially when large ureteral catheters are used. Although it is relatively simple, using small catheters, to obtain information concerning qualitative differences between the two kidneys, to gather information on quantitative differences requires the use of large-sized catheters so that no leak will occur.

The development of renography utilizing radionuclides was in a sense one of the more humane by-products of the Manhattan (atomic bomb) Project of the early 1940s. Radioactive iodine (^{131}I) was one of the readily made products of the reactor pile at Oak Ridge, Tennessee. Utilization of ^{131}I for renal studies was the by-product of prior development of an externally performed tracer test of liver function utilizing ^{131}I-labeled rose bengal. The originator of this methodology, Dr. George D. Taplin, working in cooperation with Dr. Chester Winter, performed the initial clinical studies. Thus, an exceedingly useful clinical tool known in this country as *radioisotope renography* was later developed. In some European countries, the *radioisotope renogram* is known as a *radioisotope nephrogram*.

Technic. Today, this methodology principally utilizes intravenously administered ^{131}I-labeled sodium iodohippurate. However, other tracers such as ^{197}Hg- and

^{203}Hg-labeled chlormerodrin are used also. Regardless of which tracer or radionuclide one uses, the test involves external tracing by *scintillation probes* placed in such a manner that they will detect the uptake and excretion of radionuclides by each kidney.

The illustration shows examples of such graphic recordings of uptake and excretion by normal kidneys and also shows ischemia, and both partial and complete obstruction. Many types of scintillation probes, *collimators, counters,* and other more or less sophisticated methods for interpretation of results have appeared over the years. The methodology can still be exceedingly useful; it retains the advantage of rendering exceedingly low radiation to the patient. Thus, it proves valuable for consecutive studies at frequent intervals. Additionally, the equipment is relatively inexpensive. However, in many instances the technic works to the physician's disadvantage because it records total ac-

tivity obtained over a given kidney without distinguishing between different areas of that kidney. Accurate positioning of the probes is quite critical and yet, since one cannot "see" the kidney as he can with a *gamma scintillation camera,* errors may result.

The enormous contribution made to medicine by the basic technology of radioisotope renography represents the basis for development of the *gamma scintillation camera* (see page 104). This camera supplies the information noted above and, as will be described, has the added advantage of showing the physician both kidneys and the bladder. Furthermore, it spatially depicts the differences in uptake within a kidney.

Therefore, renography, as originally developed, is now primarily of historical interest. Although there are isolated areas in which it still can serve a useful purpose, the development of new detector equipment has made standard renography obsolete. □

Renal Scintillation Scanning

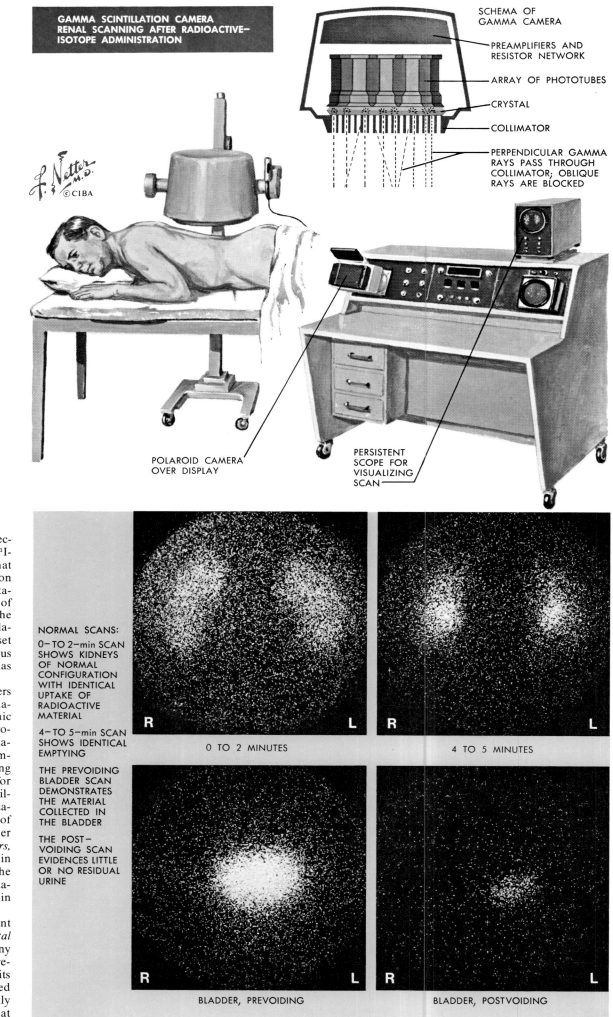

GAMMA SCINTILLATION CAMERA RENAL SCANNING AFTER RADIOACTIVE-ISOTOPE ADMINISTRATION

SCHEMA OF GAMMA CAMERA

PREAMPLIFIERS AND RESISTOR NETWORK

ARRAY OF PHOTOTUBES

CRYSTAL

COLLIMATOR

PERPENDICULAR GAMMA RAYS PASS THROUGH COLLIMATOR; OBLIQUE RAYS ARE BLOCKED

POLAROID CAMERA OVER DISPLAY

PERSISTENT SCOPE FOR VISUALIZING SCAN

NORMAL SCANS:

0- TO 2-min SCAN SHOWS KIDNEYS OF NORMAL CONFIGURATION WITH IDENTICAL UPTAKE OF RADIOACTIVE MATERIAL

4- TO 5-min SCAN SHOWS IDENTICAL EMPTYING

THE PREVOIDING BLADDER SCAN DEMONSTRATES THE MATERIAL COLLECTED IN THE BLADDER

THE POST-VOIDING SCAN EVIDENCES LITTLE OR NO RESIDUAL URINE

0 TO 2 MINUTES

4 TO 5 MINUTES

BLADDER, PREVOIDING

BLADDER, POSTVOIDING

The invention of externally placed detectors that utilize such radionuclides as ^{131}I-labeled sodium iodohippurate, and that picture dynamic events in kidneys, soon led to the development of instrumentation permitting spatial representation of morphology. This equipment utilizes the so-called *rectilinear scanner:* The scintillation probe moves mechanically, in a preset pattern, to picture radioactivity and thus form an image of an organ which has been made radioactive.

Although newer rectilinear scanners could obtain such representation in relatively short periods of time, fast dynamic events prevent such equipment from providing true representation. Thus, the stationary *gamma camera* was the next improvement in this rapidly developing field. Several kinds of gamma cameras for a survey of both kidneys are now available. These units allow rapid visualization of appearance and disappearance of radionuclides of various types. Further refinements, such as *channel analyzers,* permit more exact counts to be made in smaller areas within a kidney. Thus the physician can perform a true quantitation, knowing exactly the specific area in which counting is taking place.

Equipment. Most detector equipment now available uses a *sodium iodide crystal* activated with a trace of *thallium.* A tiny flash of light occurs when a photon, resulting from the radionuclide decay, hits the crystal. *Scintillation* is the term used to describe the multitude of practically simultaneous, tiny flashes of light that result from the release of a quantum of

Renal Scintillation Scanning

Continued

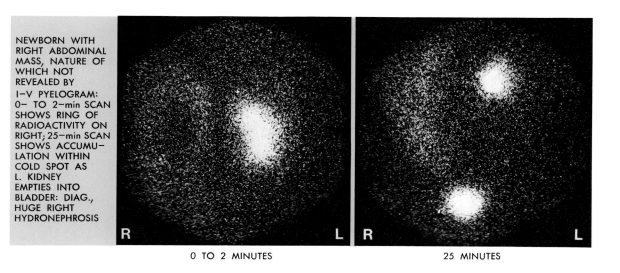

NEWBORN WITH RIGHT ABDOMINAL MASS, NATURE OF WHICH NOT REVEALED BY I–V PYELOGRAM: 0– TO 2–min SCAN SHOWS RING OF RADIOACTIVITY ON RIGHT; 25–min SCAN SHOWS ACCUMULATION WITHIN COLD SPOT AS L. KIDNEY EMPTIES INTO BLADDER: DIAG., HUGE RIGHT HYDRONEPHROSIS

R   L   R   L

0 TO 2 MINUTES   25 MINUTES

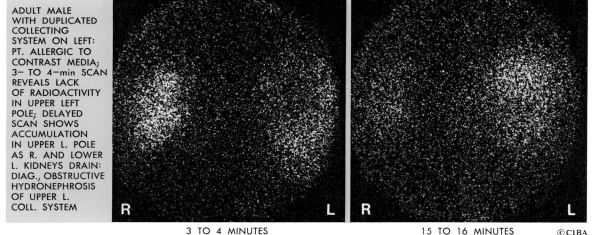

12–YEAR–OLD MALE WITH SEVERE HYPERTENSION: 1– TO 3–min SCAN, DECREASED UPTAKE IN L. LOWER POLE; 10–min SCAN, PERSISTENT ACTIVITY IN L. LOWER POLE; ANGIOGRAM REVEALED VASCULAR ABNORMALITIES IN THIS AREA; L. NEPHRECTOMY CURED HYPERTENSION

R   L   R   L

1 TO 3 MINUTES   10 MINUTES

ADULT MALE WITH DUPLICATED COLLECTING SYSTEM ON LEFT: PT. ALLERGIC TO CONTRAST MEDIA; 3– TO 4–min SCAN REVEALS LACK OF RADIOACTIVITY IN UPPER LEFT POLE; DELAYED SCAN SHOWS ACCUMULATION IN UPPER L. POLE AS R. AND LOWER L. KIDNEYS DRAIN: DIAG., OBSTRUCTIVE HYDRONEPHROSIS OF UPPER L. COLL. SYSTEM

R   L   R   L

3 TO 4 MINUTES   15 TO 16 MINUTES   ©CIBA

gamma radiation, termed an *event*. One or several *photomultiplier tubes*, coupled to the crystal, convert this light into electrical energy, permitting a quantitative assessment of the gamma radiation. The gamma radiation emanating from the organ will go in all directions, but with the use of a *collimator*, usually made of lead and having variable numbers of small channels, only the *primary* gamma rays which travel the shortest straight-line path from the tissue to the crystal will pass to be recorded during scintillation.

The original renogram scintillation probe consists of one small sodium iodide crystal and one photomultiplier tube; the stationary detector, also called a gamma camera, consists of either a large crystal *(Anger camera)* or a multitude of small crystals *(Bender and Blau autofluoroscope).* The collimator is in front of the crystal or crystals. Behind the crystal(s) one finds an array of phototubes, with optical coupling, connected to preamplifiers.

Technic. When the gamma rays strike the crystal, the intensity of each scintillation corresponds to the energy of the event. For instance, should an event occur in the upper pole of the right kidney, a flash of light will be seen in the corresponding place on the oscilloscope. By using time-exposure photography or a persistent oscilloscope, one can form a visible image of these discrete flashes.

Because rapid change of position can be made, the patient can be sitting, prone, or supine. Utilizing the persistent scope, one can view, for example, the uptake of radiohippurate as it occurs, eliminating

the chance that part of one or both kidneys will be missed. Usually an adult is given 300 microcuries of radiohippurate intravenously. In most instances, this dose will give a sufficient count over the kidneys to obtain 1-minute sequence exposure and counts.

The radioactivity delivered to a given patient who has normal kidney function is considerably less than that delivered when obtaining a roentgenogram of the abdomen insofar as the dose received by the kidney is concerned and is insignificant with respect to the gonadal dose. Sodium iodohippurate is given in exceedingly small amounts compared to the amounts of similar organic iodine compounds used for intravenous urography, and reactions to intravenously administered radiohippurate are extremely rare.

A gamma camera, which permits simultaneous viewing of both kidneys, can give the same basic information as renography. Simultaneously, it permits

the pictorial display of those dynamic events with *quantitation* possible over any area selected. This can demonstrate the possible existence of "cold spots" which would indicate renal masses or segmental renal ischemia.

Within the urinary tract, scanning and quantitation of counts over the bladder before and after voiding allow determination of residual urine. If the voided urine volume is known, exact quantitation of residual urine can be obtained without catheterization. Measurement of the radioactivity administered and recovered, and evaluation of total function can be made at the same time using a *dose calibrator.* Thus, within 30 minutes, one can evaluate the kidneys and the entire urinary tract and obtain gross information about morphologic abnormalities. Such a procedure is accurate, with a low radiation dose, and causes little or no patient discomfort. *Continued on page 106*

Renal Scintillation Scanning

Continued from page 105

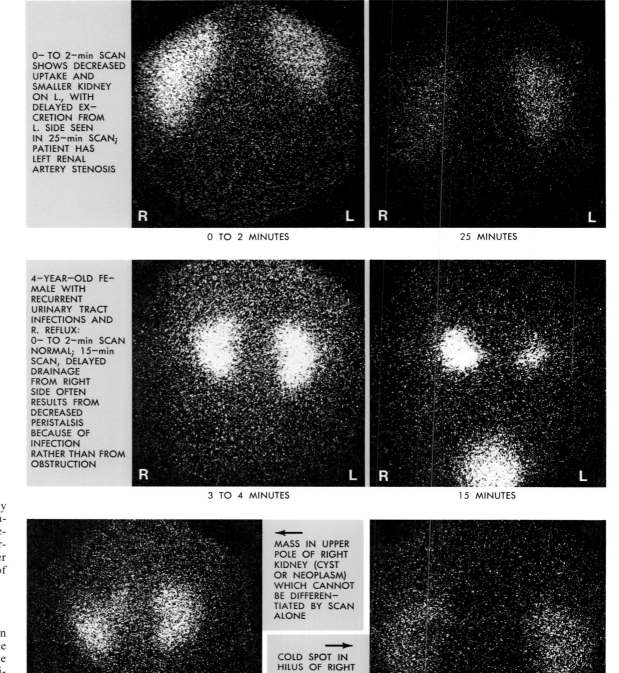

0— TO 2-min SCAN SHOWS DECREASED UPTAKE AND SMALLER KIDNEY ON L., WITH DELAYED EX-CRETION FROM L. SIDE SEEN IN 25-min SCAN; PATIENT HAS LEFT RENAL ARTERY STENOSIS

0 TO 2 MINUTES   25 MINUTES

4—YEAR—OLD FE-MALE WITH RECURRENT URINARY TRACT INFECTIONS AND R. REFLUX: 0— TO 2-min SCAN NORMAL; 15—min SCAN, DELAYED DRAINAGE FROM RIGHT SIDE OFTEN RESULTS FROM DECREASED PERISTALSIS BECAUSE OF INFECTION RATHER THAN FROM OBSTRUCTION

3 TO 4 MINUTES   15 MINUTES

MASS IN UPPER POLE OF RIGHT KIDNEY (CYST OR NEOPLASM) WHICH CANNOT BE DIFFEREN-TIATED BY SCAN ALONE

COLD SPOT IN HILUS OF RIGHT KIDNEY; REPRESENTING LARGE CALCIFIED RENAL ARTERY ANEURYSM

2 TO 3 MINUTES   2 TO 3 MINUTES   ©CIBA

The radionuclide still most commonly used is ^{131}I-labeled sodium iodohippurate, but [99m]Tc (technetium-pertechnetate-99) and [203]Hg- and [197]Hg-labeled chlormerodrin are also used widely. The latter three are valuable in the evaluation of various parameters of renal function.

Gamma Scintillation vs. Intravenous Pyelogram

In some instances, the radiohippurate scan can be of superior diagnostic importance relative to an intravenous pyelogram (see page 91). In patients having known sensitivity to radiopaque media, radiohippurate scans may provide the only diagnostic tool for accurate diagnosis.

In the screening of a hypertensive population in which only about 10 percent of the patients can be shown to have correctable renal arterial lesions, such a noninvasive procedure is of immense importance. It is particularly important to be able to recognize segmental renal ischemia, which is at best exceedingly difficult to detect by standard renography or intravenous pyelography. Utilizing the gamma scintillation camera with quantitation and counts within the renal areas, the physician can quite readily demonstrate such segmental lesions and thus improve the diagnostic yield of hypertensive patients with correctable renal lesions.

It should be emphasized at this time, however, that the emergence of the scintillation camera by no means makes radiology of the urinary tract obsolete. It is important to distinguish between utilization of the renal and urinary tract scintillation scanning, as described here for screening individuals having no particular

renal or urinary symptomatology, and utilization of such procedures for more refined diagnostic evaluation. Although renal scintillation scanning cannot now and possibly may not in the future be able to compete with radiology for more detailed morphologic studies, unquestionably additional information can be obtained by sophisticated scintillation scanning approaches. Also, scanning has applicability in those cases already mentioned in which the use of radiopaque material is contraindicated because of sensitivity.

Thus, the utilization of several radionuclides to delineate specific functional parameters may often complement both the screening procedure and radiologic investigations. In a "poor risk" patient, for instance, where even *angiography* (see page 100) may be considered a hazard, the differential diagnosis between cysts and neoplasm in a kidney can be partially resolved by the utilization of a radiohippurate scan

as well as a *technetium scan*. The radiohippurate scan will reveal a "cold spot," while the technetium scan will show the presence or absence of vascularization. Obviously, however, this methodology will at best differentiate only between a cyst or a necrotic tumor on the one hand and a vascularized neoplasm on the other.

Specific functional information which can be obtained with scintillation has also proven of value in distinguishing between rejection, obstruction, and acute tubular necrosis in renal transplant patients (see page 264). Furthermore, the procedure should be equally applicable to the scanning of patients before and after surgery and following trauma.

Although still in their developmental infancy, radionuclide scanning technics have already become valuable diagnostic tools. The future should hold new and equally valuable advances. □

Renal Biopsy

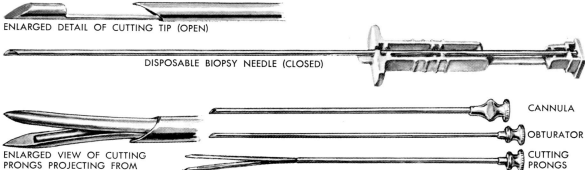

ENLARGED DETAIL OF CUTTING TIP (OPEN)

DISPOSABLE BIOPSY NEEDLE (CLOSED)

ENLARGED VIEW OF CUTTING PRONGS PROJECTING FROM END OF CANNULA

FRANKLIN MODIFICATION OF VIM–SILVERMAN NEEDLE

CANNULA
OBTURATOR
CUTTING PRONGS

Renal biopsy is used primarily to make an exact histologic diagnosis. It also provides data useful in the patient's clinical management and helps the physician assess the prognosis.

Usually the tissue is examined, after appropriate preparation, by light microscopy, electron microscopy, and immunofluorescent technics. In addition, both the renal blood on the biopsy needle and a piece of renal tissue should be cultured. If necessary, special microbiologic studies (virologic, fungal, and animal inoculations) can be done, and in rare instances, histochemical staining, quantitative chemical analysis, and ultramicrochemistry are also useful.

Patient Selection. The contraindications to a renal biopsy are the absence of a kidney, renal neoplasms, polycystic kidneys, and hemorrhagic tendency. Relative contraindications are terminal renal disease, contracted kidneys, progressive uremia, and gross hypertension. Prior to biopsy, in addition to the usual physical examination and laboratory studies, the patient's bleeding, clotting, and prothrombin times are determined. The platelet counts and thromboplastin consumption are also measured. Blood is typed and crossmatched, and compatible blood is set aside. A urine specimen is cultured. An intravenous pyelogram is performed to determine that two kidneys are present and to show their locations.

Preparation and Aftercare of the Patient. The plans for the biopsy are discussed with the patient. In cooperative adults and older children, the biopsy may be done under local anesthesia, and appropriate instructions will ensure that the patient cooperates fully, *e.g.*, by holding his breath when directed. In infants and younger children, either deep sedation or general anesthesia may be required, whereas in uncooperative or seriously ill patients, the biopsy is best performed by surgical exposure of the kidney.

After the percutaneous biopsy, the patient lies flat in bed for 24 hours, and pulse and blood pressure are closely followed. Fluids are given parenterally and orally to ensure good flow of urine. Both the first urine passed after the biopsy and a second specimen 24 hours later are cultured. Aliquots of all other urine specimens passed are saved and examined to determine if there is excessive bleeding. Prior to dis-

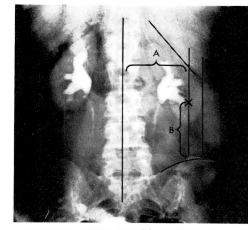

PROPOSED BIOPSY SITE (X) SELECTED ON X–RAY AND ITS TOPOGRAPHY DEFINED BY MEASUREMENT FROM LINES OF SPINOUS PROCESSES, ILIAC CREST, AND 12th RIB

THE SITE IS IDENTIFIED ON PATIENT'S BACK BY IDENTICAL MEASUREMENTS FROM SAME REFERENCE LINES DRAWN IN 1% CRYSTAL VIOLET; PT. LIES PRONE WITH SANDBAGS UNDER ABDOMEN TO FIX KIDNEY AGAINST BACK; BLOOD PRESSURE AND PULSE ARE MONITORED

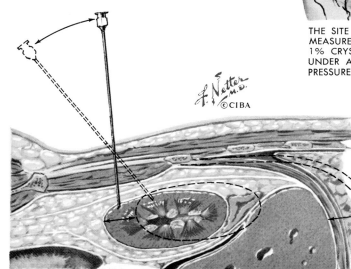

SKIN DISINFECTED, ANESTHETIC WHEAL RAISED, AND SUBCUTANEOUS TISSUES AND MUSCLES OF BACK ANESTHETIZED BELOW WHEAL; 6", 22-GAUGE EXPLORING NEEDLE INTRODUCED TOWARD KIDNEY, PASSING THROUGH BACK MUSCLES; RESISTANCE IS FELT AS NEEDLE PENETRATES RENAL CAPSULE AND NEEDLE SWINGS IN WIDE ARC WITH RESPIRATION; ITS MOTION SHOULD NOT BE RESTRICTED; DEPTH IS MARKED OFF AND NEEDLE WITHDRAWN; PROCAINE IS AGAIN INJECTED (BUT NOT IN KIDNEY SUBSTANCE) AS NEEDLE IS WITHDRAWN

charge the patient is instructed on possible short- and long-term complications and a follow-up visit with his physician is arranged. He is also instructed to report immediately should untoward symptoms occur.

Technic

Biopsy Needles. Although there are many biopsy needles available, the one most commonly used is the Franklin modification of the Vim-Silverman needle, often called the Franklin-Silverman needle. This needle is designed so that the tips of the cutting prongs are sealed. In this way the piece of renal tissue is severed free on all sides. The standard Vim-Silverman needle must not be used because renal tissue is tough, and failures will result with this instrument. A disposable needle similar in construction to the Hamburger needle is also available.

Localization of Puncture Site. Prior to the procedure, the patient empties his bladder and then lies face

down on a firm table. A thin, firm sandbag wrapped in a towel and placed between the patient's abdomen and the table pushes the kidney toward the back.

On the intravenous pyelogram film the physician measures the distances: (1) from the vertebral spinous processes to the lateral margin of the kidney; (2) from the vertebral spinous processes to the selected site of biopsy in the kidney; and (3) from the iliac crest to the proposed renal biopsy site. Next, the physician palpates the twelfth rib, the iliac crest, and the vertebral spinous processes and marks the skin over these bony landmarks with crystal violet dye. The kidney of the patient is then palpated during both inspiration and expiration.

With the three distances measured on the X-rays as a guide, the lateral border of the kidney and the selected site of puncture are drawn on the skin of the patient. *Continued on page 108*

Renal Biopsy

Continued from page 107

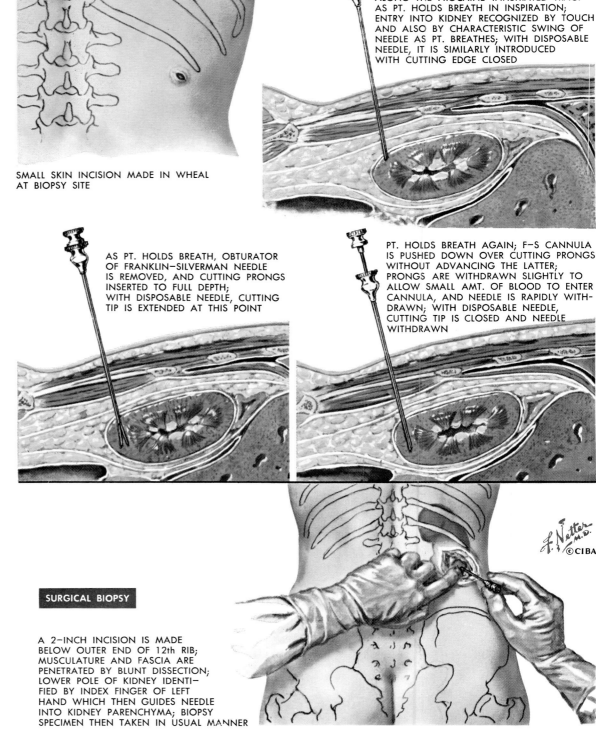

SMALL SKIN INCISION MADE IN WHEAL AT BIOPSY SITE

IF FRANKLIN–SILVERMAN NEEDLE IS USED, CANNULA, WITH OBTURATOR IN PLACE, IS INTRODUCED TO PREMEASURED DEPTH ALONG THE PROCAINE–INFILTRATED TRACT AS PT. HOLDS BREATH IN INSPIRATION; ENTRY INTO KIDNEY RECOGNIZED BY TOUCH AND ALSO BY CHARACTERISTIC SWING OF NEEDLE AS PT. BREATHES; WITH DISPOSABLE NEEDLE, IT IS SIMILARLY INTRODUCED WITH CUTTING EDGE CLOSED

AS PT. HOLDS BREATH, OBTURATOR OF FRANKLIN–SILVERMAN NEEDLE IS REMOVED, AND CUTTING PRONGS INSERTED TO FULL DEPTH; WITH DISPOSABLE NEEDLE, CUTTING TIP IS EXTENDED AT THIS POINT

PT. HOLDS BREATH AGAIN; F–S CANNULA IS PUSHED DOWN OVER CUTTING PRONGS WITHOUT ADVANCING THE LATTER; PRONGS ARE WITHDRAWN SLIGHTLY TO ALLOW SMALL AMT. OF BLOOD TO ENTER CANNULA, AND NEEDLE IS RAPIDLY WITHDRAWN; WITH DISPOSABLE NEEDLE, CUTTING TIP IS CLOSED AND NEEDLE WITHDRAWN

SURGICAL BIOPSY

A 2-INCH INCISION IS MADE BELOW OUTER END OF 12th RIB; MUSCULATURE AND FASCIA ARE PENETRATED BY BLUNT DISSECTION; LOWER POLE OF KIDNEY IDENTIFIED BY INDEX FINGER OF LEFT HAND WHICH THEN GUIDES NEEDLE INTO KIDNEY PARENCHYMA; BIOPSY SPECIMEN THEN TAKEN IN USUAL MANNER

Insertion of Exploratory Needle. The skin of the back is sterilized with appropriate solutions such as iodine followed by alcohol. With sterile gloves donned, the physician drapes the patient's back with sterile towels. If local anesthesia is desired, the site of puncture and the subcutaneous tissues are injected with lidocaine. Meanwhile, a nurse or an assistant at the head of the table monitors blood pressure and pulse.

The physician gently inserts a 6-inch, 22-gauge needle through the skin site and into the tissues of the back. At this point the patient is asked to hold his breath and the needle is passed into the kidney. The patient is now told to resume breathing, and if the needle is in the kidney, it will swing freely through an arc and may also pulsate.

The patient again holds his breath. The exploring needle is held between thumb and forefinger where it meets the skin and is withdrawn. The distance from thumb to needle tip, the depth of the kidney, is measured, and the biopsy needle is appropriately marked.

Obtaining the Biopsy. A small incision is made in the skin at the biopsy site. With the obturator in place, the cannula of the Franklin-Silverman needle is inserted through the incision and, as the patient holds his breath, is passed along the path of the exploratory needle to the premeasured depth. Entry into the kidney is recognized by the characteristic increase in resistance as the renal capsule is encountered and also by the characteristic swing with the resumption of respiration.

Again the patient holds his breath. The obturator is removed, and the cutting prongs are inserted. The cannula of the needle is now advanced deeper over the cutting prongs. The cutting prongs are slightly withdrawn, allowing a small amount of blood to enter the cannula. Finally the cannula and prongs, with the contained sliver of renal tissue, are rapidly withdrawn together.

The procedure using the disposable biopsy needle is essentially similar. This needle is inserted with the cutting edge closed. When the instrument is in the kidney, the cutting tip is extended, and the biopsy is obtained by closing the cutting tip and rapidly withdrawing the needle, as with the Franklin-Silverman needle.

After the needle is withdrawn, pressure is applied to the site of the biopsy for 3 minutes. The wound is dressed and the patient returned to bed.

As noted previously, the tissue obtained is divided into portions for various studies; it is placed in appropriate fixatives or frozen in liquid nitrogen. The needle and small amount of blood within the needle are cultured. It is stressed that the tissue requires special handling by highly trained and competent pathology technicians, and all procedures should be done by hand. Ultrathin sections of 1 to 2 micra are used for light microscopy.

Percutaneous biopsy of the kidney is much easier to do when the kidney is visualized using television-monitored fluoroscopy. The technic and both pre- and postoperative care are as described above, except that contrast material is infused into an arm vein during the procedure and a radiolucent, sausage-shaped bag is placed under the patient. Television-monitored fluoroscopic control has become the procedure of choice in most hospitals which have this equipment. Moreover, disposable renal biopsy needles have become more popular than the Franklin-Silverman type.

Surgical Biopsy. If it is necessary to obtain a renal biopsy surgically, a 2-inch incision is made inferior to the lateral end of the twelfth rib. Blunt section is sufficient to penetrate the muscle and fascial layers of the back, and the inferior pole of the kidney may be identified by the index finger; the finger is used to guide the biopsy needle into the renal parenchyma. Obtaining the actual piece of tissue is otherwise identical to the procedure described for needle biopsy. A single suture can be used to control bleeding, and the wound is closed with one or two sutures and covered by sterile dressing. □

Section IV

Diseases of the Kidney

Frank H. Netter, M.D.

in collaboration with

E. Lovell Becker, M.D.   *Plates 12-15*

D. A. K. Black, M.D., F.R.C.P.   *Plate 27*

Claus Brun, M.D. and Steen Olsen, M.D.   *Plates 1-2*

Jacob Churg, M.D., Marvin Goldstein, M.D.,
and Edith Grishman, M.D.   *Plates 19-25*

Gustave J. Dammin, M.D.   *Plates 30-31*

David P. Earle, M.D.   *Plate 26*

Robert T. McCluskey, M.D.   *Plates 16-18, 28-29*

Theodore N. Pullman, M.D. and Fredric L. Coe, M.D.   *Plates 3-11*

Acute Renal Failure

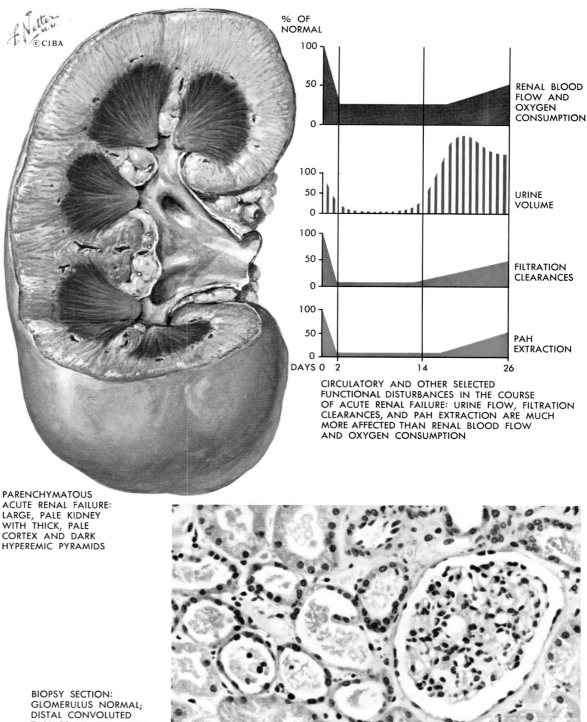

% OF NORMAL

RENAL BLOOD FLOW AND OXYGEN CONSUMPTION

URINE VOLUME

FILTRATION CLEARANCES

PAH EXTRACTION

CIRCULATORY AND OTHER SELECTED FUNCTIONAL DISTURBANCES IN THE COURSE OF ACUTE RENAL FAILURE: URINE FLOW, FILTRATION CLEARANCES, AND PAH EXTRACTION ARE MUCH MORE AFFECTED THAN RENAL BLOOD FLOW AND OXYGEN CONSUMPTION

PARENCHYMATOUS ACUTE RENAL FAILURE: LARGE, PALE KIDNEY WITH THICK, PALE CORTEX AND DARK HYPEREMIC PYRAMIDS

BIOPSY SECTION: GLOMERULUS NORMAL; DISTAL CONVOLUTED TUBULES DILATED, WITH FLATTENED EPITHELIUM, "PRETZEL—LIKE" DISTORTION, AND CONTAINING HEME CASTS (H. & E. STAIN)

Acute renal failure may be defined as a sudden reduction of renal function to a degree which is incompatible with life if continued. This corresponds to a reduction of the endogenous creatinine clearance to values below five percent of normal. With very few exceptions, *oliguria* or *anuria* is present.

There are obviously many conditions which can result in acute renal failure. On the basis of pathogenesis it is convenient to classify these conditions in three groups: *prerenal*, *postrenal*, and *parenchymatous*.

Prerenal Factors. Renal function may be *reversibly* reduced or abolished by numerous factors outside the kidney, such as hypotension, salt depletion, or dehydration. The renal failure lasts only as long as the pre- or extrarenal factors continue.

Postrenal Causes. Renal failure may be caused by obstruction to the flow of urine in the urinary tract which may result from a variety of conditions (see page 185). Frequently, when patients have complete cessation of urine excretion (anuria) as distinguished from diminished urine production (oliguria), postrenal conditions are likely causes.

Parenchymatous acute renal failure is a malfunction of the nephrons. The etiologic factors are multiple and include such widely different diseases as acute glomerulonephritis (see page 131), acute pyelonephritis (see page 189), disseminated lupus erythematosus (LED) (see page 141), polyarteritis nodosa (see page 167), myelomatosis (see page 180), amyloidosis (see page 163), toxic nephropathy (see page 168), and others.

Therapeutically and numerically important, however, is acute renal failure which follows or is associated with incompatible blood transfusions, septicemia, obstetric and gynecologic complications, crush lesions, and major surgery. (Although circulatory or septic shock is frequently associated with this type of acute renal failure, neither is an obligatory prerequisite.) An exact clinical delineation of this type of acute renal failure is not possible. However, there are many clinical features which are common to the various conditions and the histologic findings are widely uniform. Because of the multiple etiologic factors, this type of acute renal failure is known by a large number of names: crush kidney, shock kidney, lower nephron nephrosis, acute tubular necrosis, acute tubulointerstitial nephropathy, and ischemic anuria. Our preferred terminology is *acute tubulointerstitial nephropathy*.

Parenthetically, it is important to differentiate between the renal failure of the so-called "shock kidney" and the oliguria with diminished renal function which accompanies the shock itself. In the latter case, renal function is only transiently reduced and returns to normal immediately or shortly after normal blood pressure is restored. In contrast, in true "shock kidney" the renal failure persists, often for weeks after the restoration of normal circulation.

The pathogenesis of acute tubulointerstitial nephropathy has not been fully elucidated to date. Since the condition often follows shock, *renal hypoxia* has been proposed as the cause of the renal shutdown. However, the available experimental data do not support the contention that *damaging* renal hypoxia occurs during hemorrhagic shock, even though there is marked reduction in renal blood flow. Thus, a hypoxic theory regarding the initiation of acute renal failure following shock must be questioned.

Moreover, in established acute renal failure there is a poor correlation between renal function on the one hand and renal blood flow and oxygen consumption on the other. (The pooled data of several groups of investigators are shown in Plate 1.) It thus appears that the reduction in blood flow and oxygen uptake is probably not the cause of the severe renal insufficiency. Furthermore, there have been only a few observations of the *distribution* of blood flow within the kidney in established acute *Continued on page 112*

Acute Renal Failure

Continued from page 111

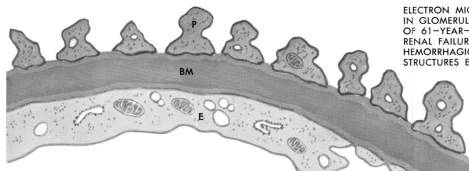

ELECTRON MICROSCOPIC FINDINGS IN GLOMERULAR CAPILLARY WALL OF 61—YEAR—OLD MAN WITH ACUTE RENAL FAILURE FOLLOWING ACUTE HEMORRHAGIC PANCREATITIS: STRUCTURES ESSENTIALLY NORMAL

P = FOOT PROCESSES OF EPITHELIUM
BM = BASEMENT MEMBRANE
E = CYTOPLASM OF ENDOTHELIAL CELL

renal failure. These observations suggest that the cortical blood flow is primarily affected. Thus it must be concluded that the noxious agent in production of acute renal failure has not yet been identified.

Pathology. Grossly, the kidney in patients who have acute anuria is large and pale. On section, the thick, pale cortex contrasts with the dark, hyperemic pyramids. Since rapid autolytic changes render the study of tubular details impossible after a few hours, the histologic structure is best studied in biopsy material. Characteristically, the glomeruli are normal even though there is severe functional reduction. The distal convoluted tubules, and to some extent the proximal tubules, are dilated, with flattened epithelium.

Casts of brownish or reddish granular material (hemecasts) are seen in both the distal and collecting tubules. Complete or widespread necrosis of tubular epithelium is absent in biopsy material, but degenerative changes are not infrequently found in the epithelium surrounding the casts in the distal tubules. The term "acute tubular necrosis" is thus not particularly appropriate.

A slight-to-moderate, focal, interstitial, cellular infiltration of lymphocytes, plasma cells, and granulocytes is present, together with a moderate interstitial edema, especially in patients with manifest clinical overhydration. Also, hydropic changes in the proximal tubular epithelium appear to be produced by infusion of solutions such as mannitol, sucrose, and dextran. In patients with renal failure combined with icterus, bile pigment may be found in the casts and tubular cells. In general, the light microscopic picture, as seen in biopsy material, is rather characteristic and permits a histologic diagnosis.

Electron microscopy of biopsy material has confirmed the normal glomerular appearance observed with light microscopy. In addition, the epithelium of the distal tubules presents lesions of the degenerative type, but necrosis is only rarely seen. In patients treated with mannitol solution or dextran, the proximal tubular epithelium often shows severe vacuolization, but no other constant lesions are observed.

It is obvious that neither the structural nor ultrastructural lesions observed in

HISTOLOGIC FINDINGS IN ACUTE RENAL FAILURE TREATED WITH LOW MOLECULAR WEIGHT DEXTRAN: HYDROPIC DEGENERATION OF TUBULAR EPITHELIUM WITH INTRUSION OF THE TRANSFORMED EPITHELIUM INTO BOWMAN'S CAPSULE

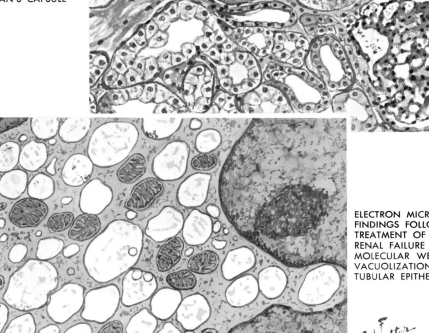

ELECTRON MICROSCOPIC FINDINGS FOLLOWING TREATMENT OF ACUTE RENAL FAILURE WITH LOW MOLECULAR WEIGHT DEXTRAN: VACUOLIZATION OF THE PROXIMAL TUBULAR EPITHELIUM

acute anuria adequately explain the pathogenesis.

The clinical picture during the first few days of renal shutdown is that of the underlying disease. Even during the first week, the only additional symptoms may be limited to lethargy and nausea. The urine is scanty, of high specific gravity, and usually contains protein, red blood cells, and reddish granular casts (hemecasts). Traces of glucose may also be found. As the condition progresses, the clinical features are related to the rising azotemia, increasing acidosis, and increasing serum potassium levels. Cardiac complications can occur even in patients who have not gained weight. Overhydration represents an additional threat to the integrity of the circulation, and patients may develop congestive cardiac failure. The cardiovascular manifestations are further complicated by potassium intoxication which may be corrected, to a certain extent, by administration of glucose, correction of acidosis, oral or rectal use of

potassium-absorbing ion exchange resins, and digitalization. However, sudden death can occur since the susceptibility of the heart to vagal stimulation is increased with elevated serum potassium levels. Thus, if hyperkalemia cannot be controlled by the measures outlined, dialysis should be used. Coma, convulsions, and anemia may occur as the renal shutdown continues.

After a period of about 14 days, diuresis begins. Usually, this signals the end of the renal shutdown. However, the prognosis is not good, and in approximately 50 percent of the cases death occurs, mainly a result of the underlying serious disease or some complication of the underlying condition. The outcome is usually favorable in young patients in whom the original disease is cured (*e.g.*, gynecologic and obstetric cases). Ordinarily if patients survive, they regain normal or nearly normal renal function, even after long-standing oliguria or anuria. □

Chronic Renal Failure

Chronic renal failure usually results from chronic intrinsic renal disease. Almost any progressive bilateral nephropathy can terminate in chronic renal failure. Even such initially nonrenal diseases as obstructive nephropathies (see page 185) may eventually produce intrinsic renal disease and chronic renal failure. However, chronic renal failure is unlike acute renal failure (see page 111) which may be caused by both nonrenal and renal factors.

The same pattern of functional derangement in renal failure can result from any number of diverse renal diseases. (Plate 3 is intended to be illustrative rather than plenary in its classifications of causes.) The functional consequences of such diverse entities as ischemia, increased intrapelvic pressure, infection with certain microorganisms, or deposition of complement-binding antigen-antibody complexes can be remarkably similar in end result. However, in man, the most common causes of chronic renal failure are the diffuse, bilateral, progressive forms of glomerulonephritis and other nephritides.

Mild impairment of renal function is usually detectable only by imposition of unusual demands upon the kidney, as during concentration tests (see page 82), or by presenting the kidney with an exogenous solute such as para-aminohippurate (PAH) for which a normal kidney exhibits a high clearance (see page 43).

As renal function progressively declines, a state of *general renal insufficiency* supervenes. However, advancing renal impairment should not be viewed as a cascade of clearly delineated stages but as a continuum of increasing restriction of homeostatic functions.

Generally, *renal insufficiency* is regarded as a moderately severe phase of functional impairment and is chiefly characterized by a marked loss of flexibility of renal homeostatic function despite absence of major alterations in body fluid composition. At times, however, unusual dietary or metabolic stress may precipitate such changes in body fluids.

Further loss in function results in *renal failure*, a term that usually connotes abnormalities in the composition of body fluids; the homeostatic powers of the kidneys are depressed beyond that point at which the kidneys can adjust appropriately for the ordinary metabolic demands of the body.

Use of the term *uremia* is more traditional than utilitarian. Generally, it refers to the constellation of clinical findings associated with terminal renal disease. It is discussed more fully on pages 121 and 122.

Water Excretion

When renal substance is lost by surgical removal, the remaining tissue undergoes

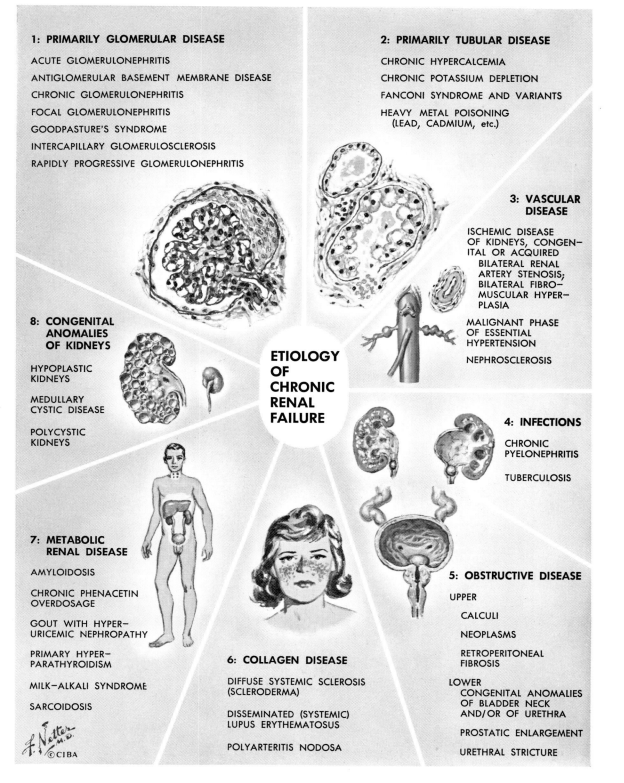

1: PRIMARILY GLOMERULAR DISEASE

ACUTE GLOMERULONEPHRITIS

ANTIGLOMERULAR BASEMENT MEMBRANE DISEASE

CHRONIC GLOMERULONEPHRITIS

FOCAL GLOMERULONEPHRITIS

GOODPASTURE'S SYNDROME

INTERCAPILLARY GLOMERULOSCLEROSIS

RAPIDLY PROGRESSIVE GLOMERULONEPHRITIS

2: PRIMARILY TUBULAR DISEASE

CHRONIC HYPERCALCEMIA

CHRONIC POTASSIUM DEPLETION

FANCONI SYNDROME AND VARIANTS

HEAVY METAL POISONING
(LEAD, CADMIUM, etc.)

3: VASCULAR DISEASE

ISCHEMIC DISEASE OF KIDNEYS, CONGENITAL OR ACQUIRED BILATERAL RENAL ARTERY STENOSIS; BILATERAL FIBROMUSCULAR HYPERPLASIA

MALIGNANT PHASE OF ESSENTIAL HYPERTENSION

NEPHROSCLEROSIS

ETIOLOGY OF CHRONIC RENAL FAILURE

8: CONGENITAL ANOMALIES OF KIDNEYS

HYPOPLASTIC KIDNEYS

MEDULLARY CYSTIC DISEASE

POLYCYSTIC KIDNEYS

7: METABOLIC RENAL DISEASE

AMYLOIDOSIS

CHRONIC PHENACETIN OVERDOSAGE

GOUT WITH HYPERURICEMIC NEPHROPATHY

PRIMARY HYPERPARATHYROIDISM

MILK–ALKALI SYNDROME

SARCOIDOSIS

4: INFECTIONS

CHRONIC PYELONEPHRITIS

TUBERCULOSIS

5: OBSTRUCTIVE DISEASE

UPPER

CALCULI

NEOPLASMS

RETROPERITONEAL FIBROSIS

LOWER
CONGENITAL ANOMALIES OF BLADDER NECK AND/OR OF URETHRA

PROSTATIC ENLARGEMENT

URETHRAL STRICTURE

6: COLLAGEN DISEASE

DIFFUSE SYSTEMIC SCLEROSIS (SCLERODERMA)

DISSEMINATED (SYSTEMIC) LUPUS ERYTHEMATOSUS

POLYARTERITIS NODOSA

hypertrophy and hyperplasia, but no new nephrons are formed. The simplest demonstration of this structural adaptation to loss of functioning nephrons is evidenced by the hypertrophy of the remaining kidney within hours after its mate has been removed.

There are also functional correlates of the well-documented *structural hypertrophy*. For instance, the remaining kidney ultimately displays an effective renal plasma flow and glomerular filtration rate of approximately 80 percent of the values obtained with two normal kidneys. The most pronounced changes occur in the proximal convolution and the loop of Henle, but the entire nephron, including the glomerulus, participates in the hypertrophy. Parenthetically, it does not seem to matter whether removal of functional renal tissue is accomplished by unilateral nephrectomy or by excision of a portion of a kidney. In excisional experiments the remnant of renal tissue shows both

functional and morphologic hypertrophy of intact nephrons.

In experimentally induced, diffuse renal disease, findings similar to those observed in excisional experiments have been repeatedly reported. Similarly, in chronic renal failure in man caused by diffuse bilateral progressive forms of glomerulonephritis and other parenchymal diseases, the unaffected nephrons show hypertrophy and hyperplasia not unlike those found in excisional experiments in animals. Therefore, from many clinical observations and animal experiments, the concept has evolved that the common structural basis for renal failure in man is a diminution in the *number* of functioning nephrons, with the remaining nephrons exhibiting hypertrophy and its functional correlate, increased work per nephron. This concept, cogently articulated by Sir Robert Platt and subsequently supported by data *Continued on page 114*

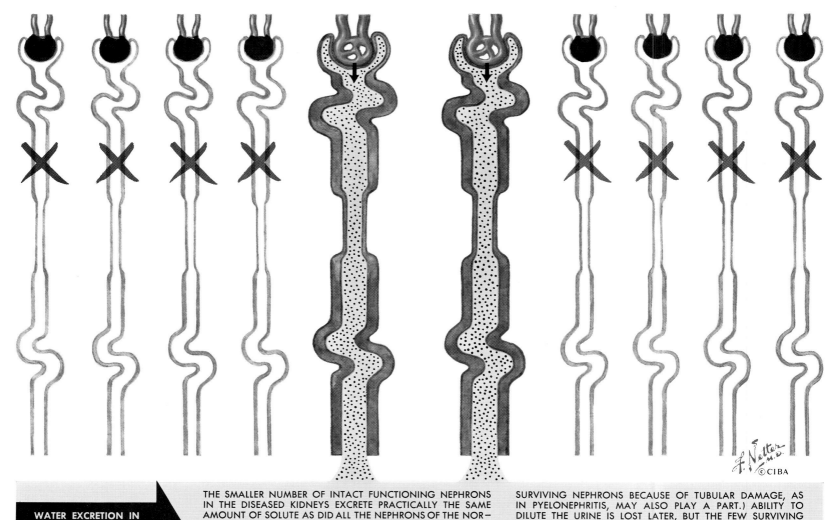

WATER EXCRETION IN RENAL INSUFFICIENCY: INTACT NEPHRON THEORY

THE SMALLER NUMBER OF INTACT FUNCTIONING NEPHRONS IN THE DISEASED KIDNEYS EXCRETE PRACTICALLY THE SAME AMOUNT OF SOLUTE AS DID ALL THE NEPHRONS OF THE NOR‑ MAL KIDNEY. THUS THE SOLUTE EXCRETED PER SURVIVING NEPHRON IS INCREASED, RESULTING IN OSMOTIC DIURESIS, i.e., RISE IN URINE FLOW AND REDUCTION IN CONCENTRA‑ TION. (DIMINISHED WATER REABSORPTION CAPACITY OF THE

SURVIVING NEPHRONS BECAUSE OF TUBULAR DAMAGE, AS IN PYELONEPHRITIS, MAY ALSO PLAY A PART.) ABILITY TO DILUTE THE URINE IS LOST LATER, BUT THE FEW SURVIVING NEPHRONS MAY NOT BE ABLE TO EXCRETE THE SAME TOTAL AMOUNT OF WATER AS DID ALL THE NEPHRONS OF THE NORMAL KIDNEY, RESULTING IN IMPAIRED ABILITY TO EXCRETE A WATER LOAD.

Chronic Renal Failure

Continued from page 113

provided by an ingenious experimental model developed by Dr. Neal Bricker, has been called the *intact nephron hypothesis.* However, it cannot be expected to offer insight into the abnormalities generated by lesions associated with nephrotoxins or by diseases which have selective actions (see *mercury* or *dichromate poisoning,* page 168, and *acute tubular necrosis,* page 111, or variants of the *Fanconi syndrome,* page 247).

It must be emphasized that nephrons are not all structurally identical and that it is only reasonable to expect an association between structure and function. For example, differences in function between nephrons with long and short loops of Henle are well known (see pages 51-59), and further differences certainly occur in disease states. Nevertheless, the concept of *filtration rate per nephron* (whether computed as an average or measured in a superficial cortical nephron) has practical usefulness just as the idea of glomerular filtration rate per kidney has meaning. In chronic renal insufficiency caused by either diffuse renal disease or surgical removal of renal tissue, the concept of a population of residual, but overworked, nephrons has utility, if a literal definition of structural integrity or normalcy is not demanded.

An increase in the number of osmotically active particles requiring excretion causes an increase in urine volume per minute, whether the kidneys

are normal or diseased. This osmotic effect, exerted primarily in the proximal convolution, decreases the rate of reabsorption of the glomerular filtrate. If the number of milliosmoles demanding excretion continues to increase, urine volume increases further and the osmolality of the urine approaches that of the glomerular filtrate.

In Plate 4, eight out of 10 nephrons are represented as nonfunctional. The remaining two of 10 are depicted as hypertrophied. Several facts immediately become apparent, and a number of deductions can be made. First, it is known that the *measured rate* of solute excretion per kidney is the same whether kidney function is normal or depressed to 20 percent of normal. Second, although total glomerular filtration rate is decreased, mean glomerular filtration rate *per functioning nephron* is greatly augmented. Third, homeostatic regulation must be achieved with 20 percent of the functional units available for this task.

Since the amount of solute presented to the tubules is directly proportional to the glomerular filtration rate, residual healthy nephrons are working in excess of their normal capacity and thereby achieve a total solute excretory rate indistinguishable from that of a normal kidney. However, this is accomplished by decreased water reabsorption, resulting in a loss of *concentrating ability* termed *hyposthenuria* (one of the early signs of chronic renal failure) and polyuria.

Somewhat later in the disease process, impairment of the ability to dilute urine appears and

results in the formation of urine of relatively *fixed osmolality*—isosthenuria. As renal insufficiency progresses and *azotemia* supervenes, the increased concentration of urea adds to the total osmotic load.

It is apparent that the common denominator of greatest importance in chronic renal failure is loss or impairment of homeostatic functions. As noted previously, the intact nephrons must perform all the work of the normal complement of nephrons, or as shown schematically, two nephrons excrete the same amount of solute as 10 nephrons of a normal kidney by excreting more solvent.

As renal disease progresses, the kidneys maintain excretion of urea, creatinine, and inorganic phosphate because the concentration of these substances in plasma is elevated. However, the ability of the residual nephrons to compensate for metabolic exigencies is sharply curtailed, since the nephrons can vary the osmolality of the urine only within narrow limits.

Acid-Base Disturbances

Loss of functioning nephrons at first produces no change in blood pH because the remaining nephrons increase their rates of acid excretion. Thus, in the early stages of renal disease, diminished acid excretion can be detected only by using acid-loading tests (see page 87). Continued loss of nephrons, however, progressively restricts acid excretion and leads to the gradual appearance of metabolic acidosis.

Chronic Renal Failure

Continued

In principle, renal disease could impair acid excretion by damaging any or all of the mechanisms that normally maintain acid-base homeostasis (see pages 60-64). However, bicarbonate reabsorption and distal tubular proton secretion are usually well preserved in renal disease, and the primary reasons for impaired acid excretion are decreased availability of ammonia and urinary buffers.

The first detectable abnormality of acid excretion is the decline in the rate of urinary ammonium excretion. At this stage, total acid excretion is usually still normal because protons that would otherwise have combined with ammonia (NH_3) are excreted in the form of titratable acid.

As renal disease progresses, ammonium excretion generally becomes quite low, and acid excretion comes to depend almost entirely upon excretion of titratable acid. (Note that Plate 5 depicts changes which occur in the later stages of renal failure.)

Titratable acid excretion usually remains relatively intact until *glomerular filtration rate* (GFR) falls to 20 percent, or even 15 percent, of normal. The stability of this mechanism results from well-preserved proton secretion in the distal tubule and continued delivery of phosphate for excretion. In turn, the maintenance of urinary phosphate excretion depends upon two factors: (1) As GFR falls, serum phosphate concentration rises reciprocally so that the filtered load—the product of GFR and serum phosphate concentration—remains reasonably constant; (2) there is a decrease in proximal tubular phosphate reabsorption. Normally, 80 percent or more of filtered phosphate is reabsorbed and does not appear in the final urine. However, as GFR declines, this fraction falls to as little as 10 percent, and urinary phosphate excretion can remain nearly normal despite a fall in the filtered load.

The decrease in tubular phosphate reabsorption, so critical to the maintenance of acid excretion in the presence of progressive renal failure, results from an increased secretion of parathyroid hormone. This is stimulated by phosphate retention and the consequent diminished absorption of calcium from the gastrointestinal tract (see page 119).

When GFR falls below 15 to 20 percent of normal, titratable acid excretion begins to fall despite the two compensatory mechanisms, and renal acid excretion becomes progressively inadequate, leading to severe systemic acidosis (as depicted in Plate 5).

This general pattern—an early fall in ammonium excretion, subsequent gradual

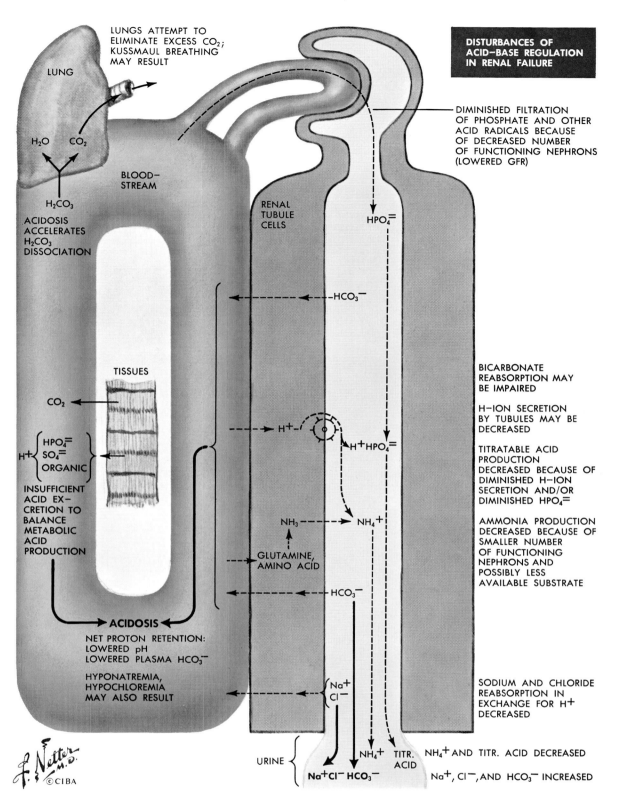

DISTURBANCES OF ACID–BASE REGULATION IN RENAL FAILURE

LUNGS ATTEMPT TO ELIMINATE EXCESS CO_2; KUSSMAUL BREATHING MAY RESULT

LUNG

H_2O CO_2

H_2CO_3

ACIDOSIS ACCELERATES H_2CO_3 DISSOCIATION

BLOOD-STREAM

TISSUES

CO_2

H^+ { $HPO_4^=$ $SO_4^=$ ORGANIC

INSUFFICIENT ACID EXCRETION TO BALANCE METABOLIC ACID PRODUCTION

ACIDOSIS

NET PROTON RETENTION: LOWERED pH LOWERED PLASMA HCO_3^-

HYPONATREMIA, HYPOCHLOREMIA MAY ALSO RESULT

RENAL TUBULE CELLS

DIMINISHED FILTRATION OF PHOSPHATE AND OTHER ACID RADICALS BECAUSE OF DECREASED NUMBER OF FUNCTIONING NEPHRONS (LOWERED GFR)

$HPO_4^=$

HCO_3^-

H^+

$H^+ HPO_4^=$

NH_3 → NH_4^+

GLUTAMINE, AMINO ACID

HCO_3^-

Na^+ Cl^-

BICARBONATE REABSORPTION MAY BE IMPAIRED

H–ION SECRETION BY TUBULES MAY BE DECREASED

TITRATABLE ACID PRODUCTION DECREASED BECAUSE OF DIMINISHED H–ION SECRETION AND/OR DIMINISHED $HPO_4^=$

AMMONIA PRODUCTION DECREASED BECAUSE OF SMALLER NUMBER OF FUNCTIONING NEPHRONS AND POSSIBLY LESS AVAILABLE SUBSTRATE

SODIUM AND CHLORIDE REABSORPTION IN EXCHANGE FOR H^+ DECREASED

URINE { NH_4^+ TITR. ACID NH_4^+ AND TITR. ACID DECREASED

$Na^+ Cl^- HCO_3^-$ Na^+, Cl^-, AND HCO_3^- INCREASED

decline of titratable acid excretion, nearly normal preservation of bicarbonate reclamation, and maintenance of proton secretion in the distal nephron—occurs in the great majority of patients suffering from renal disease. On occasion, however, patients depart from this pattern and manifest disturbances of bicarbonate reabsorption or proton secretion. In this event, acid excretion can be severely compromised in the presence of a normal or only slightly reduced glomerular filtration rate. Failure to reabsorb filtered bicarbonate completely leads to metabolic acidosis by selectively depleting the body of the conjugate base (*i.e.*, HCO_3^- of the CO_2 and H_2CO_3 buffer system). Furthermore, inability to achieve an appropriately acid fluid in the lumen of the distal tubule directly compromises the formation and excretion of ammonium ions and decreases titratable acidity.

Disorders of bicarbonate reabsorption and distal proton secretion may produce acidosis despite normal GFR. These disorders are referred to as forms of *renal tubular acidosis* (RTA) and are discussed in detail on pages 248-249.

RTA secondary to abnormal bicarbonate reabsorption often is designated *proximal RTA* because most bicarbonate reabsorption occurs in the proximal convoluted tubule; the defect is presumed to reside in the proximal tubule.

Impairment of proton secretion is called *distal RTA* for analogous reasons. Another more correct name for this abnormality is *gradient RTA*, because the principal defect is an absolute limitation, not upon the rate of proton secretion, but upon the maximum pH gradient that can be achieved by the tubular epithelium between luminal fluid and blood. Normally this gradient can be up to 1000:1. With gradient RTA, it is 100:1 or less. *Continued on page 116*

Chronic Renal Failure

Continued from page 115

Selective acidification defects (forms of RTA) have been described for many renal diseases. Proximal RTA, which is rare, is usually associated with other proximal tubular disorders constituting complete or incomplete forms of the Fanconi syndrome. Distal RTA usually is a hereditary renal disease but can occur in a variety of acquired renal diseases such as urinary tract obstruction, pyelonephritis, and interstitial nephritis and in renal abnormalities produced by such systemic disorders as hyperglobulinemic states, hypercalcemia, sickle cell anemia, hepatorenal syndrome, and phenacetin abuse.

Impact on Systemic Physiology. Whether the mechanism of acid retention is the common one of restricted ammonium excretion or the uncommon one of acidification defects, the impact upon systemic physiology is the same. Retained protons titrate all available extra- and intracellular buffer systems. Principal among the extracellular fluid buffers is bicarbonate (HCO_3^-), which in the process of titration forms carbon dioxide and water, with a resulting fall in plasma bicarbonate content (see page 61). Plasma proteins and intracellular buffers (of which hemoglobin within red cells is most important) share in the stabilization of blood pH. A fraction of the retained protons titrate bone salts, thereby liberating calcium and phosphate from bone and diminishing bone mineral content.

The respiratory center is stimulated by lowered blood pH acting on chemoreceptors in the great vessels and brain stem. The resulting increase in respiratory rate and depth lowers the partial pressure of carbon dioxide, thereby helping maintain nearly normal blood pH at the expense of a further lowering of plasma bicarbonate content. As renal failure advances and acid retention becomes more severe, this respiratory compensation becomes increasingly essential to maintenance of blood pH within a range compatible with life. At this stage, severe overventilation, often referred to as *Kussmaul breathing*, begins to appear. Usually, it is present only in patients suffering from far-advanced renal failure and uremia.

Blood and urine findings in patients who have acidosis secondary to renal failure are characteristic. Blood pH, pCO_2, and bicarbonate concentrations are all low; serum phosphate concentration is high. Other anions such as sulfate are also increased. As a result, the "anion gap"—the difference between sodium plus potassium, and chloride plus bicarbonate—increases above the usual upper limit of 15 mEq/l. Urine pH is generally quite low, and the urine contains little ammonium ion.

Findings are similar in patients who have the uncommon syndrome of RTA, except that hyperchloremia is present. Filtration and excretion of anions such as phosphate and sulfate are better preserved than proton excretion. Since plasma

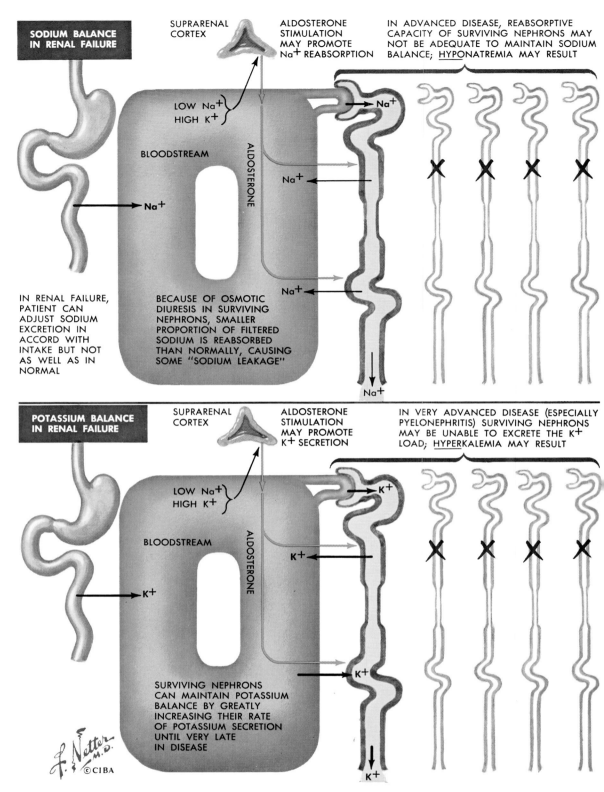

bicarbonate concentration falls, chloride (the only readily available reabsorbable anion) is conserved in order to maintain serum electroneutrality. In addition to having hyperchloremic acidosis, patients with the gradient form of RTA have alkaline or insufficiently acid urine which reflects the underlying defects.

Sodium Balance

In renal disease, an increased sodium load per residual nephron results from the increased glomerular filtration rate per nephron. The absolute rate of sodium reabsorption per nephron is thus increased, but fractional sodium reabsorption is low (see page 46). Consequently, the remaining functional tubules reabsorb sodium at a rate approaching their maximum abilities, but at the same time there is an obligatory *loss* of sodium in the urine. Therefore, the patient in chronic renal failure is particularly prone to sodium depletion

if the intake of sodium is curtailed by diet or, as is often the case, if nausea and vomiting are present.

Such a restriction in salt intake causes a common sequence of events. Because the kidney is unable to reduce sodium excretion appropriately, a small negative sodium balance occurs. This process results in a slowly developing, cumulative, severe extracellular volume depletion so that eventually glomerular filtration rate is reduced. Reduction in renal blood flow may also occur if *oligemia* develops; the symptoms and chemical abnormalities of uremia are therefore intensified.

This apparent worsening of the patient's condition is reversible upon administration of adequate amounts of salt and water. If attempts are made to correct the dehydration with water alone, a *dilutional hyponatremia* will develop.

In the later stages of renal failure there is a limited ability to augment sodium excretion. An increase in

Chronic Renal Failure
Continued

dietary sodium which would not be excessive for a normal person could then be sufficient to lead to heart failure or fluid overload.

Other factors play roles in determining net sodium balance. *Secondary hyperaldosteronism* may result from diminution of blood volume secondary to sodium depletion, or from low plasma volume when hypoalbuminemia accompanies renal failure. Patients with severe hypertension or renal artery stenosis tend to develop particularly severe manifestations of secondary hyperaldosteronism. The common denominator in secondary hyperaldosteronism involves the juxtaglomerular (JG) apparatus and the renin-angiotensin system which have been described elsewhere (see page 49 and CIBA COLLECTION, Vol. 4, pages 95–97).

Potassium Balance

Although total body potassium in a normal human adult is slightly less than total body sodium (42 mEq/kg vs. 60 mEq/kg), the differences in the function and distribution of these two ions pose radically different problems for renal homeostasis.

Roughly 50 percent of total body sodium is extracellular, 10 percent or less is in the nonosseous *intracellular* compartment, and about 40 percent of the total is associated with bone. Somewhat more than half the amount in bone is nonexchangeable.

In contrast, 98 percent of total body potassium is intracellular in a concentration of 160 mEq/l and is readily exchangeable. The remaining two percent is distributed throughout the extracellular fluid in a concentration of only 4 mEq/l, which is less than three percent of the extracellular concentration of sodium. Thus, movement of a small amount of potassium from the intracellular fluid compartment of about 35 liters (potassium concentration of 160 mEq/l) into the 20-liter extracellular compartment (potassium concentration of 4 mEq/l) could be catastrophic without a sensitive and responsive regulatory mechanism.

With the exception of a small moiety lost in gastrointestinal secretions, the kidney remains the chief organ for disposal of excess potassium. Under normal circumstances the excretory rate of potassium is independent of the rate at which potassium is filtered at the glomeruli. Much experimental evidence supports the concept that filtered potassium undergoes almost complete reabsorption in the proximal convolution, and that the excretory rate of potassium is dependent mainly upon secretory activity of the distal tubular epithelium (see page 50 for a review).

Relatively normal excretion of potassium in the earlier stages of renal failure, despite impairment of glomerular filtration rate, suggests that the tubular secretory capacity for potassium has undergone functional adaptive hypertrophy. However, as with other homeostatic functions,

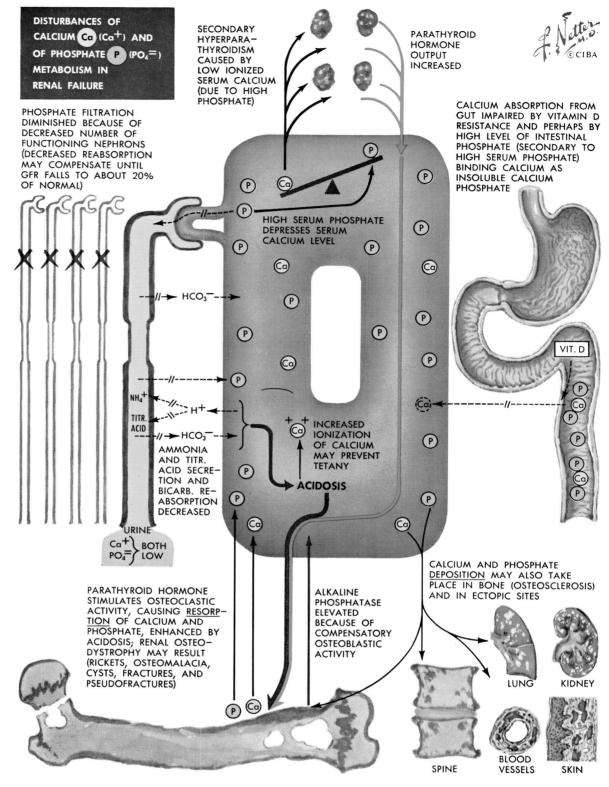

DISTURBANCES OF CALCIUM Ca (Ca⁺) AND OF PHOSPHATE P (PO₄⁼) METABOLISM IN RENAL FAILURE

PHOSPHATE FILTRATION DIMINISHED BECAUSE OF DECREASED NUMBER OF FUNCTIONING NEPHRONS (DECREASED REABSORPTION MAY COMPENSATE UNTIL GFR FALLS TO ABOUT 20% OF NORMAL)

SECONDARY HYPERPARA-THYROIDISM CAUSED BY LOW IONIZED SERUM CALCIUM (DUE TO HIGH PHOSPHATE)

PARATHYROID HORMONE OUTPUT INCREASED

CALCIUM ABSORPTION FROM GUT IMPAIRED BY VITAMIN D RESISTANCE AND PERHAPS BY HIGH LEVEL OF INTESTINAL PHOSPHATE (SECONDARY TO HIGH SERUM PHOSPHATE) BINDING CALCIUM AS INSOLUBLE CALCIUM PHOSPHATE

HIGH SERUM PHOSPHATE DEPRESSES SERUM CALCIUM LEVEL

VIT. D

HCO_3^-

NH_4^+

TITR. ACID

H^+

HCO_3^-

AMMONIA AND TITR. ACID SECRETION AND BICARB. REABSORPTION DECREASED

INCREASED IONIZATION OF CALCIUM MAY PREVENT TETANY

ACIDOSIS

URINE
Ca⁺ } BOTH
PO₄⁼ } LOW

PARATHYROID HORMONE STIMULATES OSTEOCLASTIC ACTIVITY, CAUSING RESORPTION OF CALCIUM AND PHOSPHATE, ENHANCED BY ACIDOSIS; RENAL OSTEODYSTROPHY MAY RESULT (RICKETS, OSTEOMALACIA, CYSTS, FRACTURES, AND PSEUDOFRACTURES)

ALKALINE PHOSPHATASE ELEVATED BECAUSE OF COMPENSATORY OSTEOBLASTIC ACTIVITY

CALCIUM AND PHOSPHATE DEPOSITION MAY ALSO TAKE PLACE IN BONE (OSTEOSCLEROSIS) AND IN ECTOPIC SITES

LUNG   KIDNEY

SPINE

BLOOD VESSELS   SKIN

the failing kidney exhibits marked diminution in reserve. Therefore, excretion of potassium is usually normal until the late stages of renal failure, unless there is an increase in *potassium load.* Such increased loads include catabolic response to stress, injury or tissue death, hemolytic episodes, acidosis, and the use of such drugs as spironolactone and triamterene, all of which may lead to hyperkalemia.

As described previously (see page 50), the antikaliuretic effects of decreased distal tubular sodium delivery are explained by the relation of sodium concentration to intratubular negativity and to the flow-limited characteristics of the distal potassium transport system. In salt depletion, less sodium reaches the distal tubule, and therefore, less intratubular negativity is generated by salt reabsorption. In addition, distal tubular flow rate is diminished in sodium depletion. Both of these mechanisms apparently act to diminish potas-

sium secretion and thereby induce hyperkalemia.

Hypokalemia is an uncommon event in chronic renal failure. If hypokalemia occurs, it is usually secondary to potassium losses associated with gastrointestinal disturbances. However, occasionally, patients suffering from renal failure and normokalemia will develop hypokalemia if acidosis is corrected. Also, potassium depletion may occur because of *secondary hyperaldosteronism* (see CIBA COLLECTION, Vol. 4, pages 95–97; also see page 49) which may supervene in patients in chronic renal failure.

Calcium and Phosphorus Disturbances

Normal Calcium-Phosphorus Metabolism. The serum level of ionized calcium is maintained by a variety of factors including rates of bone dissolution and renewal, overall ionic strength of the plasma, and plasma pH and by a variety of physicochemical *Continued on page 118*

Chronic Renal Failure

Continued from page 117

interactions involving calcium in solution, in solid phase, and bound to protein. However, the most potent regulator of serum calcium level is the serum level of *parathyroid hormone* (PTH).

A complete review of the mechanisms for calcium and phosphorus homeostasis may be found in the CIBA COLLECTION, Vol. 4, pages 178 and following. For convenience, a brief summary follows.

The major if not sole stimulus to parathyroid hormone secretion and release is a fall in *ionized* serum calcium levels. Conversely, parathyroid hormone secretion is suppressed by an increase in ionized serum calcium level. At any given total serum calcium concentration, ionized calcium concentration reflects the interaction between protein binding, blood pH, and serum phosphorus levels.

To a great extent, protein binding of calcium has a fixed constant. Decreased serum protein concentration may thus lead to lowered *total* serum calcium concentration, but normal *ionized* calcium concentration is maintained.

Serum phosphorus and ionized serum calcium are in equilibrium with solid phase calcium-phosphorus minerals (located primarily in bone) so that the product of the ionized serum calcium and serum phosphorus concentrations tends to remain constant. As a result, an increase in serum phosphorus concentration tends to lower ionized serum calcium levels, and a fall in serum phosphorus tends to raise ionized serum calcium levels. By virtue of this relationship, the serum phosphorus level becomes a normal determinant of parathyroid hormone secretion, and an increase in serum phosphorus concentration tends to increase circulating parathyroid hormone.

PTH increases calcium absorption from the gastrointestinal tract, mobilizes calcium from bone, and indirectly diminishes urinary calcium excretion by increasing tubular calcium reabsorption. The hormone lowers tubular reabsorption of phosphorus by a direct tubular action, thereby increasing urinary phosphorus excretion and lowering serum phosphorus.

Certain of these actions of PTH require adequate levels of vitamin D activity in the serum. Calcium absorption from the bowel and mobilization of calcium from bone are critically dependent upon vitamin D activity. It is not yet clear if the increased renal reabsorption of calcium, which is promoted by PTH, depends on vitamin D. However, it is known that the phosphaturic action of PTH is independent of vitamin D. Thus, increased levels of circulating PTH can diminish tubular reabsorption of phosphorus and maintain serum phosphorus levels at lower values, despite low or absent vitamin D activity.

In renal failure there usually exists a combination of hyperparathyroidism and some degree of vitamin D resistance

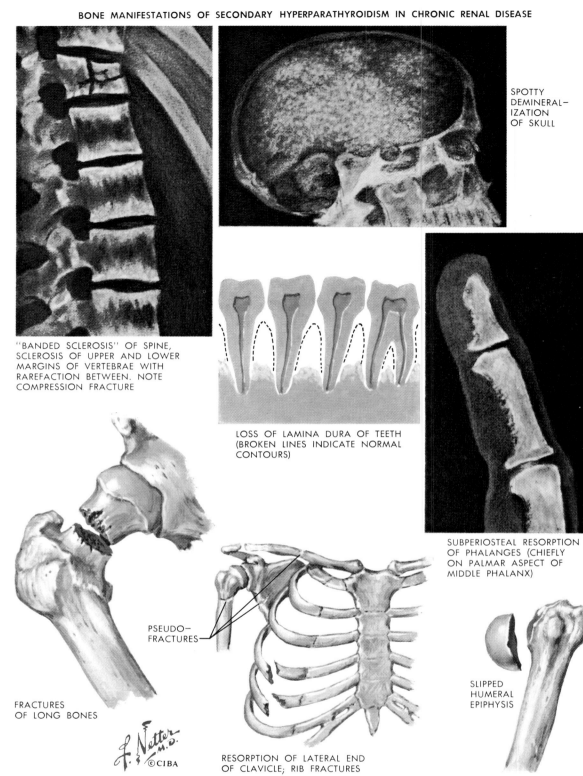

BONE MANIFESTATIONS OF SECONDARY HYPERPARATHYROIDISM IN CHRONIC RENAL DISEASE

"BANDED SCLEROSIS" OF SPINE, SCLEROSIS OF UPPER AND LOWER MARGINS OF VERTEBRAE WITH RAREFACTION BETWEEN. NOTE COMPRESSION FRACTURE

SPOTTY DEMINERAL-IZATION OF SKULL

LOSS OF LAMINA DURA OF TEETH (BROKEN LINES INDICATE NORMAL CONTOURS)

SUBPERIOSTEAL RESORPTION OF PHALANGES (CHIEFLY ON PALMAR ASPECT OF MIDDLE PHALANX)

FRACTURES OF LONG BONES

PSEUDO-FRACTURES

RESORPTION OF LATERAL END OF CLAVICLE; RIB FRACTURES

SLIPPED HUMERAL EPIPHYSIS

or insufficiency. In order to comprehend the biochemical, osseous, and soft tissue complications of renal failure, it is helpful to have a clear understanding of the effects of hyperparathyroidism and vitamin D insufficiency states when the one is not complicated by the presence of the other (see CIBA COLLECTION, Vol. 4, pages 179, 180, 190, and 191).

Hyperparathyroidism produces an elevation of serum calcium concentration through the action of PTH. Simultaneously, tubular phosphorus reabsorption is diminished with a consequent fall in serum phosphorus levels. The net effect is an increase in the calcium-phosphorus product in the blood, and this can lead to the deposition of calcium salts in the kidney—nephrocalcinosis. However, soft tissue calcification elsewhere in the body does not occur as frequently.

Although tubular reabsorption of calcium is increased, glomerular filtration of calcium is usually increased even more because of the increased serum calcium level. As a result, total urinary calcium excretion may be increased. Renal calculus formation is a common phenomenon in hyperparathyroidism and is usually ascribed to this hypercalciuric state.

Hyperparathyroidism also stimulates osteocytes to reabsorb surface bone. Osteoblastic new bone formation is increased secondarily. However, osteoclasts predominate, and as a consequence, there is a decrease in total skeletal mass.

Because resorption is particularly prominent in cortical bone immediately beneath the periosteum, the typical radiologic findings of osteitis fibrosa may be noted: radiolucency at the outer edge of bony cortex, particularly in the phalanges and metacarpals, and the disappearance of the lamina dura.

Insufficient vitamin D activity may result from either dietary deficiency or increased resistance to the actions

Chronic Renal Failure

Continued

of the vitamin. Dietary deficiency of vitamin D may be a part of total nutritional deficiency, particularly in children, or be caused by intestinal malabsorption. Increased vitamin D resistance can occur in renal tubular acidosis, renal insufficiency, and the familial syndrome of hypophosphatemic rickets.

Regardless of cause, vitamin D insufficiency produces hypocalcemia, apparently by diminishing intestinal calcium absorption. Hypophosphatemia is also present and appears to result from hyperparathyroidism secondary to hypocalcemia.

Vitamin D insufficiency causes bone disease. In childhood this takes the form of classical rickets, while in the adult, the bone disease takes the form of osteomalacia. Although total bone mass is generally normal or increased, bone composition is radically altered. The fraction of bone in the form of uncalcified osseous tissue is much higher than normal, and the amount of mineralized bone is usually decreased.

Histologically, the osteoid seams are widened, but this can be detected only when bone sections are studied in the uncalcified state. Radiologically, pseudofractures represent the primary manifestation of osteomalacia. These appear as linear fracture lines in long bones and the scapulae and are similar to ordinary fractures except for the thinness of the bone and the absence of bony reaction.

Renal Insufficiency. Ionized serum calcium levels fall because of hyperphosphatemia and vitamin D resistance. The hyperphosphatemia is secondary to phosphate retention, in turn caused by diminished filtration. The cause of vitamin D resistance is unsettled but may, in part, be based upon failure of the kidney to convert vitamin D to its active form.

Hypocalcemia stimulates parathyroid hormone secretion; PTH partially restores serum ionized calcium and phosphorus levels by causing increased intestinal calcium absorption, bone calcium mobilization, and diminished tubular phosphate reabsorption. However, as GFR decreases further, increasing levels of circulating PTH are required to maintain normal serum calcium and phosphorus levels. Overt hypocalcemia and hyperphosphatemia result when GFR becomes very low.

Clinical Features. Specific biochemical and clinical features in any patient depend upon the balance between degree of hyperparathyroidism and that of vitamin D resistance. In patients having mild vitamin D resistance, the effects of hyperparathyroidism predominate. Serum calcium levels are maintained relatively high even as hyperphosphatemia supervenes. As a result, the serum calcium-phosphorus product becomes extremely high. This increased calcium-phosphorus product can lead to deposition of calcium salts in

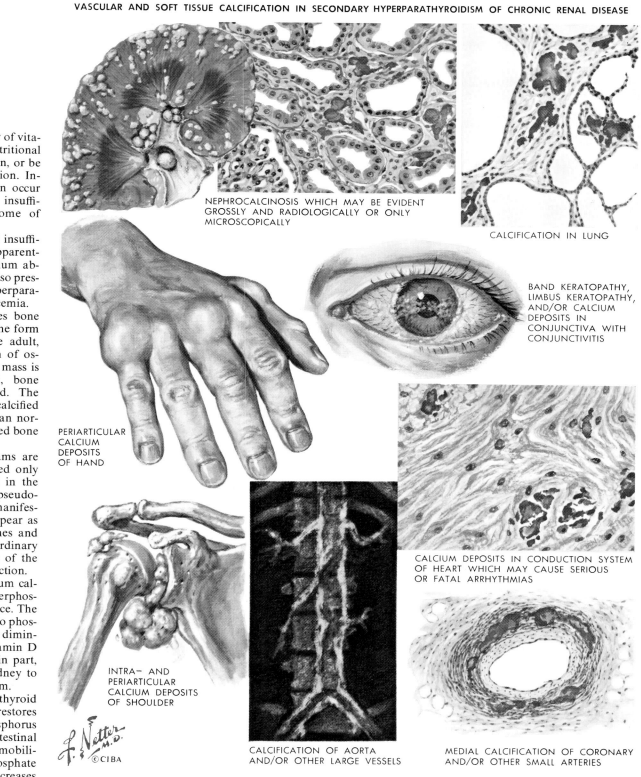

NEPHROCALCINOSIS WHICH MAY BE EVIDENT GROSSLY AND RADIOLOGICALLY OR ONLY MICROSCOPICALLY

CALCIFICATION IN LUNG

BAND KERATOPATHY, LIMBUS KERATOPATHY, AND/OR CALCIUM DEPOSITS IN CONJUNCTIVA WITH CONJUNCTIVITIS

PERIARTICULAR CALCIUM DEPOSITS OF HAND

CALCIUM DEPOSITS IN CONDUCTION SYSTEM OF HEART WHICH MAY CAUSE SERIOUS OR FATAL ARRHYTHMIAS

INTRA— AND PERIARTICULAR CALCIUM DEPOSITS OF SHOULDER

CALCIFICATION OF AORTA AND/OR OTHER LARGE VESSELS

MEDIAL CALCIFICATION OF CORONARY AND/OR OTHER SMALL ARTERIES

soft tissues such as the kidneys, lungs, joints, bursae, blood vessels, and conduction system of the heart. Calcium deposition in vessels and the heart can further compromise circulatory status.

Bony abnormalities in these patients (in whom the hyperparathyroidism predominates) consist primarily of *osteitis fibrosa*, of which bone pain will be the only symptom. Radiologically, findings typical of osteitis fibrosa will include subperiosteal resorption, resorption of the ends of the clavicles and of areas around fractures, and loss of lamina dura. On biopsy, features typical of osteitis fibrosa are usually present.

At the other end of the spectrum are patients whose course will be dominated primarily by Vitamin D resistance. Although circulating levels of parathyroid hormone may be extremely high, serum calcium levels will tend to be quite low and the calcium-phosphorus product will not be very high. In general, soft tissue

calcium deposition will not be a feature in this type of patient. Instead, osteomalacia, the bone disease of mild vitamin D resistance, will be the predominant bony abnormality. Clinically, bone pain and pelvic girdle weakness can be found. However, instead of subperiosteal bone resorption, the primary findings will be pseudofractures, and on biopsy, undecalcified sections will reveal widened osteoid seams.

Many patients fall between the two extremes. In these patients the calcium-phosphorus product is variable, and soft tissue calcification occurs in a more irregular manner. Most importantly, bony lesions include a mixture of osteitis fibrosa and osteomalacia, and features of both diseases may be present radiologically and on biopsy.

Overt hypercalcemia may occur in some patients even though all the mechanisms producing hyperparathyroidism in renal insufficiency are *Continued on page 120*

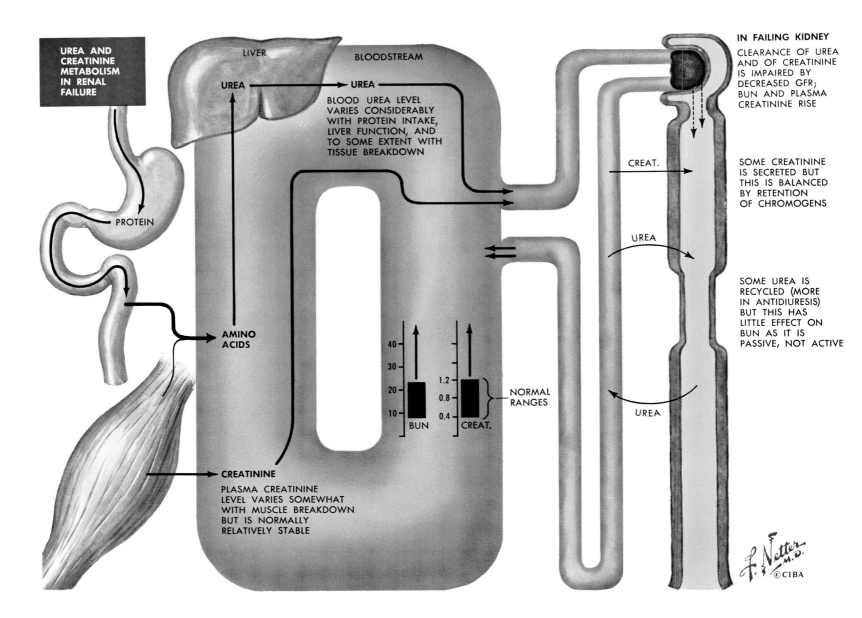

UREA AND CREATININE METABOLISM IN RENAL FAILURE

LIVER

BLOODSTREAM

UREA

UREA

BLOOD UREA LEVEL VARIES CONSIDERABLY WITH PROTEIN INTAKE, LIVER FUNCTION, AND TO SOME EXTENT WITH TISSUE BREAKDOWN

PROTEIN

AMINO ACIDS

CREATININE

PLASMA CREATININE LEVEL VARIES SOMEWHAT WITH MUSCLE BREAKDOWN BUT IS NORMALLY RELATIVELY STABLE

CREAT.

UREA

UREA

NORMAL RANGES

BUN   CREAT.

IN FAILING KIDNEY

CLEARANCE OF UREA AND OF CREATININE IS IMPAIRED BY DECREASED GFR; BUN AND PLASMA CREATININE RISE

SOME CREATININE IS SECRETED BUT THIS IS BALANCED BY RETENTION OF CHROMOGENS

SOME UREA IS RECYCLED (MORE IN ANTIDIURESIS) BUT THIS HAS LITTLE EFFECT ON BUN AS IT IS PASSIVE, NOT ACTIVE

Chronic Renal Failure

Continued from page 119

based upon a tendency toward hypocalcemia. One explanation, true in certain patients, is that *primary* hyperparathyroidism occurs and the renal damage results from hypercalcemia. In other patients this clearly is not an appropriate explanation, for hypercalcemia can be shown to develop long after renal insufficiency occurs. In such cases, the parathyroid glands act as though they had undergone adenomatous transformation, perhaps as a result of the original constant stimulus of hypocalcemia. Thus, these glands apparently secrete parathyroid hormone in great excess, and the hormone in turn produces hypercalcemia.

When hypercalcemia appears during the course of renal failure, the calcium-phosphorus product in the serum is invariably high and depositional disease is usually present. Bone disease, often severe, is usually and primarily osteitis fibrosa.

Treatment. A general rule that applies to nearly all patients with renal failure is that serum phosphorus levels should be maintained low or normal by decreasing phosphorus absorption from the bowel, which can be done most effectively by the use of nonabsorbable antacid gels. This treatment should be started early, long before overt hyperphosphatemia appears, because it is in the early stages that hyperparathyroidism begins.

Later in the course of renal failure, especially when bone disease is present, therapy depends entirely upon the relative effects of hyperpara-

thyroidism and vitamin D resistance. To assess the clinical situation accurately, bone biopsy must be done. In patients who have bone disease primarily as a result of hyperparathyroidism, subtotal parathyroidectomy may be beneficial. Parathyroidectomy may also be beneficial in patients who have severe depositional disease in the soft tissues.

Patients who primarily have osteomalacia may benefit from treatment with vitamin D. This treatment requires highly specialized laboratory measurements because most vitamin D preparations cannot be used without standardization. Vitamin D should never be used in the absence of careful patient evaluation, including bone biopsy, because its use can accelerate the course of bone disease in patients who primarily have osteitis fibrosa. Similarly, unless carefully controlled, vitamin D treatment may result in severe hypercalcemia and accelerated depositional disease.

Virtually all of the small group of patients in whom hypercalcemia develops during the course of renal insufficiency require surgical parathyroidectomy (also see page 179).

Disturbances of Urea and Creatinine

The theoretical and practical considerations of creatinine metabolism and creatinine clearance have been described (see pages 45 and 83).

Similarly, urea, the chief end product of protein catabolism, is formed in the liver by a complex chain of chemical reactions, for which the free energy is derived largely from adenosine triphosphate. (Urea has also been discussed, in relation to

urea clearance, on pages 44 and 83.) After a series of enzymatically catalyzed reactions, nitrogen from deaminated amino acids enters the arginine-ornithine-citrulline cycle. Urea released from arginine is discharged into the systemic circulation and, at equilibrium, is distributed throughout total body water. Since the rate of urea production is directly related to the rate of protein catabolism, the blood urea nitrogen (BUN) varies directly with the protein content of the diet in states of nitrogen balance and under ordinary circumstances.

Azotemia, the increased concentration of nonprotein nitrogenous compounds in blood, is one of the historical hallmarks of renal failure. However, because urea and creatinine have been considered the final compounds in their respective metabolic pathways, each has received much emphasis in the literature on the pathophysiology of renal failure. Moreover, although it is natural that similarities between the physiologic origins, dispositions, and ultimate fates of these compounds should attract interest, it is their corresponding differences that are more informative, and these will be considered.

Creatinine. A normal, hypothetical subject produces 1.70 gm of creatinine a day, or 1.18 mg/min. At an assumed normal creatinine clearance of 120 ml/min and an assumed steady state, the clearance formula predicts a plasma concentration of 0.98 mg percent, because plasma concentration plotted against clearance yields a rectangular hyperbola. If this subject now undergoes an abrupt tenfold reduction in glomerular filtration rate, but no other changes occur, it can again be predicted from the clearance formula that the plasma concentration of creatinine will rise tenfold to 9.8 mg percent. (Although the clearance formula does not provide the time during which this rise occurs, the time can nonetheless be calculated from theoretical considerations. Such calculations agree closely with clinical observations.)

Furthermore, it is apparent that a glomerular filtrate which is one tenth of normal will contain creatinine at a concentration 10 times normal, and so will achieve the same excretory rate of creatinine as obtained before the theoretical reduction in renal function. The creatinine excretory rate is thus preserved, but creatinine homeostasis is not.

The osmotic contribution of creatinine is minor. A blood creatinine of 34 mg percent represents only 3 mM/l. Also, the urine/plasma ratios of creatinine fall during osmotic diuresis, which may occur in renal failure. As a result, creatinine contributes less than 30 mOsm/l to the urinary osmolality.

Urea. An average man, in steady state and consuming average amounts of dietary protein, daily forms and excretes about 30 gm of urea (corresponding to 14 gm of urea nitrogen). With a normal urea clearance of 75 ml/min, the predicted blood urea nitrogen will be 13 mg percent. If renal function were to cease entirely and protein metabolism were not to change, 14,000 mg of urea nitrogen would be added per day to total body water, which measures about 50,000 ml. The BUN would thus rise 28 mg percent in 24 hours—the additional amount being slightly more than double the normal BUN level. In contrast, creatinine would increase by 3.4 mg percent which represents nearly four times the normal creatinine level.

However, when renal function is reduced but not absent, the same considerations hold for urea as described for creatinine. A new steady state is achieved whereby elevation of the blood urea compensates for the fall in filtration rate, and a normal urea excretion rate is achieved.

Although on a weight basis about 18 times as much urea is produced and excreted per day as creatinine, on an osmotic basis, 33 times as much urea is produced and excreted as creatinine—urea excretion is roughly 500 mOsm/day. Therefore, unlike creatinine, urea contributes substantially to the osmotic load responsible for the osmotic diuresis of renal failure.

Another important difference between urea and creatinine is the fact that a substantial portion of urea is reabsorbed in the tubules and that this reabsorption is flow dependent (see page 44). Under conditions of average hydration, the normal individual reabsorbs about 60 percent of filtered urea. During water diuresis the fraction reabsorbed falls to 40 percent or less, while during osmotic diuresis reabsorption as low as 15 and 20 percent has been reported. On the other hand, at very low urinary flow rates such as occur in oliguria, the fractional reabsorption of urea may rise even higher than 60 or 70 percent.

This flow-dependence of urea reabsorption provides an explanation for the disproportionate changes in blood urea and creatinine seen in certain clinical situations. The dynamics of a previously normal kidney with reduced glomerular filtration rate because of nonintrinsic renal disease, such as occurs in shock or heart failure, are markedly different from those of a kidney with an equally low glomerular filtration rate because of loss of functioning nephrons. In the first situation the filtration rate per nephron is lower than normal; in the second condition GFR per functioning nephron is much higher than normal. Therefore, although the creatinine clearance per kidney is the same in the two clinical states, the urea clearance per kidney will be low in proportion to

filtration rate in the first instance (low GFR per nephron) because of the greatly augmented tubular reabsorption.

On the other hand, when the GFR per nephron is high, urea clearance per kidney will be high in proportion to the GFR because of the greatly reduced tubular reabsorption under conditions of osmotic diuresis. Thus, when the urea-to-creatinine ratio in blood exceeds its usual range of about 10 to 15, the possibility of a prerenal cause for azotemia should be considered (see page 111). Other causes of a BUN disproportionately high compared to serum creatinine include increased tissue catabolism caused by stress, injury, or suprarenal corticosteroids, a marked increase in dietary protein, sequestration within the gastrointestinal tract or within body cavities of a large volume of blood, and obstructive uropathy of recent onset.

Parenthetically, it is not generally appreciated that variable but significant quantities of urea diffuse into the gastrointestinal tract in amounts proportional to the level of BUN. Almost all of this urea undergoes hydrolysis, presumably because of the action of urease-producing microorganisms. The ammonia derived from this ureolysis is absorbed from the gastrointestinal tract and rapidly removed from the hepatic portal circulation by the liver. In the liver, it reenters the urea cycle. Recent evidence indicates that this ammonia nitrogen may, under certain circumstances, be incorporated into amino acids and proteins, and this observation has stimulated interest in new approaches to nutritional problems in renal failure.

Uremia

Uremia is a constellation of clinical findings associated with severe renal failure. Many or all of its manifestations may be present in varying degrees. The known chemical abnormalities generated by diminution in homeostatic function have been presented on the previous pages, and it only remains to classify the various clinical manifestations of the uremic state.

Biochemical Features. In Plate 11, page 122, the *biochemical* abnormalities of uremia are summarized. Knowledge of the mechanisms underlying such changes is far more complete than in other areas. Although the search for a uremic "toxin" still goes on, the toxin theory is probably too simplistic. Instead, the manifestations of uremia are ultimately best explained by compositional and volume changes secondary to derangement of the homeostatic function, in turn resulting from what the diseased kidney does, as much as from what it fails to do.

The gastrointestinal manifestations of uremia, although neither many nor varied, can cause the uremic patient great distress and, by dehydration, threaten to compromise an already minimal renal blood flow. Anorexia, nausea, and vomiting are extremely common, although the mechanism of their causation remains obscure.

Some of the normal flora of the oral cavity are urease-containing—and therefore urea-splitting—organisms. The ammonia generated thereby is thought to play a role in the pathogenesis of uremic stomatitis; it also contributes to the uriniferous odor of the breath.

Ulcerations, often multiple, may occur any place in the gastrointestinal tract. Erosion of blood vessels in the ulceration may lead to occult melena, to hemorrhagic shock, or to any intermediate state of blood loss. Shock and oligemia constitute further threats to the life of the uremic patient. As noted above, a high urea-to-creatinine ratio in blood should arouse suspicion of a prerenal component to the uremic state, and gastrointestinal hemorrhage is a common cause of such a clinical situation.

The neurologic symptoms of uremia are protean and poorly understood. Although lassitude is common, alternating periods of somnolence and excitement may occur. Convulsions, when present, are usually a result of hypertensive encephalopathy, although they are sometimes seen in the absence of hypertension. Eventually, confusion and coma appear in the untreated patient.

Usually there is an increase in muscular irritability which, occasionally, but not usually, is explained by hypocalcemia or hypomagnesemia. Also, hyperparathyroidism has been known to produce a poorly understood form of central muscle wasting. When asterixis is not obviously present, it can often be elicited by careful testing.

With the advent of hemodialysis, many of the central nervous system manifestations of uremia have been found to be reversible. However, too rapid normalization of body fluid composition has led to the recognition of what has been termed a *disequilibrium syndrome,* presumably caused by the time lag involved in obtaining equilibrium across the blood-brain barrier. Dialysis has also focused attention on the frequency with which peripheral neuropathy develops in uremia. Sensory neuropathy is partially reversible in some patients after intensive prolonged dialysis, but with motor neuropathy, improvement is the exception rather than the rule.

Successful renal transplantation (see page 264) ameliorates the peripheral neuropathy, often many months later. Other treatment of neuropathy has been singularly disappointing. However, a resurgence of interest in substances which may have an inhibitory effect on normal neural metabolism and which are not adequately excreted in uremia offers new avenues of therapy. Present examples include guanidosuccinate and an as yet unidentified low molecular weight substance which inhibits erythrocyte transketolase.

Cardiovascular Manifestations. Hypertension occurs, sooner or later, during the course of most forms of renal failure. It is less common in renal amyloidosis (see page 163), lupus nephritis (see page 141), and obstructive uropathy (see page 185). The salt-losing propensities of some forms of chronic pyelonephritis (see page 191) and particularly of medullary cystic disease (see page 229) could explain the reduced frequency of hypertension in these disorders (see also CIBA COLLECTION, Vol. 5, page 225).

Sterile fibrinous pericarditis was, prior to dialysis, an ominous sign in uremia. Pericardial effusions, which also may occur and are often sanguineous in nature, respond to intensive dialysis. Nevertheless, cardiac tamponade is a constant and real danger during the acute episode.

The anemia of uremia may further compromise an already impaired myocardial reserve. At least in the chronic state, hemolysis is not a feature of uremic anemia which is caused by diminished erythrocyte production and decreased red cell survival. Erythropoietin, a polypeptide normally manufactured in the kidney (see page 65), is diminished or absent, and although there are extrarenal sources of erythropoietin which may undergo functional adaptive hypertrophy, they are inadequate to correct the anemia.

In addition to the usual physiologic disadvantages of anemia, there is an additional threat to the patient undergoing chronic hemodialysis in preparation for, and awaiting the arrival of, a cadaveric allograft. Such patients usually require an average of two units of blood a month and, despite meticulous care in washing donor red cells, there is the possibility of leukocyte antigens' gaining access to the patient's circulation. These could stimulate antibody formation which would easily lead to diminution in the number of histocompatible donors. *Continued on page 122*

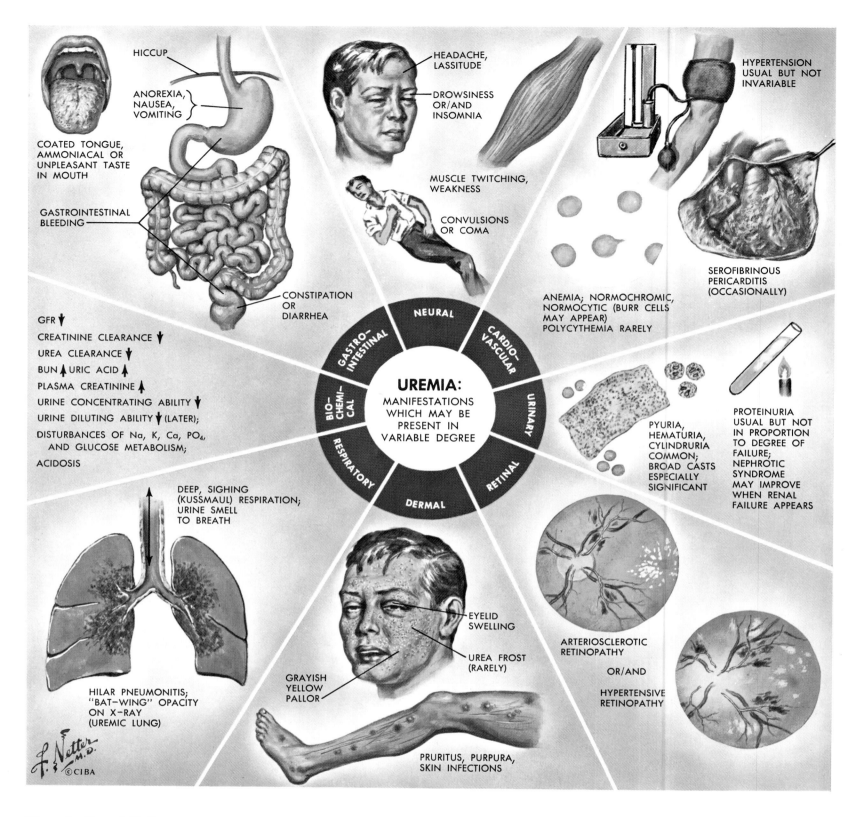

UREMIA:
MANIFESTATIONS WHICH MAY BE PRESENT IN VARIABLE DEGREE

NEURAL
CARDIO-VASCULAR
URINARY
RETINAL
DERMAL
RESPIRATORY
BIO-CHEMI-CAL
GASTRO-INTESTINAL

HICCUP

ANOREXIA, NAUSEA, VOMITING

COATED TONGUE, AMMONIACAL OR UNPLEASANT TASTE IN MOUTH

GASTROINTESTINAL BLEEDING

CONSTIPATION OR DIARRHEA

GFR ↓
CREATININE CLEARANCE ↓
UREA CLEARANCE ↓
BUN ↑ URIC ACID ↑
PLASMA CREATININE ↑
URINE CONCENTRATING ABILITY ↓
URINE DILUTING ABILITY ↓ (LATER);
DISTURBANCES OF Na, K, Ca, PO_4, AND GLUCOSE METABOLISM;
ACIDOSIS

HEADACHE, LASSITUDE

DROWSINESS OR/AND INSOMNIA

MUSCLE TWITCHING, WEAKNESS

CONVULSIONS OR COMA

HYPERTENSION USUAL BUT NOT INVARIABLE

ANEMIA; NORMOCHROMIC, NORMOCYTIC (BURR CELLS MAY APPEAR) POLYCYTHEMIA RARELY

SEROFIBRINOUS PERICARDITIS (OCCASIONALLY)

PYURIA, HEMATURIA, CYLINDRURIA COMMON; BROAD CASTS ESPECIALLY SIGNIFICANT

PROTEINURIA USUAL BUT NOT IN PROPORTION TO DEGREE OF FAILURE; NEPHROTIC SYNDROME MAY IMPROVE WHEN RENAL FAILURE APPEARS

DEEP, SIGHING (KUSSMAUL) RESPIRATION; URINE SMELL TO BREATH

HILAR PNEUMONITIS; "BAT-WING" OPACITY ON X-RAY (UREMIC LUNG)

GRAYISH YELLOW PALLOR

EYELID SWELLING

UREA FROST (RARELY)

PRURITUS, PURPURA, SKIN INFECTIONS

ARTERIOSCLEROTIC RETINOPATHY
OR/AND
HYPERTENSIVE RETINOPATHY

Chronic Renal Failure

Continued from page 121

The urinary findings of uremia are essentially those of the underlying disease. Short, dark, broad casts (renal failure casts) and waxy casts usually signify long-standing chronic renal disease and are seen with somewhat greater frequency in renal failure than in the early stages of renal pathology without failure. When the nephrotic syndrome (see page 123) is part of the disease picture, it is not uncommon for proteinuria to diminish as renal failure supervenes. This change in proteinuria is attributable to fibrosis and scarring of the glomeruli and to a diminished rate of glomerular filtration. For the same reason, the sediment usually improves in appearance as the disease enters its final stages.

The retinopathy of uremia is identical to that of hypertensive disease. Arteriolosclerosis is associated with hypertension of moderate severity and duration and may also be seen. The eyeground changes have been described in detail elsewhere (see CIBA COLLECTION, Vol. 5, page 227). Those changes resulting from hypertension are entirely reversible if blood pressure is brought under control.

Dermatologic Manifestations. The skin of a uremic patient often has a peculiar, pale yellow color resulting from a combination of anemia and alleged accumulation of urochrome pigments.

A crust of urea crystals, representing the residual solute after evaporation of sweat, is known as *uremic frost.* This condition is not seen as often as previously and, when it does occur, largely reflects inadequate nursing hygiene.

One of the most distressing symptoms of uremia

is intractable pruritus, which often poses difficult problems in management. The unremitting itching leads to scratching, with its attendant excoriations and subsequent infection. Recently, pruritus has been reported to disappear following parathyroidectomy for secondary hyperparathyroidism. Other skin manifestations include ecchymoses, purpura, and a variety of drug-induced eruptions.

The respiratory findings in uremia are variable. Acidosis may lead to the hyperpnea known as *Kussmaul breathing* (see page 116). Uremic pneumonitis is usually described as a hilar radiopacity extending outward in a fluffy fashion and having a "butterfly" or "bat-wing" appearance. However, it is a controversial subject because many such radiologic findings disappear after digitalization or relief of fluid overload by dialysis. Others disappear after appropriate antibiotic therapy. □

Nephrotic Syndrome

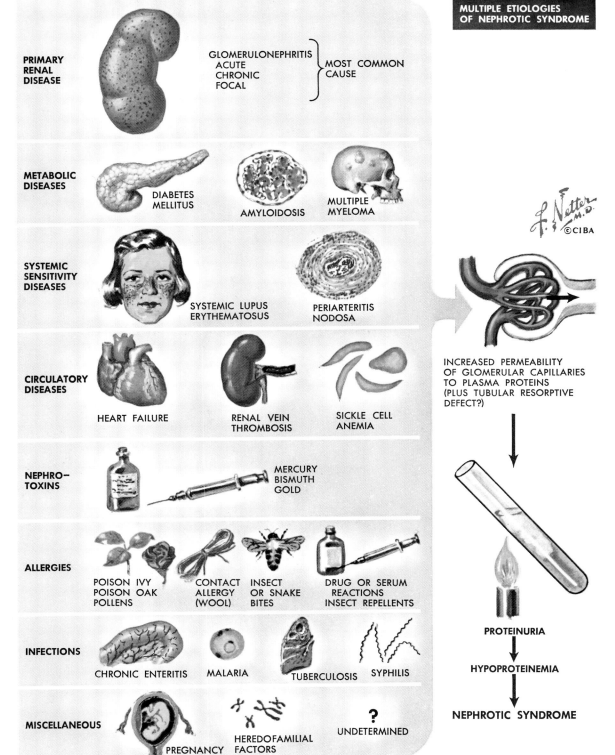

In 1827, Richard Bright described the association of *edema* (dropsy), *proteinuria,* and renal disease. Later, *hypoalbuminemia* and *hyperlipemia* were reported in association with renal disease. With time, the presence of all four of these findings has come to be considered necessary for the diagnosis of the *nephrotic syndrome.*

The definition is rather rigid, and some patients who have characteristic pathologic alterations in the kidney may not meet such clinical criteria. Therefore, Kark and his co-workers have defined the nephrotic syndrome as the metabolic, nutritional, and clinical consequences of continued massive *proteinuria.* To establish the diagnosis, Berman and Schreiner require that proteinuria exceed 3.5 gm/24 hours/1.73 m² of body surface area in the absence of reduced glomerular filtration rate, and that the urine contain doubly refractile oval fat bodies.

It would seem that the criteria suggested by Kark, Berman, and Schreiner are more apt to include all forms of the nephrotic syndrome, whereas the usual textbook definition may be restrictive.

Etiology

The causes of the nephrotic syndrome may be listed in seven major groups and one miscellaneous category. By far the most common cause of the nephrotic syndrome is *glomerulonephritis,* a primary renal disease. The pathology of glomerulonephritis may be of five types: (1) lipoid nephrosis (minimal disease, "nil" disease, or foot-process disease); (2) lipoid nephrosis with glomerulosclerosis; (3) membranous glomerulonephritis (membranous nephropathy); (4) membranoproliferative (mesangiocapillary or lobular) glomerulonephritis; and (5) focal glomerulonephritis. These categories are based upon pathologic descriptions. Clinically, all five types can be somewhat similar, although their courses are often different.

The second group of diseases causing massive proteinuria includes *diabetes mellitus* (see page 149), *amyloidosis* (see page 163), and *multiple myeloma* (see page 180). In all instances, proteinuria results from direct involvement of the kidney by the primary disease.

A third group of systemic diseases complicated by the nephrotic syndrome includes *lupus erythematosus* (see page 141) and *periarteritis nodosa* (see page 167).

Renal vein thrombosis (see page 173), *right heart failure* (see page 175), and *sickle cell disease* are also known to cause massive proteinuria. Researchers are not entirely sure of the mechanisms involved, but increased renal venous pressure, clotting abnormalities and/or thrombi, and ischemia may all play roles.

Many *nephrotoxins* (see page 168) such as gold, bismuth, trimethadione, paramethadione, and ammoniated mercury ointment may produce the nephrotic syndrome.

Allergic reactions make up the sixth etiologic group. For example, insect and snake bites, serum sickness, and reactions to poison ivy all have been described as causing proteinuria.

Infections such as malaria, syphilis, tuberculosis (see page 196), and chronic enteritis may produce the nephrotic syndrome directly, or secondarily, by intrarenal deposition of amyloid.

The *miscellaneous group* includes such entities as a familial nephrotic syndrome (see page 245) and pregnancy.

Common to all types of massive proteinuria is *increased permeability of the glomerular capillary membrane to plasma proteins.* Possibly there is also a defect in tubular reabsorption of proteins. It is this large protein loss which initiates the chain of events resulting in hypoalbuminemia, edema, and ultimately the "nephrotic syndrome." *Continued on page 124*

Nephrotic Syndrome

Continued from page 123

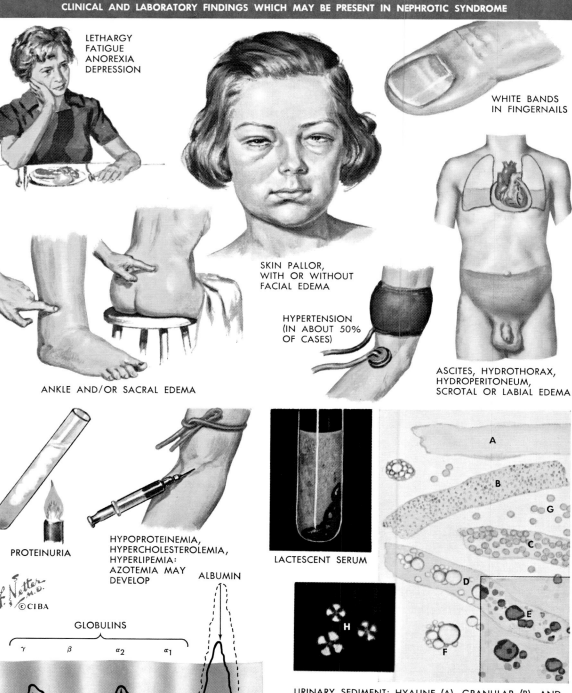

LETHARGY
FATIGUE
ANOREXIA
DEPRESSION

WHITE BANDS IN FINGERNAILS

SKIN PALLOR, WITH OR WITHOUT FACIAL EDEMA

HYPERTENSION (IN ABOUT 50% OF CASES)

ANKLE AND/OR SACRAL EDEMA

ASCITES, HYDROTHORAX, HYDROPERITONEUM, SCROTAL OR LABIAL EDEMA

PROTEINURIA

HYPOPROTEINEMIA, HYPERCHOLESTEROLEMIA, HYPERLIPEMIA: AZOTEMIA MAY DEVELOP

LACTESCENT SERUM

ALBUMIN

GLOBULINS

γ β α_2 α_1

SERUM ALBUMIN DECREASED, α_2–GLOBULIN INCREASED (BROKEN LINE INDICATES NORMAL)

URINARY SEDIMENT: HYALINE (A), GRANULAR (B), AND BLOOD (C) CASTS, AND CASTS CONTAINING FAT DROPLETS (D) WHICH STAIN RED WITH SUDAN III (E); FREE FAT DROPLETS (F) AND RED BLOOD CELLS (G); ALSO CHOLESTEROL ESTER CRYSTALS (MALTESE CROSSES) (H) DEMONSTRATED BY POLARIZED LIGHT

Clinical and Laboratory Observations

On physical examination, patients exhibiting the nephrotic syndrome appear pale, have swollen features, and frequently complain of lethargy, fatigue, anorexia, and depression. These symptoms may be caused, in part, by the associated depressed thyroid activity.

Although thyroid function in patients with nephrotic syndrome has been intensively investigated, specific alterations are not well understood. It has been suggested that both the function of the thyroid and the supply of hormone to the tissue are normal, while the low protein-bound iodine (PBI) reflects change in the concentration (or binding capacity) of the plasma proteins. Other suggested explanations of depressed thyroid function include abnormal loss of thyroid hormone in the urine and possible specific glandular abnormality. The truth probably encompasses all possibilities, but to date the entire story remains unexplained.

Edema is present at some point during the course of the disease in about 66 percent of adults who exhibit the nephrotic syndrome. With more severe degrees of edema, *ascites* and *hydrothorax* may also occur. Although the fingernails may show white bands, these are not pathognomonic for the nephrotic syndrome and may occur in any condition which produces edema of the nail bed, as in cirrhosis of the liver with ascites.

Hypertension does not occur frequently in patients with nephrotic syndrome but can be found more often than is appreciated. This observation has little significance in studies of general groups of patients. However, when the presence of hypertension is related to specific forms of the nephrotic syndrome, as described pathologically, it becomes very meaningful. Approximately 50 percent of patients exhibiting membranous glomerulonephritis have hypertension. In

those patients with chronic proliferative glomerulonephritis (see pages 135 and 136), intercapillary glomerulosclerosis (see page 152), or systemic lupus erythematosus (see page 141), the incidence of hypertension can rise to 75 percent or higher.

Proteinuria. Massive *proteinuria* and resultant hypoproteinemia (chiefly hypoalbuminemia) have long been recognized as part of the nephrotic syndrome. Until recent years, practically all authorities had considered the nephrotic syndrome as a single entity and had not recognized that different pathologic alterations may produce the same effects of massive proteinuria and hypoproteinemia.

Recently, a correlation was shown to exist between the molecular weights of plasma proteins excreted and both the underlying pathology and the expected response to immunosuppressive therapy. A process referred to as *glomerular selectivity* defines these rela-

tionships. The glomerulus is considered to be *highly selective* if predominantly low molecular weight proteins are excreted, and *nonselective* if predominantly high molecular weight proteins are passed. Patients exhibiting high selectivity usually respond well to immunosuppressive therapy and show minimal change in the kidney under examination by light microscopy. Those exhibiting nonselective glomerular filtration respond very poorly and have marked renal pathology.

In an effort to quantitate this phenomenon, the U/P ratios of several different molecular weight proteins (transferrin, IgG, α_2M) have been determined by an immunodiffusion technic. For example, clearance of the test protein is related to clearance of transferrin ($C_{\alpha_2M}/C_{Trans} \times 100$). This relation is plotted logarithmically against the molecular weight of the protein, making it possible to construct a line; the angle between this line and the abscissa of the graph is called

Nephrotic Syndrome
Continued

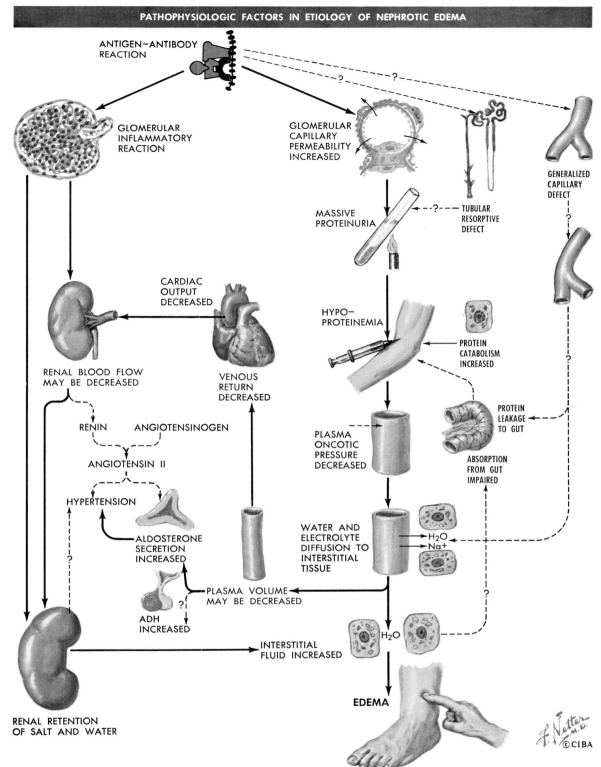

theta (Θ) and is a measure of the glomerular selectivity. Theta greater than 67° is considered highly selective; theta below 54° is nonselective. This selectivity is constant, irrespective of the amount of protein excreted, be it 2 gm/24 hours or 20 gm/24 hours.

The increased serum level of α_2-macroglobulin is difficult to explain although it certainly is present in almost all patients who exhibit massive proteinuria. There may be a variable elevation in other proteins, *e.g.*, γ, β, and α_1.

Lipid Metabolism. The serum is *lactescent* owing to *hyperlipidemia,* and in addition, *hypercholesterolemia* will be evident. These alterations are not fully understood. Generally, the primary alteration of lipid metabolism in the nephrotic syndrome is an elevation of triglycerides and high density lipoproteins. Apparently, there is a defect in the rate of interconversion from large to small lipoprotein fractions. Whether or not this results from lack of a specific substance is not known, but albumin is considered to be important as an *acceptor* in the transport chain required for interconversion. Occasionally, in the presence of low serum albumin, less-marked interconversion may be noted, a phenomenon which is possibly secondary to changes in the protein fraction. Clinically, the observation has been made that the hyperlipidemia improves when albumin is administered, or if the patient responds to immunosuppressive therapy with decreased proteinuria and increased serum albumin concentration.

The urinary sediment (see pages 75-76) found in patients who exhibit the nephrotic syndrome secondary to intrinsic renal disease or glomerulonephritis is of interest, although it is not too helpful for suggesting the pathologic alterations. In these patients the urine will have fat bodies and cholesterol esters which appear as maltese crosses under polarized

light (see page 76). Further, use of the fat stain Sudan III will reveal red droplets. The presence of fat has given rise to the term *lipoid nephrosis of childhood.*

Microscopic hematuria and occasional red cell casts (see page 75) are present in all forms of nephritis which produce the nephrotic syndrome. However, these urinary findings are more prominent in patients who have proliferative glomerulonephritis (see page 135) and, for all practical purposes, are not seen in patients with minimal or "foot-process" disease (see page 127). Granular casts also may be seen in patients who have proliferative disease but usually are not present in patients who have membranous disease (see page 136) or minimal disease.

Pathophysiology of Nephrotic Edema

Glomerulonephritis which produces the nephrotic syndrome is thought to be an *antigen-antibody reaction* (see

pages 131-136). This reaction produces an inflammatory response in the glomerulus which is evident as proliferation of cells and changes in the basement membrane. In some cases, only minimal changes are noted as seen by light microscopy. Whether this latter form—described as minimal disease, lipoid nephrosis, or "foot-process" disease—is an antigen-antibody reaction has not been well established. However, patients who exhibit this form do respond to immunosuppressive therapy.

All patients who suffer from the glomerular inflammatory reaction can exhibit salt and water retention, particularly if they show decreases in glomerular filtration rate. This direct effect on the glomeruli may produce a decrease in renal blood flow, and through the *renin-angiotensin mechanism*, angiotensin II is elaborated. The resultant hypertension can set up a vicious cycle within the kidney. *Continued on page 127*

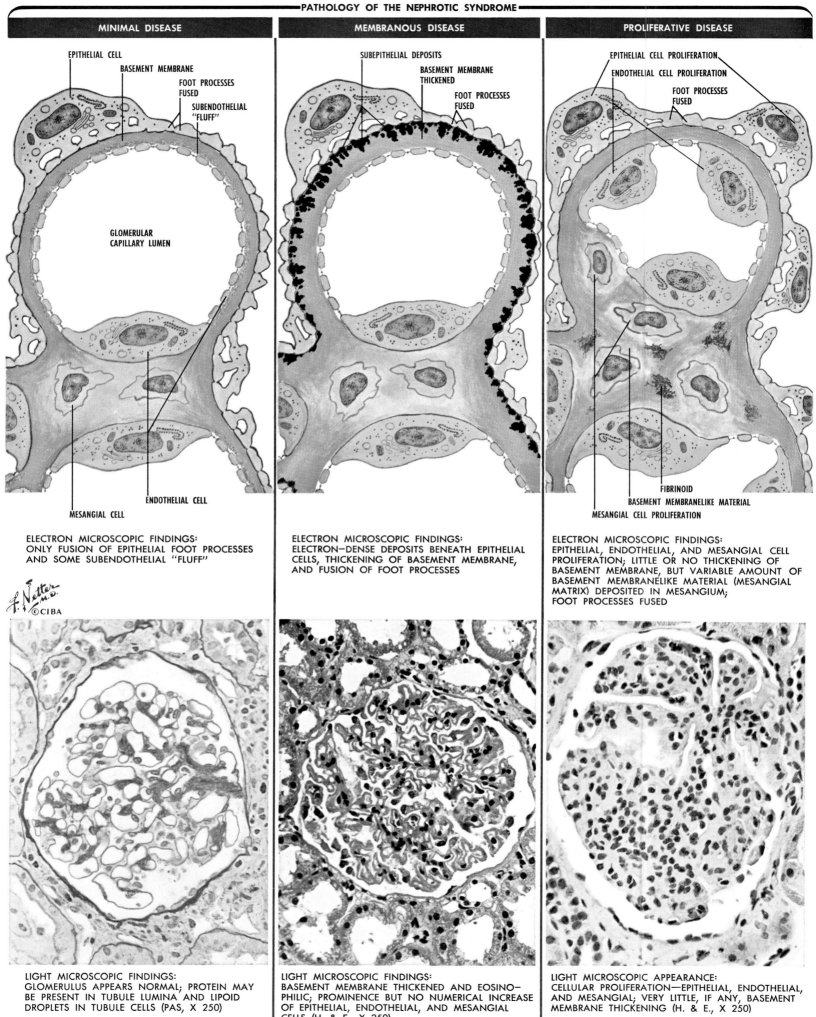

MINIMAL DISEASE

EPITHELIAL CELL
BASEMENT MEMBRANE
FOOT PROCESSES FUSED
SUBENDOTHELIAL "FLUFF"

GLOMERULAR CAPILLARY LUMEN

ENDOTHELIAL CELL

MESANGIAL CELL

ELECTRON MICROSCOPIC FINDINGS:
ONLY FUSION OF EPITHELIAL FOOT PROCESSES AND SOME SUBENDOTHELIAL "FLUFF"

LIGHT MICROSCOPIC FINDINGS:
GLOMERULUS APPEARS NORMAL; PROTEIN MAY BE PRESENT IN TUBULE LUMINA AND LIPOID DROPLETS IN TUBULE CELLS (PAS, X 250)

MEMBRANOUS DISEASE

SUBEPITHELIAL DEPOSITS
BASEMENT MEMBRANE THICKENED
FOOT PROCESSES FUSED

ELECTRON MICROSCOPIC FINDINGS:
ELECTRON–DENSE DEPOSITS BENEATH EPITHELIAL CELLS, THICKENING OF BASEMENT MEMBRANE, AND FUSION OF FOOT PROCESSES

LIGHT MICROSCOPIC FINDINGS:
BASEMENT MEMBRANE THICKENED AND EOSINO-PHILIC; PROMINENCE BUT NO NUMERICAL INCREASE OF EPITHELIAL, ENDOTHELIAL, AND MESANGIAL CELLS (H. & E., X 250)

PROLIFERATIVE DISEASE

EPITHELIAL CELL PROLIFERATION
ENDOTHELIAL CELL PROLIFERATION
FOOT PROCESSES FUSED

FIBRINOID
BASEMENT MEMBRANELIKE MATERIAL
MESANGIAL CELL PROLIFERATION

ELECTRON MICROSCOPIC FINDINGS:
EPITHELIAL, ENDOTHELIAL, AND MESANGIAL CELL PROLIFERATION; LITTLE OR NO THICKENING OF BASEMENT MEMBRANE, BUT VARIABLE AMOUNT OF BASEMENT MEMBRANELIKE MATERIAL (MESANGIAL MATRIX) DEPOSITED IN MESANGIUM; FOOT PROCESSES FUSED

LIGHT MICROSCOPIC APPEARANCE:
CELLULAR PROLIFERATION—EPITHELIAL, ENDOTHELIAL, AND MESANGIAL; VERY LITTLE, IF ANY, BASEMENT MEMBRANE THICKENING (H. & E., X 250)

Nephrotic Syndrome

Continued from page 125

Furthermore, there will be alterations in glomerular capillary permeability, allowing the loss of large amounts of protein. It is this prolonged *massive proteinuria* and resultant *hypoproteinemia* which provide the common denominator for all consequent metabolic and nutritional defects.

A *tubular reabsorptive defect* has been suggested for low molecular weight proteins. Studies in patients exhibiting massive proteinuria, using lysozyme as a marker for low molecular weight protein (17,000 molecular weight), suggest that this protein is filtered at the glomerulus but is not reabsorbed to a normal degree in the proximal tubule. Although this source of proteinuria may not have much effect quantitatively, it does contribute to the total amount of protein in the urine.

The hypoproteinemia ultimately gives rise to a decreased plasma oncotic pressure which allows water and electrolytes to diffuse into the interstitial tissue. This diffusion of fluid into the interstitial tissue is recognized clinically as *edema*. The reduction in plasma oncotic pressure produces a reduction in plasma volume. Therefore, cardiac output conceivably can be decreased, further decreasing the function of the kidney. When the plasma volume is markedly decreased, there is an elevation of aldosterone. Clinically, the elevated aldosterone levels are treatable by the use of aldosterone-blocking agents. However, such agents are not as effective in patients with nephrotic syndrome as they are in other diseases.

Another alteration found in glomerulonephritis and nephrotic syndrome is the *generalized capillary defect*, suggested many years ago as one of the explanations for edema formation and for the lack of absorption of water or electrolytes from the gut. It also has been shown that in children exhibiting nephrotic syndrome of the glomerulonephritis type there is a leakage of protein into the gut. This would further suggest the operation of a generalized capillary defect. *Protein catabolism* has also been implicated in this condition as a contributing factor to the pathophysiology of edema formation. Protein degradation provides

tissue water secondary to cellular breakdown, producing more interstitial fluid.

Consideration of these various factors in the formation of edema in the nephrotic syndrome can pinpoint those mechanisms at which specific antiedemic therapy may be directed most judiciously. The first is *hypoproteinemia*. In this situation, such agents as salt-poor albumin are administered in order to increase plasma volume, thereby increasing oncotic pressure and drawing fluid from the interstitial tissues into the vascular volume. This reaction will decrease aldosterone release and increase the plasma volume available to the kidneys for the ultimate excretion of salt and water. The increase in plasma volume will lead to an increase in the glomerular filtration rate and will further allow for salt and water excretion. Moreover, it is possible to block aldosterone with pharmacologic diuretics, which will further enhance the diuresis. Also, the retention of salt and water found in patients with nephrotic syndrome can be directly affected by pharmacologic agents such as the standard diuretics, furosemide, ethacrynic acid, and thiazides (see page 253).

While we are not yet aware of the complete story regarding edema formation, the factors mentioned are implicated at all, or nearly all, times; no one factor causes clinical edema, which must be the result of a combination of many factors.

Renal Pathology

The pathologic changes found in kidney biopsies of patients who have nephrotic syndrome secondary to glomerulonephritis may be divided into five categories.

Lipoid Nephrosis. Specimens from patients with lipoid nephrosis show little or no change when examined by light microscopy. However, electron microscopy reveals fused foot processes of the epithelial cells (see facing Plate 15, Minimal Disease). Immunofluorescent studies add little information except to demonstrate the presence of IgE (γe). These patients respond very well to immunosuppressive therapy.

Lipoid Nephrosis with Focal Glomerulosclerosis. In patients with this pathologic condition, light

microscopy shows focal and segmental sclerosis. With electron microscopy, fused foot processes, capillary collapse, and mesangial expansion are observed. Immunofluorescence occasionally shows gamma globulin deposits. These patients respond very poorly to therapy.

Membranous Nephropathy. In biopsies from this group of patients, the glomerular capillary walls are thickened. Electron microscopy shows "spikes" in the basement membrane caused by the presence of antigen-antibody complexes beneath the epithelial cells (see facing Plate 15, Membranous Disease). With immunofluorescence, these antigen-antibody complexes are found to be diffuse granular deposits of IgG and C3 (β_1C) (complement). These patients also have a poor response to therapy (see also page 136).

Mesangiocapillary Glomerulonephritis. The fourth group of patients with intrinsic renal disease and massive proteinuria have been variously diagnosed as having membranoproliferative glomerulonephritis, mesangiocapillary (lobular) glomerulonephritis, or hypocomplementemic nephritis (see page 135). The pathologic alterations include thickening of the glomerular capillary walls, mesangial proliferation, and sclerosis. Further, on electron microscopy there is an ingrowth of mesangium into the capillary walls and subendothelial deposits. Immunofluorescent studies show the presence of C3 (β_1C) and IgG in a lumpy, nonlinear pattern (see page 129). Properdin is also present. There is no known therapy for patients with this condition.

Focal Glomerulonephritis. This is a condition in which segmental inflammatory necrosis and crescent formation are seen with both light microscopy and electron microscopy. The findings with immunofluorescence are quite variable. The response to therapy in patients with this pathologic lesion is quite poor (see page 139).

In summary, nephrotic syndrome (massive proteinuria) secondary to intrinsic glomerular renal disease (glomerulonephritis) probably is an antigen-antibody disease. However, at the present time, definite data are lacking in many areas to help elucidate the etiology of this condition. □

Immunologic Mechanisms in Glomerular Diseases (Experimental Hypersensitivity Glomerular Diseases)

Knowledge concerning glomerular diseases associated with hypersensitivity has increased rapidly in recent years, largely because of the development of several experimental models and through elucidation of the immunologic mechanisms involved in these models. This experimental work has made possible identification of the immunologic mechanisms involved in certain human glomerular diseases.

There are two main categories of experimental, immunologically induced glomerular diseases:

1. Antiglomerular basement membrane disease in which antibody is directed against the glomerular basement membrane—the antigen is a normal

constituent of the glomerulus.

2. Immune complex disease in which there is deposition in glomeruli of antigen-antibody complexes formed in the circulation—the antigen is *not* a part of the glomerulus.

Frequently, these two major types can be recognized on the basis of certain immunofluorescent and electron microscopic findings.

Antiglomerular Basement Membrane (Anti-GBM) Disease

This disease may be produced by either *heterologous antibodies* or *autoantibodies*. The former is the best known and most extensively studied form and will be discussed first.

Heterologous Antibody Disease (Masugi Nephritis; Nephrotoxic Serum Nephritis). Although various species combinations may be used, one example—the disease produced in rabbits by sheep antiserum—will be discussed. Sheep are immunized with preparations of rabbit kidney. These may range from crude extracts of renal tissue to highly purified preparations of glomerular basement membrane. After immunization, the sheep serum is collected, absorbed with rabbit red cells, and injected intravenously into rabbits. With potent antiserum, a relatively small amount (<1 ml) will consistently result in severe glomerulonephritis.

The *first (heterologous) phase* of the disease begins immediately after injection and is a result

of the combination of sheep antibodies with rabbit glomerular basement membrane (Plate 16, A). The *second (autologous) phase* begins after several days, when rabbit antibodies against sheep gamma globulin are produced and unite with the sheep antibody fixed in the glomeruli.

Of the two phases, the second (autologous) is generally more severe; a diffuse proliferative glomerulonephritis typically occurs, often with conspicuous *crescent* formation and rapidly developing glomerular obliteration. (The heterologous phase is shown in Plate 16, A. The antibodies attaching to the glomerular basement membrane are sheep antibodies; the attachment of rabbit antibodies formed against the sheep gamma globulin is not shown. Plate 16, B depicts the tissue reaction which occurs in the autologous phase.)

This model is produced in a highly artificial way and hardly serves as the basis for spontaneously occurring disease. Nevertheless, it provides some very useful information which helps to differentiate anti-GBM disease from immune complex disease. First, this model shows that glomerular disease can be produced by *circulating* antibodies, in contrast to the situation usually found with other solid tissues. Second, it demonstrates that gamma globulin, representing the antibodies responsible for the disease, can be readily detected within the glomeruli by immunofluorescence: these antibodies are *Continued on page 128*

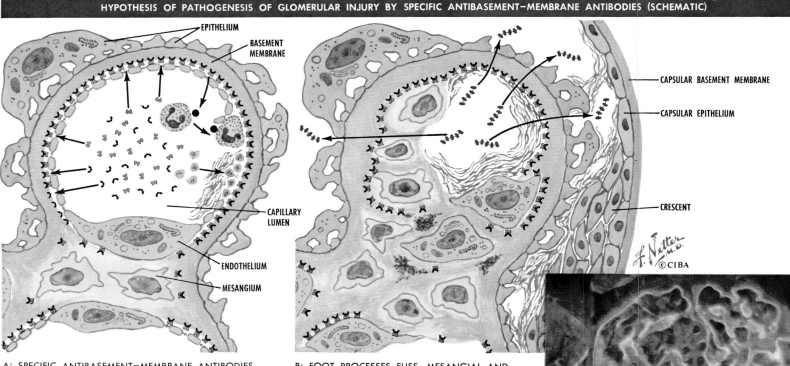

A: SPECIFIC ANTIBASEMENT–MEMBRANE ANTIBODIES PENETRATE ENDOTHELIUM OF GLOMERULAR CAPILLARIES AND ATTACH TO RECEPTOR SITES ON BASEMENT MEMBRANE; COMPLEMENT ATTACHES TO ANTIBODY AND BASEMENT MEMBRANE; COMPLEMENT COMPONENTS C'5, C'6, AND C'7 FORM A COMPLEX WHICH IS CHEMOTACTIC AND ATTRACTS POLYMORPHONUCLEAR LEUKOCYTES; THE LATTER ATTACK ENDOTHELIUM AND BASEMENT MEMBRANE BY RELEASING PROTEOLYTIC ENZYMES; PLATELETS ADHERE TO CAPILLARY WALL, AND FIBRIN IS DEPOSITED

B: FOOT PROCESSES FUSE; MESANGIAL AND ENDOTHELIAL CELLS SWELL AND PROLIFERATE, INVADING CAPILLARY LUMEN; FIBRINOID AND BASEMENT MEMBRANELIKE MATERIAL (MESANGIAL MATRIX) ARE DEPOSITED; DAMAGED CAPILLARY WALL PERMITS ESCAPE OF PLASMA PROTEINS, RESULTING IN PROTEINURIA; FIBRINOUS CAPSULAR ADHESIONS AND EPITHELIAL CRESCENTS DEVELOP

KEY

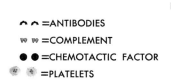

∧ ∧ =ANTIBODIES

w w =COMPLEMENT

● ● =CHEMOTACTIC FACTOR

=PLATELETS

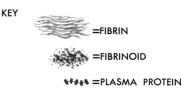

=FIBRIN

=FIBRINOID

=PLASMA PROTEIN

IMMUNOFLUORESCENT PREPARATION, ANTIBASEMENT–MEMBRANE DISEASE (MASUGI NEPHRITIS): "LINEAR," NONGRANULAR DEPOSITION OF ANTIBODY AND COMPLEMENT ALONG BASEMENT MEMBRANE

Immunologic Mechanisms in Glomerular Diseases (Experimental Hypersensitivity Glomerular Diseases)

Continued from page 127

distributed along the basement membrane of every glomerulus in a highly distinctive, continuous ("linear") pattern. Third, electron microscopy usually reveals only inconspicuous deposits along the *endothelial* side of the basement membrane.

The study of Masugi nephritis has also yielded information about some of the pathogenic mechanisms involved after the initial combination of antibody with antigen in the glomerular basement membrane. For instance, *complement,* as detected by immunofluorescence, is deposited along the basement membrane. Furthermore, depletion of circulating complement, which is possible for several hours, partially prevents *proteinuria* during the first phase.

One way by which the complement system may lead to damage is through the production of a *chemotactic factor (C' 5, 6, 7).* This is a mechanism which is probably involved in neutrophil accumulation in glomeruli—a feature sometimes conspicuous, especially during the first phase. Experimentally, it has been shown that neutrophil accumulation may lead to glomerular damage, and that depletion of circulating leukocytes results in

diminished proteinuria during the first phase. The damage produced by leukocytes is presumably caused by the release of lysosomal enzymes.

In the second phase, the most serious aspect of the disease is glomerular obliteration which results from swelling and proliferation of endothelial and mesangial cells, accumulation of basement membranelike material, and crescent formation. However, a pathogenic role for leukocytes in the second phase is less firmly established. Furthermore, it is not known whether complement contributes to glomerular damage in other ways, such as by a process analogous to cell lysis.

It is known that fibrin and other fibrinogen derivatives produced during the coagulation process are involved. Electron microscopy and immunofluorescence show large amounts of fibrin, or fibrinogen derivatives, within or between proliferating cells and in Bowman's space, where they appear to stimulate crescent formation. Thus, anticoagulant therapy will prevent crescent formation and a large part of the proliferative and sclerosing changes.

Autoantibody Disease (Steblay Nephritis). Another form of experimental antiglomerular basement membrane disease is produced in an entirely different way. If heterologous glomerular basement membrane preparations are injected into animals (usually sheep), some of the resulting antibodies are *autoantibodies* which will react with the animal's own glomerular basement membrane. Although the initiating immunologic events are

different from those of Masugi nephritis, the glomerulonephritis produced is quite similar: Both diseases basically result from antibodies against the glomerular basement membrane; in both, immunofluorescence shows gamma globulin and complement within the glomeruli in a highly characteristic, continuous ("linear") pattern along the basement membranes; both diseases are typically severe proliferative glomerulonephritis with conspicuous crescents, often rapidly leading to glomerulosclerosis. Presumably, similar pathogenic mechanisms (leukocytes, complement, and coagulation factors) operate in both diseases.

Importantly, investigation of experimental autoimmune glomerulonephritis has shown that autoantibodies against glomerular basement membrane cannot always be demonstrated in the circulation as long as the animal's kidneys are in place. However, within a few days after bilateral nephrectomy, such autoantibodies appear in the circulation. These observations indicate that generally autoantibodies are continuously and rapidly removed from the circulation by combination with the glomerular basement membrane.

It is also possible to produce autoantibodies against glomerular basement membrane by stimulation with other exogenous antigens containing similar antigenic determinants (*e.g.,* infectious agents). In addition, altered autologous basement membrane material can provide the stimulus. Either mechanism could operate in naturally occurring disease in man, although proof is lacking.

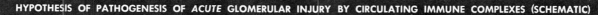
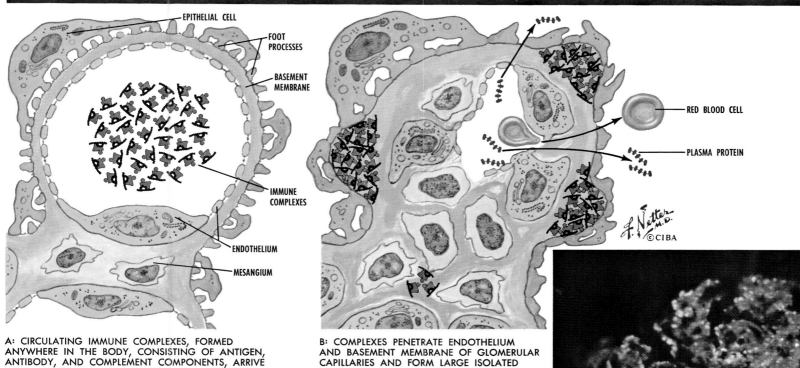

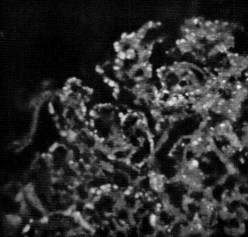

A: CIRCULATING IMMUNE COMPLEXES, FORMED ANYWHERE IN THE BODY, CONSISTING OF ANTIGEN, ANTIBODY, AND COMPLEMENT COMPONENTS, ARRIVE AT GLOMERULAR CAPILLARIES IN *LARGE AMOUNTS OVER A SHORT PERIOD OF TIME*

B: COMPLEXES PENETRATE ENDOTHELIUM AND BASEMENT MEMBRANE OF GLOMERULAR CAPILLARIES AND FORM LARGE ISOLATED DEPOSITS (HUMPS); FOOT PROCESSES FUSE; MESANGIAL AND ENDOTHELIAL CELLS SWELL AND PROLIFERATE, INVADING CAPILLARY LUMEN; FIBRILLAR BASEMENT MEMBRANELIKE MATERIAL (MESANGIAL MATRIX) IS DEPOSITED BETWEEN CELLS; INCREASED POROSITY OF CAPILLARY WALLS PERMITS ESCAPE OF PLASMA PROTEINS AND BLOOD CELLS, CAUSING PROTEINURIA AND HEMATURIA

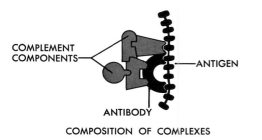

COMPOSITION OF COMPLEXES

IMMUNOFLUORESCENT PREPARATION, ACUTE GLO-MERULONEPHRITIS: IRREGULAR LUMPY DEPOSITS OF GAMMA GLOBULIN AND COMPLEMENT, RESEMBLING EXPERIMENTAL ACUTE IMMUNE COMPLEX DISEASE

Immune Complex Diseases

The second major category of immunologically induced glomerular disease is caused by deposition of immune complexes from the circulation. In contrast to antibodies against glomerular basement membrane, circulating complexes do not localize in glomeruli because of any immunologic specificity. Instead, their deposition in glomeruli appears to be related to certain physical properties of the complexes themselves.

Exogenous Antigen Diseases. Experimentally induced, immune complex disease produced by exogenous antigen may be one of several types.

ACUTE SERUM SICKNESS is the classic form of immune complex disease. In rabbits, this is produced by a single intravenous injection of a large amount of heterologous serum or heterologous plasma protein. During the ensuing first few days, the serum concentration of injected protein declines very slowly, reflecting a normal turnover rate for the protein. After several days the rabbit produces antibodies against the foreign protein; when these are first released into the circulation, they encounter an excess of antigen and accordingly form soluble antigen-antibody complexes. Most of these complexes are rather quickly removed from the circulation by cells of the reticuloendothelial system, within which they are rapidly degraded. However, some complexes also deposit within glomeruli and arteries, where they stimulate an inflammatory response.

The glomerular lesions are characterized by diffuse, fairly uniform swelling and proliferation of endothelial and mesangial cells with slight neutrophil infiltration. Immunofluorescence will usually demonstrate antibody and antigen (*i.e.,* immune complexes) in glomeruli in the form of scattered, granular deposits along the basement membrane. This pattern contrasts strikingly with the continuous accumulation seen in anti-GBM disease. Electron microscopy will show a few dense deposits along the epithelial side of the basement membrane, corresponding to the deposits seen by immunofluorescence. If no further injections of antigen are given, the glomeruli rapidly return to normal.

CHRONIC SERUM SICKNESS is experimentally produced by giving rabbits daily intravenous injections of moderate amounts of foreign protein over a period of many weeks or months. In those rabbits which produce moderate amounts of antibody, the resulting complexes persist in the circulation for several hours or more each day, and these animals usually develop characteristic glomerular lesions.

In histologic sections, only slight, fairly uniform thickening of the glomerular capillary walls is usually seen. However, both electron microscopy and immunofluorescence show innumerable deposits of immune complexes along the epithelial side of the basement membrane. In some animals, proliferative and sclerosing changes are seen.

VIRAL-INDUCED IMMUNE COMPLEX DISEASE is another type produced by exogenous antigen. Mice

injected at birth with lymphocytic choriomeningitis virus often develop glomerular lesions similar to those of chronic serum sickness. The glomerular disease appears to be caused by immune complexes formed between circulating viral material and antiviral antibody. An interesting aspect of this condition is that there is frequently no other manifestation of viral disease.

Autologous immune complex disease is represented by two forms, one experimentally induced and the other occurring naturally in certain strains of mice.

HEYMANN NEPHRITIS is an immune complex disease which develops from the formation of circulating complexes between autoantibodies and autologous material. This type of disease is produced by repeated injections into rats of homologous renal tissue. The glomerular lesions, which develop several weeks after the start of the injections, are quite similar to those of chronic serum sickness.

It was first thought that the disease was a form of autoimmune glomerulonephritis (*i.e.,* caused by autoantibodies against glomerular basement membrane—Steblay nephritis). However, it is now clear that the autoantibodies are directed against a protein normally present in the renal tubular epithelial cells. This protein is continuously released into the circulation in small amounts and combines with autoantibodies. As with the complexes of exogenous antigen, the complexes of autologous antigen localize in *Continued on page 130*

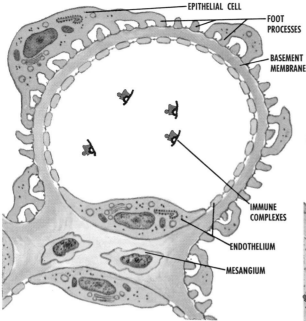

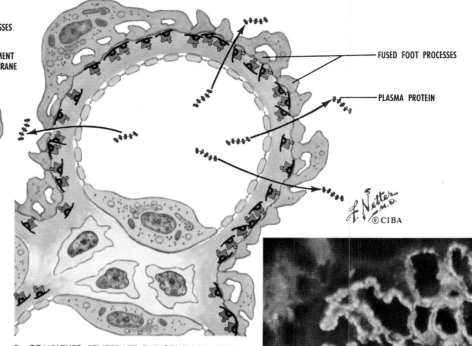

A: CIRCULATING IMMUNE COMPLEXES, FORMED ANYWHERE IN THE BODY, CONSISTING OF ANTIGEN, ANTIBODY, AND COMPLEMENT COMPONENTS, ARRIVE AT GLOMERULAR CAPILLARIES IN *SMALL AMOUNTS OVER A PROLONGED PERIOD OF TIME*

B: COMPLEXES PENETRATE ENDOTHELIUM AND BASEMENT MEMBRANE OF GLOMERULAR CAPILLARIES AND FORM DIFFUSE GRANULAR DEPOSITS; BASEMENT MEMBRANE PROLIFERATES TO ENCOMPASS DEPOSITS; FOOT PROCESSES FUSE; LITTLE OR NO ENDOTHELIAL CELL OR MESANGIAL CELL PROLIFERATION OCCURS, BUT POROSITY OF CAPILLARY WALL IS INCREASED, PERMITTING ESCAPE OF PLASMA PROTEINS AND CAUSING PROTEINURIA

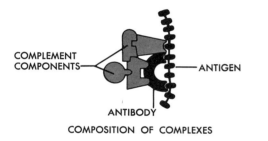

COMPOSITION OF COMPLEXES

IMMUNOFLUORESCENT PREPARATION, MEMBRANOUS NEPHROPATHY: DIFFUSE GRANULAR DEPOSITS ON BASEMENT MEMBRANE, RESEMBLING FINDINGS IN EXPERIMENTAL CHRONIC SERUM SICKNESS

Immunologic Mechanisms in Glomerular Diseases (Experimental Hypersensitivity Glomerular Diseases)

Continued from page 129

the glomeruli because of physical properties, not because of any immunologic specificity directed against a glomerular constituent.

Autologous immune complex disease can probably be produced with many other autologous antigens; however, autoantibody formation must be stimulated and the autologous antigens must be present in the circulation.

GLOMERULAR DISEASE—NZB MICE. In addition to the experimentally induced forms of immune complex disease, a spontaneous disease occurs in New Zealand Black (NZB) and related strains of mice. The glomerular lesions are caused by circulating immune complexes, and some of the antigens involved appear to be autologous material.

The cause of this disease is unknown, although it is apparent that genetic factors and viral infection are involved. In many respects, the disease resembles systemic lupus erythematosus (see page 141).

Immunologic Mechanisms in Human Glomerular Diseases

There is impressive evidence that several human glomerular diseases are caused by hypersensitivity.

Also, it now appears possible to determine the type of immunologic mechanism involved by a comparison with the described experimental models.

Anti-GBM Disease in Man. Convincing evidence has been obtained in a few patients exhibiting glomerulonephritis that the disease resulted from antiglomerular basement membrane antibodies. These patients reflected either a clinical picture of rapidly progressive renal disease (pathologically classified as subacute glomerulonephritis, see page 133) or Goodpasture's syndrome, characterized by lung hemorrhage and severe and rapidly progressive glomerulonephritis (see page 177).

In the patients studied, immunofluorescent technics showed a pattern of linear accumulation of immunoglobulins along the glomerular basement membranes. These findings are indistinguishable from those of experimentally induced anti-GBM disease. Furthermore, gamma globulin eluted from the glomeruli was shown to combine with glomerular basement membrane.

Circulating antiglomerular basement membrane antibodies have been demonstrable, but in some cases only after bilateral nephrectomy in preparation for renal transplantation. Thus, as in the experimental model, autoantibodies are continuously removed from the circulation by combination with glomerular basement membrane.

Immune Complex Disease in Man. Several glomerular diseases appear to be caused by deposition of circulating antigen-antibody complexes, and these diseases are much more common than those

caused by anti-GBM antibodies. This mechanism is most thoroughly documented in systemic lupus erythematosus (see page 141).

Poststreptococcal glomerulonephritis (see page 131) is also presumed to represent immune complex disease since it closely resembles experimental acute serum sickness in the rabbit; electron microscopy shows both to be diffuse proliferative glomerulonephritis with focal granular accumulation of immunoglobulins along the epithelial surface of the basement membrane. The latter corresponds to the typical *dense deposits* ("humps"). Parenthetically, it is likely that the antigen involved is a streptococcal product, but this has not yet been established.

Another disease for which an immune complex basis seems probable is the glomerulonephritis associated with subacute bacterial endocarditis since the vegetation is a source of repeated release of antigens into the circulation. However, immunofluorescent and electron microscopic observations which might support this interpretation apparently are not available. Evidence has also been obtained that a form of glomerulonephritis seen in some patients with malaria is caused by immune complexes containing malarial antigens.

Other diseases in which an immune complex pathogenesis may operate include membranous nephritis, membranoproliferative glomerulonephritis (mesangiocapillary glomerulonephritis), and the nephritis associated with anaphylactoid purpura. □

Acute Glomerulonephritis

Acute glomerulonephritis is a nonsuppurative inflammatory process involving the glomeruli of both kidneys. In the classic course of the disease, a streptococcal infection of the respiratory tract precedes by 10 to 14 days the abrupt onset of edema, hypertension, and abnormal urinalysis.

Although the disease occurs most often in children and young adults, it is now recognized that older adults also are frequently affected. In this latter group, however, the onset is more apt to be insidious, with few or no clinical findings to suggest a preceding streptococcal infection.

The pathogenesis of acute glomerulonephritis, in most cases, can be considered a renal inflammatory response to infection with several types of group A β-hemolytic streptococci (types 12, 4, 25, and, rarely, others). Occasionally, pneumococcal, staphylococcal, and viral infections have been implicated. An immunologic mechanism appears to be the cause of the inflammatory response of the glomeruli. This view is supported by the occurrence, early in the course of the disease, of a low serum complement and deposition of γ-globulin in the capillary wall. However, in spite of the considerable experimental data to support an immunologic etiology, this has not been definitely established.

The common presenting features of acute glomerulonephritis include hematuria, proteinuria, edema, and hypertension.

Hematuria occurs at some time in virtually every patient and is gross in about 40 percent of the cases. Reduction in the amount of blood in the urine is usually a reliable sign of recovery, although microscopic hematuria may persist for months.

Proteinuria, at times marked, is also characteristic at the onset of the disease process and may continue for years after the other findings have disappeared. A nephrotic syndrome rarely occurs. Cylindruria, in the form of hyaline, hemoglobin, and red blood cell casts, is also commonly found. In a few cases, however, urinalysis may be entirely normal, so that diagnosis can be established only by renal biopsy.

Edema, the hallmark of excess total body salt and water, may be moderate to severe. The extent of the edema depends upon both the severity of the glomerular inflammation (with attendant renal insufficiency) and the time interval between recognition of the disease process and institution of dietary salt restriction.

Hypertension almost always occurs, although the rise in blood pressure may be only moderate. In about five percent of patients with markedly elevated blood pressure, encephalopathy (with severe headache, convulsions, and coma) may occur. The elevated blood pressure usually subsides with the onset of a diuresis which marks the beginning of clinical improvement.

Because of the hypertension and fluid and salt retention, a number of cardiovascular findings are usually noted. Symptoms of dyspnea and orthopnea, with physical findings of rales, a gallop rhythm,

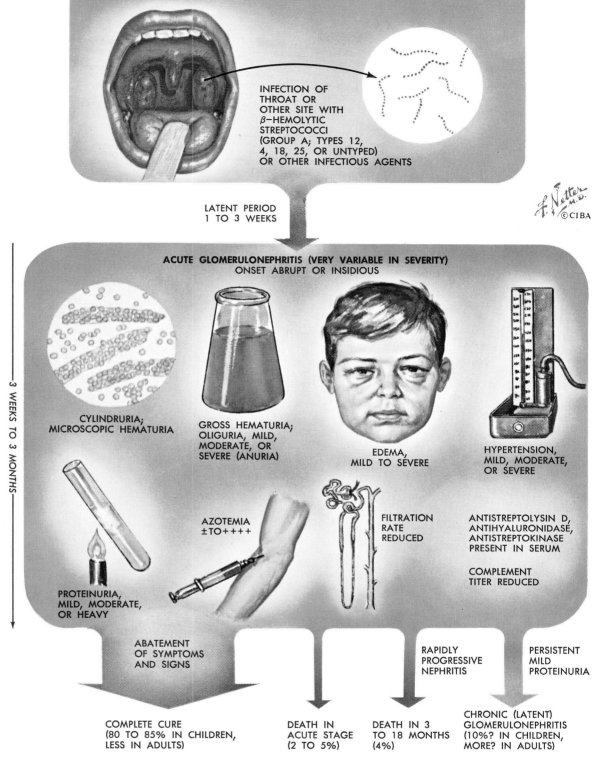

CLINICAL COURSE OF ACUTE GLOMERULONEPHRITIS

INFECTION OF THROAT OR OTHER SITE WITH β–HEMOLYTIC STREPTOCOCCI (GROUP A; TYPES 12, 4, 18, 25, OR UNTYPED) OR OTHER INFECTIOUS AGENTS

LATENT PERIOD 1 TO 3 WEEKS

3 WEEKS TO 3 MONTHS

ACUTE GLOMERULONEPHRITIS (VERY VARIABLE IN SEVERITY) ONSET ABRUPT OR INSIDIOUS

CYLINDRURIA; MICROSCOPIC HEMATURIA

GROSS HEMATURIA; OLIGURIA, MILD, MODERATE, OR SEVERE (ANURIA)

EDEMA, MILD TO SEVERE

HYPERTENSION, MILD, MODERATE, OR SEVERE

PROTEINURIA, MILD, MODERATE, OR HEAVY

AZOTEMIA ±TO++++

FILTRATION RATE REDUCED

ANTISTREPTOLYSIN D, ANTIHYALURONIDASE, ANTISTREPTOKINASE PRESENT IN SERUM

COMPLEMENT TITER REDUCED

ABATEMENT OF SYMPTOMS AND SIGNS

RAPIDLY PROGRESSIVE NEPHRITIS

PERSISTENT MILD PROTEINURIA

COMPLETE CURE (80 TO 85% IN CHILDREN, LESS IN ADULTS)

DEATH IN ACUTE STAGE (2 TO 5%)

DEATH IN 3 TO 18 MONTHS (4%)

CHRONIC (LATENT) GLOMERULONEPHRITIS (10%? IN CHILDREN, MORE? IN ADULTS)

and an elevated venous pressure, may appear.

Usually renal function is moderately reduced. As might be expected, glomerular filtration rate is affected to the greatest degree. Mild retention of urea is chiefly associated with oliguria and a sodium-free urine having a high specific gravity. Five to 10 percent of the patients experience severe oliguria (less than 200 ml/day) and impaired renal function. The clinical picture in these patients is often indistinguishable from that seen in acute renal failure from any cause, especially if the onset of the disease has been insidious (see page 111). Death occurs in 50 percent of patients with severe oliguria and apparently more frequently in elderly patients.

The onset of improvement is usually marked by the development of diuresis with a rapid decrudescence of the edema, hypertension, and the cardiovascular manifestations. However, microscopic hematuria and

proteinuria (particularly the latter) may continue for months to several years.

Complete recovery occurs in the vast majority of patients. After a variable period of time, ranging from weeks to months, 80 to 85 percent of affected children show normal urinalysis and no clinical manifestations of disease. The prospect for recovery in adults is less favorable. The overall death rate in all ages during the *acute stage* ranges between two and five percent. Approximately four percent of patients show continuous clinical manifestations and abnormal urinalyses. In this group, *progressive renal insufficiency* develops over a period of 3 to 18 months. Another small number of patients do not heal completely and enter a so-called latent phase of glomerulonephritis in which there are no clinical manifestations of disease and the only abnormalities are hematuria, proteinuria, and cylindruria. *Continued on page 132*

Acute Glomerulonephritis

Continued from page 131

After many years of good health, this type of patient begins to suffer from gradually deteriorating renal function and eventually dies because of uremia.

No specific therapy has been shown to influence either the acute inflammation or the healing process. Thus, treatment is directed toward control of the pathophysiologic complications of the disease. Edema and circulatory congestion are managed by dietary salt restriction and, occasionally, by the administration of diuretics. Hypertension usually responds to bed rest, sedation, and salt restriction. However, on rare occasions, antihypertensive agents are required. When acute renal failure occurs in the course of acute glomerulonephritis, conservative management (fluid, sodium, and potassium restriction) usually suffices. Only rarely is it necessary to employ dialysis (see page 258).

Pathologic Changes

Although much controversy and ignorance still exist regarding the pathogenesis and pathologic features of chronic glomerulonephritis (see pages 134-137), there seems to be general agreement with regard to *acute diffuse glomerulonephritis,* especially the so-called poststreptococcal type.

The morphology of this disease was first described by Volhard and Fahr in 1914. Although their description is based entirely on autopsy material, it agrees surprisingly well with recent findings in large biopsy series. Only some details have been added to that original description, owing to the introduction of such new technics as electron and immunofluorescent microscopy.

Grossly, the kidneys in acute diffuse (poststreptococcal) glomerulonephritis exhibit moderate-to-marked enlargement and pallor. There may be occasional punctate hemorrhages.

Microscopically, the most important changes take place in the glomeruli which appear large and cellular. All glomeruli are rather evenly affected. They contain few red blood cells because of the proliferation and swelling of the glomerular cells and consequent narrowing of the capillary lumina. There is a distinct, though variable, increase in polymorphonuclear leukocytes which is especially marked in the early stages of the disease.

The nature of the proliferating cells has been clarified mainly by the use of the thin section technic, serial sections (Jones), and electron microscopy. While there is some swelling and a slight increase in endothelial cells, the most marked proliferation takes place in the mesangium.

The mesangium, it will be recalled, is a specialized form of connective tissue found only in the glomerulus and located in the center of each lobule. Normally, it consists of a few cells and a small amount of matrix (produced by these cells) which, on light microscopy, appears as PAS-positive, fibrillar, or membrane-like material (see pages 7-9).

In acute glomerulonephritis, the mesangial cells proliferate to varying degrees, depending on the severity of the process,

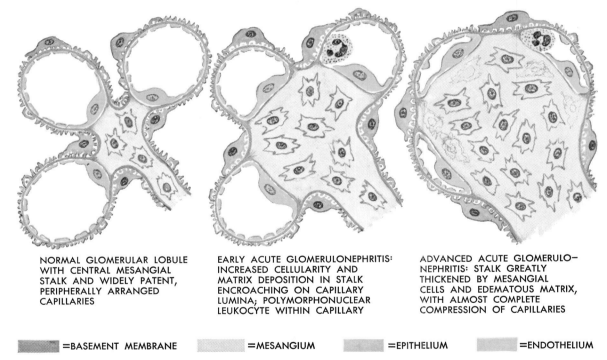

ACUTE GLOMERULONEPHRITIS

GLOMERULUS WITH GREATLY INCREASED CELLULARITY AND MESANGIAL MATRIX AND ALMOST COMPLETE OBLITERATION OF CAPILLARY LUMINA; THE CELLS ARE CHIEFLY MESANGIAL IN TYPE, WITH SOME POLYMORPHONUCLEAR LEUKOCYTES AND A FEW EOSINOPHILS

SCHEMA OF PROGRESSIVE CHANGES IN GLOMERULAR LOBULES IN ACUTE GLOMERULONEPHRITIS

NORMAL GLOMERULAR LOBULE WITH CENTRAL MESANGIAL STALK AND WIDELY PATENT, PERIPHERALLY ARRANGED CAPILLARIES

EARLY ACUTE GLOMERULONEPHRITIS: INCREASED CELLULARITY AND MATRIX DEPOSITION IN STALK ENCROACHING ON CAPILLARY LUMINA; POLYMORPHONUCLEAR LEUKOCYTE WITHIN CAPILLARY

ADVANCED ACUTE GLOMERULO-NEPHRITIS: STALK GREATLY THICKENED BY MESANGIAL CELLS AND EDEMATOUS MATRIX, WITH ALMOST COMPLETE COMPRESSION OF CAPILLARIES

=BASEMENT MEMBRANE =MESANGIUM =EPITHELIUM =ENDOTHELIUM

and lay down thin layers of matrix, thus filling the lobular centers. The enlargement of the mesangial portion of the lobule causes gradual compression of the capillaries which interferes with glomerular functions, especially with the glomerular filtration rate.

Usually the epithelial cells also swell, contain hyaline droplets, and may show focal proliferation which leads to the formation of cellular *crescents.* Occasionally, fibrin thrombi may be found in the capillary lumina. (The presence of crescents and fibrin thrombi is regarded as a poor prognostic sign.) If the number of polymorphonuclear leukocytes is excessive, some authors talk about an *exudative* type of acute glomerulonephritis as opposed to the described *proliferative* type.

The tubules often contain red blood cells (sometimes as casts), polymorphonuclear leukocytes, or hyaline casts. Also frequently seen are hyaline droplets in tubular epithelial cells.

The interstitial stroma shows edema and focal infiltration with polymorphonuclear leukocytes, lymphocytes, or histiocytes. Blood vessels usually are not affected.

All changes described are reversible and usually do reverse since most patients with acute glomerulonephritis, especially children, heal completely. A considerable degree of mesangial proliferation and matrix deposition may, eventually, be completely resorbed. Polymorphonuclear leukocytic exudation and small crescents may disappear, while large crescents, adhesions, and fibrinous exudate tend to become organized by fibrous tissue.

Electron microscopy discloses that all cells appear enlarged. The endothelial cells lose their normal fenestration and show large vacuoles. Mesangial cells are increased in number and are surrounded by mesangial matrix with a density similar to that of basement

Acute Glomerulonephritis
Continued

membrane but is slightly more fibrillar. Mesangial cells are also separated from the capillary lumina by a more or less complete membrane composed of the mesangial matrix. In early stages, only thin membranelike areas of matrix are visible; these become thicker as the disease progresses. The basement membrane itself is little changed except for focal thickening, while the epithelial cells may show focal fusion of foot processes. Polymorphonuclear leukocytes are present in the capillary lumina.

An important electron microscopic finding, and the only one not previously recognized under light microscopy, consists of the so-called "humps"—protein deposits of roughly semicircular or triangular shape, located between the basement membrane and epithelial cells. The deposits are believed to be diagnostic for acute poststreptococcal glomerulonephritis, although on occasion they may also be found in serum sickness and in acute exacerbations of chronic glomerulonephritis. These "humps" appear early in the disease and disappear after several weeks. There are claims that a thorough search made during the early stage will reveal "humps" in virtually all patients.

Immunofluorescent microscopy shows varied morphologic patterns in acute glomerulonephritis. Most authors agree now that a granular pattern along the capillary wall is the usual finding. The granules represent deposition of γ-globulin and correspond to the sites of electron-dense subepithelial nodules seen with electron microscopy. Human complement (C′3) has been demonstrated (Burkholder) at the same glomerular sites and, occasionally, in the walls of blood vessels.

To prove the presence of antigen-antibody complexes at these sites, it would be necessary to find the antigen also. However, localization and identification of the antigen have proved to be extremely difficult. By using immunofluorescence and immunoelectron microscopic technics, Seegal *et al.* observed the presence of focally distributed antigens of the cell wall of type-12 streptococci along the capillary wall, a finding which has not yet been confirmed.

Possibly, streptococcal antigens cross-react with basement membrane antigens. However, although the presence in glomeruli of antigen-antibody complexes has been definitely established in experimental serum sickness (see page 130), an analogous situation can only be postulated for acute glomerulonephritis.

Rapidly Progressive Glomerulonephritis

Lately, one type of acute glomerulonephritis has been distinguished from acute poststreptococcal disease because it differs clinically, morphologically, and probably etiologically. It is the so-called *rapidly progressive* or *extracapillary glomerulonephritis.*

Previously, when only postmortem tissue was available to pathologists for interpretation, the disease was called *subacute glomerulonephritis* because it was

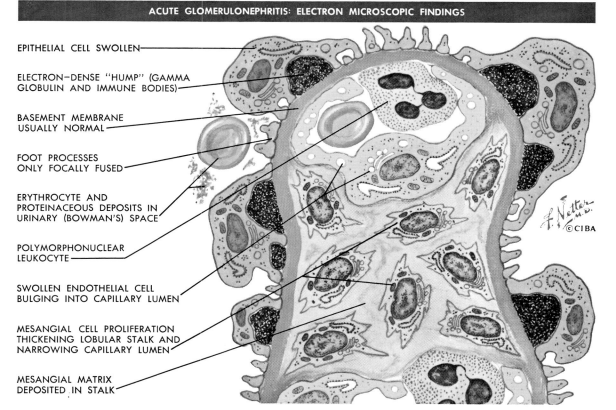

ACUTE GLOMERULONEPHRITIS: ELECTRON MICROSCOPIC FINDINGS

EPITHELIAL CELL SWOLLEN

ELECTRON—DENSE "HUMP" (GAMMA GLOBULIN AND IMMUNE BODIES)

BASEMENT MEMBRANE USUALLY NORMAL

FOOT PROCESSES ONLY FOCALLY FUSED

ERYTHROCYTE AND PROTEINACEOUS DEPOSITS IN URINARY (BOWMAN'S) SPACE

POLYMORPHONUCLEAR LEUKOCYTE

SWOLLEN ENDOTHELIAL CELL BULGING INTO CAPILLARY LUMEN

MESANGIAL CELL PROLIFERATION THICKENING LOBULAR STALK AND NARROWING CAPILLARY LUMEN

MESANGIAL MATRIX DEPOSITED IN STALK

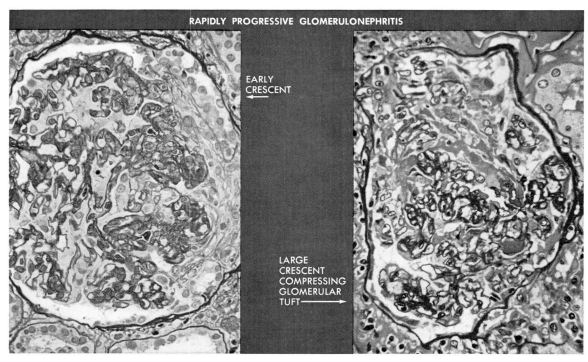

RAPIDLY PROGRESSIVE GLOMERULONEPHRITIS

EARLY CRESCENT

LARGE CRESCENT COMPRESSING GLOMERULAR TUFT

believed that development of crescents required considerable time. However, with the use of renal biopsies, it has been learned that cellular crescents can be found in early stages of the disease.

Microscopically, rapidly progressive glomerulonephritis is characterized by the presence of many, large, cellular crescents consisting of proliferated epithelial cells of Bowman's capsule. All glomeruli are involved to a similar degree. The severe epithelial proliferation causes compression of the glomerular capillaries which simply collapse. Clinically, this leads to oliguria or anuria and to rapidly developing renal failure. In the pure form of this disease, there is practically no proliferation of the mesangium or endothelial cells and no exudation of polymorphonuclear leukocytes. Fibrin, however, may be present between the cells of the crescent. The tubules, stroma, and blood vessels behave as in acute poststreptococcal glomerulonephritis.

Electron microscopic findings correspond to those of light microscopy. There is marked epithelial proliferation, and fibrin, with typical fibrillar structure and periodicity, has been identified within the crescents. Capillaries appear collapsed but lack the subepithelial "humps" found in acute poststreptococcal glomerulonephritis. With immunofluorescent microscopy, linear or, more often, irregular deposits of γ-globulin may be found along the capillary walls.

As the disease progresses, the crescents rapidly become organized by fibrous tissue. This fibrosis prevents the capillaries from reexpanding so that after a short time (a few weeks to a few months) one finds many large, fibrous crescents surrounding remnants of compressed capillaries. This feature explains the rapidly developing and irreversible renal failure. The tubules also atrophy rapidly, signaling the development of marked interstitial fibrosis. □

Chronic Glomerulonephritis

Chronic glomerulonephritis is a disease process, probably of multiple etiology, characterized pathologically by sclerotic and obsolescent glomeruli and clinically by the manifestations of renal insufficiency.

In the majority of patients there is no apparent history of preceding renal disease. About 10 percent of the cases are presumed to arise as a late manifestation of *acute poststreptococcal glomerulonephritis,* but this association is controversial (see page 131). Also in some patients, there is a preceding focal glomerulonephritis (see pages 138–139).

Clinical Course

The disease characteristically begins insidiously without any obvious inciting factor. The patient usually has no physical disability, or rarely will note intermittent edema, and during a routine examination evidence of renal disease is discovered fortuitously. Moderate hypertension and persistent proteinuria may be the only abnormal findings. Not infrequently, however, the disease is heralded by the abrupt onset of a full-blown nephrotic syndrome (see page 123). Finally, there are those rare cases in which the patient presents with signs of uremia (see pages 121–122).

The clinical picture and course of the disease depend upon the severity of the renal insufficiency. If azotemia is only moderate, hypertension and edema may be mild. As renal function deteriorates, hypertension becomes severe, resulting in cardiac enlargement and congestive heart failure which further aggravates renal function (see page 175).

During the course of the disease, heavy proteinuria may develop, leading to a nephrotic syndrome. (As mentioned, patients may present with the nephrotic syndrome.) The nephrotic phase may vary in both intensity and duration, apparently remitting spontaneously, only to recur weeks or months later. However, as renal function declines, the quantity of protein lost in the urine gradually diminishes, and the nephrosis clears.

In a small percentage of patients, there are acute exacerbations of glomerulonephritis characterized by sudden onset of hematuria, an increase in proteinuria and cylindruria, and an abrupt decrease in renal function. Such episodes, often preceded by an upper respiratory tract infection caused by group A hemolytic streptococci, are usually transitory and do not appear to contribute to the ultimate progression of the disease.

When renal insufficiency becomes advanced and glomerular filtration rate is markedly reduced, the clinical picture is one of variable edema, sustained diastolic hypertension, increasing azotemia, anemia, and metabolic acidosis. Terminally there is frank uremia.

From the time the diagnosis is first made there is a variable, but usually long (10- to 30-year) period of time during which the patient enjoys good health. No known therapy, however, will significantly alter the natural course of chronic glomerulonephritis. Thus, treatment should attempt to prevent complications and relieve

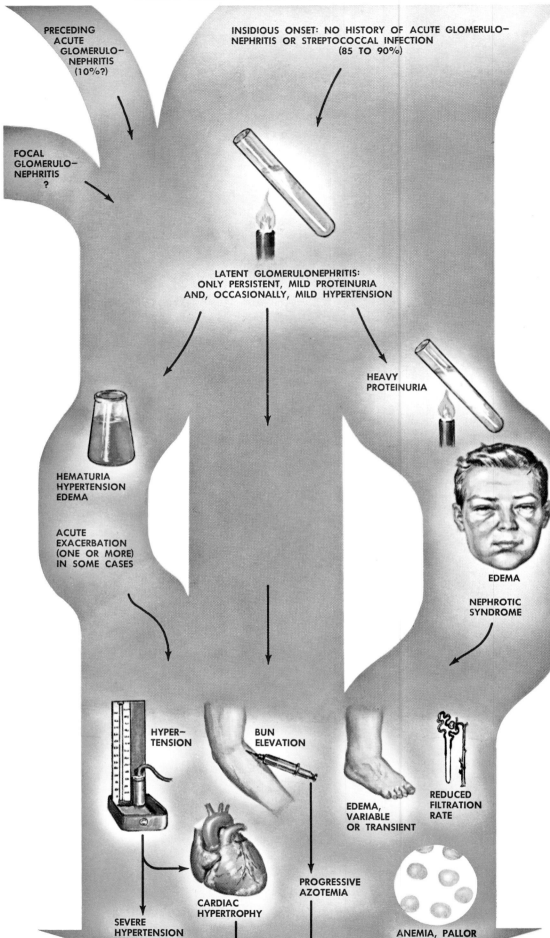

CLINICAL COURSE OF CHRONIC GLOMERULONEPHRITIS

PRECEDING ACUTE GLOMERULO-NEPHRITIS (10%?)

INSIDIOUS ONSET: NO HISTORY OF ACUTE GLOMERULO-NEPHRITIS OR STREPTOCOCCAL INFECTION (85 TO 90%)

FOCAL GLOMERULO-NEPHRITIS ?

LATENT GLOMERULONEPHRITIS: ONLY PERSISTENT, MILD PROTEINURIA AND, OCCASIONALLY, MILD HYPERTENSION

HEAVY PROTEINURIA

5 TO 30 YEARS

HEMATURIA HYPERTENSION EDEMA

ACUTE EXACERBATION (ONE OR MORE) IN SOME CASES

EDEMA

NEPHROTIC SYNDROME

HYPER-TENSION

BUN ELEVATION

EDEMA, VARIABLE OR TRANSIENT

REDUCED FILTRATION RATE

SEVERE HYPERTENSION

CARDIAC HYPERTROPHY

PROGRESSIVE AZOTEMIA

ANEMIA, PALLOR

FAILURE

UREMIA

DEATH

Chronic Glomerulonephritis

Continued

symptoms of renal failure. When hypertension becomes sustained, antihypertensive therapy may tend to slow progression of the vascular lesions. Steroid and/or immunosuppressive therapy may temporarily diminish the protein loss in the nephrotic subject, but it does not appear to influence renal function.

Because streptococcal infection may precede acute exacerbations of glomerulonephritis, routine prophylactic penicillin has been advocated. However, there is no evidence that such therapy slows the progression of the disease.

When renal failure becomes abject and the uremic syndrome supervenes, life can be prolonged only by means of chronic dialysis or renal transplant. The long-range results of these technics are not known, but the procedures sustain patients suffering from end-stage kidney disease.

Early Chronic Glomerulonephritis

Chronic glomerulonephritis, by definition, is an inflammatory process of the glomeruli which is no longer expected to revert to normal. On the contrary, it tends to progress, and the inflammatory lesions become replaced by sclerosis and scarring.

Some patients are first seen when the lesions have progressed to a point where it is no longer possible to determine the nature of the initial inflammatory lesion, the stage of *late* chronic glomerulonephritis. The late stage will be discussed subsequently, after the various gross and histologic features of *early* chronic glomerulonephritis are presented.

Pathology. Grossly, the kidneys may be enlarged, normal, or slightly reduced in size, and often pale yellow in color. The surfaces may be smooth, particularly in kidneys of normal size, or finely granular in smaller sized organs. On cut section the cortex may appear pale and swollen while the pyramids are usually darker than normal. The cortical pallor is caused both by lipid in the tubules and by interstitial edema which collapses the capillaries.

Histologically, the glomeruli exhibit two essential features: (1) proliferation of cells, and (2) deposition of intercellular material (proliferative and sclerosing glomerulonephritis). Some authorities also include membranous glomerulonephritis (membranous nephropathy), but in this disease, cell proliferation and sclerosis are absent, and the histologic changes are limited to the capillary walls, at least in the early stages.

In proliferative and sclerosing glomerulonephritis there is a fairly even balance between cell proliferation and sclerosis. The cells are mainly mesangial, although some participation of the endothelial cells may be seen. Sclerosis is caused chiefly by excessive formation of mesangial matrix. These two processes expand the mesangial stalk and enlarge the lobular centers so that glomeruli often become larger than normal. There may be proliferation of the epithelial cells with formation of epithelial (and later, fibroepithelial) crescents and adhesions, but this varies from patient to patient (and from glomerulus to glomerulus) and may be completely absent. At first, the tubules

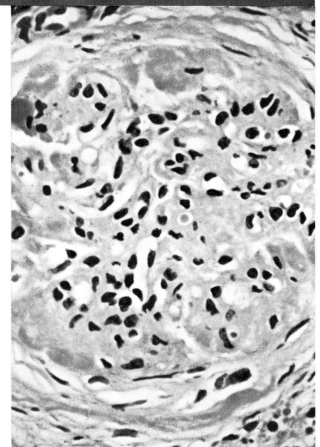

GLOMERULUS SHOWING MODERATE CELL PROLIFERATION AND RATHER EXTENSIVE SCLEROSIS

LARGE, PALE YELLOW KIDNEY, WITH SMOOTH OR ONLY SLIGHTLY GRANULATED SURFACE

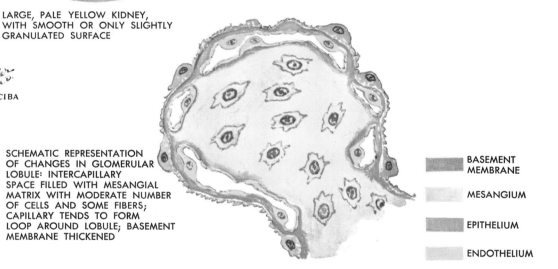

SCHEMATIC REPRESENTATION OF CHANGES IN GLOMERULAR LOBULE: INTERCAPILLARY SPACE FILLED WITH MESANGIAL MATRIX WITH MODERATE NUMBER OF CELLS AND SOME FIBERS; CAPILLARY TENDS TO FORM LOOP AROUND LOBULE; BASEMENT MEMBRANE THICKENED

BASEMENT MEMBRANE

MESANGIUM

EPITHELIUM

ENDOTHELIUM

are preserved and often large; the tubular cells may contain hyaline droplets, probably reabsorbed protein, and appreciable amounts of lipid.

Progression of the disease is characterized by a decrease in the number of cells in the glomeruli and an increase in the amount of intercellular material leading to collapse and compression of the capillaries and sclerosis of the glomeruli. Hypertension and related vascular sclerosis frequently occur in patients with chronic glomerulonephritis; the narrowing of the arteries and arterioles further impairs the glomerular circulation and accelerates the glomerular sclerosis. In turn, constriction of the glomerular capillary bed is followed by tubular ischemia and progressive atrophy.

Mesangiocapillary Glomerulonephritis

This form of chronic glomerulonephritis is known by a variety of names including *membranoproliferative*, *lobular,* and *hypocomplementemic glomerulonephritis.* Although classified as a type of proliferative nephritis by many authorities, mesangiocapillary glomerulonephritis deserves special mention because of certain clinical and pathologic features.

Although rather uncommon, this form of the disease accounts for an appreciable number of cases of nephrotic syndrome among older children and young adults, especially teenage girls.

The onset is usually insidious, and edema is often the first symptom that brings the patient to the physician. The edema may have been shortly preceded by a minor nonspecific infection, especially a mild sore throat. However, in some patients, especially children, the onset is acute and indistinguishable from poststreptococcal glomerulonephritis. Though not yet confirmed, there is a suggestion that some of the more severe cases of acute diffuse Continued on page 136

Chronic Glomerulonephritis

Continued from page 135

proliferative glomerulonephritis progress to mesangiocapillary glomerulonephritis.

The main clinical manifestation is *heavy proteinuria.* In the majority of patients, but not in all, *hypoalbuminemia* and *nephrotic syndrome* are present at the onset or develop later. *Hematuria,* an important finding, is usually microscopic. *Hypertension* is common.

A characteristic, though not invariable, feature is depression of serum complement (C3 [β_1C] component) which is seen in 60 to 80 percent of patients at one time or another. The reduced complement may result from its consumption in an immunologic process related to the disease, or from the instability and precipitation in the tissues of some of the complement components.

As with other forms of chronic glomerulonephritis, mesangiocapillary disease is slowly progressive, with gradual deterioration of renal function. Many patients survive 10 years or longer, but the use of steroids and other immunosuppressants has little apparent effect. Also, patients with concomitant hypertension often do not tolerate steroids.

Histology. The picture is characteristic. Glomeruli are enlarged and moderately cellular, lobular centers are expanded, and capillary walls thickened. The enlargement is caused by proliferation of the mesangial cells and matrix, often leading to striking "lobulation" of the glomerulus *(lobular glomerulonephritis).* Ingrowth of the mesangium into the capillary wall causes capillary wall thickening, separates the endothelium from the basement membrane and narrows the lumen. Best demonstrated by electron microscopy, these features appear as a tissue response to some forms of glomerular injury. Use of PAS or silver methenamine stains often produces the picture of a "railroad track," with one track representing the basement membrane, the other representing a layer of mesangial matrix, and the lighter space in between representing the mesangial cell cytoplasm. In addition, protein may be densely deposited in the mesangial matrix and surround the mesangial cells. However, even though the basement membrane may appear duplicated because of the "railroad track" appearance, it nevertheless is usually thin and unchanged. Also, the proliferating mesangial cells encroach upon and partially surround the capillary endothelial cells and separate them from the basement membrane.

Immunofluorescent microscopy reveals that the deposits within the mesangial matrix consist mainly of complement (β_1C), although small amounts of γ-globulin (IgG, IgM) may also be present. The deposits tend to obscure the basement membrane and the mesangial matrix and render them nonargyrophilic. Bowman's capsule usually shows no change, but epithelial cells often exhibit extensive fusion of foot processes—a common finding in patients with nephrotic syndrome.

Within the tubules, changes characteristic of the nephrotic syndrome are found. These consist of casts, hyaline droplets, and lipid vacuoles.

As the disease progresses, crescents, capsular adhesions, and diffuse sclerosis lead to total obliteration of the glomeruli, with consequent tubular atrophy and interstitial fibrosis.

The histology of mesangiocapillary glomerulonephritis may resemble that of diabetic nodular glomerulosclerosis. Both conditions are characterized by bulbous thickening of glomerular lobules, but usually in diabetic glomerulosclerosis there is also a marked thickening of capillary basement membranes. In addition, in diabetic glomerulosclerosis there are frequently exudative (or insudative) changes with hyaline deposits in the glomeruli and marked hyaline arteriolosclerosis involving both the afferent and efferent arterioles. These findings are rare in mesangiocapillary glomerulonephritis. Furthermore, diabetic nodules are usually acellular or hypocellular, variable in size, and tend to be located in the peripheral lobules away from the hilus (see pages 149–152).

Membranous Glomerulonephritis (Membranous Nephropathy)

The clinical presentation and gross appearance of the kidneys in patients with membranous glomerulonephritis are similar to those in patients with mesangiocapillary glomerulonephritis. Membranous nephropathy is rare in childhood but is relatively frequent in teenagers and reaches maximum incidence between the ages of 40 and 60 years, in both men and women.

In early stages of the disease, standard histologic stains often show only minimal alterations in the glomeruli, much like those observed in lipoid nephrosis (minimal or "nil" disease, see pages 126 and 127). (However, there is no evidence that lipoid nephrosis ever develops into membranous nephropathy.)

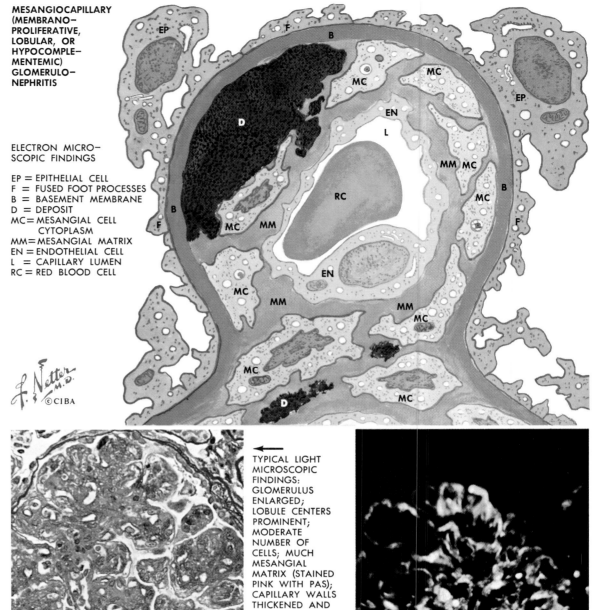

MESANGIOCAPILLARY (MEMBRANO-PROLIFERATIVE, LOBULAR, OR HYPOCOMPLEMENTEMIC) GLOMERULONEPHRITIS

ELECTRON MICROSCOPIC FINDINGS

EP = EPITHELIAL CELL
F = FUSED FOOT PROCESSES
B = BASEMENT MEMBRANE
D = DEPOSIT
MC = MESANGIAL CELL CYTOPLASM
MM = MESANGIAL MATRIX
EN = ENDOTHELIAL CELL
L = CAPILLARY LUMEN
RC = RED BLOOD CELL

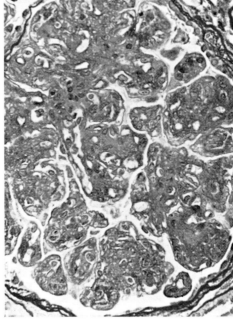

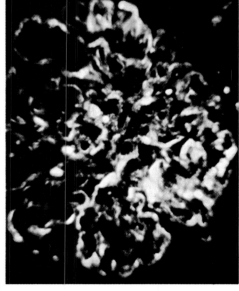

TYPICAL LIGHT MICROSCOPIC FINDINGS: GLOMERULUS ENLARGED; LOBULE CENTERS PROMINENT; MODERATE NUMBER OF CELLS; MUCH MESANGIAL MATRIX (STAINED PINK WITH PAS); CAPILLARY WALLS THICKENED AND LUMINA NARROWED

IMMUNOFLUORESCENT PREPARATION STAINED FOR COMPLEMENT: IRREGULAR DEPOSITION ALONG WALLS OF CAPILLARIES

Chronic Glomerulonephritis
Continued

Light microscopy (silver stains) and more especially electron microscopy reveal characteristic changes in and around the capillary basement membranes. Small, dense, protein deposits which appear between the basement membrane and the overlying, fused foot processes (see page 126) contain γ-globulin and complement ($\beta_1 C$) and are interrupted by focal thickening, or projections ("spikes"), of the basement membrane. Eventually the deposits are surrounded by, and incorporated into, the markedly thickened basement membrane.

Late Chronic Glomerulonephritis

Late chronic gomerulonephritis is characterized clinically by progressive renal insufficiency and pathologically by the predominance of scarring and atrophy. The disease is really a late common pathway of many glomerular processes, such as acute diffuse glomerulonephritis (rarely), mesangiocapillary (or lobular) glomerulonephritis, and occasionally membranous nephropathy. It may also represent the end result of focal glomerular diseases, such as recurrent attacks of acute focal glomerulonephritis of bacterial or viral origin, or an insidious process called focal and segmental glomerulosclerosis often seen in patients with lipoid nephrosis.

Systemic diseases such as lupus erythematosus may also lead to a nonspecific picture of late chronic glomerulonephritis (see page 141). Moreover, the very advanced stages of chronic glomerulonephritis ("end-stage kidney") may be difficult to differentiate from end-stage kidney of renal arteriolosclerosis or of chronic pyelonephritis.

Grossly, in late chronic glomerulonephritis the kidneys are small, tannish gray, finely or coarsely granular, weigh under 100 gm each, sometimes as low as 50 gm. Cut surfaces show marked reduction in width, especially of the pale cortex.

Histologically, the vast majority of glomeruli are altered, although an occasional glomerulus appears normal. The outstanding feature is disorganization of the normal lobular architecture which may appear as irregular thickening and distortion of lobules, interlobular adhesions, or adhesions between the lobules and Bowman's capsule. In some glomeruli, early changes of cellular proliferation of the mesangium and cellular crescents may be seen, but in many glomeruli late changes are apparent. The glomeruli may be large with fibrous crescents and hyalinization of the tufts, or small because of the collapse of capillaries. The latter change probably is caused by ischemia and corresponds to obsolete glomeruli in arteriolosclerotic kidneys. There is a diminution in the number of glomeruli, many apparently having been resorbed.

Many tubules show atrophy, with thickened basement membranes and flat epithelium, while a few are hypertrophied and show tall epithelial cells. Other tubules are markedly dilated and filled with protein precipitate. Small areas of atrophied and hypertrophied tubules usually alternate beneath the renal capsule.

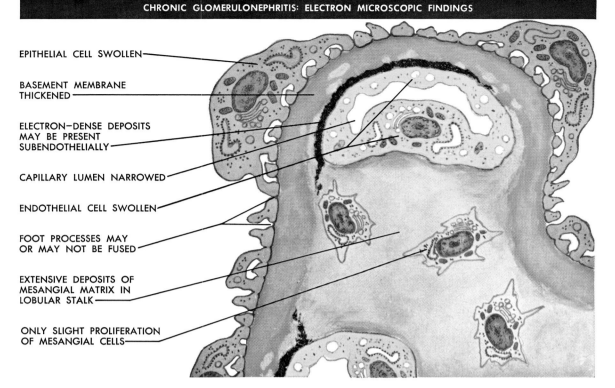

CHRONIC GLOMERULONEPHRITIS: ELECTRON MICROSCOPIC FINDINGS

- EPITHELIAL CELL SWOLLEN
- BASEMENT MEMBRANE THICKENED
- ELECTRON-DENSE DEPOSITS MAY BE PRESENT SUBENDOTHELIALLY
- CAPILLARY LUMEN NARROWED
- ENDOTHELIAL CELL SWOLLEN
- FOOT PROCESSES MAY OR MAY NOT BE FUSED
- EXTENSIVE DEPOSITS OF MESANGIAL MATRIX IN LOBULAR STALK
- ONLY SLIGHT PROLIFERATION OF MESANGIAL CELLS

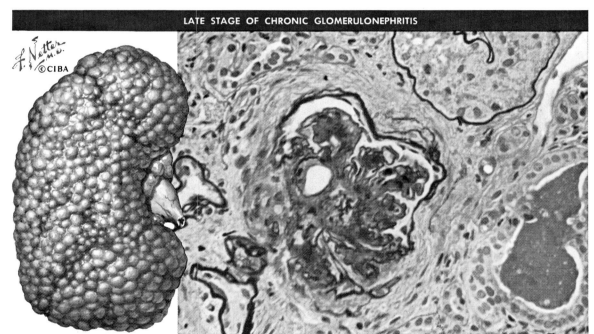

LATE STAGE OF CHRONIC GLOMERULONEPHRITIS

CONTRACTED, PALE, COARSELY GRANULAR KIDNEY

GLOMERULI IN VARIOUS STAGES OF OBSOLESCENCE; DEPOSITION OF PAS-STAINING MATERIAL, HYALINIZATION, FIBROUS CRESCENT FORMATION, TUBULAR ATROPHY, INTERSTITIAL FIBROSIS

Blood vessels often show all changes seen in arterio- and arteriolosclerosis, including fibrous thickening of the intima, hyalinization of the media, and duplication of the elastica. Occasionally, changes of accelerated nephrosclerosis may be present. Undoubtedly, some of the glomerular collapse is secondary to these vascular changes, and it may be difficult to differentiate, on histologic grounds, chronic glomerulonephritis from primary arterio- and arteriolosclerotic kidneys.

In general, if proliferative and sclerosing glomerular changes outweigh those of ischemic collapse, it is reasonable to assume that one is dealing with chronic glomerulonephritis. On the other hand, vascular changes, especially accelerated arteriolosclerosis, also may lead to focal glomerular proliferation. Thus, it can be seen that the diagnosis may, at times, become a subjective matter, a fact particularly true for the so-called end-stage kidney, which is characterized by dif-

fuse scarring, shrinkage of all parenchymal elements, and marked interstitial fibrosis and lymphocytic infiltration of the stroma. This type of picture is now seen more frequently in patients who have undergone prolonged hemodialysis.

Histologically, the differentiation of chronic glomerulonephritis from chronic pyelonephritis is based on the fact that chronic pyelonephritis shows changes predominantly in tubules and interstitial tissue, while the glomeruli remain relatively intact for a long time. However, vascular changes also can be very severe in chronic pyelonephritis.

Neither immunofluorescence nor electron microscopy has been of much help in the differential diagnosis or in the understanding of chronic glomerulonephritis, and it is likely that only by means of serial renal biopsies will the development of this disease be elucidated. □

CLINICAL COURSE AND PATHOLOGY OF FOCAL GLOMERULONEPHRITIS

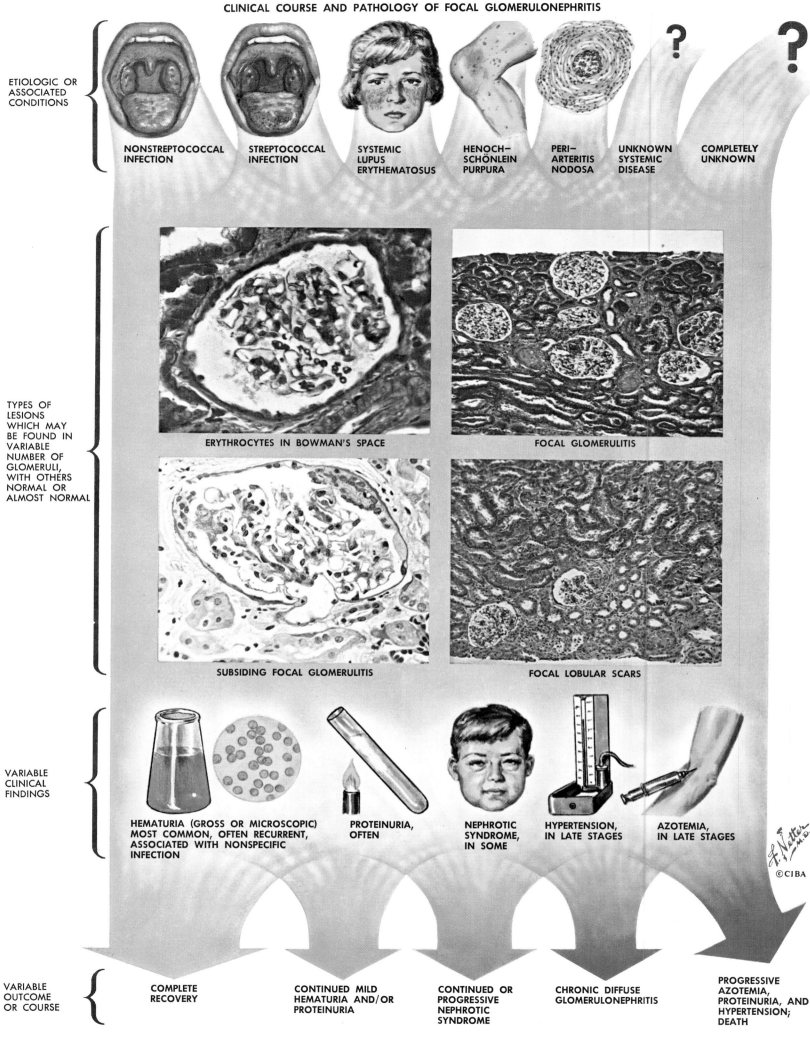

ETIOLOGIC OR ASSOCIATED CONDITIONS

NONSTREPTOCOCCAL INFECTION | STREPTOCOCCAL INFECTION | SYSTEMIC LUPUS ERYTHEMATOSUS | HENOCH-SCHÖNLEIN PURPURA | PERI-ARTERITIS NODOSA | UNKNOWN SYSTEMIC DISEASE | COMPLETELY UNKNOWN

TYPES OF LESIONS WHICH MAY BE FOUND IN VARIABLE NUMBER OF GLOMERULI, WITH OTHERS NORMAL OR ALMOST NORMAL

ERYTHROCYTES IN BOWMAN'S SPACE

FOCAL GLOMERULITIS

SUBSIDING FOCAL GLOMERULITIS

FOCAL LOBULAR SCARS

VARIABLE CLINICAL FINDINGS

HEMATURIA (GROSS OR MICROSCOPIC) MOST COMMON, OFTEN RECURRENT, ASSOCIATED WITH NONSPECIFIC INFECTION | PROTEINURIA, OFTEN | NEPHROTIC SYNDROME, IN SOME | HYPERTENSION, IN LATE STAGES | AZOTEMIA, IN LATE STAGES

VARIABLE OUTCOME OR COURSE

COMPLETE RECOVERY | CONTINUED MILD HEMATURIA AND/OR PROTEINURIA | CONTINUED OR PROGRESSIVE NEPHROTIC SYNDROME | CHRONIC DIFFUSE GLOMERULONEPHRITIS | PROGRESSIVE AZOTEMIA, PROTEINURIA, AND HYPERTENSION; DEATH

©CIBA

Focal Glomerulonephritis

The term "focal glomerulonephritis" implies that some, but not all, glomeruli are diseased. In some instances, however, portions of all glomeruli are diseased, and the term "local glomerulonephritis" has been used to designate this situation.

The occurrence of focal glomerular lesions in association with several systemic diseases has been recognized for many years. The focal "embolic" glomerulonephritis of subacute bacterial endocarditis (see CIBA COLLECTION, Vol. 5, page 187) is perhaps the best known. Likewise, association of focal lesions with systemic lupus erythematosus (see page 141), arteritis (see page 167), diabetes (see page 149), and other systemic diseases is well recognized. Moreover, renal biopsies have revealed a focal distribution of glomerular lesions in rare cases of poststreptococcal acute glomerulonephritis (see page 131) and in patients who have developed urinary abnormalities subsequent to several types of infections. Finally, on renal biopsy, focal glomerular lesions have been found in a number of patients who had evidence of chronic renal disease and in whom no etiologic clues were obvious.

Focal glomerular lesions may have proliferative, exudative, or membranous features, alone or in combination. The lesions may be so focal that the only evidence for glomerular disease is the presence of erythrocytes in Bowman's space or in scattered tubules. In contrast, lesions which initially are focal may become so extensive that all glomeruli may be seriously compromised, leading to renal insufficiency and possibly obscuring the original focal nature of the disease. Focally distributed exudative lesions, necrosis, or capillary loop thromboses may lead to scarring and hyalinized glomeruli or lobules. In retrospect, establishment of the original cause of such lesions is rarely possible on the basis of histology alone. This problem becomes even more difficult when the focal nature of vascular nephrosclerosis and pyelonephritis is considered. These and related diseases may result in total or local hyalinization of some glomeruli. Thus, although renal biopsy can establish the presence of focal glomerular disease, only rarely can it supply a specific or etiologic diagnosis. Ancillary information is most essential in the analysis and diagnosis of patients with focal glomerular lesions.

Poststreptococcal Acute Glomerulonephritis

On renal biopsy, patients who have poststreptococcal acute glomerulonephritis typically have diffuse proliferative or exudative glomerular lesions. However, in some mild and in most subclinical cases renal biopsy has revealed focal distribution of lesions, at least by light microscopy. Much painstaking work with the electron microscope is necessary, however, to establish whether or not these instances are truly focal in nature.

Benign Acute (Nonstreptococcal) Hemorrhagic Nephritis

A "benign and curable form of acute hemorrhagic nephritis" was first described in 1926 by George Baehr. In 1957 an outbreak of acute hemorrhagic nephritis at a naval training station was shown to be associated with infections unequivocally of nonstreptococcal origin. In 14 patients, transient gross hematuria followed pharyngitis by 8 days or less. Rapid, complete recovery was the rule. Similar sporadic cases have been reported subsequently, and renal biopsies revealed focal glomerulitis. Although the etiology was not established, the associated infections appeared to be of viral origin.

Recurrent Glomerulitis

From time to time, instances have been described of recurrent gross hematuria associated with a variety of nonspecific infections. Many of these undoubtedly were considered to be exacerbations in poststreptococcal chronic glomerulonephritis. However, evidence of acute or chronic renal insufficiency is extremely rare in these patients. Usually, the urine returns to normal between acute attacks although biopsies show the continued presence of some severely damaged glomeruli. The antecedent infections appear to be caused by a number of organisms. Immunofluorescence, electron microscopy, and other means of study have not yet been applied to a sufficient volume of cases to define the pathogenetic relationships. The prognosis appears to be excellent.

Chronic Focal Glomerulonephritis

A number of patients who show signs or symptoms of chronic glomerulonephritis, with or without evidence of renal insufficiency, with or without the nephrotic syndrome, and with no etiologic clues, have been found, on biopsy, to have focal glomerular proliferative lesions. These cases undoubtedly represent a number of different diseases whose etiologic and pathogenetic mechanisms have not yet been established. Some appear to be progressive, with the nephrotic syndrome and renal insufficiency characterizing their progress. Again, more careful observations of the natural history and pathogenesis will be essential to properly classify these cases.

Focal Glomerular Lesions in Systemic Diseases

Subacute Bacterial Endocarditis. For many years, focal "embolic" glomerulonephritis classically has been a frequent part of this form of endocarditis. At times, the glomerular lesions may be focal while on other occasions they are quite diffuse.

The lesions probably represent an antigen-antibody response, and the focal type of distribution may represent a response to embolic deposition of the antigen. This concept could also easily include instances of diffuse glomerulonephritis in association with subacute bacterial endocarditis if the process were to involve either more prevalent antigen-antibody complexes or a wider distribution of bacterial antigen (see CIBA COLLECTION, Vol. 5, page 187).

Systemic Lupus Erythematosus. Experimental work on animals and correlated studies with man suggest that lupus glomerulonephritis is an expression of immune response to circulating DNA-anti-DNA complexes. Why the attendant glomerular lesions should be focally distributed is not clear; perhaps large complexes of limited number are involved (see page 141).

Arteritis. Although involvement of arteries of the kidney may be obvious in periarteritis, why this condition should result in focal glomerulitis is as yet unclear. Ischemia *per se* may lead to focal glomerular lesions, but these are generally quite bland and usually are associated with vascular lesions (see page 167).

Nephrosclerosis. Arteriosclerotic changes in larger blood vessels may eventually lead to partial occlusion, which can result in focally ischemic glomeruli. Diabetes can contribute to this general process and, at times, may also lead to focal glomerulosclerotic changes (see page 149). □

Photomicrographs courtesy of Dr. Robert B. Jennings, Department of Pathology, Northwestern University Medical School.

Nephropathy in Anaphylactoid Purpura (Henoch-Schönlein Disease)

The occurrence of renal involvement in hypersensitivity disorders is particularly important not only because it contributes materially to the ultimate mortality of such disorders but because it possesses general significance relative to the more common syndrome of poststreptococcal glomerulonephritis (see page 131).

The similarity of renal involvement in the two conditions supports the view, arrived at on other grounds, that poststreptococcal glomerulonephritis also represents a hypersensitivity response of the glomerulus to some component of the original streptococcal insult. That analogy, although it can never constitute absolute proof, is at least more firmly based when it concerns human disease known to have an allergic basis than when it is derived from the studies of experimental nephritis reviewed by Unanue and Dixon. We have selected the renal involvement in allergic purpura (Henoch-Schönlein disease) as an example of this important general phenomenon.

Anaphylactoid purpura is a disorder which affects children predominately, although not exclusively. The association of cutaneous purpura with arthralgia was described by Schönlein in 1837 and, with visceral manifestations, by Henoch in 1874. The platelets and other factors concerned in coagulation are normal, and bleeding is secondary to angiitis, with a perivascular infiltrate of both polynuclear and mononuclear cells.

The similarity between anaphylactoid purpura and serum sickness was recognized by Osler, and the lesions of anaphylactoid purpura can be mimicked in experimental animals by allergic insult.

Although the clinical attack may follow a respiratory infection and be associated with an elevated serum antistreptolysin titer, these associations are by no means constant. Multiple allergens may be involved in different patients.

Skin lesions include urticaria, maculopapular swelling, petechiae, and purpura. Affected joints are painful and swollen, the edema being mainly periarticular although there may be a serous synovial effusion. The most common gastrointestinal manifestation is colicky abdominal pain. However, vomiting, hematemesis, and melena also occur. Even in the absence of frank melena, chemical tests may show blood in the stools. Cerebral hemorrhage is a rare complication.

The great majority of patients recover after a few weeks, but death can occur in the acute attack from gastrointestinal bleeding, renal failure, or hypertensive encephalopathy; delayed mortality results from established and progressive renal damage.

Renal Involvement

Association of anaphylactoid purpura with nephritis was emphasized by Henoch

NEPHROPATHY IN ANAPHYLACTOID PURPURA (HENOCH–SCHÖNLEIN DISEASE)

ANTECEDENT STREPTOCOCCAL ? INFECTION

FOOD OR DRUG ? ALLERGY

INSECT BITES ?

NO KNOWN ANTECEDENT OR POSSIBLE ETIOLOGIC FACTOR

CNS SIGNS

FEVER

ABDOMINAL DISTRESS, NAUSEA, VOMITING, BLOODY STOOLS

PURPURA

ANEMIA

ARTHRALGIA

HYPERTENSION

IN SEVERE CASES

AZOTEMIA

HEMATURIA, OFTEN GROSS; HYALINE, GRANULAR, & BLOOD CASTS

PROTEINURIA

EDEMA; NEPHROTIC SYNDROME OCCASIONALLY

EARLY: FOCAL AMORPHOUS EOSINOPHILIC DEPOSITS, HYPERCELLULARITY, AND CRESCENT FORMATION

LATE: GLOMERULUS DIFFUSELY INVOLVED WITH EOSINOPHILIC DEPOSIT AND EPITHELIAL PROLIFERATION, CRESCENT FORMATION, AND CAPSULAR ADHESIONS

COMPLETE RECOVERY IN MANY CASES (PROGNOSIS BETTER IN CHILDREN)

PERSISTENT MILD HEMATURIA AND/OR PROTEINURIA IN SOME

DEATH (MORTALITY VARIABLE LOWER IN CHILDREN)

but had already been recognized by Johnson. The clinical picture closely resembles that of acute glomerulonephritis, with hematuria, edema, and hypertension. The most important differential feature is the occurrence of nonrenal manifestations of anaphylactoid purpura. In addition, gross hematuria may be more persistent than in ordinary acute glomerulonephritis.

A minor degree of nitrogen retention is frequent, and severe renal failure may occur in the acute attack. In various small series of patients, e.g., those of Gairdner, there has been a higher incidence of progressive renal damage than is usual in acute glomerulonephritis, but the generality of this observation has not been established. In some patients, the course appears to have been favorably influenced by immunosuppressive agents, but in others, these drugs often have failed to arrest progression.

Renal biopsies have shown striking variations in the degree of glomerular involvement, in contrast to the uniform involvement of glomeruli in ordinary acute glomerulonephritis. Between 20 and 50 percent of the glomeruli appeared normal. Others showed endothelial proliferation with accumulations of amorphous PAS-positive material within the tuft. The less severely involved glomeruli showed only hypercellularity; the more severely involved showed adhesions to the parietal layer of Bowman's capsule and even some formation of epithelial crescents. Proliferation of mesangial cells also has been described. When the renal lesion of anaphylactoid purpura becomes progressive, the focal character of the glomerular lesion is lost and the appearances merge into those of chronic glomerulonephritis (see page 134). □

Photomicrographs courtesy of Dr. G. Williams, Department of Pathology, University of Manchester, England, and Dr. G. Berlyne, Central Negev Hospital, Israel.

Lupus Nephritis

f. Netter ©CIBA

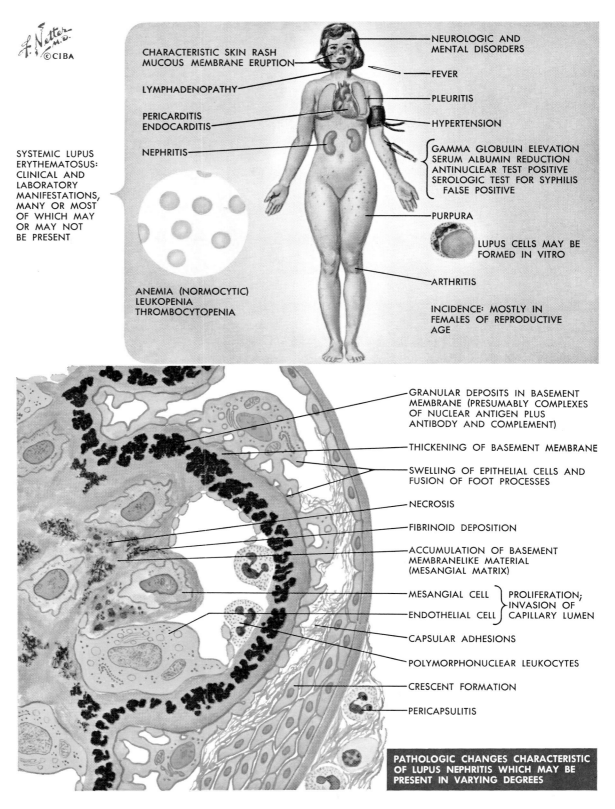

SYSTEMIC LUPUS ERYTHEMATOSUS: CLINICAL AND LABORATORY MANIFESTATIONS, MANY OR MOST OF WHICH MAY OR MAY NOT BE PRESENT

CHARACTERISTIC SKIN RASH MUCOUS MEMBRANE ERUPTION

LYMPHADENOPATHY

PERICARDITIS ENDOCARDITIS

NEPHRITIS

NEUROLOGIC AND MENTAL DISORDERS

FEVER

PLEURITIS

HYPERTENSION

GAMMA GLOBULIN ELEVATION SERUM ALBUMIN REDUCTION ANTINUCLEAR TEST POSITIVE SEROLOGIC TEST FOR SYPHILIS FALSE POSITIVE

PURPURA

LUPUS CELLS MAY BE FORMED IN VITRO

ARTHRITIS

ANEMIA (NORMOCYTIC) LEUKOPENIA THROMBOCYTOPENIA

INCIDENCE: MOSTLY IN FEMALES OF REPRODUCTIVE AGE

GRANULAR DEPOSITS IN BASEMENT MEMBRANE (PRESUMABLY COMPLEXES OF NUCLEAR ANTIGEN PLUS ANTIBODY AND COMPLEMENT)

THICKENING OF BASEMENT MEMBRANE

SWELLING OF EPITHELIAL CELLS AND FUSION OF FOOT PROCESSES

NECROSIS

FIBRINOID DEPOSITION

ACCUMULATION OF BASEMENT MEMBRANELIKE MATERIAL (MESANGIAL MATRIX)

MESANGIAL CELL ⎫ PROLIFERATION; INVASION OF
ENDOTHELIAL CELL ⎭ CAPILLARY LUMEN

CAPSULAR ADHESIONS

POLYMORPHONUCLEAR LEUKOCYTES

CRESCENT FORMATION

PERICAPSULITIS

PATHOLOGIC CHANGES CHARACTERISTIC OF LUPUS NEPHRITIS WHICH MAY BE PRESENT IN VARYING DEGREES

Systemic lupus erythematosus (SLE) is a rather uncommon disease of unknown etiology which occurs principally in young women. Although many tissues and organs are affected in SLE, renal involvement is one of the most serious aspects of the disease. The reported incidence of clinically apparent renal involvement in SLE ranges from 50 to 80 percent; if minor glomerular abnormalities detectable only by electron microscopy or immunofluorescence were also counted, the incidence would be even higher.

Certain pathologic features are characteristic of lupus nephritis, but none is pathognomonic (with the dubious exception of the rarely seen *hematoxylin bodies*). The most important abnormalities involve the glomeruli and include swelling and proliferation of endothelial and mesangial cells, necrosis, fibrinoid deposits, thrombi, neutrophil infiltration, crescent formation, increased basement membranelike material (mesangial matrix), and thickening and abnormal deposits associated with the basement membrane, some of which give the appearance of *"wire-loop"* lesions. By electron microscopy, the deposits appear as dense granular material which may be seen along either side of or within the basement membrane; the basement membrane itself may show irregular thickening or splitting. Additionally, interstitial infiltration with various kinds of leukocytes, principally lymphocytes and plasma cells, may be seen.

Typically, the glomerular abnormalities are irregularly distributed within and among the glomeruli and are seen in various combinations. Both the extent and severity of glomerular involvement vary. Nevertheless, there appears to be value in subdividing lupus nephritis on the basis of histologic findings, particularly since the clinical features and course of the renal disease correlate, to some extent, with the pathologic picture. One classification which has been found useful divides lupus nephritis into three types: *focal proliferative, diffuse proliferative,* and *membranous.* "Proliferative" is used for the sake of convenience and because proliferation of endothelial and mesangial cells is conspicuous; however, other features are also present. Although the distinction between these types is often arbitrary and overlap may be apparent, most cases can readily be classified even

on the basis of examination of biopsy material.

Focal Proliferative Lupus Nephritis

Those cases in which only portions of some glomeruli are involved are classified as *focal proliferative lupus nephritis.* Usually, many of the glomeruli appear histologically normal, and in most of the abnormal glomeruli only relatively small portions are affected. Although involved areas may show any of the features of lupus nephritis mentioned above, the most frequent findings include swelling and proliferation of endothelial and mesangial cells, neutrophil accumulation, and necrosis.

The clinical features of focal proliferative lupus nephritis usually parallel the pathologic findings and are generally mild and reversible. In most instances, microscopic hematuria is present and a minimal amount of proteinuria is characteristic, although, in

rare instances, heavy proteinuria may occur. Moderate hypertension may be found, but elevation of blood urea nitrogen is uncommon.

These signs of renal disease usually appear only during phases when active involvement of other organs is apparent. They generally disappear when the activity of the systemic disease subsides, either spontaneously or following steroid therapy.

Biopsies performed during periods of remission show either no glomerular abnormalities or such minimal residual changes as mild, focal increase in basement membranelike material. Recurrences of systemic and renal disease activity are not uncommon but generally respond to increased doses of corticosteroids administered for short periods. Patients who have focal proliferative lupus nephritis usually do not develop diffuse glomerular disease with progressive renal insufficiency. Usually, they survive *Continued on page 142*

Lupus Nephritis

Continued from page 141

for many years or die of their disease for reasons unrelated to renal involvement.

Diffuse Proliferative Lupus Nephritis

Instances in which most glomeruli are severely involved may be classified as the *diffuse proliferative* form of *lupus nephritis*. Most of the individual pathologic features are similar to those seen in patients classified as having the focal form. However, accumulation of basement membrane material in the glomeruli generally is much greater, widespread abnormalities of basement membranes are more frequent, and interstitial inflammation is more severe and widespread.

The clinical manifestations of diffuse proliferative lupus nephritis include marked proteinuria—almost always with the nephrotic syndrome—gross hematuria, hypertension, and renal insufficiency. The course is generally characterized by persistent evidence of severe renal disease with progressive renal insufficiency, although partial remission may rarely occur.

It is not clear whether adrenocorticosteroid therapy significantly retards progression of the glomerular disease. Histologically, signs of active damage persist, usually in association with increasing glomerular obliteration resulting principally from the progressive accumulation of basement membranelike material. Death usually occurs within several years and is generally caused by a combination of factors, principally renal insufficiency, active SLE, infections, and complications secondary to steroid therapy.

Membranous Lupus Nephritis

Patients who show diffuse abnormalities of the basement membranes as the major findings are categorized as having *diffuse membranous lupus nephritis*. The histologic picture closely resembles that of idiopathic membranous nephropathy (see pages 127 and 136). In H. and E. sections there is diffuse, fairly uniform thickening of the capillary wall with relatively little proliferation of endothelial or mesangial cells. Use of special stains, such as azocarmine, shows that most of the thickening of the glomerular capillary walls reflects abnormal deposits. Electron microscopy reveals that, in addition to thickening and splitting of the basement membrane, the

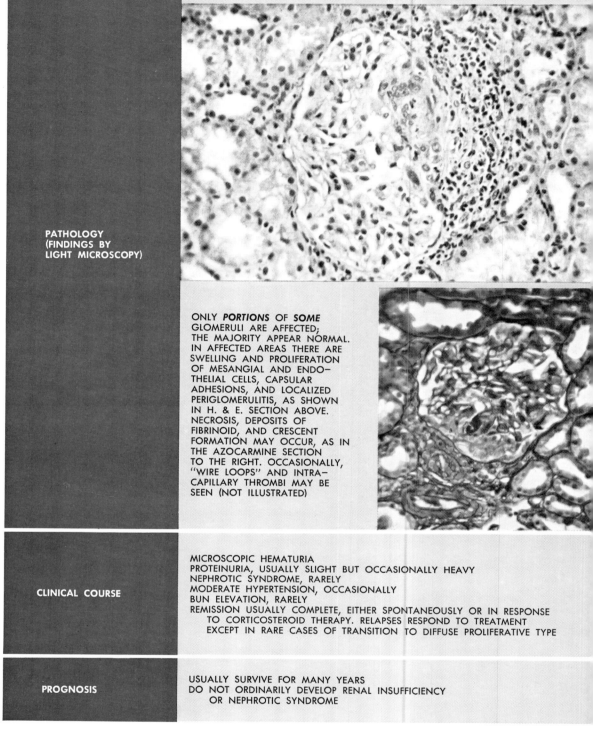

PATHOLOGY (FINDINGS BY LIGHT MICROSCOPY)

FOCAL PROLIFERATIVE

ONLY **PORTIONS** OF **SOME** GLOMERULI ARE AFFECTED; THE MAJORITY APPEAR NORMAL. IN AFFECTED AREAS THERE ARE SWELLING AND PROLIFERATION OF MESANGIAL AND ENDO-THELIAL CELLS, CAPSULAR ADHESIONS, AND LOCALIZED PERIGLOMERULITIS, AS SHOWN IN H. & E. SECTION ABOVE. NECROSIS, DEPOSITS OF FIBRINOID, AND CRESCENT FORMATION MAY OCCUR, AS IN THE AZOCARMINE SECTION TO THE RIGHT. OCCASIONALLY, "WIRE LOOPS" AND INTRA-CAPILLARY THROMBI MAY BE SEEN (NOT ILLUSTRATED)

CLINICAL COURSE

MICROSCOPIC HEMATURIA
PROTEINURIA, USUALLY SLIGHT BUT OCCASIONALLY HEAVY
NEPHROTIC SYNDROME, RARELY
MODERATE HYPERTENSION, OCCASIONALLY
BUN ELEVATION, RARELY
REMISSION USUALLY COMPLETE, EITHER SPONTANEOUSLY OR IN RESPONSE TO CORTICOSTEROID THERAPY. RELAPSES RESPOND TO TREATMENT EXCEPT IN RARE CASES OF TRANSITION TO DIFFUSE PROLIFERATIVE TYPE

PROGNOSIS

USUALLY SURVIVE FOR MANY YEARS
DO NOT ORDINARILY DEVELOP RENAL INSUFFICIENCY OR NEPHROTIC SYNDROME

deposits are composed of dense granular material found within or along the basement membrane, often principally on the epithelial side. These deposits correspond to the sites of granular staining for immunoglobulins and complement seen by immunofluorescence. Although such deposits are present in all forms of lupus nephritis, they are more numerous in the membranous type and are more uniformly distributed along the basement membranes of all glomeruli.

Clinically, membranous lupus nephritis usually is manifested by heavy proteinuria with the nephrotic syndrome, although in some instances only mild proteinuria is found. Hematuria generally is present, and hypertension is frequent. Usually, renal function is normal. However, in occasional instances progressive renal insufficiency may develop. Most patients survive for many years, either with persistent heavy proteinuria or with remission apparently induced by steroid therapy.

It should be emphasized that the primary value of this classification is that it aids in assessing prognosis. As a rule, patients tend to remain in the same category into which they fit when first classified. Furthermore, there is general agreement that patients afflicted with SLE who do not develop renal disease early usually will not develop it later.

Etiology

Although the etiology of SLE is unknown, recent investigations have shown that the glomerular lesions (and probably certain other lesions) are produced by circulating antigen-antibody complexes. It has been known for some time that patients with SLE have numerous circulating autoantibodies many of which are directed against nuclear constituents. It is not clear how these autoantibodies can lead to tissue damage since they are unable to enter normal cells *in vivo.*

DIFFUSE PROLIFERATIVE

MEMBRANOUS

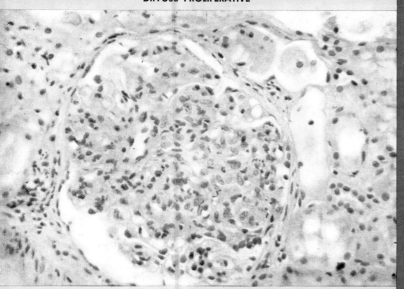

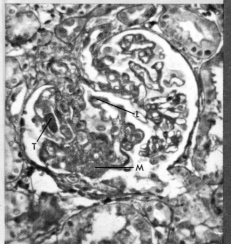

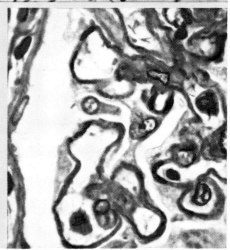

GLOMERULAR ABNORMALITIES ARE SIMILAR TO THOSE OF FOCAL PROLIFERATIVE, BUT *ALL OR ALMOST ALL GLOMERULI ARE INVOLVED*, AND LARGER PORTIONS OF GLOMERULI ARE AFFECTED. IN H. & E. SECTION ABOVE, THERE ARE SEVERE, IRREGULAR SWELLING AND PRO-LIFERATION OF ENDOTHELIAL AND MESANGIAL CELLS, WITH OBLITERATION OF CAPILLARIES, NECROSIS, AND KARYORRHEXIS. HEMATOXYLIN BODIES AND CRESCENTS MAY SOMETIMES BE SEEN. AZOCARMINE SECTION TO RIGHT SHOWS "WIRE LOOP" (L), THROMBUS (T), AND HEAVY DEPOSIT OF BASEMENT-MEMBRANELIKE MATERIAL (M)

CHARACTERIZED BY *DIFFUSE, FAIRLY UNIFORM THICKENING OF GLOMERULAR CAPILLARY WALLS*, AS ILLUSTRATED IN H. & E. SECTION ABOVE. NECROSIS, NEUTROPHIL INFIL-TRATION, OR CRESCENTS ARE *NOT FOUND*, AND ONLY MES-ANGIAL CELL PROLIFERATION IS PRESENT. IF INTRACAPIL-LARY CELL PROLIFERATION IS PROMINENT, THE CONDITION IS CLASSIFIED AS "DIFFUSE PROLIFERATIVE." IN AZOCAR-MINE SECTION AT RIGHT, DIFFUSE THICKENING OF CAPILLARY WALL IS SEEN TO BE DUE MAINLY TO DEPOSITS OF CARMINOPHILIC MATERIAL ALONG OUTER SIDE OF BASE-MENT MEMBRANE

GROSS HEMATURIA
HEAVY PROTEINEMIA
NEPHROTIC SYNDROME, USUALLY
HYPERTENSION, USUALLY
RENAL INSUFFICIENCY AND AZOTEMIA, USUALLY
REMISSIONS MAY OCCUR BUT ARE RARELY COMPLETE
RELAPSES COMMON
USUALLY DOES *NOT* RESPOND TO TREATMENT

GROSS HEMATURIA
HEAVY PROTEINURIA
NEPHROTIC SYNDROME, ALMOST INVARIABLY
HYPERTENSION, USUALLY
RENAL INSUFFICIENCY, OCCASIONALLY
MAY REMIT WITH TREATMENT BUT USUALLY RELAPSES
USUALLY CHARACTERIZED BY HEAVY PROTEINURIA WITH LITTLE OR NO
   RENAL INSUFFICIENCY

RENAL INSUFFICIENCY AND NEPHROTIC SYNDROME PROGRESS
DEATH COMMONLY OCCURS WITHIN 5 YEARS BUT MAY COME MUCH
   EARLIER; DEATH USUALLY DUE TO OTHER ASPECTS OF SLE OR ITS
   COMPLICATIONS RATHER THAN TO UREMIA

MOST CASES SURVIVE FOR MANY YEARS
IN SOME, COMPLETE REMISSION MAY BE MAINTAINED FOR LONG PERIODS
DEATH IN UREMIA RARE

©CIBA

However, antibodies are able to combine with antigen in the circulation to form immune complexes. Evidence that these autologous immune complexes are responsible for the glomerular lesions can be summarized:

1. The immunofluorescent and electron microscopic findings in lupus nephritis are often very similar to those found in experimental immune complex disease (see page 129). In both diseases there are granular deposits of electron-dense material along or within the basement membrane. Immunofluorescence demonstrates that these deposits contain immunoglobulins and complement.

2. Gamma globulin eluted from glomeruli in lupus nephritis possesses a high concentration of antinuclear antibodies; this observation is consistent with the interpretation that γ-globulin is present in the form of immune complexes rather

than as the result of nonspecific trapping. Furthermore, this finding eliminates the possibility that lupus nephritis could represent the other major type of immunologically induced glomerular disease, anti-GBM disease.

3. Some patients exhibiting lupus nephritis are found to have free DNA in their circulation; since at other times these patients have circulating anti-DNA, immune complexes must be repeatedly formed.

4. Finally, it has been possible to demonstrate DNA *within* the glomerular deposits of a few patients. This can be considered a direct demonstration of the antigen portion of the complex. It seems likely that in some cases autoantibodies directed against constituents other than DNA also participate in the pathogenesis of the glomerular lesions.

Presumably, some of the secondary pathogenic

mechanisms elucidated in the experimental models operate in the human disease; these include factors derived from leukocytes, complement, and the coagulation process. Most of these mechanisms cannot be directly explored in human disease. However, it has been shown by immunofluorescence that fibrin or other fibrinogen derivatives are present in the active glomerular lesions. This observation indicates that the coagulation process may contribute to the proliferative and sclerotic changes as it has been shown to do in experimental nephrotoxic serum nephritis.

Although considerable progress has been made in elucidation of the immunologic mechanisms underlying the glomerular damage, nothing conclusive has been learned about the cause of the disease or the manner of initiation of autoantibody formation. □

Acute Diffuse Interstitial Nephritis

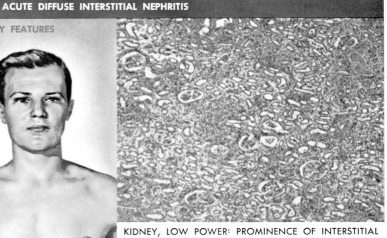

CLINICAL AND LABORATORY FEATURES

HISTORY OF DRUG EXPOSURE

103°
101°
99°
FEVER

EOSINOPHILIA

BUN ELEVATION

RENAL ENLARGEMENT

OLIGURIA

HEMATURIA

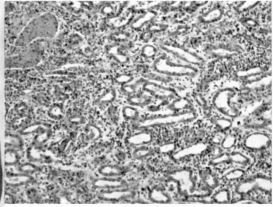

KIDNEY, LOW POWER: PROMINENCE OF INTERSTITIAL TISSUE DUE TO CLUSTERED FOCI OF CELLS; NECROTIC TUBULES IN UPPER RIGHT CORNER (H. & E. STAIN)

KIDNEY, MEDIUM POWER: UNIFORM INTERSTITIAL EDEMA AND CELLULAR INFILTRATION, CHIEFLY OF LYMPHOCYTES; TUBULES RELATIVELY NORMAL EXCEPT NECROTIC TUBULES AT UPPER LEFT (H. & E. STAIN)

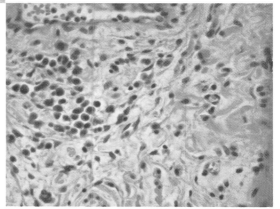

URETER, LOW POWER: EXTENSIVE EDEMA RESULTING IN MARKED NARROWING OF LUMEN; CELLULAR INFILTRATION IN SUBMUCOSA AND IN MUSCULATURE (H. & E. STAIN)

URETER, HIGH POWER: CLUSTER OF EOSINOPHILS IN SUBMUCOSA ADJACENT TO BAND OF SMOOTH MUSCLE (H. & E. STAIN)

Acute diffuse interstitial nephritis is an uncommon disorder, but one which must be considered among the important causes of acute oliguric renal failure (see page 111). The renal lesion was first described in detail by Councilman in 1898 when he reported his observations on 42 cases and reviewed those in the literature. It was recognized then, and during the succeeding four decades, as a lesion that occurred largely in children with acute febrile infections, particularly streptococcal infections or diphtheria. With the control and decline of diphtheria, streptococcal infection became the dominant cause of acute diffuse interstitial nephritis.

The introduction of chemotherapeutic agents led to a decline in the number of cases which could be related to streptococcal infection. This decline was soon followed by the appearance of cases believed to be caused by drug reactions. Sulfonamides, and later penicillin and methicillin, became identified with acute diffuse interstitial nephritis as the use of these drugs increased.

Acute diffuse interstitial nephritis is a well-defined but uncommon pattern of *clinical and pathologic* responses to streptococcal infections or to drugs. The more common forms of such untoward responses are acute glomerulonephritis (see page 131) and/or disseminated arteritis (see page 167).

The essential clinical features are fever, rash, eosinophilia, hematuria, oliguria, and nitrogen retention. The kidneys are enlarged, occasionally to almost three times their normal weight—a degree of enlargement readily recognized radiologically.

Microscopically, the prominent features are pronounced edema and cellular infiltration of the interstitial tissue by lymphocytes, eosinophils, and occasionally, plasma cells. Dramatic as this pattern is, there is little parenchymal damage, so that by sustaining the patient through a period of oliguria or anuria, one can expect the recovery of appreciable renal function.

Usually the only parenchymal lesion is focal tubular necrosis. The glomeruli are little affected, usually manifesting only a slight increase in cellularity. Also, there is no arteritis.

As noted, neither glomerulonephritis nor arteritis is a component of the interstitial nephritis pattern of reaction to the penicillins, yet both glomerular and vascular lesions may be manifestations of other forms of penicillin hypersensitivity. The principal pathogenetic mechanism in interstitial nephritis is believed to be a drug hypersensitivity characterized by, for instance, the deposition of penicillin haptens and IgG in glomerular and tubular basement membranes, in tubular epithelium, and in the interstitium.

Because the histologic pattern is a characteristic one and is readily distinguishable from glomerulonephritis and/or periarteritis, renal biopsy can be useful both as a diagnostic and also as a prognostic procedure. □

Balkan Endemic Nephropathy

Balkan endemic nephropathy was first recognized about 20 years ago as a chronic, slowly progressive, renal insufficiency which affects populations in well-defined areas of Yugoslavia, Bulgaria, and Rumania. The clinical picture is one of gradually advancing uremia, with no recognizable episodes of acute illness. There is progressive anemia, a yellow-to-tan pallor of the skin, weakness, and weight loss. The blood pressure is usually normal and there is little or no edema even in the later stages of the disease. Pulmonary and other systemic infections usually appear terminally.

The amount of proteinuria is small, usually less than 2 gm/day, and there are few casts, leukocytes, or erythrocytes in the urinary sediment. The electrophoretic pattern of urinary protein is "tubular" in type and thus reflects the principal anatomic abnormality, a tubulointerstitial lesion.

Grossly, the lesion usually presents as a concentric atrophy without scarring, and is distinguished from pyelonephritis and arterionephrosclerosis. Microscopically, there is profound atrophy of renal tubules, especially in the outer cortex, and interstitial fibrosis without cellular infiltration. In its developing stages, Balkan endemic nephropathy can be distinguished from the more common renal lesions which may result in progressive insufficiency and parenchymal atrophy. Later, however, focal parenchymal damage secondary to pyelonephritis and/or arteriosclerosis may be superimposed. The glomeruli and blood vessels appear normal until late in the disease. By the time tubular atrophy and interstitial fibrosis are far advanced, glomerulosclerosis and arteriosclerosis with medial atrophy can be observed.

Etiology. The demonstration of tubular damage by renal function studies, the identification of a "tubular" pattern of urinary protein, and the tubulointerstitial lesion observed histologically point to a tubular nephrotoxin as the causal agent(s).

The endemic nephropathy appears to have been present for a generation or longer, although it has received concentrated attention only in the last decade or so. No new geographic foci of the disease have appeared, and cases continue to occur in those areas originally identified. Therefore, it seems unlikely that the pathogenesis is related to the use of newer chemical fertilizers, pesticides, industrial wastes, food additives, fuels, or similar environmental influences.

Attempts to explain the disease on the basis of heredity, infectious agents, diet, drug use, and other factors have been unrewarding. The populations affected live largely in agricultural areas adjacent to large rivers, namely, the Danube, Sava, and their tributaries. Few cases have been identified in such areas at elevations higher than 400 feet above sea level, except in Bulgaria, where most cases have

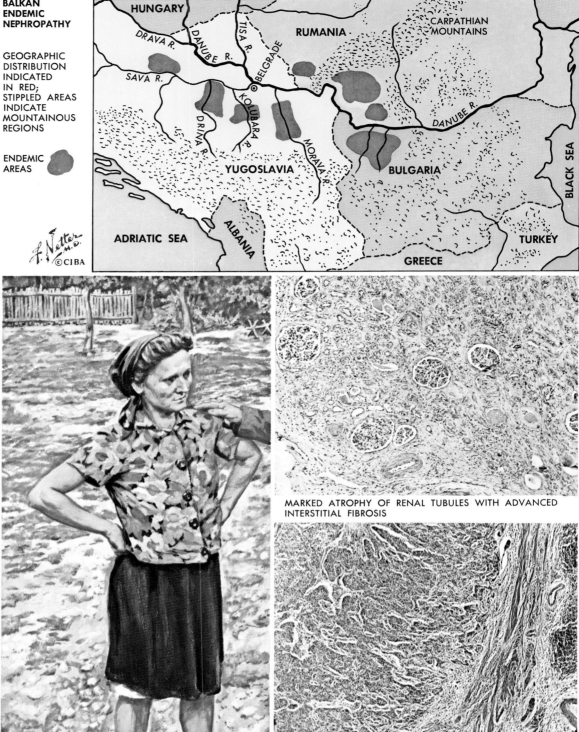

BALKAN ENDEMIC NEPHROPATHY

GEOGRAPHIC DISTRIBUTION INDICATED IN RED; STIPPLED AREAS INDICATE MOUNTAINOUS REGIONS

ENDEMIC AREAS

MARKED ATROPHY OF RENAL TUBULES WITH ADVANCED INTERSTITIAL FIBROSIS

TYPICAL APPEARANCE OF PATIENT: YELLOWISH PALLOR WITH MODERATE WEAKNESS AND WEIGHT LOSS

PAPILLARY CARCINOMA OF THE URETER FROM A CASE OF BALKAN ENDEMIC NEPHROPATHY

been found at elevations from 500 to 1500 feet.

Endemic nephropathy appears to be a "place disease," seen primarily in those who work in certain farming areas but not afflicting those who work in other areas. In some highly endemic communities, almost half of the adult population may have chronic uremia.

In his initial studies of endemic nephropathy, Hall demonstrated that the excreted urinary proteins had molecular weights in the range of 10,000 to 50,000—a characteristic of classic tubular proteinuria associated with primary renal tubular disorders. More recently, Hall has shown that another type of tubular proteinuria precedes the classic form and has as its major component a β_2-microglobulin with a molecular size of 11,800. The presence of this microglobulin is now the basis for detecting early cases.

From Belgrade, Petkovic has reported a high incidence of papillary carcinoma of the renal pelvis and ureter in the endemic nephropathy areas of Yugoslavia. An increased frequency of *bilateral* ureteral and renal pelvic papillary cancers and papillomas is also notable in the cases studied by Petkovic.

The observations of Puchlev and Tancev in the Vraca area of Bulgaria indicate the overall cancer morbidity is higher in the endemic nephropathy villages than in control localities. Furthermore, mortality from malignant tumors of the urinary tract in the endemic area equaled 20 percent of the total number of cancer deaths compared to five percent in control areas. Also, the association of endemic nephropathy with papillomatosis of the urinary tract is high (about 70 percent), as is the association of endemic nephropathy with urinary tract cancer (about 30 percent). Such figures are reflected in the overall mortality of urinary tract disease, which in some communities exceeds that resulting from cardiovascular disease. □

Section V

The Kidney and Systemic Diseases

Frank H. Netter, M.D.

in collaboration with

D. A. K. Black, M.D., F.R.C.P.   *Plate 27*

Jacob Churg, M.D.   *Plates 10-11*

Alan S. Cohen, M.D.   *Plates 14-16*

John L. Duffy, M.D.   *Plates 28-29*

David P. Earle, M.D.   *Plate 31*

Edwin R. Fisher, M.D.   *Plate 30*

H. O. Heinemann, M.D.   *Plate 25*

Paul Kimmelstiel, M.D.   *Plates 1-3*

Willy Mautner, M.D.   *Plate 22*

F. K. Mostofi, M.D.   *Plates 12-13*

Conrad L. Pirani, M.D.   *Plates 17-18, 23*

Solomon Papper, M.D. and Carlos A. Vaamonde, M.D.   *Plate 26*

George E. Schreiner, M.D.   *Plates 19-21*

Gerald S. Spear, M.D.   *Plate 24*

Victor Vertes, M.D.   *Plates 4-9*

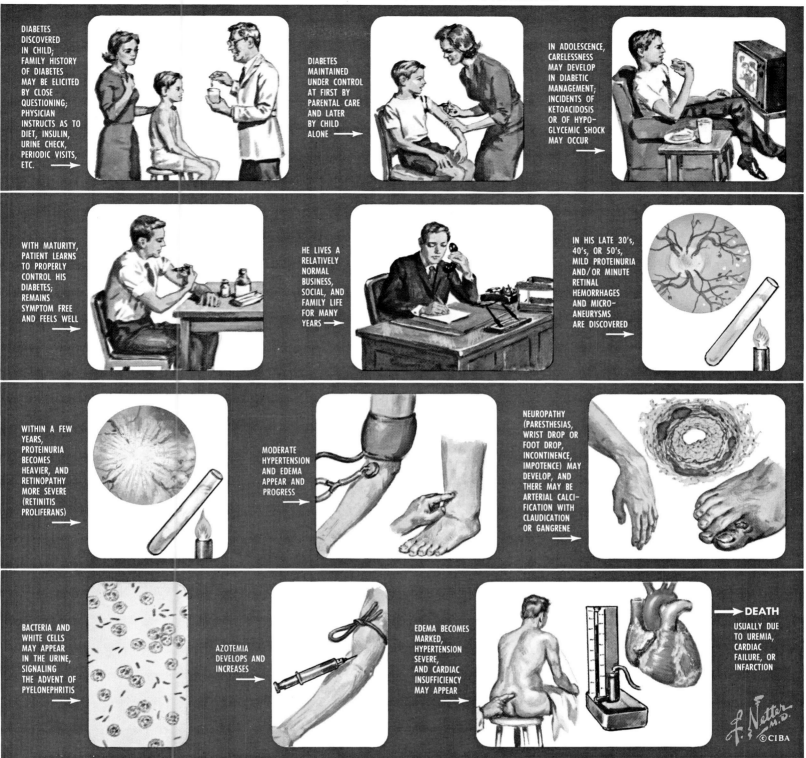

Diabetic Nephropathy

Diabetes mellitus may affect all anatomic elements of the kidney but with varying degrees of severity. Structural changes can be seen in the arteries, arterioles, glomeruli, tubules, and interstitial tissues. Several of the lesions have been described in a previous book (see CIBA COLLECTION, Vol. 4, pages 164, 166, and 167). As predicted, additional research performed during the interim with renal biopsies and electron microscopy has added considerable information and has changed some of the older concepts.

Arterio- and Arteriolosclerosis

Arterio- and arteriolosclerosis of the kidney are found much more frequently and in more severe degrees in diabetics than in nondiabetics. However, the morphologic vascular changes seem to be the same as those in nondiabetics. The only significant difference is involvement of the glomerular efferent arteriole *(vas efferens)*. Hyalinization of the afferent arteriole *(vas afferens)* is frequently seen in both diabetics and nondiabetics, but the same process is rarely, if ever, seen in the efferent arteriole *(vas efferens)* unless the patient is diabetic. Although probably not specific, hyalinization of the vas efferens thus constitutes a helpful histologic criterion for the diagnosis of diabetes.

Diabetic Intercapillary Glomerulosclerosis

Diabetic glomerulosclerosis has been recognized as a characteristic lesion, and a distinction has been made between nodular and diffuse forms. Although both have been shown to be manifestations of the same pathogenic process, they should be discussed separately since the nodular form is, by itself, virtually specific for diabetes. The diffuse form is not.

Nodular glomerulosclerosis originally was described as a deposit of "hyalin" in the intercapillary tissue of the glomerular tufts. This rather striking histologic lesion was thought to be a manifestation of a clinical triad—namely, diabetes, hypertension, and a nephrotic *Continued on page 150*

Continued on page 150

Diabetic Nephropathy

Continued from page 149

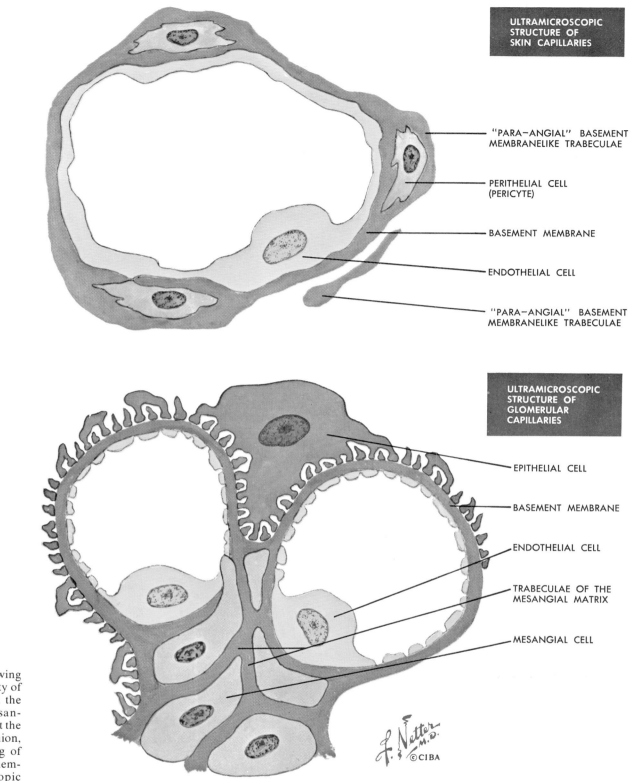

ULTRAMICROSCOPIC STRUCTURE OF SKIN CAPILLARIES

"PARA–ANGIAL" BASEMENT MEMBRANELIKE TRABECULAE

PERITHELIAL CELL (PERICYTE)

BASEMENT MEMBRANE

ENDOTHELIAL CELL

"PARA–ANGIAL" BASEMENT MEMBRANELIKE TRABECULAE

ULTRAMICROSCOPIC STRUCTURE OF GLOMERULAR CAPILLARIES

EPITHELIAL CELL

BASEMENT MEMBRANE

ENDOTHELIAL CELL

TRABECULAE OF THE MESANGIAL MATRIX

MESANGIAL CELL

syndrome. During the 25 years following the original description, the specificity of this lesion was widely accepted, but the existence of an intercapillary "mesangium" was denied. It was assumed that the nodule, in a somewhat nebulous fashion, was formed by preceding thickening of the peripheral capillary basement membrane. However, electron microscopic studies of renal biopsies and quantitative analyses have failed to confirm this hypothesis. Thus, the following thesis has evolved.

The existence of an intercapillary mesangium is now firmly established (see pages 8 and 9). It is a tissue structurally and functionally distinct from the endothelial cells which line the inner surface of the glomerular capillaries. (The endothelial cells have an attenuated porous cytoplasm.) The mesangium, situated in the center of the glomerular lobule, is composed of cells, with abundant cytoplasm, that lie in a spongy network of basement membranelike trabeculae called *mesangial matrix*. These trabeculae merge imperceptibly with the overlying capillary basement membrane.

The relationship of mesangial matrix and peripheral basement membrane is still under discussion. One school believes that the peripheral basement membrane is produced by epithelial cells and that it sends branches into the axial portion of the glomerular lobule, thus forming the mesangial matrix. The other school proposes that there is ample indirect evidence to support the concept that the matrix is laid down by the mesangial cells, the only living cells in direct contact with it.

Excessive deposition of matrix can be found under different circumstances, particularly if there is mesangial cell proliferation. Such a process can, for instance, be demonstrated in certain forms and stages of glomerulonephritis in human and in animal experiments (see pages 127-137).

Diabetic glomerulosclerosis has been shown to result from an increased deposit of mesangial matrix. The

trabeculae appear in greater numbers than normal, become more plump, and finally merge into a discrete nodular mass. The mesangial cells become atrophic in the center and disappear. Some of the adjacent capillaries may become part of the nodule as it expands.

Quantitative analyses have demonstrated that an increased number of the nuclei seen in the periphery of nodules in diabetic glomerulosclerosis result from mesangial proliferation; only a few such nuclei are endothelial in origin and belong to capillaries engulfed in the mesangial nodule.

The nodule is rich in glycoproteins and lipids and contains an increased amount of hydroxyproline and, rarely, collagen fibrils. Characteristically, the nodule is surrounded by a patent, occasionally distended, capillary whose basement membrane may be normal or increased in thickness.

Diabetic Nephropathy

Continued

Diffuse diabetic glomerulosclerosis was originally described as a primary thickening of the peripheral capillary basement membrane with similarly stained, poorly defined deposits through the axial portion of the lobules. However, later studies, including electron microscopy, revealed that this form of glomerulosclerosis differs from the nodular sclerosis. An excessive deposit of mesangial matrix is more diffusely distributed in each glomerulus and is less discrete. There is also more thickening of the peripheral basement membrane.

Although not fundamental, these differences account for the fact that the lesion of diffuse glomerulosclerosis resembles many other glomerular lesions and does not permit a reliable identification of its diabetic origin without additional criteria. Both forms of glomerulosclerosis are basically of the same nature and more often than not occur concurrently in the same patient and even in the same glomeruli. It is the exception to find either lesion in pure form.

Additional lesions that are highly suggestive of diabetes and found in conjunction with glomerulosclerosis are:

(1) *Hyalinization of vas efferens* (discussed previously).

(2) *Parietal deposits on Bowman's capsule.* These may appear as waxy, homogeneous material which stains with H. and E., and PAS. This sudanophilic material may be foamy in appearance and contain much lipid. The deposits, which may be small and rounded like droplets, or large like crescents, are situated beneath the parietal epithelium which is lifted up from the capsular membrane. If the deposits lack nuclei, they can be considered to be highly suggestive of diabetes, whether or not the capillary tufts show either form of sclerosis.

(3) *Thickening of the tubular basement membrane, especially in the proximal convoluted tubules.* The basement membrane may be so thick that it resembles amyloid. Such thickening occurs in many conditions other than diabetes, the most common being ischemia. Therefore little diagnostic specificity can be claimed for this change. Thickening of the tubular basement membrane suggests diabetes only if it is seen in the absence of epithelial atrophy. Tubular atrophy secondary to ischemia or any other cause is evidenced by a wrinkled basement membrane that is often markedly thickened.

(4) *Lipohyaline deposits in glomeruli.* These consist of homogeneous "hyaline" deposits in the walls of peripheral capillaries and often contain fat droplets. This change has little diagnostic value because it frequently occurs in advanced glomerular hyalinization seen with chronic glomerulonephritis and nephrosclerosis.

Pathogenesis of Glomerulosclerosis

Since diabetic glomerulosclerosis is most likely only one manifestation of so-called diabetic microangiopathy, a discussion of the pathogenesis of the renal lesions must take into consideration the systemic vascular pathology. It has become customary to identify systemic diabetic microangiopathy as a thickening of capillary basement membranes in many organs. The retina, skin, and striated muscles have been the most extensively studied.

Using electron microscopy, one finds that the glomerular capillaries most closely resemble skin capillaries. The latter possess an almost continuous basement membrane which, at its outer surface, appears to be surrounded by, and in direct continuity with, irregularly laminated basement membranelike trabeculae. *Perithelial cells* are embedded in the meshwork of trabeculae. The function of these cells is not well understood, but it is widely assumed that they play an important role in the production and maintenance of the basement membrane. In other organs, capillaries vary considerably in regard to the density or relative paucity of perithelial cells and "para-angial" trabeculae, but their structural pattern is basically the same as that of skin capillaries.

The structural complexity of capillaries is greatest in the glomeruli. In this context one may refer to glomerular "perithelial cells" as being concentrated on one side of the capillary wall, in the center of an overlying lobule of convoluted capillaries. These cells have previously been referred to as mesangial cells, and they are in equally intimate contact with the capillary basement membrane as other pericytes, either directly or through the trabeculae of the matrix. Insofar as position and relationship to capillary basement membrane are concerned, the mesangial cells are essentially the same as the pericytes in skin or other capillaries; the mesangial cells, however, differ in that their position also permits direct contact of the basement membrane with epithelial cells on the opposite side of the capillary wall (see facing Plate 2 and pages 8 and 9).

Obviously, glomerular mesangial cells can be identified with perithelial cells of other capillaries only by inference. Moreover, this inference accounts for the generally parallel involvement, in diabetes, of basement membranes in many capillaries of the body, including those of the glomeruli, providing one accepts the thesis that glomerular perithelial cells (mesangial cells) are largely responsible for maintenance and thickness of the basement membrane. Opinions on this problem remain divided, yet the alternate hypothesis, that epithelial cells are responsible for the thickness of the basement membrane, is difficult to reconcile with the many analogous observations.

Diabetes may be associated with massive deposition of mesangial matrix, without or with thickening of basement membrane. However, increased thickening of the basement membrane in the absence of an increase of mesangium has not been demonstrated. Moreover, the mesangial cells show increased activity under these circumstances, as evidenced by proliferation, whereas the epithelial cells are diminished in number. Under the same circumstances, one may observe basement membrane thickening of the capillaries in the skin, retina, and striated muscle. In skin capillaries, this thickening may be confined to the outer layer of basement membranelike trabeculae, leaving the basement membrane proper of normal width—findings comparable to those seen in glomeruli.

These observations suggest that the pericytes, including those of the glomeruli, are the primary site of injury in diabetes. While the nature of the injury is not yet known, quantitative studies imply that it induces the cells not only to proliferate but also to deposit excessive matrix which may result in basement membrane thickening at an early stage. Most frequently, however, this thickening occurs late in the development of glomerulosclerosis.

Factors other than systemic disturbance of carbohydrate metabolism may enter the pathogenesis. Some authorities have proposed that capillary angiopathy in diabetes is hereditary. Measurements of capillaries in striated muscles have indicated that thickening of the basement membrane occurs only in hereditary diabetes, and that it is absent in nonhereditary diabetes caused by destruction of the pancreas.

Proliferation of the mesangium, excessive deposition of the matrix, and thickening of the basement membrane in glomeruli or other capillaries are nonspecific processes which frequently occur in conditions other than diabetes. Why these changes sometimes take the peculiar and almost pathognomonic nodular form in glomeruli is unknown.

The observation that the nodular lesion had a rather high degree of specificity in diabetes was based on autopsy observations, yet nodular glomerulosclerosis has been reported in isolated instances in which the clinical examination prior to death did not indicate diabetes. In these cases, of course, no special studies could be made retrospectively to rule out diabetes. Eventually, our ever expanding experience with renal biopsies will give us final assessment of the specificity of this lesion, for an unexpected diagnosis of diabetic glomerulosclerosis warrants pursuance by a complete and refined clinical study.

Tubular Changes

If diabetes is associated with a nephrotic syndrome, the epithelial cells of proximal convoluted tubules are likely to contain sudanophilic material. However, the only tubular lesion virtually pathognomonic for diabetes is the Armanni-Ebstein cell. This glycogen-filled epithelial cell characteristically occurs in the distal, straight portion of the proximal tubule. It can be recognized as an empty, plantlike cell in conventional preparations stained with hematoxylin and eosin. This type of cell can also be found in the kidneys of rats with experimental alloxan diabetes, but its pathogenesis is not clearly understood. The Armanni-Ebstein cell seems to occur less frequently in diabetic patients whose carbohydrate metabolism is well regulated, but a controlled study had not been performed for more than two decades. *Continued on page 152*

Diabetic Nephropathy

Continued from page 151

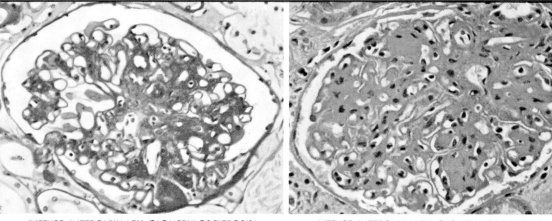

DIFFUSE INTERCAPILLARY GLOMERULOSCLEROSIS;
PAS STAIN

DIFFUSE INTERCAPILLARY GLOMERULOSCLEROSIS;
H. AND E. STAIN

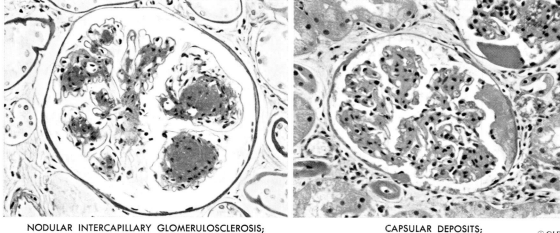

NODULAR INTERCAPILLARY GLOMERULOSCLEROSIS;
PAS STAIN

CAPSULAR DEPOSITS;
H. AND E. STAIN

 ©CIBA

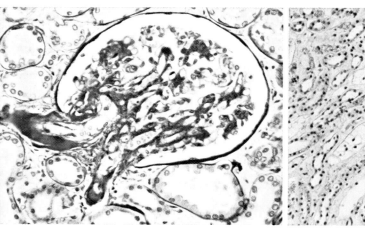

ARTERIOLOSCLEROSIS WITH HYALINIZATION OF EFFERENT
AND AFFERENT ARTERIOLE; ANILINE BLUE STAIN

ARMANNI–EBSTEIN CELLS IN RENAL TUBULES;
H. AND E. STAIN

Interstitial Tissues

Pyelonephritis and other infectious diseases have been thought to occur more frequently in diabetic patients than in the population at large. However, in more recent years this hypothesis has been challenged. As pointed out previously, the clinical and morphologic diagnoses are difficult to substantiate unless pyelonephritis is encountered in the acute stage or during a recurrent episode. Controlled studies of bacteriuria in diabetics and nondiabetics have produced conflicting results.

Clinicopathologic Correlation

Diabetic glomerulosclerosis has been described as a lesion found in diabetics who have hypertension and a nephrotic syndrome. Frequently, and inaccurately, this has been designated as the Kimmelstiel-Wilson (K-W) syndrome, but extensive studies have shown that the association of nodular glomerulosclerosis with the clinical triad was a serendipitous observation. We know now that the hypertension is more closely related to the arterio- and arteriolosclerosis than to the glomerular lesion, and also that less than 50 percent of the cases of diabetic glomerulosclerosis develop nephrotic syndrome. Moreover, the nephrotic syndrome occurs more frequently in association with the diffuse or mixed form of glomerulosclerosis than with the nodular form.

The pathogenesis of the nephrotic syndrome which occurs with diabetic glomerulosclerosis, however, remains unclear. Although it has been thought that membranous changes in the glomerular capillary basement membrane can be found in all such cases, this has not been confirmed. In addition, there is no evidence that such changes in the basement membrane are indeed the cause of an increased permeability to protein; they could just as well be a result of continuous passage of protein through the basement membrane. Similarly, there is no certainty that the systemic capillary angiopathy causes functional abnormalities.

The frequency of these described lesions in diabetes is indeed striking, but there is no proof, statistical or otherwise, that they are the basis of functional disturbances in the various organs in which they occur. For instance, in skin biopsies, vascular changes are observed to extend far beyond the areas of specific dermal and epidermal lesions. Generally, the angiopathy occurs most frequently without any other lesions, and it cannot be related specifically to hemodynamic abnormalities.

If there is progressive glomerulosclerosis in conjunction with severe and widespread arterio- and arteriolosclerosis, hypertension, and gradually deteriorating renal function, the prognosis is grave. Moreover, there is still no assurance that proteinuria and progressive renal disease can be attenuated or prevented by early and continuous treatment of the metabolic disorder of diabetes. □

Renovascular Hypertension

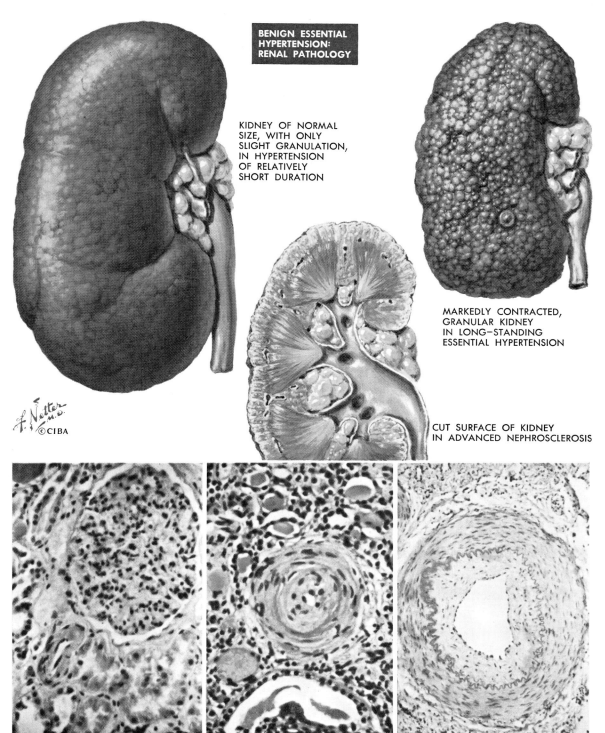

BENIGN ESSENTIAL HYPERTENSION: RENAL PATHOLOGY

KIDNEY OF NORMAL SIZE, WITH ONLY SLIGHT GRANULATION, IN HYPERTENSION OF RELATIVELY SHORT DURATION

MARKEDLY CONTRACTED, GRANULAR KIDNEY IN LONG–STANDING ESSENTIAL HYPERTENSION

CUT SURFACE OF KIDNEY IN ADVANCED NEPHROSCLEROSIS

FIBROSIS AND HYALINIZATION OF PRE–GLOMERULAR ARTERIOLE WITH STENOSIS OF LUMEN (WALL CUT ON BIAS); GLOMERULUS STILL UNALTERED (X 160)

OBLITERATIVE FIBROSIS AND HYALINIZATION (SCLEROSIS) OF SMALL INTRARENAL ARTERY (X 160)

OBLITERATIVE FIBROSIS AND HYALINIZATION (SCLEROSIS) OF INTRARENAL ARTERY OF MODERATE SIZE (X 160)

There is general agreement that significant obstruction or compression of one or both main renal arteries, or their immediate branches, results in an elevation of blood pressure *(extrarenal renovascular hypertension)*. Also, there is increasing evidence that intrarenal arterial and arteriolar sclerosis produces hypertension *(intrarenal renovascular hypertension)*. Thus, both conditions will be discussed.

Intrarenal Renovascular Hypertension

Benign Essential Hypertension. Because of the variable, slow progression of intrarenal vascular lesions, a broad spectrum of gross and microscopic alterations has been reported in intrarenal renovascular hypertension. In some cases the kidneys appear grossly normal. However, in most instances the surfaces are finely granular to varying degrees because of focal cortical atrophy and fibrosis resulting from obliterative vascular disease.

On occasion, changes consistent with the presence of pyelonephritis (shrinkage, scarring, or cyst formation) are found. As a result of progressive vascular disease, the shrinkage and scarring increase so that finally each kidney may weigh less than 75 gm. Such organs show

great reduction in the thickness of the cortex. Grossly, the kidney may at this time be indistinguishable from the end-stage kidney that results from long-standing chronic glomerulonephritis.

The microscopic appearance, like the gross appearance, is variable. Early in the course of the vascular disease only minimal sclerosis of preglomerular arterioles, with some degree of obliterative sclerosis of larger intrarenal arterial branches, may be observed. The vascular lesions consist of intimal fibrosis, proliferation, and variable degrees of hyalinization. Intimal thickening produces stenosis of the lumen and may well be occlusive.

A preglomerular arteriole (cut on the bias) with some fibrosis and hyalinization of its wall and moderate stenosis of the lumen is shown in Plate 4. Note particularly that the glomerulus remains unaffected in this instance.

A more advanced degree of arteriolar nephrosclerosis is also shown in Plate 4. There are marked hyalinization and fibrosis of the intima and media of the vessel, and the lumen is virtually obliterated. The same process is depicted in a larger vessel, and again the marked obliterative fibrosis and hyalinization are apparent.

Clinically, the onset of the benign phase of intrarenal renovascular disease usually occurs between the ages of 30 and 50, and the course is variable. For as many as 20 to 30 years, only an elevated blood pressure may be detected. The diastolic blood pressure is usually between 90 and 120 mm of mercury. While there may be headache, palpitations, and ill-defined anxiety, usually there are no consistent complaints that correspond to the progress of the condition.

Although a few patients may lead perfectly normal lives despite the elevated blood *Continued on page 154*

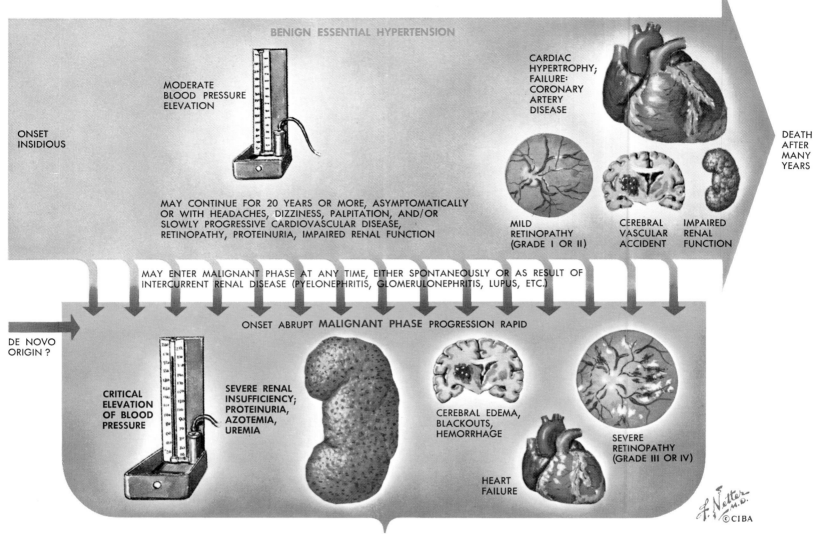

BENIGN ESSENTIAL HYPERTENSION

ONSET INSIDIOUS

MODERATE BLOOD PRESSURE ELEVATION

CARDIAC HYPERTROPHY; FAILURE: CORONARY ARTERY DISEASE

DEATH AFTER MANY YEARS

MAY CONTINUE FOR 20 YEARS OR MORE, ASYMPTOMATICALLY OR WITH HEADACHES, DIZZINESS, PALPITATION, AND/OR SLOWLY PROGRESSIVE CARDIOVASCULAR DISEASE, RETINOPATHY, PROTEINURIA, IMPAIRED RENAL FUNCTION

MILD RETINOPATHY (GRADE I OR II)

CEREBRAL VASCULAR ACCIDENT

IMPAIRED RENAL FUNCTION

MAY ENTER MALIGNANT PHASE AT ANY TIME, EITHER SPONTANEOUSLY OR AS RESULT OF INTERCURRENT RENAL DISEASE (PYELONEPHRITIS, GLOMERULONEPHRITIS, LUPUS, ETC.)

DE NOVO ORIGIN ?

ONSET ABRUPT MALIGNANT PHASE PROGRESSION RAPID

CRITICAL ELEVATION OF BLOOD PRESSURE

SEVERE RENAL INSUFFICIENCY; PROTEINURIA, AZOTEMIA, UREMIA

CEREBRAL EDEMA, BLACKOUTS, HEMORRHAGE

SEVERE RETINOPATHY (GRADE III OR IV)

HEART FAILURE

DEATH IN 3 TO 6 MONTHS (UNTREATED)

Renovascular Hypertension

Continued from page 153

pressure, most develop some changes associated with hypertensive cardiovascular disease as the benign phase progresses. The brain, kidneys, and heart usually are eventually affected.

Generally, the degree of involvement of the central nervous system can be determined by funduscopic examination. However, even in patients who have only Grade I or Grade II retinopathy, cerebrovascular accidents can occur and actually account for 14 percent of deaths in patients who have benign essential hypertension.

Approximately seven percent of patients suffering from benign essential hypertension develop renal insufficiency. The renal involvement is manifested by proteinuria, decreased renal clearances, azotemia, and, terminally, uremia.

However, the primary effect of elevated blood pressure is on the heart, where either coronary artery disease or congestive heart failure may dominate the picture. Available statistics indicate that 43 percent of patients expire as a result of myocardial infarction and that 36 percent die from

congestive heart failure. Physical examination, chest X-ray, and electrocardiogram are all helpful in assessing the degree of involvement in an individual patient (see CIBA COLLECTION, Vol. 5, pages 232 and 233).

The benefit and value of control of blood pressure in the early period of the benign phase have recently been demonstrated. However, there is no unequivocal evidence that blood pressure control will prevent the further development of arteriolar nephrosclerosis. Nevertheless, once hypertensive cardiovascular disease has developed, antihypertensive therapy can be of immense value in controlling the manifestations of end-organ failure.

Malignant Phase. Less than 10 percent of patients who suffer from intrarenal renovascular disease develop a malignant or accelerated form, either early in the course of the benign phase or at any time during its progression. The malignant phase may result from renal ischemia caused by either severe obliterative extrarenal or severe intimal vascular sclerosis. However, it may be secondary to glomerulitis or interstitial inflammation complicating the moderately obliterative renal vascular disease observed in the benign phase.

Clinically, a number of specific signs and symptoms are associated with the malignant phase, in contrast to the benign phase in which specific symptoms are not apparent until end-organ in-

volvement is present. Diagnosis of the malignant phase can be made if the following triad is present: (1) diastolic blood pressure greater than 120 mm of mercury; (2) Grade IV retinopathy; (3) evidence of renal excretory dysfunction, ranging from proteinuria or hematuria to marked azotemia or uremia.

Most patients with malignant hypertension either have long-standing hypertension or have previously been treated for some other chronic nephropathy. On occasion, however, development of the malignant phase is so explosive that no past history of elevated blood pressure is available, and the disease appears to have developed *de novo.*

Headaches are common, are usually most severe in the morning, occipital in location, and constant. Anorexia, nausea, and vomiting may accompany the headaches, and there may be a severe and unexplained weight loss. Although a Grade IV retinopathy has been considered essential for a positive diagnosis, the explosive nature of the disease may bring the patient under care at a time when only a Grade III retinopathy (characterized by white exudates and flame-shaped hemorrhages) is present. Some patients develop fatal cerebral vascular lesions, while others may die of uremia.

The gross and microscopic appearances of the kidneys in patients who have malignant hypertension depend in large part upon the type and

Renovascular Hypertension

Continued

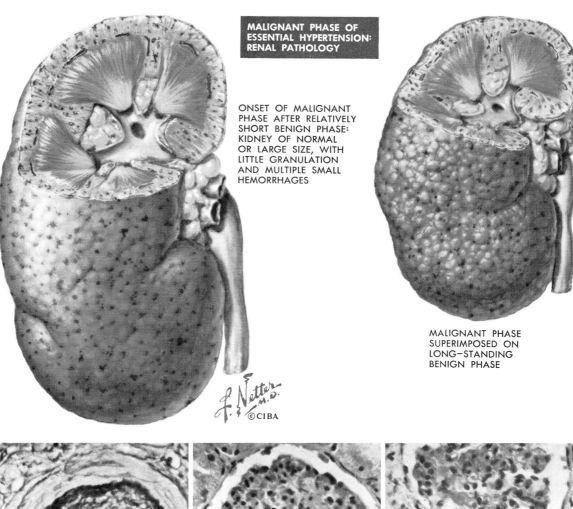

ONSET OF MALIGNANT PHASE AFTER RELATIVELY SHORT BENIGN PHASE: KIDNEY OF NORMAL OR LARGE SIZE, WITH LITTLE GRANULATION AND MULTIPLE SMALL HEMORRHAGES

MALIGNANT PHASE SUPERIMPOSED ON LONG-STANDING BENIGN PHASE

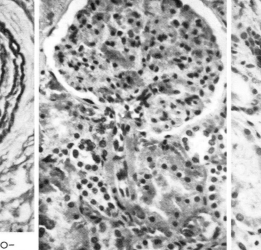

OBLITERATIVE, ENDARTERIAL FIBRO-ELASTOSIS OF INTRARENAL ARTERY OF MODERATE SIZE, USUALLY ASSOCIATED WITH CHRONIC PYELONEPHRITIS BUT MORE COMMONLY WITH MALIGNANT PHASE OF HYPERTENSION (X 160)

EARLY STAGE OF MALIGNANT HYPERTENSION: SUBENDOTHELIAL DEPOSIT OF FIBRIN IN PREGLOMERULAR ARTERIOLE (X 160)

LATER STAGE: NECROSIS OF WALL OF PREGLOMERULAR ARTERIOLE (X 160)

extent of the underlying renal disease. The kidney may be of normal size with minimal granularity and some petechiae from arteriolar rupture, or it may be shrunken and scarred.

Microscopically, one of the characteristic, but not specific, changes is a proliferative endarterial fibroelastosis frequently associated with complicating chronic pyelonephritis. The obliterative vascular disease may progress rapidly and produce both pronounced vascular stenosis and parenchymal changes secondary to the ischemia. Plasmatic arteriolosis, another change commonly seen in the malignant phase, is caused by the subendothelial transudation of blood plasma and the deposition of fibrin in the preglomerular arterioles as well as in the glomeruli. This lesion is the so-called fibrinoid degeneration or necrosis of the arterioles and glomerular capillaries. The vessels may thrombose and often rupture, producing hemorrhagic lesions within or on the surface of the kidney.

The glomeruli supplied by affected blood vessels may also show subendothelial precipitation of fibrin within the glomerulus, and this eventually leads to glomerular hyaline degeneration.

The early stages of deposition of subendothelial fibrin are evident in a pre-glomerular arteriole shown in Plate 6. The more advanced stage of this process reveals a "smudgy" appearance of the vessel, owing to necrosis and some involvement of the glomerulus in the region close to the arteriole. In addition, the process has extended into the proximal part of the glomerulus.

Almost all untreated patients who have malignant hypertension die within 2 years of the presumable onset of the condition, and approximately 66 percent succumb within the first 9 months. Thus, it is mandatory to treat promptly all those patients in whom the diagnosis of malignant hypertension has been made on the basis of the clinical picture described before. Blood pressure must be reduced immediately in order to avoid cerebrovascular accidents or acute congestive heart failure. Once the pressure has been reduced, maintenance therapy is required to help prevent further endorgan failure.

A number of patients who suffer from malignant hypertension develop uremia and marked reduction of renal excretory function to less than five percent of normal. They also may be oliguric. If patients who have superimposed renal failure do not respond to antihypertensive drug therapy and if elevated plasma renin levels are found, then bilateral nephrectomy should be considered.

Extrarenal Renovascular Hypertension

Arteriographic studies have revealed various stenosing or obstructing lesions of the extrarenal vasculature which often result in hypertension. Such lesions include arteriosclerotic plaques (more common in the older age group), fibromuscular hyperplasia and intimal fibroplasia (more common in the younger age group), obstruction (because of pressure or cicatrization), and abnormalities of the *Continued on page 156*

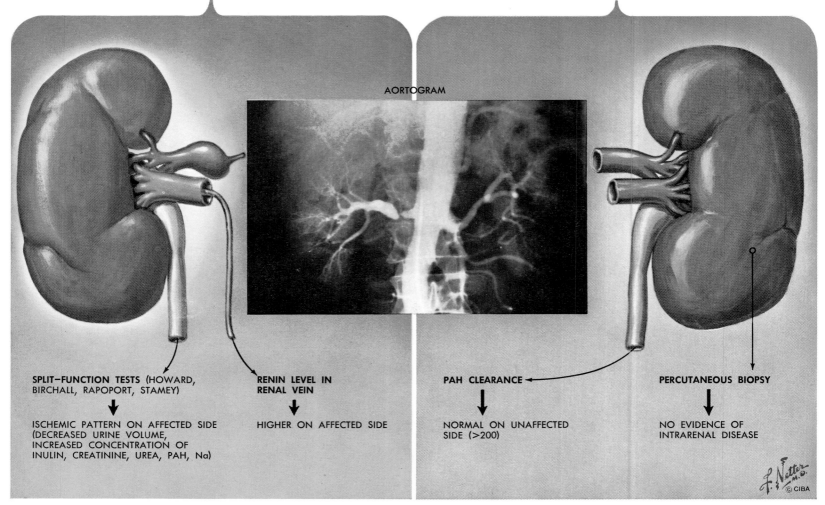

AFFECTED KIDNEY
EVIDENCE OF <u>SIGNIFICANT</u> ANATOMIC LESION

CONTRALATERAL KIDNEY
ABSENCE OF SIGNIFICANT INTRARENAL DISEASE

AORTOGRAM

SPLIT–FUNCTION TESTS (HOWARD, BIRCHALL, RAPOPORT, STAMEY)

ISCHEMIC PATTERN ON AFFECTED SIDE (DECREASED URINE VOLUME, INCREASED CONCENTRATION OF INULIN, CREATININE, UREA, PAH, Na)

RENIN LEVEL IN RENAL VEIN

HIGHER ON AFFECTED SIDE

PAH CLEARANCE

NORMAL ON UNAFFECTED SIDE (>200)

PERCUTANEOUS BIOPSY

NO EVIDENCE OF INTRARENAL DISEASE

Renovascular Hypertension

Continued from page 155

renal arterial tree secondary to trauma to perirenal tissues.

Probably less than one percent of all hypertensive patients exhibit any of the above conditions. Nevertheless, the possible need for corrective surgery demands investigation in those patients in whom the history, physical findings, or laboratory data suggest an extrarenal cause for hypertension. The following should be considered suggestive: (1) onset of diastolic hypertension before age 30 or after age 50; (2) sudden onset or worsening of preexistent hypertension; (3) hypertension which cannot be controlled with drugs or is controlled only with many side effects; (4) a history of trauma to tissues in the renal area; and (5) a history of thromboembolic disease.

An abdominal bruit in the region of a main renal artery may be the only physical finding which suggests extrarenal renovascular disease as the cause of the hypertension. This finding is somewhat unreliable, since a bruit may be heard when any vessel within the abdomen is diseased.

In all patients in whom extrarenal renovascular hypertension is suspected, a "hypertensive" intravenous pyelogram should be employed as the initial laboratory screening procedure (see page 95). This procedure utilizes specific timing in the obtaining of films. It can thus reveal both significant variations in renal size and disparity in the appearance and disappearance of dye in the kidneys. Up to 85 percent of extrarenal obstruction can be detected by this procedure.

Transfemoral aortography (see pages 100 and 101) must be performed in those individuals in whom history and physical findings are suggestive of extrarenal renovascular disease and in whom the "hypertensive" IVP is abnormal (see page 95). Careful assessment of the results can lead to verification of the presence, location, and type of lesion. For instance, stenosis and poststenotic dilatation of the right renal artery are shown in the radiograph in Plate 7. However, the mere presence of an anatomic lesion is not sufficient evidence on which to make a prognosis. Incidental renal artery lesions are commonly found in normotensive patients, and therefore the *functional* significance of any lesion must be established (see pages 85 and 86).

Perhaps the simplest method for assessing the significance of a lesion is determination of a plasma renin level: an elevated renin level suggests significant obstruction (renal ischemia). A

second, more reliable (but more formidable) method for establishing the significance of a lesion is determination of renin levels in the renal vein from each kidney. A disparity between the renin levels on the two sides positively confirms the functional significance of a lesion.

Indications for Surgery. If the history and/or physical findings suggest an extrarenal cause for the hypertension, and if the IVP and aortogram are abnormal and the functional significance of the lesion has been confirmed, the chances are good that at least some reduction in blood pressure will occur should corrective surgery be attempted. However, if the goal is permanent cure of the hypertension by surgery, a precise assessment of both the excretory function and the structural integrity of the intrarenal vasculature is also essential. It has been shown that correction of the extrarenal lesion will not result in a long-term cure of the hypertension if significant intrarenal disease is present.

The status of the intrarenal vasculature can be assessed most accurately by a renal biopsy (see pages 107 and 108). However, there is some degree of morbidity associated with either an open or a closed biopsy. As an alternative to biopsy, one may employ the split-function test described by Stamey, utilizing in particular the para-aminohippurate (PAH) clearance values (see page 86). Although the Stamey test was developed primarily to

Renovascular Hypertension

Continued

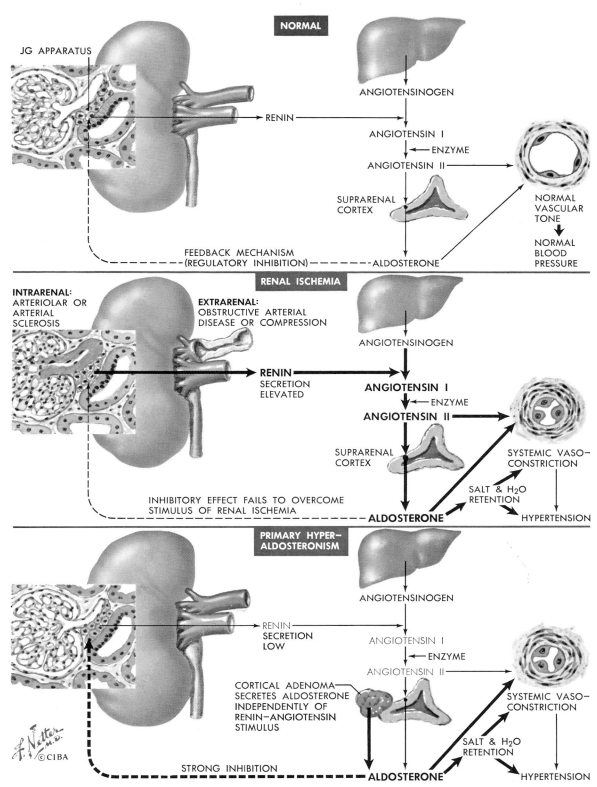

NORMAL

JG APPARATUS

ANGIOTENSINOGEN

RENIN

ANGIOTENSIN I

ENZYME

ANGIOTENSIN II

SUPRARENAL CORTEX

NORMAL VASCULAR TONE

NORMAL BLOOD PRESSURE

FEEDBACK MECHANISM (REGULATORY INHIBITION) — ALDOSTERONE

RENAL ISCHEMIA

INTRARENAL: ARTERIOLAR OR ARTERIAL SCLEROSIS

EXTRARENAL: OBSTRUCTIVE ARTERIAL DISEASE OR COMPRESSION

ANGIOTENSINOGEN

RENIN SECRETION ELEVATED

ANGIOTENSIN I

ENZYME

ANGIOTENSIN II

SUPRARENAL CORTEX

SYSTEMIC VASO-CONSTRICTION

SALT & H_2O RETENTION

INHIBITORY EFFECT FAILS TO OVERCOME STIMULUS OF RENAL ISCHEMIA — ALDOSTERONE

HYPERTENSION

PRIMARY HYPER-ALDOSTERONISM

ANGIOTENSINOGEN

RENIN SECRETION LOW

ANGIOTENSIN I

ENZYME

ANGIOTENSIN II

CORTICAL ADENOMA SECRETES ALDOSTERONE INDEPENDENTLY OF RENIN-ANGIOTENSIN STIMULUS

SYSTEMIC VASO-CONSTRICTION

SALT & H_2O RETENTION

STRONG INHIBITION — ALDOSTERONE

HYPERTENSION

establish the functional significance of an anatomic lesion (and can be so employed), it can also provide information on the vascular status of the kidney which has no lesion.

Documentation of the presence of vascular disease in one kidney is adequate because in most instances the progression is symmetrical. If the PAH clearance on the side without the lesion is less than 200cc per minute, considerable intrarenal vascular disease is present in that kidney and probably in both kidneys. Surgery will not result in a long-term cure. On the other hand, if the PAH clearance is greater than 200 cc per minute, the presence of intrarenal disease cannot be ruled out by this test, and a renal biopsy must be performed. Should the biopsied kidney be found essentially normal, a permanent cure can be anticipated if the affected kidney is removed surgically.

Occasionally, bilateral lesions are demonstrated in hypertensive patients by aortography. In these instances, bilateral renal vein levels of renin are of questionable value in determining the functional significance of the lesions. Also, the PAH clearance cannot be employed to assess the vascular status of either kidney in these patients because the flow rate is reduced bilaterally. Therefore, a renal biopsy must be performed. In the absence of intrarenal disease, corrective surgery should be attempted.

Unilateral intrarenal disease also represents a form of surgically correctable renal hypertension. The "hypertensive" IVP, in unilateral renal disease, will be abnormal, but aortography will be normal. Split-function studies or bilateral renal vein renin values will confirm the functional disparity. Assessment of the status of the *contralateral kidney* is again of utmost importance, and if it is essentially normal, the hypertension can be cured by unilateral nephrectomy.

Renin-Angiotensin System in Renovascular Hypertension

Among the many factors potentially involved in renovascular hypertension, the renin-angiotensin system is thought to play an important role. The juxta glomerular (JG) apparatus (see pages 6 and 7) appears to be the source of the enzyme *renin.* Although the precise stimulus involved in the production and release of renin has not been established, baroreceptors, chemoreceptors, mean arterial pressure, and altered pulse pressure have been suggested as possible factors. Clinically, variations in sodium intake or in plasma volume are known to inhibit or stimulate renin production. Also, it has been definitely established that a feedback mechanism is initiated in the normal individual following renin release.

The substrate *angiotensinogen* is converted by renin to a decapeptide, *angiotensin I,* which enters the venous circulation. A converting enzyme, thought to be produced in the lung, changes angiotensin I to *angiotensin II,* which then enters the arterial circulation and produces *Continued on page 158*

Continued on page 158

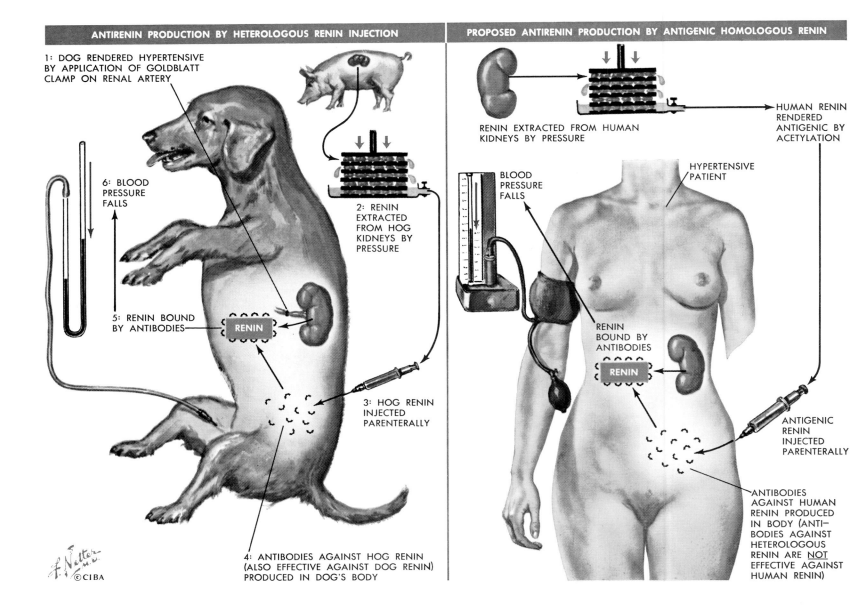

1: DOG RENDERED HYPERTENSIVE BY APPLICATION OF GOLDBLATT CLAMP ON RENAL ARTERY

6: BLOOD PRESSURE FALLS

5: RENIN BOUND BY ANTIBODIES

RENIN

2: RENIN EXTRACTED FROM HOG KIDNEYS BY PRESSURE

3: HOG RENIN INJECTED PARENTERALLY

4: ANTIBODIES AGAINST HOG RENIN (ALSO EFFECTIVE AGAINST DOG RENIN) PRODUCED IN DOG'S BODY

RENIN EXTRACTED FROM HUMAN KIDNEYS BY PRESSURE

HUMAN RENIN RENDERED ANTIGENIC BY ACETYLATION

HYPERTENSIVE PATIENT

BLOOD PRESSURE FALLS

RENIN BOUND BY ANTIBODIES

RENIN

ANTIGENIC RENIN INJECTED PARENTERALLY

ANTIBODIES AGAINST HUMAN RENIN PRODUCED IN BODY (ANTI-BODIES AGAINST HETEROLOGOUS RENIN ARE NOT EFFECTIVE AGAINST HUMAN RENIN)

Renovascular Hypertension

Continued from page 157

vasoconstriction of the systemic arterioles. Also, angiotensin II stimulates the suprarenal cortex to produce the mineralocorticoid aldosterone which, in turn, causes retention of sodium and water and elevation of blood pressure in a normal individual. These effects decrease the stimulus for renin production by the JG apparatus, thus completing the feedback cycle (see CIBA COLLECTION, Vol. 4, page 95, and Vol. 5, pages 224-226).

Alterations to this cycle have been documented in two disease states. In *primary hyperaldosteronism,* the feedback mechanism is altered by the presence of a suprarenal tumor autonomously producing increased amounts of aldosterone. This excessive aldosterone inhibits the release of renin, and therefore plasma renin levels are characteristically low.

In contrast, in the second disease, *extrarenal renovascular hypertension,* the presence of a significant lesion of a main renal artery or arteries results in an increased production of renin by the affected

kidney, and plasma renin values are high. Initially, the increased amounts of renin trigger the normal sequence of events, including increased production of aldosterone. However, the continuing presence of the lesion interferes with the normal feedback mechanism, and renin continues to be produced in excessive amounts.

In intrarenal renovascular hypertension, alterations in the renin-angiotensin system have not been documented. Plasma renin titers are almost uniformly within the normal range, despite the fact that the many stenotic or obstructive lesions in the arterioles should simulate the effects of one large obstruction in the main renal artery, since both are proximal to the JG apparatus.

Antirenin

To resolve the seemingly contradictory findings, an experiment originally designed to demonstrate the importance of the renin-angiotensin system in extrarenal renovascular hypertension was adapted for intrarenal renovascular disease. In the original experiment, dogs were made hypertensive by constriction of the main renal arteries by means of Goldblatt clamps. This procedure resulted in a functionally significant extrarenal obstruction. The subcutaneous or intramuscular injection of heterologous (hog) or acetylated homologous (dog) renin resulted in the development of *antirenin* and a fall in blood pressure to normal. When the injections of renin were discontinued, the con-

centration of antirenin in the blood decreased to a low level, and the blood pressure gradually returned to hypertensive levels. These results could be obtained repeatedly on the same animal.

Unfortunately, arteriolar nephrosclerosis does not exist in experimental animals, so that the above described procedure could not be used in animal studies to establish the role of renin and angiotensin in intrarenal disease. Therefore, injections of heterologous (hog) renin were made in humans. A high titer of antirenin to heterologous (hog) renin was produced in human hypertensives, but this antirenin was not effective against human renin, and hypertension persisted. Subsequently, it has been found that acetylated human renin is antigenic in humans and stimulates antirenin production. However, since the production of acetylated human renin is limited by both the availability of human kidneys and the need for further purification, only preliminary results are available. The subcutaneous or intramuscular injections of acetylated human renin into a few hypertensive humans have resulted in the development of low titers of antirenin to human renin, and slight decreases in blood pressure.

Although additional renal factors may contribute to the development of hypertension, these experiments appear to confirm the importance of the renin-angiotensin system in renovascular hypertension of either extrarenal or intrarenal origin. □

Hemolytic-Uremic Syndrome (Intravascular Coagulation and Thrombotic Microangiopathy)

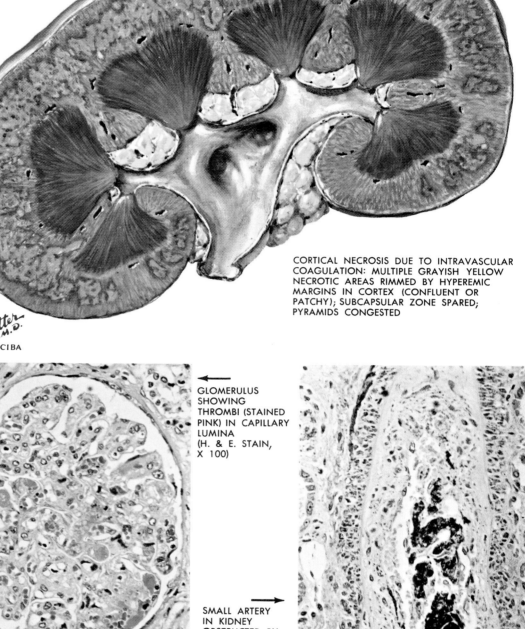

INTRAVASCULAR COAGULATION, HEMOLYTIC–UREMIC SYNDROME, AND THROMBOTIC MICRO–ANGIOPATHY

CORTICAL NECROSIS DUE TO INTRAVASCULAR COAGULATION: MULTIPLE GRAYISH YELLOW NECROTIC AREAS RIMMED BY HYPEREMIC MARGINS IN CORTEX (CONFLUENT OR PATCHY); SUBCAPSULAR ZONE SPARED; PYRAMIDS CONGESTED

GLOMERULUS SHOWING THROMBI (STAINED PINK) IN CAPILLARY LUMINA (H. & E. STAIN, X 100)

SMALL ARTERY IN KIDNEY OBSTRUCTED BY FIBRIN THROMBUS (STAINED PURPLE) (PHOSPHOTUNG–STIC ACID, HEMA–TOXYLIN STAIN, X 100)

Intrarenal coagulation frequently accompanies renal disease. Small amounts of fibrin and clumps of platelets may be found in the glomerular capillaries in a variety of renal diseases, such as acute diffuse glomerulonephritis (see page 131) and lipoid nephrosis (see page 123), and may contribute to the progression of the glomerular damage. Coagulation is also an important factor in certain forms of focal glomerulonephritis (see page 139) and extracapillary glomerulonephritis (see page 133) and leads to segmental necrosis of the glomerular tuft and crescent formation.

In acute defibrination syndrome, which may occur in conjunction with various complications of pregnancy and delivery (dead fetus, amniotic fluid embolism, abruptio placentae), glomerular thrombosis occurs rapidly. Lysis of the thrombi usually follows, with depletion of various coagulation factors and a hemorrhagic tendency.

Hemolytic-Uremic Syndrome (HUS)

In a syndrome characterized by various combinations of hemolysis, thrombocytopenia, hypertension, and renal failure, thrombosis is more insidious and more persistent. The complete syndrome is known as *hemolytic-uremic syndrome* (HUS), and it occurs either as an idiopathic disease or during the course of a variety of systemic diseases including malignant hypertension, eclampsia, and disseminated carcinomatosis.

Idiopathic HUS occurs mainly in infants and young children but can also be found in older children and adults. Often it is preceded by a febrile episode with gastrointestinal disturbances or respiratory manifestations. Hemolytic anemia with

*See Glossary

distorted red blood cells *(schistocytes), reticulocytosis, thrombocytopenia,* and varying degrees of renal failure and hypertension follow in a few days. Deficiencies of coagulation factors are inconstant and may be totally absent. Mortality is high—30 to 50 percent in children and even higher in adults. Many who survive eventually develop severe hypertension and chronic renal failure.

Because the renal lesions are somewhat similar to those produced by endotoxin in the generalized Shwartzman phenomenon, gram negative infection may be suspected as a possible mechanism. Etiologic agents such as viruses, rickettsiae, and allergic reactions to vaccines have been suggested. Pregnancy appears to predispose to HUS, which frequently complicates eclampsia. However, HUS may also follow a normal gestation, days, weeks, or even months after delivery.

The effectiveness of presently available therapy is

difficult to evaluate because the natural course of the disease is variable. Some successes have been reported with heparin, but it must be administered as soon as possible after the onset. Prolonged dialysis will often sustain the patient through the acute episode but may not prevent the development of chronic renal damage.

Pathology. At one time HUS was thought to represent a nonspecific manifestation of various unrelated kidney diseases. However, it appears now that the pathologic picture is unique and quite specific. In the acute stage, the kidneys are enlarged and edematous. If patients die, diffuse or patchy cortical necrosis is almost invariably seen but may be minimal or absent in patients who recover. Thrombi are found in small arteries, arterioles, and glomerular capillaries. They are sometimes accompanied by fibrinoid necrosis of the vessel walls which is probably the result of insudation* of blood proteins, including *Continued on page 160*

Hemolytic-Uremic Syndrome (Intravascular Coagulation and Thrombotic Microangiopathy)

Continued from page 159

INTRAVASCULAR COAGULATION, HEMOLYTIC-UREMIC SYNDROME, AND THROMBOTIC MICRO-ANGIOPATHY (CONTINUED)

COMMON ELECTRON MICROSCOPIC FINDINGS: DEPOSITS (D) AND MESANGIAL CELL CYTOPLASMIC PROCESSES (M) IN THE SUBENDOTHELIAL SPACE; ENDOTHELIUM (E) SWOLLEN; BOTH MESANGIAL (MC) AND ENDOTHELIAL CELLS (EN) CONTAIN MANY VACUOLES AND DILATED ROUGH ENDOPLASMIC RETICULUM; LUMEN (L) NARROWED (MAY BE "SLITLIKE"); RED BLOOD CELLS (RC) MAY OR MAY NOT BE PRESENT; BASEMENT MEMBRANE (B) OFTEN WRINKLED; EPITHELIAL FOOT PROCESSES (F) PARTLY FUSED

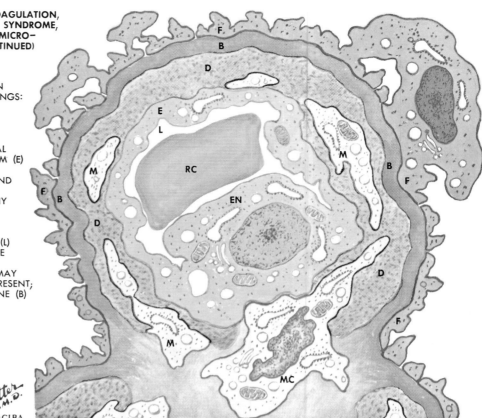

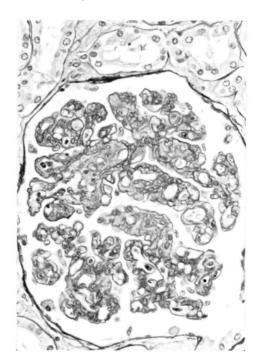

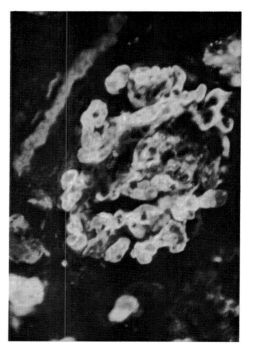

GLOMERULUS SHOWING THICKENING OF CAPILLARY WALLS AND PARTIAL CAPILLARY COLLAPSE (PAS STAIN, X 160)

FIBRINOGEN DEPOSITION ALONG CAPILLARY WALLS OF GLOMERULUS (IMMUNO-FLUORESCENT PREPARATION, TAGGED ANTI-FIBRINOGEN SERUM, X 100)

fibrinogen, into the wall. The damaged vessel may dilate to form a small aneurysm.

The accumulation of pale, finely granular or fibrillar material between the endothelium and the basement membrane of the glomerular capillaries is an important feature. This material does not stain with the usual fibrin stains but on immunofluorescence gives strong reaction with antifibrinogen serum, at least in the early stages of the disease. It probably consists of fibrinogen or its incompletely polymerized derivatives. Other proteins, such as globulins, are usually absent.

The affected capillary walls become thick and the lumina correspondingly narrow. This combination of arteriolar thrombosis and capillary wall thickening is known as *thrombotic microangiopathy.* It interferes with glomerular perfusion and filtration and leads to collapse of the tuft and eventual sclerosis with little if any cellular reaction.

In patients who develop severe hypertension, vascular necrosis may predominate over thrombosis, and the distinction from primary malignant hypertension (see page 155) is very difficult.

The pathogenesis of the hemolysis and thrombocytopenia is unknown, but it has been suggested that cells are damaged while passing through vessels lined with sticky fibrin. Alternatively, hemolysis may cause fibrin deposition by liberating thromboplastin from the damaged cells.

HUS is sometimes difficult to distinguish from *thrombotic thrombocytopenic purpura (TTP, Moschcowitz's disease),* which is seen mainly in adults. Both HUS and TTP have very similar hematologic manifestations and histologic changes, and possibly both are produced by the same mechanisms. However, in HUS the vascular lesions are almost completely limited to the kidneys, whereas in TTP they are widely disseminated and cause multisystem manifestations. While renal symptoms are common in TTP, renal failure is infrequent.

Malignant hypertension is frequently associated with HUS. In a recent report, hemolysis and thrombocytopenia were documented in 16 of 24 such patients. Also, in experimental rats with DOCA-induced hypertension, HUS has been observed. Nevertheless, the sequence of events when HUS and malignant hypertension occur concomitantly is not entirely clear. Destruction of red blood cells and platelets could be explained by the previously mentioned mechanism—the passage of cells through damaged blood vessels. On the other hand, it is entirely possible that in a certain number of patients, idiopathic or primary malignant hypertension represents the sequela of HUS. In such patients, the syndrome of HUS may have been recognized or may have passed undetected.

In systemic lupus erythematosus, hemolysis and thrombocytopenia are known accompaniments, and the complete syndrome, either HUS or TTP, is not infrequent. Also, in a fair proportion of cases of TTP or HUS in adults, positive LE preparations are found. In fact, sometimes one or the other syndrome is the initial event and precedes other manifestations of lupus by months or years (see page 141).

In patients having such advanced debilitating diseases as disseminated carcinomatosis or severe inflammatory processes, secondary HUS may be seen. Often these patients are already anemic, but their most obvious problem is renal failure. Investigation may reveal a hemolytic component to the anemia and the presence of thrombocytopenia. Diagnosis can be confirmed, as in all cases of HUS, by finding pure fibrinogen deposits in renal glomeruli. □

Radiation Effects on the Kidney

Only recently has it been realized that the kidneys are probably the most radiosensitive of abdominal organs. Confusion still cloaks the pathology and pathogenesis of the radiation-produced lesions, and many diagnostic terms are used: clinically, acute and chronic radiation nephritis and radiation nephropathy; pathologically, glomerulosclerosis, arterial and arteriolar nephrosclerosis, necrotizing vasculitis and glomerulonephritis, *nephroendotheliosis, sclerosing nephrosis,* and *nephroglomerulosis.*

The diverse terminology has resulted because almost all the pathologic observations in man have been based on end-stage studies and only rarely have been correlated with well-controlled, serial, experimental findings. However, designations must reflect the dose and the time interval which has elapsed after exposure to radiation. Also, individual variations and preexisting renal lesions which may affect the type of response should be considered.

The kidneys are not usually exposed to radiation because they are shielded by the abdominal wall. However, if patients receive radiotherapy of malignant tumors of the upper abdomen, the pelvis, or the testis, or if they receive either total body irradiation or heavy metal radioisotopes, the kidneys may receive radiation. This discussion will be limited to the effects on the kidneys of therapeutic radiation applied regionally.

Nephroendotheliosis

Although it has long been maintained that the renal areas may be given radiation doses less than 2500 r without concern, many patients receiving radiation to the kidney region will manifest proteinuria during the course of therapy. Disturbances of renal plasma flow (see page 43), glomerular filtration rate (see page 39), and tubular function (see page 41) have been reported beginning at 400 r and continuing through the course of irradiation. Although no histologic findings have been described in man in conjunction with the physiologic changes, the author suggests that there are endothelial and tubular epithelial injuries in association with transient edema and congestion. The condition is called *nephroendotheliosis.* Whether these changes are reversible or irreversible depends on the total amount of radiation and possibly other factors.

Sclerosing Nephrosis

Mild Forms. Several months to years after irradiation patients may be asymptomatic except for mild proteinuria. When these patients die of other causes, the kidneys become available only incidentally. Such kidneys are smaller than normal, but their architecture is well preserved. Microscopically, tubules and vessels appear normal with conventional H. and E. stain. However, using silver, trichrome, and PAS stains, the author has reported that the tubules, although normal in contour, are small and collapsed. There are varying but mild degrees of interstitial fibrosis and vascular sclerosis (Plate 12, A).

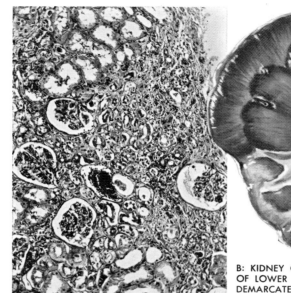

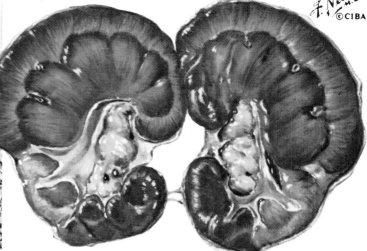

B: KIDNEY OF EXPERIMENTAL ANIMAL 5 MONTHS AFTER X−IRRADIATION OF LOWER SEGMENT (TOTAL DOSE 2500 R); IRRADIATED AREA SHARPLY DEMARCATED, GRAYISH, FIBROTIC, AND COLLAPSED

A: MILD SCLEROSING NEPHROSIS: COLLAPSE OF RENAL CORTEX; TUBULES SMALL AND LINED BY LOW CUBOIDAL EPITHELIUM (MASSON TRICHROME STAIN, X 115)

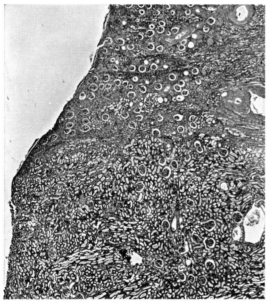

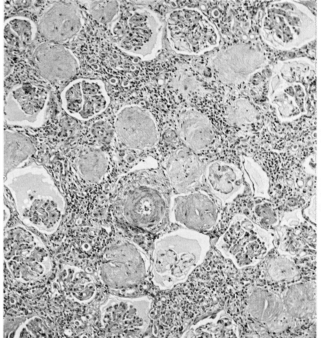

C: SEVERE SCLEROSING NEPHROSIS: SHARP LINE OF DEMARCATION SEPARATING IRRADIATED FROM NON-IRRADIATED AREA (MASSON TRICHROME STAIN, X 11)

D: SEVERE SCLEROSING NEPHROSIS: MARKED ATROPHY OF TUBULES AND COLLAPSE OF RENAL PARENCHYMA; MANY GLOMERULI HYALINIZED, OTHERS NORMAL; SCLEROSIS OF THE ARTERIES (H. & E. STAIN, X 80)

Severe Forms. In some patients, because of either higher radiation dosage or increased sensitivity of certain kidneys to irradiation, more severe involvement of renal tissue will be apparent. In addition to proteinuria, these patients will manifest progressive weakness, anemia, and gradually progressive impairment of renal function. About half the patients manifest hypertension. Depending on the extent of renal involvement, patients may live for many years with chronic renal failure and/or hypertension.

The gross and microscopic changes in the kidney represent more advanced stages of the lesions described for asymptomatic, mild sclerosing nephrosis. The extent of renal tissue involvement corresponds to the irradiated field, and one or both kidneys or the lower segment of one or both kidneys may be involved. If the entire kidney is affected, it is small and scarred; if only a segment, the irradiated area is sharply demarcated (Plate 12, B and C). Histologically, there is severe tubular atrophy and interstitial fibrosis but no appreciable inflammatory infiltration (Plate 12, D). Although some glomeruli are hyalinized, the majority appear normal. Vascular sclerosis, usually moderate to severe in degree, is present.

The pathogenesis, described in detail in the literature, may be briefly summarized: The vascular response is similar to that induced in other sites by radiation; most of the tubular damage is directly induced by radiation, although some is secondary to vascular impairment; the glomerular changes, which appear quite late in the disease process, are secondary to tubular and vascular changes; the interstitial fibrosis is probably in response to tubular damage, stromal collapse, or direct effect of radiation on the fibrous stroma.

In man, the lesion has generally been designated as chronic radiation nephritis *Continued on page 162*

Radiation Effects on the Kidney

Continued from page 161

and considered primary if it develops initially or secondary if it follows so-called acute radiation nephritis. However, this terminology is unsatisfactory since there is no evidence of inflammation.

For the lesions observed in experimental animals, the term nephrosclerosis has been employed. This also is a misnomer because in the usual nephrosclerosis, the glomerular, tubular, and interstitial changes follow the vascular lesions. Furthermore, the vascular lesions of true nephrosclerosis may exist alone, while the glomerular changes coincide with vascular sclerosis and tubular atrophy. Also, in kidneys damaged by radiation, the tubular atrophy precedes sclerosis of the vessels and there is a considerable time lag between tubular loss and the development of glomerular hyalinization. Consequently, the term *sclerosing nephrosis* is used to categorize tubular necrosis, interstitial fibrosis, and sclerosis.

Nephroglomerulosis

The previously described sclerosing nephrosis, usually with vascular sclerosis, is the renal lesion observed most frequently in association with radiation. Superimposed on this basic pathology is a third manifestation, designated as *nephroglomerulosis* by the author, but generally called acute radiation nephritis.

Clinically, patients show renal involvement approximately 3 to 12 months after irradiation. In addition to proteinuria, there are anemia, weakness, progressive ankle or facial edema, exertional dyspnea, headache, hypertension, and uremia.

Grossly, the large, swollen kidneys have smooth cortices and numerous cortical petechiae (Plate 13, E). Microscopically, the glomeruli are large and hypocellular with fusion of capillary loops and apparent thickening of capillary walls by an eosinophilic fibrillary material which suggests a smudgy thickening of the basement membrane (Plate 13, F).

In thin sections stained with PAS, Masson trichrome, or PAMS*, the basement membrane is distinctly delicate. The thickening appears to involve the capillary endothelium. The cytoplasm of the endothelial cells and, to a lesser extent, that of the epithelial cells, appear swollen with vacuolization. Electron microscopy has shown that considerable amounts of basement membranelike material are present on the endothelial side of the capillaries, and the endothelial cells appear surrounded by and even contained in material similar to *lamina densa* (Plate 13, G).

Sclerosing nephrosis is virtually always present in those patients diagnosed as having nephroglomerulosis. However, neither tubular atrophy nor interstitial fibrosis is as advanced as in patients who die of sclerosing nephrosis. For instance, although tubular cells show cloudy swelling and fatty and hyaline droplets, these findings are sparse. Similarly, vascular sclerosis may be present, but endothelial changes like those seen in the early stages of radiation-induced vascular damage are more frequently observed.

*See Glossary

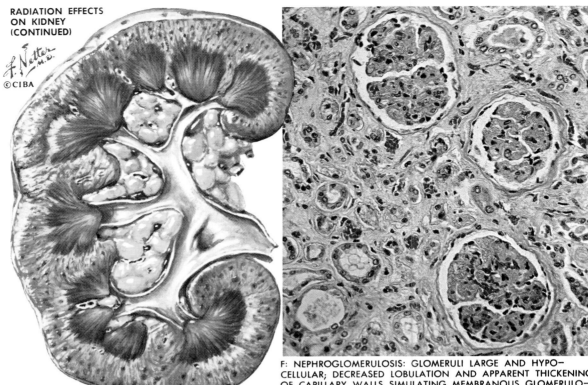

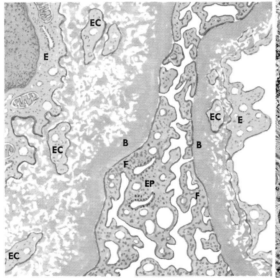

E: NEPHROGLOMERULOSIS: KIDNEY SWOLLEN; NUMEROUS PETECHIAE

F: NEPHROGLOMERULOSIS: GLOMERULI LARGE AND HYPO-CELLULAR; DECREASED LOBULATION AND APPARENT THICKENING OF CAPILLARY WALLS SIMULATING MEMBRANOUS GLOMERULO-NEPHRITIS; MILD DEGREE OF SCLEROSING NEPHROSIS MANIFESTED BY TUBULAR ATROPHY AND INTERSTITIAL FIBROSIS (H. & E. STAIN, X 180)

G: NEPHROGLOMERULOSIS, ELECTRON MICROSCOPIC FINDINGS: ENDOTHELIAL CYTOPLASMIC PROCESSES (EC) ENMESHED IN MATERIAL SIMILAR TO LAMINA DENSA AND OF VARYING THICKNESS, ON ENDOTHELIAL SIDE OF BASEMENT MEMBRANE (B); FOOT PROCESSES (F) FUSED; E = ENDOTHELIUM; EP = EPITHELIUM

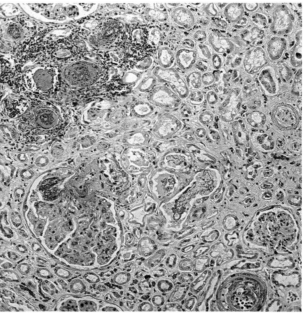

H: NEPHROGLOMERULOSIS WITH MILD SCLEROSING NEPHROSIS AND SEVERE NECROTIZING VASCULITIS; INTERSTITIAL HEMORRHAGE (H. & E. STAIN, X 180)

The pathogenesis and even the exact time of onset of nephroglomerulosclerosis remain unknown. It has been hypothesized, however, that the changes may represent a reaction of endothelial cells to an abnormal stimulus, with the formation of excessive amounts of basement membranelike material. Alternatively, a deposition of blood protein, which causes a breakdown of some cellular protein molecules, may represent the stimulus. A third possibility is that the lesions represent direct effects of radiation on the capillary basement membrane.

As indicated previously, nephroglomerulosis has been designated as acute radiation nephritis or as membranous glomerulonephritis. However, these terms are both misleading since the lesion is not acute. (There is an interval of 3 or more months before the onset of clinical symptoms.) There is no nephritis and the basement membranes are delicate. Moreover, these terms do not account for the endothelial and tubular alterations observed.

Necrotizing vasculitis, as manifested clinically by malignant hypertension, may be superimposed on either sclerosing nephrosis with nephrosclerosis or nephroglomerulosis. It has a serious impact on the prognosis.

Luxton has related the immediate prognosis in patients with nephroglomerulosis to the occurrence and severity of malignant hypertension. In a series of 20 patients, eight developed hypertension and six of these died within 3 to 12 months. Including these six patients with malignant hypertension, a total of 10 patients died of renal disease: three with chronic renal failure from 7 to 11 years after irradiation, and one, 4 years after irradiation, from cerebral hemorrhage secondary to hypertension. Another patient died with widespread metastatic disease. Thus, 10 years after onset, nine patients were still living but had chronic renal failure. □

Amyloidosis

HEREDOFAMILIAL

FAMILIAL AMYLOID NEUROPATHY

    PORTUGUESE TYPE — — — — — — — — — — — — NEUROPATHY (LOWER LIMBS), GASTROINTESTINAL AND CARDIAC

    OTHER TYPES (RUKAVINA ET AL., ETC.) — — — VITREOUS DISORDERS, CARPAL TUNNEL SYNDROME

AMYLOID NEPHROPATHY OF FAMILIAL — — — — NEPHROPATHY (PLUS WIDESPREAD BLOOD VESSEL
MEDITERRANEAN FEVER   INVOLVEMENT)

FAMILIAL AMYLOID CARDIOPATHY — — — — — — SEVERE CARDIAC AMYLOID (SOME SYSTEMIC INVOLVEMENT)

FAMILIAL AMYLOID NEPHROPATHY — — — — — — URTICARIA, DEAFNESS, RENAL DISEASE (PES CAVUS, GLAUCOMA)

FAMILIAL CUTANEOUS AMYLOID — — — — — — — FOCAL ONLY

FAMILIAL MEDULLARY THYROID CARCINOMA — — ASSOCIATED PHEOCHROMOCYTOMA
PRODUCING AMYLOID

LATTICE CORNEAL DYSTROPHY — — — — — — — PAINLESS PROGRESSIVE LOSS OF VISION

PRIMARY

    LOCAL — — — — — — — — — — — — — — — — — FOCAL LESIONS IN ALMOST ANY SITE

    SYSTEMIC — — — — — — — — — — — — — — — — HEART OFTEN INVOLVED BUT OTHER ORGANS ALSO
    AFFECTED AND MAY BE WIDESPREAD

AMYLOID OF AGED — — — — — — — — — — — — — HIGH INCIDENCE, ESPECIALLY IN HEART OF THOSE OVER 65;
SENILE PLAQUES OF CENTRAL NERVOUS SYSTEM

**DISORDERS COMPLICATED BY AMYLOIDOSIS
(SECONDARY AMYLOIDOSIS)**

CHRONIC INFECTIONS

    TUBERCULOSIS

    LEPROSY

    SYPHILIS

    OSTEOMYELITIS

    BRONCHIECTASIS

CHRONIC INFLAMMATORY DISEASES

    RHEUMATOID ARTHRITIS AND VARIANTS

    OTHER CONNECTIVE TISSUE DISEASES

NEOPLASMS   USUALLY WIDESPREAD IN DISTRIBUTION;
KIDNEY INVOLVEMENT OFTEN THE MOST SERIOUS

    HODGKIN'S DISEASE

    MULTIPLE MYELOMA

    RENAL CELL CARCINOMA

    MEDULLARY THYROID CARCINOMA

    OTHERS

METABOLIC DISEASES

    DIABETES MELLITUS

© CIBA

Amyloidosis is a disease characterized by the presence of a fibrous protein deposited in increased amounts in the connective tissue of the body. These deposits occur spontaneously *(primary amyloid)* or in association with a wide variety of infectious or inflammatory disorders *(secondary amyloid)*. In about 25 percent of autopsied rheumatoid arthritis patients this complication has been found, and it also has been reported in association with other connective tissue disorders. Amyloidosis is a common complication of chronic caseating tuberculosis, chronic osteomyelitis, and leprosy.

With regard to leprosy, amyloidosis recently was found to be present in more than 33 percent of the patient population of the United States Public Health Service Hospital, Carville, Louisiana. It also has been found in about 40 percent of paraplegic patients who survived their initial year but who ultimately died and were autopsied; amyloidosis can also be found in 10 to 20 percent of patients who die of multiple myeloma, and it has an increased association with Hodgkin's disease, renal carcinoma, and medullary carcinoma of the thyroid. Amyloidosis often is the cause of death in patients with these diseases because there may be renal involvement (and progressive uremia), gastrointestinal involvement (and massive bleeding), or cardiac arrhythmias (and sudden death).

Primary Amyloidosis. In addition to this increasing association of secondary amyloidosis with known disease, increasing numbers of cases of primary amyloidosis are being found in hospital populations. Furthermore, several interesting heredofamilial types of amyloidosis have been described. Clinically significant deposits of amyloid can be seen in very high incidence in the tissues of aged individuals, particularly in the heart, pancreas, and brain. It has become apparent that the hyaline changes seen in the pancreas in the majority of patients with diabetes mellitus provide unequivocal evidence of amyloid infiltration.

The finding of amyloid is not always incidental, and often its presence may be a contributing if not a major cause of death. A recent study of amyloid in the hearts of aged individuals revealed that cardiac amyloid apparently caused congestive heart failure and death in approximately 25 percent of elderly patients who had the disease.

Finally, amyloid has been reportedly found in a startlingly large percentage of patients exhibiting dementias of various types. If the figures are correct, and if, as suspected, the amyloid in some way contributes to the dementia, amyloidosis may be regarded as one of the most common causes of hospitalization.

Diagnosis

Clinical suspicion is obviously of the utmost importance to establish a diagnosis of *Continued on page 164*

Amyloidosis

Continued from page 163

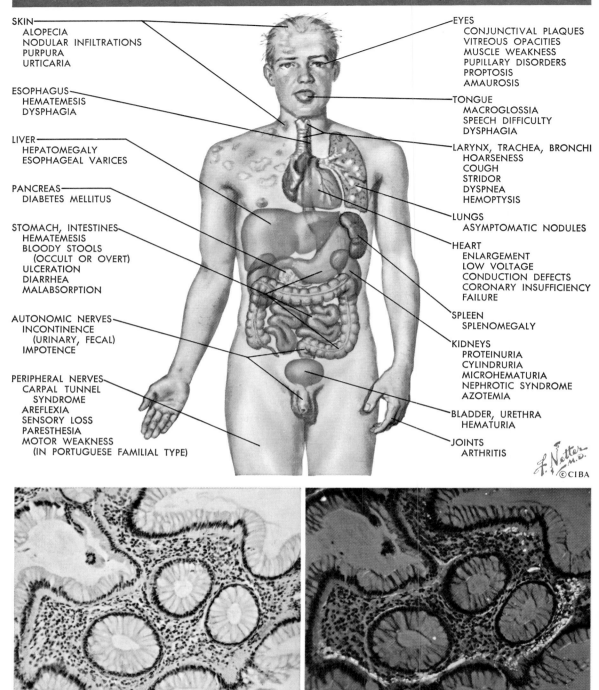

SKIN
ALOPECIA
NODULAR INFILTRATIONS
PURPURA
URTICARIA

ESOPHAGUS
HEMATEMESIS
DYSPHAGIA

LIVER
HEPATOMEGALY
ESOPHAGEAL VARICES

PANCREAS
DIABETES MELLITUS

STOMACH, INTESTINES
HEMATEMESIS
BLOODY STOOLS
(OCCULT OR OVERT)
ULCERATION
DIARRHEA
MALABSORPTION

AUTONOMIC NERVES
INCONTINENCE
(URINARY, FECAL)
IMPOTENCE

PERIPHERAL NERVES
CARPAL TUNNEL
SYNDROME
AREFLEXIA
SENSORY LOSS
PARESTHESIA
MOTOR WEAKNESS
(IN PORTUGUESE FAMILIAL TYPE)

EYES
CONJUNCTIVAL PLAQUES
VITREOUS OPACITIES
MUSCLE WEAKNESS
PUPILLARY DISORDERS
PROPTOSIS
AMAUROSIS

TONGUE
MACROGLOSSIA
SPEECH DIFFICULTY
DYSPHAGIA

LARYNX, TRACHEA, BRONCHI
HOARSENESS
COUGH
STRIDOR
DYSPNEA
HEMOPTYSIS

LUNGS
ASYMPTOMATIC NODULES

HEART
ENLARGEMENT
LOW VOLTAGE
CONDUCTION DEFECTS
CORONARY INSUFFICIENCY
FAILURE

SPLEEN
SPLENOMEGALY

KIDNEYS
PROTEINURIA
CYLINDRURIA
MICROHEMATURIA
NEPHROTIC SYNDROME
AZOTEMIA

BLADDER, URETHRA
HEMATURIA

JOINTS
ARTHRITIS

RECTAL BIOPSY STAINED WITH CONGO RED AND HEMATOXYLIN, VIEWED WITH LIGHT MICROSCOPE, SHOWING AMYLOID DEPOSITS

IDENTICAL AREA, VIEWED THROUGH POLARIZING MICROSCOPE, REVEALING GREEN BIREFRINGENCE, DIAGNOSTIC OF AMYLOID

amyloidosis. The patient with a chronic inflammatory or infectious disease who develops *hepatomegaly, splenomegaly,* or abnormalities of the urine (especially *proteinuria*) is highly suspect. Because (1) no specific clinical or laboratory abnormality is diagnostic of amyloidosis, (2) Congo red dye removal studies have certain inherent disadvantages, and (3) the diagnosis of amyloidosis ultimately rests on the finding of amyloid in tissue, there is little doubt that biopsy and utilization of appropriate stains is the best way by which to establish a diagnosis of amyloidosis.

Biopsies for the diagnosis of amyloidosis were first performed in 1925. Since then they have been utilized in such sites as the skin, rectum, gingiva, liver, kidney, spleen, respiratory tract, and small intestine. When considering biopsy, one must be aware of the potential hazard of bleeding from friable amyloid tissue, the limited accessibility of certain suspected sites of involvement, and the fact that a negative biopsy does not necessarily rule out the presence of

amyloid. There are, however, readily accessible sites, *e.g.,* the rectal mucosa, where the procedure is simple and painless, the incidence of bleeding is minimal, and the chance of involvement (if amyloid of any type is present in the body) is high.

Biopsy sections should be stained with Congo red and observed with a polarizing microscope which will indicate the presence of amyloid as a unique bright green birefringence. This positive form of birefringence characterizes amyloid of all types (primary, secondary, amyloid associated with multiple myeloma, heredofamilial, etc.). In addition to its diagnostic significance, the birefringence indicates that amyloid has an organized molecular structure. This concept has been verified with the electron microscope, which shows that amyloid of all types is made up of fine fibrils composed of thin rigid filaments.

The light microscope often shows amyloid depos-

ited subendothelially in blood vessels throughout the body, in close approximation to the mesangial area of the kidney, or between the Kupffer and parenchymal cells of the liver (see CIBA COLLECTION, Vol. 3/III, page 85). Amyloid is eosinophilic and refractile, stains with Congo red, and shows crystal violet metachromasia.

Clinical Manifestations

Because any body organ can be a site of amyloid deposition, the manifestations are protean. Amyloidosis may occur in individuals of either sex or racial background, and at almost any age, though the peak incidence usually occurs in people between 50 and 60 years old. Heavy proteinuria is the predominant mode of presentation, and a frank nephrotic syndrome occurs in 60 percent of the cases. Microscopic hematuria is not rare. Although radiologic studies of the kid-

Amyloidosis

Continued

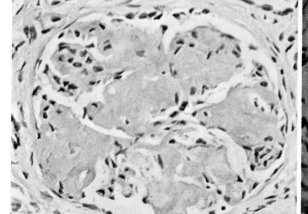

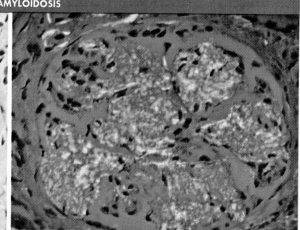

EXTENSIVE AMYLOID DEPOSITS IN GLOMERULUS OF HUMAN KIDNEY (CONGO RED & HEMATOXYLIN STAIN)

SAME SECTION, VIEWED UNDER POLARIZING MICROSCOPE, DEMONSTRATING GREEN BIREFRINGENCE

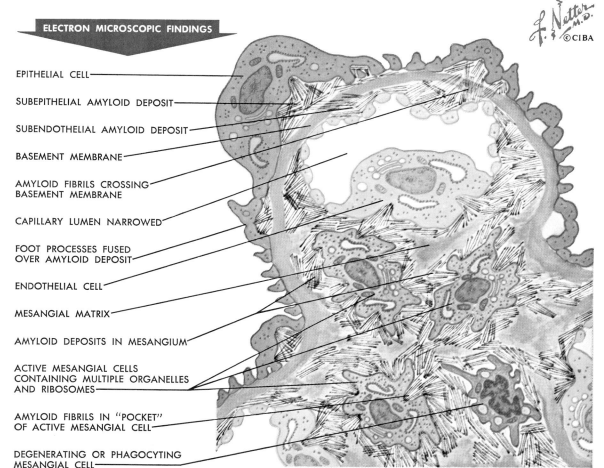

ELECTRON MICROSCOPIC FINDINGS

EPITHELIAL CELL

SUBEPITHELIAL AMYLOID DEPOSIT

SUBENDOTHELIAL AMYLOID DEPOSIT

BASEMENT MEMBRANE

AMYLOID FIBRILS CROSSING BASEMENT MEMBRANE

CAPILLARY LUMEN NARROWED

FOOT PROCESSES FUSED OVER AMYLOID DEPOSIT

ENDOTHELIAL CELL

MESANGIAL MATRIX

AMYLOID DEPOSITS IN MESANGIUM

ACTIVE MESANGIAL CELLS CONTAINING MULTIPLE ORGANELLES AND RIBOSOMES

AMYLOID FIBRILS IN "POCKET" OF ACTIVE MESANGIAL CELL

DEGENERATING OR PHAGOCYTING MESANGIAL CELL

ney often demonstrate enlargement, this is not an invariable finding. Only rarely is blood pressure elevated.

Gastrointestinal involvement may be manifested by diarrhea, constipation, and bleeding in the upper or lower gastrointestinal tract. Macroglossia may be the most striking manifestation (see CIBA COLLECTION, Vol. 3/I, page 113). Malabsorption has been described. Hepatomegaly frequently occurs in either the primary or secondary form of the disease, but most liver function tests are normal. Exceptions, however, are the sulfobromophthalein test (BSP) which may show elevated retention, and the serum alkaline phosphatase which may be elevated.

Cardiac disease is common in any type of amyloidosis and may be manifested by symptoms and signs associated with myocardial failure, conduction disturbance, or coronary vascular disease. Skin involvement may be local and isolated, or widespread (especially in primary amyloidosis). Other manifestations include abnormalities in sympathetic nervous system activity and sphincter tone, car-

pal tunnel syndrome, and various other symptoms.

Recent data suggest that the 5-year survival rate among patients suffering from amyloid disease (except that with associated myeloma) has improved with increasing use of generally supportive measures. However, there is no specific treatment for any variety of amyloidosis except eradication of any associated disease (for instance, osteomyelitis).

Pathogenesis

It is now generally accepted that the major constituent of an amyloid deposit is a fibrous glycoprotein having a unique ultrastructure, chemical composition, and crystallographic pattern. Viewed in isolation under the electron microscope, the fibril measures about 75 Å and shows a subunit structure. Compared to other fibrous extracellular proteins, it is a very poor antigen.

The relationship between immunoglobulins and

amyloid has been uncertain in the past. While patients with primary amyloidosis not infrequently develop a monoclonal gammopathy and patients with myeloma are prone to develop amyloid deposits, no specific or consistent immunoglobulin abnormalities have been found in patients with secondary or heredofamilial amyloidosis. It has also been shown that a protein isolated from primary amyloid has an amino acid sequence consistent with a portion of the variable part of immunoglobulin light chain while that from secondary amyloid has the sequence of a new and possibly unique protein.

A second component (the pentagonal unit, or "P" component) with different electron microscopic, chemical, and immunologic properties has been found in human amyloid tissues in very small and variable amounts. As of now, its nature and role in the genesis of amyloid remain to be defined. □

Progressive Systemic Sclerosis (Scleroderma) and Rheumatoid Arthritis

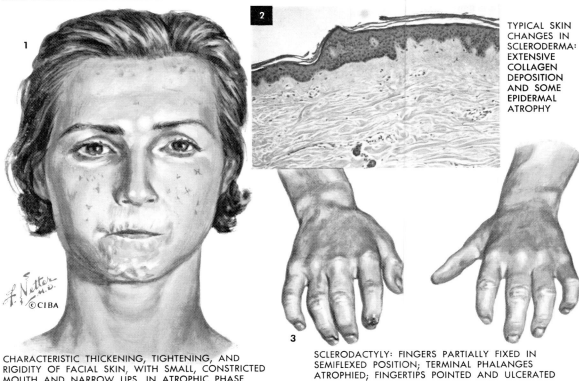

Progressive systemic sclerosis (scleroderma) is a systemic disease characterized by hypertrophy and hyperplasia of collagen fibers, by vascular lesions, and (to a much lesser extent) by inflammation. Widespread changes are present in the skin, heart, lungs, kidneys, muscles, synovial membranes, and gastrointestinal tract, especially the esophagus. Vascular lesions have been described in a number of organs and are particularly striking in the kidneys (see CIBA COLLECTION, Vol. 5, page 205).

Clinically, progressive systemic sclerosis appears in one of two forms: (a) the acute typified by fever, weight loss, polyarteritis, severe skin changes, and early visceral involvement with rapidly progressive renal disease; or (b) the chronic dominated by cutaneous manifestations (see 1 and 2 in illustration), with visceral involvement developing only after several years. Once renal involvement becomes clinically apparent, it progresses rapidly, even in the chronic form, with the development of malignant hypertension, retinopathy, encephalopathy, and, eventually, renal failure.

It is interesting to note that, even in patients having no clinical evidence of renal involvement, autopsy and biopsy studies often reveal renal vascular changes (see 4 in illustration). In patients exhibiting severe hypertension, the kidneys are usually normal in size and have mottled reddish yellow surfaces with small hemorrhages or infarcts—an appearance indistinguishable from that of malignant nephrosclerosis (see page 155).

Microscopically, striking changes are seen in the arteries. The arcuate arteries exhibit marked thickening of the walls (see 6 in illustration). This is caused primarily by mucoid swelling of the intima (see 4 in illustration) associated with various degrees of fibrosis and elastic fiber duplication (see 6 in illustration). As a result, the lumina of these vessels are severely narrowed. In patients suffering from severe hypertension and renal failure, arteriolar necrosis usually is present (see 5 in illustration). This process may extend into the glomeruli, with formation of fibrin thrombi in the capillaries and development of focal proliferative and/or sclerotic changes. Immunohistologic studies have revealed the presence of fibrinogen and gamma globulin in the walls of the altered vessels. However, these findings do not differ from those observed in malignant nephrosclerosis.

The etiology and pathogenesis of progressive systemic sclerosis appear to be related to an abnormal immune state as evidenced by the elevation of serum gamma globulin and antinuclear antibody levels, and by the demonstration of

CHARACTERISTIC THICKENING, TIGHTENING, AND RIGIDITY OF FACIAL SKIN, WITH SMALL, CONSTRICTED MOUTH AND NARROW LIPS, IN ATROPHIC PHASE OF SCLERODERMA

TYPICAL SKIN CHANGES IN SCLERODERMA: EXTENSIVE COLLAGEN DEPOSITION AND SOME EPIDERMAL ATROPHY

SCLERODACTYLY: FINGERS PARTIALLY FIXED IN SEMIFLEXED POSITION; TERMINAL PHALANGES ATROPHIED; FINGERTIPS POINTED AND ULCERATED

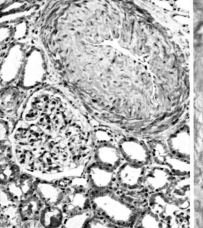

MUCOID SWELLING OF INTIMA IN MEDIUM–SIZED ARTERY OF KIDNEY, MOST OFTEN SEEN IN ACUTE CASES

COLLOIDAL IRON STAIN, DEMONSTRATING THAT INTIMAL SWELLING IS COMPOSED LARGELY OF MUCOPOLYSACCHARIDES

ARCUATE ARTERY IN CHRONIC SCLERODERMA: MARKED INTIMAL THICKENING, CONSISTING OF DENSE, LAMINATED MATRIX, RICH IN ELASTIC FIBERS, AND SMALL AMOUNT OF COLLAGEN

positive antinuclear reactions of the involved tissues.

Rheumatoid Arthritis. Renal involvement in this disease is much less common, and usually considerably less severe, than in systemic lupus erythematosus (SLE), polyarteritis nodosa, or progressive systemic sclerosis. Although the basic anatomic change in rheumatoid arthritis is now recognized to be a vasculitis involving small arteries and veins, this process does not affect the kidneys to a significant degree.

Clinically, mild proteinuria and abnormalities of the urinary sediment are not uncommon in patients who exhibit rheumatoid arthritis. However, when marked proteinuria and a significant degree of renal insufficiency are found in a patient, other possibilities must be considered. These include amyloidosis, which has been reported to occur in 10 to 20 percent of the cases (see page 163), lupus nephritis, because SLE is not uncommonly associated with rheumatoid arthritis (see

page 141), necrotizing vasculitis, possibly related to corticosteroid therapy or occurring as part of the abnormal immune status of these patients, interstitial nephritis, possibly related to phenacetin abuse (see page 144), and membranous glomerulonephropathy, related to gold therapy (see page 136).

Morphologically, slight glomerular hypercellularity resulting primarily from mesangial cell proliferation has been observed in some of the cases in which renal involvement is clinically mild or absent. Of the possibilities mentioned above, amyloidosis is by far the most frequently occurring. When amyloidosis is present, the distribution and histochemical properties follow the pattern of the secondary type. The amount of amyloid found in the kidneys may be extremely small, and the presence of this abnormal protein must be carefully looked for, utilizing special stains and polarization microscopy. □

Polyarteritis Nodosa

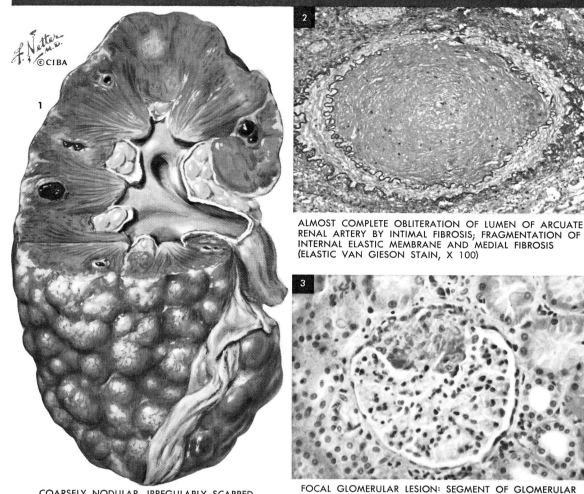

1 COARSELY NODULAR, IRREGULARLY SCARRED KIDNEY: CUT SECTION REVEALS ORGANIZING INFARCTS AND THROMBOSED ANEURYSMS IN CORTICOMEDULLARY REGION

2 ALMOST COMPLETE OBLITERATION OF LUMEN OF ARCUATE RENAL ARTERY BY INTIMAL FIBROSIS; FRAGMENTATION OF INTERNAL ELASTIC MEMBRANE AND MEDIAL FIBROSIS (ELASTIC VAN GIESON STAIN, X 100)

3 FOCAL GLOMERULAR LESION: SEGMENT OF GLOMERULAR TUFT DESTROYED BY NECROTIC PROCESS WITH MUCH FIBRIN AND SOME CELLULAR REACTION; PATIENT DIED FROM INTESTINAL PERFORATION (H. & E. STAIN, X 200)

RENAL INVOLVEMENT IN HYPERSENSITIVITY TYPE OF POLYARTERITIS NODOSA

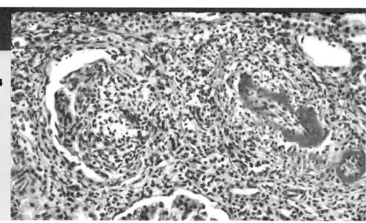

4 NECROTIZING (FIBRINOID) CHANGES IN SMALL ARTERY AT RIGHT OF SECTION, WITH INFILTRATION OF ALL LAYERS BY ACUTE AND CHRONIC INFLAMMATORY CELLS; THE INFLAMMATORY PROCESS HAS EXTENDED TO THE INTERSTITIUM AND TO THE ADJACENT GLOMERULUS (H. & E. STAIN, X 100)

Those inflammatory and necrotizing disease processes that involve medium-sized and small arteries throughout the body are included in the general term polyarteritis nodosa. These diseases are referred to as *periarteritis, hypersensitivity angiitis,* and *necrotizing angiitis.* The kidneys, gastrointestinal tract, and heart (in decreasing order of frequency) are the organ systems more commonly involved. Polyarteritis nodosa is characterized by remissions and exacerbations. As a result, all stages of the disease process may be present in the same tissue, often in the same artery. The disease is almost invariably fatal within a period of a few months to several years.

Clinically, the patient suffering from polyarteritis nodosa presents with manifestations of multisystem involvement. The urinary sediment contains red and white blood cells and a variety of casts (the so-called telescoped appearance), but proteinuria is not usually pronounced. Oliguria, renal insufficiency, and, eventually, failure are common. Hypertension is a frequent manifestation and may be "malignant" in type, with papilledema and encephalopathy.

Pathologically, when polyarteritis nodosa involves medium-sized or larger arteries, the kidneys may be coarsely nodular and irregularly scarred as a result of large areas of ischemia and infarctions which are in various stages of organization. Grossly, small aneurysms may be recognized, especially near the corticomedullary junctions. When small arteries are primarily involved, numerous small hemorrhages are present on the relatively smooth renal surfaces. Microscopically, in the acute phase, the arteries exhibit fibrinoid changes, necrosis of the media, and inflammatory cell infiltration, all of which are located primarily in the adventitia. The inflammatory exudate consists of polymorphonuclear leukocytes, includ-

ing eosinophils, and plasma cells. Occasionally, granulomatous features are present. In the chronic phase, the changes consist of fibroblastic cell proliferation, granulation, and eventually, fibrosis with intimal thickening and obliteration of the lumen. A glomerulonephritic process is almost invariably associated with vasculitis. It may be segmental and focal in distribution but, not uncommonly, may be diffuse and generalized. Necrotizing and granulomatous features are frequently seen in the glomeruli.

Overwhelming clinical and experimental evidence suggests that polyarteritis nodosa is a hypersensitivity disease. Clinically, the disease is not uncommonly associated with asthma, hay fever, and urticaria, as well as with infections — especially of the respiratory tract or of the middle ear — and with drug hypersensitivity. Among the many drugs which have been implicated are sulfonamides, sulfathiazole, penicillin, io-

dides, and diphenylhydantoin. Experimentally, the disease has been reproduced by repeated injections of heterologous proteins. Furthermore, the not infrequent association of polyarteritis nodosa with other collagen diseases suggests an immunologic mechanism in the pathogenesis.

Wegener's Granulomatosis. This disease is characterized by necrotizing granulomatous lesions in the nasal sinuses and respiratory tract associated with systemic focal necrotizing vasculitis. In the kidney, segmental and focal necrotizing glomerular lesions often are found together with a granulomatous and necrotizing arteriolitis. Wegener's granulomatosis has a rapidly progressive course and is invariably fatal. Clinically and histologically, differentiation of this disease from the hemorrhagic pulmonary-renal syndrome and from other collagen diseases may be extremely difficult. □

Toxic Nephropathy

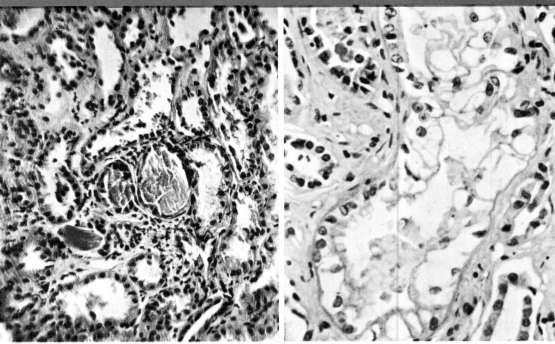

ACUTE TUBULAR NECROSIS AND DEPOSITS IN TUBULAR LUMINA IN BIOPSY TAKEN IN EARLY DIURETIC PHASE OF MERCURY POISONING

MARKED PROXIMAL TUBULAR DEGENERATION AND EXTENSIVE VACUOLIZATION IN MERCURY POISONING

©CIBA

Toxic nephropathy includes any adverse functional or structural change in the kidney because by a chemical or biologic product. The concept is also applied to well-recognized effects on the kidney of substances which normally circulate in the body, and are therefore physiologic, but which may be circulating in abnormal concentrations. This situation, for example, obtains in the nephropathies associated with hypercalcemia, hyperuricemia (secondary gout), hypokalemia, and hypomagnesemia.

The kidney is peculiarly susceptible to circulating toxins and overdoses of drugs and biologically active material. It receives a very high proportion of the blood supply relative to its weight (20 to 25 percent of the cardiac output), has the largest endothelial vascular surface of any organ of the body, and has a very high oxygen consumption and glucose production.

The reabsorption of salt and water in the tubules serves to concentrate non-reabsorbable solutes along the luminal surface of the tubular cells. Also, many toxins and chemicals unfamiliar to man's evolutionary process of filtration and reabsorption are, in fact, secreted by the kidney (e.g., uric acid, penicillin, iodinated contrast agents). Such molecules occupy an intracellular position for a time, as they are transported across the epithelium.

In the medulla of the kidney, the interstitial fluid is hyperosmotic, with a high sodium concentration, as the result of the physiologic operation of the counter-current concentration mechanism (see page 52). Thus, drugs entering the medullary interstitial fluid may be concentrated to levels far beyond those encountered in the bloodstream, lymph, or other body fluids. Few drugs have been studied for such effects except for the first metabolite of phenacetin, N-acetyl-p-aminophenol (APAP), which appears in

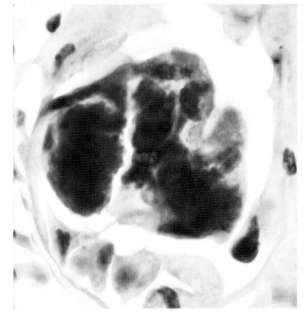

DENSE CALCIFICATION IN A NECROTIC TUBULE FROM KIDNEY OF A 61–YEAR–OLD MAN WHO DIED 10 DAYS AFTER INGESTION OF INORGANIC MERCURY

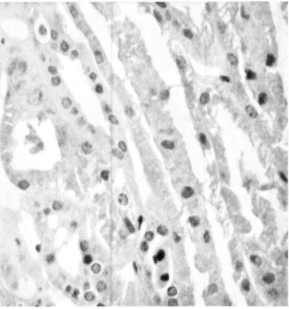

RENAL TUBULAR DEGENERATION AND NUCLEAR INCLUSION BODIES IN LEAD POISONING

higher concentrations in the medulla than in the bloodstream.

Just recently there has been clinical recognition of various ways in which toxic materials can affect the kidney. Often, the resulting diseases have gone unrecognized until their late stages or have been considered as forms of metabolic or chronic renal disease. As an example, some hospitals have recently found that as many as 75 percent of their annual admissions for gout actually have chronic plumbism, with the nephrotoxic effects of lead playing a primary pathogenetic role in the development of saturnine gout. Moreover, during the past 20 years, nephrotoxins have accounted for about 20 percent of the patients with acute renal failure who have comprised our experience at Georgetown University Hospital. Table 1, page 171, classifies the ways in which toxins can produce nephropathy.

Mercury acts as a Class 1, 2, and 4 poisoning, pro-

ducing tubular necrosis with renal insufficiency, nephrotic syndrome, and chronic renal damage. Bichloride of mercury, or mercuric chloride, is the most soluble form and most often produces tubular necrosis. Other mercuric compounds are the iodide, oxide, cyanide, and salicylate.

Mercurous compounds include the chloride, iodide, and oxide and are widely available as abortifacients, in scientific instruments, in the hat-manufacturing industry, in paints, in bronzing and marine antifouling materials, in photoengraving solutions, and in mirror-silvering material. Mercurous compounds may also contaminate foods, particularly those in the biologic food chains of marine life. Urinary excretion normally ranges from 0.1 to 1.0 $\mu g/1$ in nonexposed subjects and may go to values in excess of 300 $\mu g/1$ in patients subject to chronic industrial exposure.

The biopsy lesion shown in Plate 19 consists of

Toxic Nephropathy
Continued

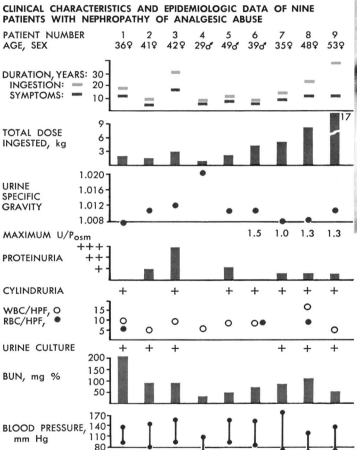

NEPHROPATHY OF ANALGESIC ABUSE

SEVERE INTERSTITIAL INFLAMMATORY REACTION WITH HYALINIZATION OF GLOMERULI AND MARKED THICKENING OF THE TUBULAR BASEMENT MEMBRANE

CLINICAL CHARACTERISTICS AND EPIDEMIOLOGIC DATA OF NINE PATIENTS WITH NEPHROPATHY OF ANALGESIC ABUSE

PATIENT NUMBER	1	2	3	4	5	6	7	8	9
AGE, SEX	36♀	41♀	42♀	29♂	49♂	39♂	35♀	48♀	53♀

DURATION, YEARS: 30
INGESTION: —
SYMPTOMS: ▬

TOTAL DOSE INGESTED, kg

URINE SPECIFIC GRAVITY 1.020 / 1.016 / 1.012 / 1.008

MAXIMUM U/P$_{osm}$ — 1.5 1.0 1.3 1.3

PROTEINURIA +++ / ++ / +

CYLINDRURIA

WBC/HPF, O — 15 / 10 / 5
RBC/HPF, ●

URINE CULTURE

BUN, mg % — 200 / 150 / 100 / 50

BLOOD PRESSURE, mm Hg — 170 / 140 / 110 / 80

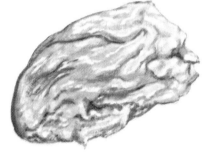

FILLING DEFECT IN LOWER URETER DUE TO OBSTRUCTION BY SLOUGHED PAPILLA

SLOUGHED PAPILLA REMOVED BY JOHNSON BASKET FROM SITE INDICATED IN ABOVE X-RAY

---

granular or vacuolar degeneration in the proximal tubule, and fragmentation and necrosis of epithelial cells. Mitotic figures and basophilic cytoplasm may be seen during the early phases of healing. Early calcification at the site of necrosis may occur and has been demonstrated in dogs within 24 hours. The degenerating renal epithelial cells contain fewer mitochondria, as observed under electron microscopy, have a lower concentration of enzymes, and are resistant to repeated doses of nephrotoxins. All segments of the tubule may be involved, and in severe cases, patchy tubular necrosis may occur. Extrarenal autopsy findings include induration of surface membranes of the pharynx, esophagus, and stomach, erosive gastritis, softening of the muscular coats of the intestine, severe colitis, congestion of the liver and spleen, degeneration of the myocardium, and focal hemorrhages at the base of the cortex of the brain.

Clinical features which may be observed are a lingering, bitter, metallic taste, followed by sensations of throat constriction and substernal burning, a feeling of suffocation, abdominal pain, nausea, vomiting, and diarrhea. Esophagitis, gastritis, overt shock, oliguria, and anuria may occur. There may also be stomatitis, erethism, tremors, hyperkinetic states, incoordination, illegible handwriting, and frank psychosis. Leukocytosis is common because of tissue necrosis. Also, an excessive rise in urea over creatinine is a prominent feature of the laboratory profile of patients with mercury poisoning. The treatment of choice is administration of dimercaprol (BAL) and hemodialysis for removal of the dimercaprol-mercury complex. Additional loading doses of dimercaprol may be used after dialysis. Both peritoneal dialysis and hemodialysis (see page 258) are useful for the maintenance of life in acute tubular

necrosis caused by mercury. Adrenocorticosteroids, such as prednisone, are useful in the treatment of the nephrotic syndrome secondary to organic mercurials and ammoniated mercury ointment.

Analgesic Agents. For the past 20 years, mixed analgesic tablets, especially those containing phenacetin, have been implicated in sectional increases in interstitial nephritis (see page 144) and in a high incidence of medullary necrosis in patients without diabetes or urinary tract obstruction (see page 194). The pathologic lesions emphasize chronic interstitial nephritis with fibrosis, cellular infiltration, and a histologic picture difficult to distinguish from that of chronic pyelonephritis (see page 191). However, there is a greater tendency toward papillary necrosis, which may be sterile in some cases, and which may range from superficial erosion to necrosis of the base of the pyramid. Calcium salts and casts may be seen in the collecting

tubule. (We have observed 11 patients who exhibited this particular disease.)

Extrarenal pathologic manifestations include yellow granular pigment in epithelial cells, particularly in the liver.

The pathogenesis of the lesions found in patients with analgesic abuse is not specifically known, although extremely large doses of the implicated drugs produce changes in the papillae of animals similar to those in humans. There may be a relationship between the lesions and the concentration of the first metabolite of phenacetin in the hypertonic interstitial fluid achieved via the countercurrent mechanism. Other metabolites of phenacetin (such as paraphenetidin) are potent formers of methemoglobin and may bear a relationship to the disease. Also, hemoglobin is in itself a nephrotoxin.

The highest incidence of this *Continued on page 170*

Continued on page 170

Toxic Nephropathy

Continued from page 169

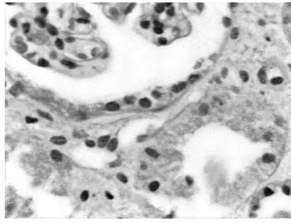

RENAL TUBULAR NECROSIS DUE TO CARBON TETRA-CHLORIDE INGESTION

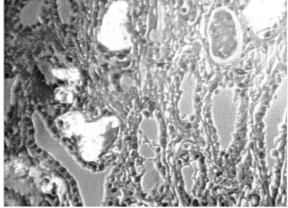

ETHYLENE GLYCOL POISONING: BIREFRINGENT CALCIUM OXYLATE CRYSTALS IN TUBULAR EPITHELIUM, VIEWED UNDER POLARIZED LIGHT

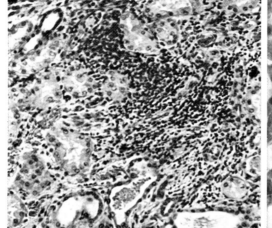

SEVERE INTERSTITIAL INFLAMMATORY REACTION AND TUBULAR NECROSIS IN ACUTE RENAL FAILURE DUE TO SULFATHIAZOLE INTOXICATION

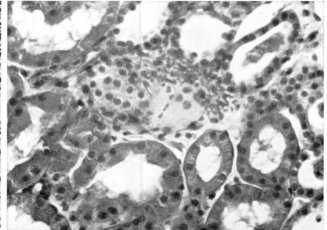

INTERSTITIAL HEMORRHAGE AND EARLY LOCAL REACTION IN AN ATHLETE WHO COMBINED 6 gm OF SULFADIAZINE WITH THE METABOLIC ACIDOSIS OF EXERCISE

disease has occurred in Scandinavia, Australia, and South Africa. Treatment consists of withdrawal of the drug, appropriate psychotherapy for patients who chronically ingest tablets (sometimes taking thousands), hydration, correction of acidosis, antibiotic therapy for the superimposed infection, and support with hemodialysis and peritoneal dialysis for those patients who have progressed to renal failure.

Plate 20 shows the clinical features and epidemiologic data of nine patients suffering from analgesic nephropathy and shows the interstitial nephritis seen on biopsy. The X-ray insert is from a patient who experienced total anuria during an airplane flight. She had been a chronic abuser of analgesics and had had a kidney removed for pyelonephritis. The filling defect in the terminal ureter was produced by a sloughed subpapilla, subsequently removed with a Johnson basket. The procedure was followed by diuresis and recovery of function in the solitary kidney.

Chronic Carbon Tetrachloride Intoxication. Inhalation or ingestion of carbon tetrachloride can cause severe damage to the kidney. In nonindustrial areas such as Washington, D.C., the wide use of the compound as a household cleaning agent, as a vermifuge, and in fire extinguishers has led to its being the most frequently encountered form of nephrotoxin. A volatile liquid, carbon tetrachloride is heavier than air and therefore difficult to ventilate.

Poisoning often occurs in low areas such as basements. Exposure to concentrations above 100 parts per million is toxic. Absorption occurs through the lungs, skin, and small intestine and is potentiated by the concomitant ingestion of alcohol or fats. Alcohol, even in relatively low doses such as may be obtained with a beer or

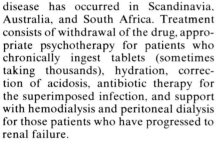

SALICYLATE INTOXICATION; RESULTS OF HEMODIALYSIS

Chart: SALICYLATE BLOOD LEVEL mg/100 ml (y-axis left) vs HOURS OF DIALYSIS (x-axis); SALICYLATE RECOVERY IN BATH, gm (y-axis right).
— COMATOSE, HYPERPNEIC
— RESPIRATION LESS FORCED
— AWAKE, ATTEMPTS AT SPEECH, DRINKING WATER
— SPEAKING RATIONALLY
— REMEMBERS EVENTS

a cocktail, markedly potentiates the nephrotoxic effect of carbon tetrachloride inhalation.

The initial symptoms of carbon tetrachloride intoxication are irritation at the site of exposure (*e.g.*, eyes or skin), burning sensation in the mouth and esophagus, headache, mental confusion, coma, and convulsions. Renal involvement is often insidious in its onset. The onset of anuria may be delayed for as long as a week, and the gastrointestinal symptoms may mislead the pursuit of the cause. Anuria persists from a day to several weeks, averaging 8 days in our series, with the longest duration being 67 days. The urinalysis is typical of acute renal failure (see page 111), with proteinuria, cylindruria, pyuria, hematuria, and renal tubular epithelial cell changes. Associated hepatic failure may be reflected by ammonia intoxication and impaired urea synthesis. Bleeding manifestations are frequent; scleral and periorbital hemorrhages are seen,

along with epistaxis and gastrointestinal hemorrhage.

Pathologically, the lesions occur primarily in the proximal tubule, although distal necrosis has been noted. The tubules are dilated, with swollen epithelium, and contain sudanophilic material. Coagulation necrosis of the proximal tubule may occur and is most prominent in the outermost zone of the cortex. There may be either pyknosis or absence of nuclei, and fragmentation of lightly eosinophilic cytoplasm. The basement membrane remains intact. Casts are noted distally and occasionally contain fat. The glomeruli usually appear normal, but protein may be present in Bowman's space. (Plate 21 illustrates, as an example, a renal biopsy from a patient with carbon tetrachloride poisoning.)

A very high rate of patient salvage is possible if life can be supported with peritoneal dialysis or hemodialysis until the lesions heal. □

TABLE I: Compounds Producing Toxic Nephropathy

Class	Description	Model
1	Nephrotoxins, direct chemical effect on the nephron	Bichloride of mercury
2	Sensitivity disease presenting as the nephrotic syndrome or nephritis	Aminonucleoside and nephroallergens
3	Sensitivity reactions presenting as angiitis or vasculitis	Sulfonamides
4	Chronic slow nephrotoxicity	Chronic lead nephropathy
5	Toxins which aggravate preexisting or coexisting kidney diseases of other etiology, or which predispose to other renal diseases such as pyelonephritis	Diuretics precipitating hypokalemia or hyperuricemic nephropathy; cathartics precipitating hypokalemia and pyelonephritis

TABLE II: Types of Nephrotoxins

Types	Examples
Heavy metals and their compounds	Mercury (organic and inorganic); bismuth; uranium; cadmium; lead; gold; arsenic and arsine; iron; silver; antimony; copper; thalium; beryllium
Organic solvents	Carbon tetrachloride; tetrachloroethylene; 2-ethoxyethanol; methanol
Glycols	Ethylene glycol; ethylene glycol dinitrate; ethylene dichloride; diethylene glycol
Physical agents	Radiation; heat stroke; electroshock therapy
Diagnostic agents	Agents used in high concentration for pyelography and aortography; sodium bunamiodyl
Therapeutic agents	Antibiotics (sulfonamides, penicillin, cephalosporin, cephaloridine, streptomycin, kanamycin, amphotericin, vancomycin, bacitracin, polymyxin, colistin, neomycin sulfate, tetracycline, amphotericin B, puromycin); analgesics (salicylates, aminosalicylic acid, phenacetin, phenylbutazone); anticoagulants (phenindione); anticonvulsants (trimethadione, paramethadione); antihypertensives (hydralazine hydrochloride); miscellaneous medications (pressor agents, diuretics, cathartics, cantharides, methoxyflurane anesthetic, penicillamine, paraquat, cyclophosphamide)
Miscellaneous chemicals	Carbon monoxide; ether; snake, spider, bee, and other venom; mushroom poison; poison ivy; "nephroallergens"; creosol; aniline and some other methemoglobin-producing chemicals; hemolysins
Pesticides	Diphenyl, chlorinated hydrocarbons; phosphorus
Abnormal concentration of physiologic substances	Calcium (hypercalcemia); uric acid (hyperuricemia); potassium (hypokalemia)

Toxemia of Pregnancy

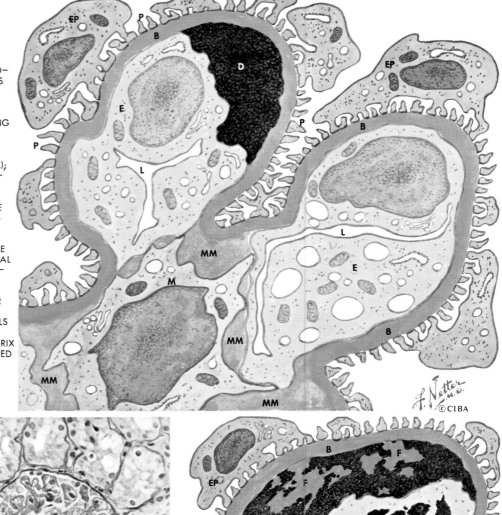

PRE–ECLAMPSIA; CHARACTERISTIC ELECTRON MICRO- SCOPIC FINDINGS IN RENAL GLOMERULAR CAPILLARIES: MARKED SWELLING OF ENDOTHELIAL CELLS (E) COM- PRESSING CAP- ILLARY LUMEN (L); BASEMENT MEM- BRANE (B) ESSENTIALLY NORMAL; DENSE PROTEINACEOUS DEPOSITS (D) BETWEEN BASE- MENT MEMBRANE AND ENDOTHELIAL CELL; FOOT PRO- CESSES (P) OF EPITHELIAL CELLS (EP) NORMAL OR FOCALLY FUSED; MESANGIAL CELLS (M) SWOLLEN, MESANGIAL MATRIX (MM) UNCHANGED

Toxemia of pregnancy, as the name implies, denotes a condition unique to pregnancy. Classically, it has been divided into an early stage, designated *pre-eclampsia*, in which there is edema, albuminuria, and hypertension, and a later stage, called *eclampsia*, in which there are also convulsions (see CIBA COLLECTION, Vol. 2, pages 235-238). However, the development of convulsive symptoms reflects the adequacy of treatment rather than the severity of the pathologic changes. Thus, the division into nonconvulsive and convulsive stages is of clinical rather than pathologic significance.

Clinicopathologic Features. The first symptom of toxemia of pregnancy is excessive weight gain, reflecting the onset of edema. In this early phase, the only pathologic alteration in the kidney is a swelling of the endothelial cells of the glomerular capillaries. As the endothelial cytoplasm swells, the endothelial pores disappear. The progressively thickening endothelial cytoplasm narrows the capillary lumina which eventually may be completely occluded or, at best, be represented by slitlike remnants. Simultaneously, there is swelling of the mesangial cell. This enlarges the mesangial stalk causing additional encroachment on the lumina. The mesangial matrix is dispersed in such a way as to give a fibrillar appearance to histologic sections stained with PAS.

As would be expected, the reduction in size of the glomerular capillary lumina causes a decrease in renal blood flow. This ischemia, which gives the toxemic glomerulus its bloodless appearance on light microscopy, may be one of the causes of hypertension frequently associated with this syndrome.

In fairly severe cases, albuminuria develops either before or after the onset of hypertension. The glomerular capillaries in patients with albuminuria show subendothelial deposits (between the basement membrane and the swollen endothelial cell) of a granular material. These deposits contain serum proteins as demonstrated by fluorescent microscopy. These proteinaceous deposits also help to reduce the size of the glomerular capillary lumina, thus further impeding blood flow. Occasionally, granular material similar to the subendothelial deposits can be found within the endothelial cells.

No matter how severe the endothelial and mesangial swelling, the glomerular basement membrane appears essentially normal in patients with toxemia uncompli-

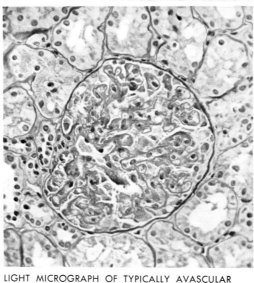

LIGHT MICROGRAPH OF TYPICALLY AVASCULAR GLOMERULUS WITH CYTOPLASMIC SWELLING AND PROMINENCE OF MESANGIUM; NO CELLULAR PROLIFERATION; URINARY SPACE DIMINISHED BUT NOT OBLITERATED; CAPILLARY WALLS, BOWMAN'S CAPSULE, AND SURROUNDING TUBULES NORMAL (PAS STAIN)

OCCASIONAL DENSE PROTEINACEOUS DEPOSITS (D) BOTH WITHIN ENDOTHELIAL CELLS AND BETWEEN ENDOTHELIUM AND BASEMENT MEMBRANE; VERY RARE FATTY DEPOSITS (F) WITHIN SUBENDOTHELIAL PROTEINACEOUS DEPOSITS

cated by other renal or systemic diseases. Also, the epithelial foot processes remain normal unless there is severe proteinuria, in which case there is focal fusion of foot processes. This preservation of the membrane and the foot processes usually makes it possible to distinguish the changes of toxemia, which are entirely reversible, from underlying and preexisting renal diseases aggravated by pregnancy, most of which are progressive and irreversible.

Differential Diagnosis. It may be difficult to distinguish essential hypertension from the hypertension associated with the early stages of pre-eclampsia. Like toxemia of pregnancy, essential hypertension does not produce membranous or epithelial changes. However, except in the 25 percent of patients in whom there is superimposed pre-eclampsia, the glomerular capillary endothelial cells are not swollen in patients who have essential hypertension.

Chronic glomerulonephritis (which may mimic pre-eclampsia), acute glomerulonephritis (which is exceedingly rare in pregnancy), and lupus nephritis all have cellular proliferation and basement membrane changes and thus may be distinguished from toxemia of pregnancy. Pyelonephritis occurring in pregnancy is usually distinguishable by clinical evidence of infection and by an examination of the urinary sediment.

The treatment of pre-eclampsia consists primarily of diet, diuretics, sedation, and rest. A low salt, low calorie diet, intermittent diuretic therapy, and bed rest, with sedation as necessary, usually control 80 to 90 percent of cases. Rarely, antihypertensive agents may be required in those patients with persistently high blood pressure. However, if conservative measures fail to control the hypertension and albuminuria, termination of pregnancy should be considered since otherwise eclampsia with convulsive seizures may supervene. □

Renal Vein Thrombosis

Renal vein thrombosis is one of the well-recognized although less frequent causes of the nephrotic syndrome (see page 123). It may occur as a primary disease or as a complication of previously existing renal disease.

In the primary form, the disease is more likely to occur in patients predisposed to venous thrombosis, following acute or chronic trauma to the lumbar region, or as a result of compression of the renal veins by tumors or adhesions.

In the secondary form, renal vein thrombosis complicates other renal diseases. Amyloidosis (see page 163) and idiopathic membranous glomerulonephritis (see page 136) are the more frequently observed underlying conditions, although lipoid nephrosis (see page 127), acute glomerulonephritis (see page 131), and various other diseases have been reported in association with renal vein thrombosis.

Renal vein thrombosis is relatively more frequent in children and usually causes cortical necrosis. Therefore, it is more likely to produce renal insufficiency rather than the nephrotic syndrome. Dehydration, secondary to a variety of causes, seems to play an important role in the pathogenesis of the infantile form.

The clinical findings more commonly associated with renal vein thrombosis are massive proteinuria (which is occasionally transient but usually persistent and accompanied by other features of the nephrotic syndrome), epigastric and costovertebral angle pain and tenderness, evidence of thromboembolism, and the urinary findings of microscopic hematuria, pyuria, hyaline and granular casts, and oval fat bodies.

Radiologic studies are most important to establish a clinical diagnosis. Intravenous urograms (see page 91) may reveal markedly enlarged kidneys as well as a scalloped or notched appearance of the pelves and ureters because of pressure by the dilated collateral periureteric veins on those structures. Properly performed phlebography of the inferior vena cava and renal veins (see page 102) can definitely establish the presence or absence of renal vein thrombosis.

Percutaneous renal biopsy (see page 107) often reveals a nonspecific pattern of histologic changes which nevertheless are strongly suggestive of renal vein thrombosis. The glomeruli are slightly enlarged and exhibit mild thickening of the capillary wall. Stasis or margination of leukocytes often is seen within the capillary lumina. Interstitial edema, often marked, results in wide separation and mild to moderate atrophy of the convoluted tubules. The interstitial and tubular changes are out of proportion to those observed in the glomeruli. In more chronic cases, interstitial fibrosis and more severe tubular atrophy develop.

At postmortem examination, the kidneys may be extremely enlarged, and their surfaces may exhibit small dilated veins.

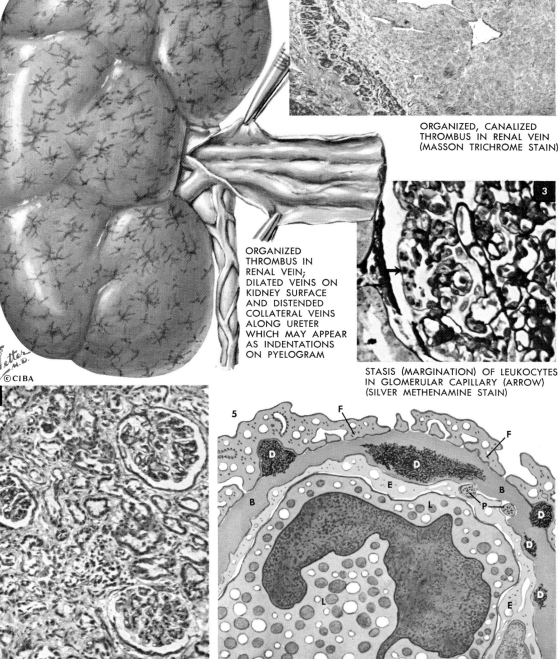

RENAL VEIN THROMBOSIS

ORGANIZED THROMBUS IN RENAL VEIN; DILATED VEINS ON KIDNEY SURFACE AND DISTENDED COLLATERAL VEINS ALONG URETER WHICH MAY APPEAR AS INDENTATIONS ON PYELOGRAM

ORGANIZED, CANALIZED THROMBUS IN RENAL VEIN (MASSON TRICHROME STAIN)

STASIS (MARGINATION) OF LEUKOCYTES IN GLOMERULAR CAPILLARY (ARROW) (SILVER METHENAMINE STAIN)

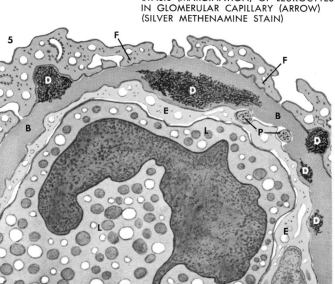

MARKED INTERSTITIAL EDEMA (MASSON TRICHROME STAIN)

ELECTRON MICROSCOPIC FINDINGS: FOOT PROCESSES (F) PARTIALLY FUSED, DEPOSITS (D) IN BASEMENT MEMBRANE (B), LEUKOCYTE (L) IN LUMEN, ENDOTHELIUM (E) SWOLLEN, PLATELET DEPOSITION (P)

Recent thrombi can easily be recognized in the renal veins and are often associated with mural thrombosis in the inferior vena cava. In chronic cases the kidneys may be smaller than normal.

The presence of organized and recanalized thrombi may not be readily recognized by the prosector, since the thrombi are represented by longitudinal fibrous thickening or cords in the walls of the veins. Large new channels in the organized thrombus, if opened longitudinally, appear to represent the original vein. Interestingly, thrombosis usually is limited to the main renal veins and their major branches and only rarely involves the small parenchymal veins. Electron microscopic studies of the glomeruli have revealed, in addition to fusion of foot processes, the presence of dense osmiophilic deposits on both sides of and, less commonly, within the basement membrane. By immunofluorescent studies, the deposits have been shown to consist of IgG, IgM, β_1C, and fibrin-fibrinogen.

The pathogenesis of renal vein thrombosis is obscure. Hemodynamic, coagulative, and immunologic factors may all play a role. The mechanism of proteinuria in this disorder is also uncertain, but increased pressure in the renal veins would seem to be of primary importance since, in other human and experimental conditions leading to severe passive congestion of the kidneys, the nephrotic syndrome has occurred. It seems likely that increased glomerular protein filtration and decreased tubular reabsorption are responsible for the severe proteinuria.

Recurrent thromboembolism is the most common and serious complication of renal vein thrombosis. Therefore, long-term treatment with anticoagulant drugs is generally recommended. However, the prognosis is poor, especially in those cases associated with renal failure and/or thromboembolic manifestations. □

Glomerular Lesions in Cyanotic Congenital Heart Disease

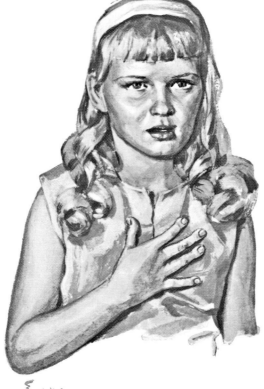

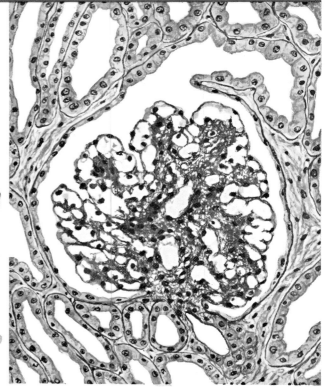

DEPOSITION OF EXCESSIVE FIBRILLAR MATERIAL IN THE MESANGIUM, PARTICULARLY IN THE AXIAL STALK; PERIPHERAL CAPILLARIES DILATED; SOME AXIAL HYPERCELLULARITY (PAS STAIN, X 350)

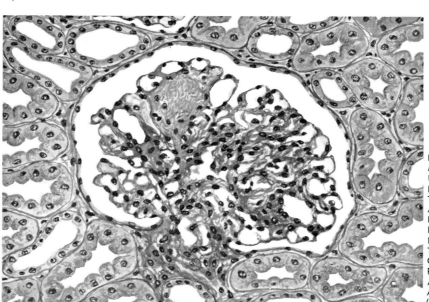

EXCESSIVE INTERCAPILLARY MATERIAL AND HYPERCELL-ULARITY PREDOMINANTLY IN THE AXIAL STALK; THE TUFTS ARE UNEQUALLY AFFECTED; THERE IS HYALINIZATION OF THE INTERCAPILLARY REGION IN THE UPPERMOST TUFT TO LEFT OF CENTER; OUTER WALLS OF PERIPHERAL CAPILLARY LOOPS APPEAR SPLIT; JUXTAGLOMERULAR APPARATUS PROMINENT (H. & E. STAIN, X 350)

In addition to the effects of thrombosis, embolism, and bacterial endocarditis, abnormalities of glomerular and renal vascular structure (with associated changes in renal function) occur in some patients with cyanotic congenital heart disease. Neither the pathogenesis nor the course of these changes is known.

Structural Abnormalities. Some patients with cyanotic congenital heart disease have no renal lesions. In others, however, there may be glomerular enlargement and capillary dilatation or engorgement with possibly an increased number of glomerular capillary loops. Within the mesangium there is hypercellularity and excessive amounts of granulofibrillar material. In addition, the glomeruli may show generalized hypercellularity. Focal glomerular sclerosis may be seen, as may thickening or duplication of glomerular capillary walls. The afferent arterioles at times are dilated and both the afferent and efferent arterioles are, on occasion, hyalinized. Prominence or scarring of the

juxtaglomerular apparatus may be present, but tubular changes are minor or incidental. Although it is generally thought that tubules are not enlarged, this concept is not certain.

As noted above, some patients with cyanotic congenital heart disease have no lesions, and the occurrence or coexistence of the various glomerular and vascular lesions is inconstant and unpredictable. Patients with primary pulmonary hypertension may have similar glomerular congestion, enlargement, or mesangial lesions. The differential diagnosis based upon histologic grounds includes subsiding acute and latent chronic glomerulonephritis (see page 132), lobular glomerulonephritis (see page 135), minimal change nephrotic syndrome (see page 123), lupus nephritis (see page 141), diabetic nephropathy (see page 149), healed focal glomerulonephritis (see page 138), focal glomerular sclerosis (see page 139), and the glomerular

lesions seen with cirrhosis of the liver (see page 176).

Functional Abnormalities. The frequency with which abnormal renal function occurs in cyanotic congenital heart disease has not been established. However, proteinuria is common. Effective renal plasma flow is decreased and the filtration fraction is increased. There may be slight hypertension, and both azotemia and hematuria also may be seen. However, even when the glomeruli are markedly abnormal, patients do not die of renal failure. Studies on glomerular filtration rate and renal blood flow have yielded inconstant data.

Pathogenesis. The cause of the renal lesions remains unclear. Various facets of the lesions have been attributed to, or correlated with, hypoxia, hypercapnia, increased postglomerular resistance, "degree of cyanosis," polycythemia, patient age, or increased pressure in the right side of the cardiac circuit. Nevertheless, the pathogenesis has not yet been determined. □

The Kidneys in Congestive Heart Failure

NORMAL

MEDULLA • CORTEX

20 TO 25% OF CARDIAC OUTPUT FLOWS THROUGH KIDNEYS: BLOOD FLOWS LARGELY THROUGH CORTICAL GLOMERULI, PARTIALLY THROUGH JUXTAMEDULLARY GLOMERULI

FILTRATION RATE MODIFIED WITHIN NORMAL RANGE BY VASCULAR RESISTANCE ACROSS GLOMERULAR CAPILLARY BED

PROTEIN CONCENTRATION AND CONSEQUENT COLLOID OSMOTIC PRESSURE IN PERITUBULAR CAPILLARIES MODIFIED WITHIN NORMAL RANGE BY FILTRATION FRACTION

H_2O Na^+

$\begin{Bmatrix} Na^+ \\ H_2O \end{Bmatrix}$

Na^+ H_2O

CAPILLARY   TUBULE CELLS
INTERCELLULAR SPACE
INTERSTITIAL SPACE

Na^+ AND H_2O ENTER TUBULE CELLS PASSIVELY; Na^+ "PUMPED" INTO INTER-CELLULAR SPACES, FOLLOWED BY H_2O, PASSING THENCE INTO INTERSTITIAL FLUID; SOME ENTERS CAPILLARIES AND SOME "LEAKS" BACK INTO CELLS TO RECYCLE

CONGESTIVE HEART FAILURE

MEDULLA • CORTEX

< 10% OF CARDIAC OUTPUT FLOWS THROUGH KIDNEYS: REDISTRIBUTION OF BLOOD FLOW FROM CORTICAL TO JUXTAMEDULLARY NEPHRONS

INCREASED VASCULAR RESISTANCE ACROSS GLOMERULAR CAPILLARY BED MAINTAINS GLOMERULAR FILTRATION RATE DESPITE REDUCED TOTAL BLOOD FLOW

INCREASED FILTRATION FRACTION RAISES PROTEIN CONCENTRATION AND THEREFORE COLLOID OSMOTIC PRESSURE IN PERI-TUBULAR CAPILLARIES THUS FACILITATING REABSORPTION IN PROXIMAL TUBULES

H_2O Na^+

$\begin{Bmatrix} Na^+ \\ H_2O \end{Bmatrix}$

Na^+ H_2O

CAPILLARY   TUBULE CELLS
INTERCELLULAR SPACE
INTERSTITIAL SPACE

INCREASED COLLOID OSMOTIC PRESSURE IN PERITUBULAR CAPILLARIES PLUS INCREASED INTERSTITIAL HYDROSTATIC PRESSURE SECONDARY TO AUGMENTED SODIUM TRANSPORT INTO THIS SPACE FAVOR REABSORPTION IN CONTRAST TO REENTRY INTO TUBULE CELLS

Normally, 20 to 25 percent of the cardiac output circulates through the kidneys. This high perfusion rate reflects the primary function of the kidneys to reconstitute continuously the extracellular fluid and is not dictated by the metabolic activity of renal tissue. It is maintained by the so-called autoregulatory mechanism of the kidneys despite wide variations in systemic blood pressure. However, in situations in which the oxygen supply to other tissues becomes inadequate (as during exercise, or in patients with congestive heart failure), the blood flow to tissues with low oxygen extraction (skin, kidneys, splanchnic area) is restricted in favor of tissues with high oxygen extraction (brain, heart, skeletal muscle). In these situations renal blood flow may decline to 10 percent or less of the total cardiac output.

Such a reduction in total renal perfusion is accompanied by intrarenal redistribution of the remaining blood flow so that relatively less blood reaches the cortical areas of the kidneys. Normally, the cortical nephrons with short loops of Henle receive most of the renal blood flow, but in congestive heart failure, a higher proportion of juxtamedullary nephrons with long loops of Henle is perfused. Since the sodium reabsorptive capacity of juxtamedullary nephrons is more effective than that of cortical nephrons, the redis-

tribution of blood flow contributes to the regulation of overall sodium balance (see page 56).

The reduction of the total renal blood flow is accompanied by increased vascular resistance across the glomerular capillary bed. This increased glomerular capillary resistance tends to maintain glomerular filtration rate. However, the resulting higher filtration fraction elevates the protein concentration, and therefore the colloid osmotic pressure, in blood reaching the postglomerular capillaries. The higher colloid osmotic pressure favors the reabsorption of proximal tubular fluid independently of active transport mechanisms. In addition, there is increased active sodium reabsorption by proximal tubular cells.

Current concepts of renal physiology maintain that augmented active sodium transport in the contraluminal area of the proximal tubular cells leads to accumulation of sodium in the peritubular interstitial fluid. This

increased interstitial sodium concentration in turn promotes the transfer of water from the cell into the intercellular space (see page 48). The increased fluid transfer raises the hydrostatic pressure in both the intercellular and interstitial spaces and favors the entry of fluid into the peritubular capillaries. Thus, both the increased intravascular colloid osmotic pressure and the increased interstitial fluid pressure facilitate the reabsorption of proximal tubular fluid.

As a consequence of increased proximal reabsorption, less fluid reaches the more distal portions of the nephron where, under normal conditions, absorption and secretion further alter tubular fluid composition before the formation of the final urine. Limited delivery of fluid to the distal segments of the nephron imposes limitations in the secretion rate of some body fluid constituents such as potassium; it also reduces the volume and raises the concentration of the final urine. □

Renal Failure in Liver Disease

Certain clinical circumstances, such as carbon tetrachloride poisoning (see page 168), Weil's disease, yellow fever, toxemia of pregnancy, and circulatory collapse, result in simultaneous injury to both the liver and the kidney (see CIBA COLLECTION, Vol. 3/III, page 76). In addition, patients suffering from liver disease may develop renal failure of unknown cause during the course of their illness.

These clinical situations, as well as the less well defined observation that renal failure may follow surgery of the biliary tract, have been included in the broad term *hepatorenal syndrome*. However, since this term implies undocumented common pathogenesis, we prefer to consider each of the above circumstances separately and refer to the condition which occurs in patients with cirrhosis as *renal failure of cirrhosis*.

Although progressive and severe oliguria is the hallmark of the syndrome, we have observed several patients who did not suffer from oliguria. Renal failure may develop very rapidly—in months, weeks, or days—without any apparent precipitating event. It may also occur following abdominal paracentesis, surgery, or gastrointestinal hemorrhage, whether gross or minimal (guaiac-positive stool). Ascites, edema, and jaundice are usually present, but they are variable in degree. Renal failure may develop when jaundice is actually decreasing. There is a modest but definite reduction in blood pressure, and tachycardia. More than 50 percent of patients develop hepatic coma, which is a common cause of death.

There are striking decreases in the glomerular filtration rate and renal plasma flow, with renal afferent vasoconstriction and preferential cortical hypoperfusion. Sodium and water retention, secondary to enhanced tubular reabsorption, are marked.

The inability to excrete a water load is most characteristic and may in part be responsible for the commonly observed hyponatremia. The blood urea nitrogen (BUN) and creatinine elevation are of variable magnitude. However, they do not generally reach the levels observed in the terminal stages of primary renal disease.

Urine generally is acid and frequently contains small amounts of protein, red

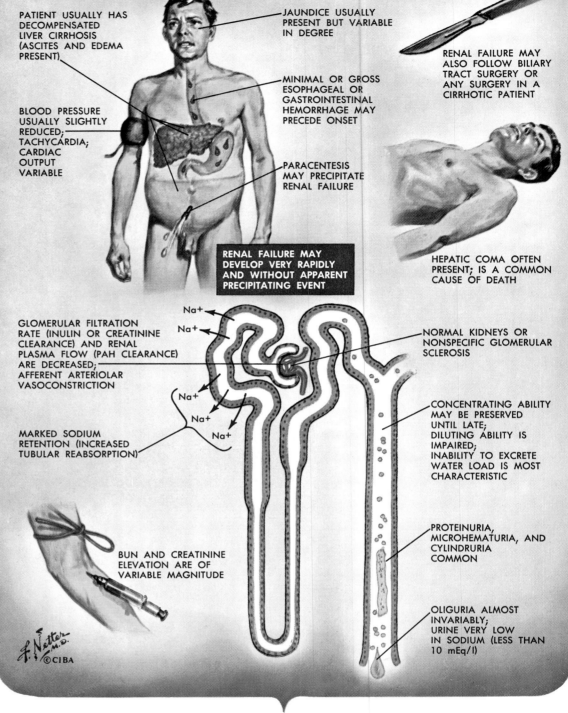

RENAL FAILURE IN LIVER DISEASE

PATIENT USUALLY HAS DECOMPENSATED LIVER CIRRHOSIS (ASCITES AND EDEMA PRESENT)

JAUNDICE USUALLY PRESENT BUT VARIABLE IN DEGREE

RENAL FAILURE MAY ALSO FOLLOW BILIARY TRACT SURGERY OR ANY SURGERY IN A CIRRHOTIC PATIENT

BLOOD PRESSURE USUALLY SLIGHTLY REDUCED; TACHYCARDIA; CARDIAC OUTPUT VARIABLE

MINIMAL OR GROSS ESOPHAGEAL OR GASTROINTESTINAL HEMORRHAGE MAY PRECEDE ONSET

PARACENTESIS MAY PRECIPITATE RENAL FAILURE

RENAL FAILURE MAY DEVELOP VERY RAPIDLY AND WITHOUT APPARENT PRECIPITATING EVENT

HEPATIC COMA OFTEN PRESENT; IS A COMMON CAUSE OF DEATH

GLOMERULAR FILTRATION RATE (INULIN OR CREATININE CLEARANCE) AND RENAL PLASMA FLOW (PAH CLEARANCE) ARE DECREASED; AFFERENT ARTERIOLAR VASOCONSTRICTION

NORMAL KIDNEYS OR NONSPECIFIC GLOMERULAR SCLEROSIS

CONCENTRATING ABILITY MAY BE PRESERVED UNTIL LATE; DILUTING ABILITY IS IMPAIRED; INABILITY TO EXCRETE WATER LOAD IS MOST CHARACTERISTIC

MARKED SODIUM RETENTION (INCREASED TUBULAR REABSORPTION)

BUN AND CREATININE ELEVATION ARE OF VARIABLE MAGNITUDE

PROTEINURIA, MICROHEMATURIA, AND CYLINDRURIA COMMON

OLIGURIA ALMOST INVARIABLY; URINE VERY LOW IN SODIUM (LESS THAN 10 mEq/l)

PROGNOSIS VERY GRAVE
DEATH MAY BE DUE TO FACTORS OTHER THAN OR IN ADDITION TO RENAL FAILURE PER SE

blood cells, and hyaline and granular casts. In many instances, urine is scanty and quite concentrated early in the course of renal failure, remaining so until death. However, most patients show a gradual decrease in urinary concentration. Urine sodium concentration is characteristically very low, generally less than 10 mEq/l.

At autopsy, the kidneys either are entirely normal or show nonspecific "bile nephrosis," glomerulosclerosis, or lesions of doubtful functional significance. When these kidneys are transplanted into patients exhibiting terminal renal disease, they function promptly.

The development of renal failure in the course of cirrhosis is of grave prognostic significance. Only one in almost 100 of our patients has had a spontaneous recovery. Few recoveries have been reported by others. Patients die *in* renal failure rather than *of* renal failure. It seems that renal failure may be the reflection of

or a part of a broader, more fundamental disturbance. Moreover, renal failure in itself is not the most important determinant of how long the patient will survive.

The pathogenesis of renal failure in patients with cirrhosis is not known. However, available evidence supports the concept of a circulatory mechanism with impairment of effective renal perfusion secondary to renal vasoconstriction. Although it is certainly possible that a reduction in effective plasma volume is a hemodynamically significant factor in some patients, the effects of volume expansion are only transient and do not appear to alter the unfavorable courses of these patients. Thus, other mechanisms such as abnormalities in intrarenal circulation deserve consideration.

In our experience, all forms of treatment have been unsuccessful in altering the outcome of this syndrome. Even repeated attempts to expand plasma volume and dialysis have been unsuccessful. □

Lung Purpura with Nephritis (Goodpasture's Syndrome)

During the 1918 pandemic of influenza, Goodpasture observed a patient with striking hemoptysis which occurred 2 months after a classic influenzal attack. Clinically, there was no renal involvement, but at autopsy the kidneys showed "a few small hemorrhages in the cortex and moderate edema." There was a glomerular nephropathy "with a fibrinous exudate in Bowman's capsule, and cellular proliferation of glomerular tufts." The pulmonary condition and indeed the whole illness was regarded as inflammatory.

Nomenclature

Parkin and his associates described seven similar patients, four of whom had polyarteritis nodosa but in whom the pulmonary lesion was still considered inflammatory. Stanton and Tange reported on nine patients and suggested the use of the name *Goodpasture's syndrome* since the etiology of the condition was obscure.

Although the term has since become widely accepted, it is uninformative and may even be a misnomer in view of the scanty evidence available on what really ailed Goodpasture's patient. The term *lung purpura with nephritis* proposed by Rusby and Wilson is preferable to the picturesque eponym.

Another problem in terminology arises from the use of the term *idiopathic pulmonary hemosiderosis* (IPH) to denote massive hemoptysis with associated radiopaque hemosiderin deposits in the lung. Although often associated with glomerulonephritis, this syndrome can occur without renal involvement. It would seem reasonable to reserve the term IPH for such uncomplicated illnesses, and limit the term Goodpasture's syndrome or, preferably, lung purpura with nephritis to those patients who have both pulmonary and renal involvement, though these are not necessarily concurrent.

Hamburger and associates stress that "the autonomy of Goodpasture's syndrome lies principally in the absence of any vascular lesions." In view of the difficulty of rigorously proving negative evidence, many would prefer to regard the syndrome as a variant of necrotizing angiitis or the polyarteritic group of diseases; there is no doubt that patients exhibiting the typical histology of polyarteritis nodosa (see page 167) also show all the clinical features of the syndrome.

General Clinical Features

The most characteristic manifestation is profound *hemoptysis*, leading to severe anemia and to virtually total disappearance of iron available for transport, the serum iron being very low indeed. Cough may persist even when there is no active bleeding, in which case the sputum is commonly purulent. Breathlessness is usual, mainly because of pulmonary involvement, but no doubt it is aggravated by the presence of anemia.

The chest film generally shows both

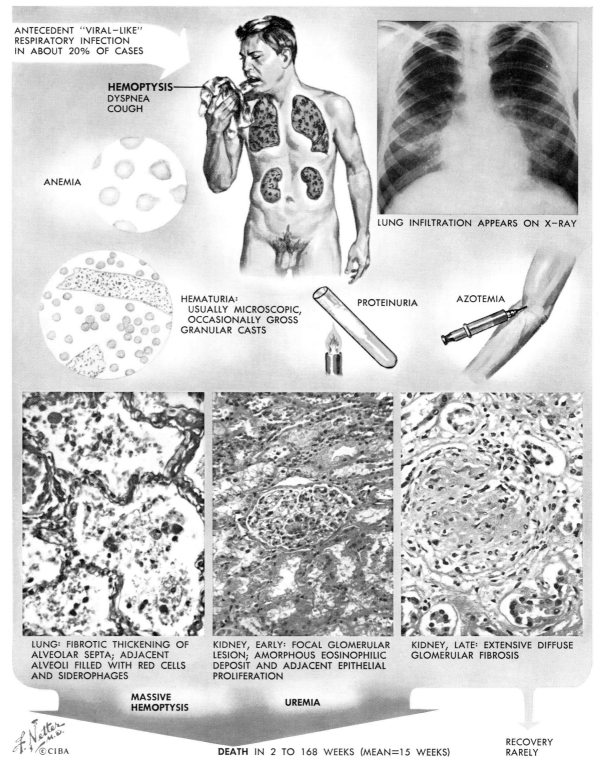

LUNG PURPURA WITH NEPHRITIS (GOODPASTURE'S SYNDROME)

ANTECEDENT "VIRAL–LIKE" RESPIRATORY INFECTION IN ABOUT 20% OF CASES

HEMOPTYSIS
DYSPNEA
COUGH

ANEMIA

LUNG INFILTRATION APPEARS ON X–RAY

HEMATURIA: USUALLY MICROSCOPIC, OCCASIONALLY GROSS GRANULAR CASTS

PROTEINURIA

AZOTEMIA

LUNG: FIBROTIC THICKENING OF ALVEOLAR SEPTA; ADJACENT ALVEOLI FILLED WITH RED CELLS AND SIDEROPHAGES

KIDNEY, EARLY: FOCAL GLOMERULAR LESION; AMORPHOUS EOSINOPHILIC DEPOSIT AND ADJACENT EPITHELIAL PROLIFERATION

KIDNEY, LATE: EXTENSIVE DIFFUSE GLOMERULAR FIBROSIS

MASSIVE HEMOPTYSIS

UREMIA

DEATH IN 2 TO 168 WEEKS (MEAN=15 WEEKS)

RECOVERY RARELY

cardiomegaly and very striking *pulmonary opacities*, either patchy or confluent. Most patients die within a year either from massive hemoptysis or from renal failure. At autopsy, the lungs show a *hemorrhagic alveolitis*, with many macrophages laden with iron pigment. Prednisone, azathioprine, and other immunosuppressive agents have been used in treatment. However, lasting remissions are very unusual, although some patients have survived for several years.

Renal Involvement

In some patients, the pulmonary symptoms may precede any evidence of renal involvement by weeks or even longer, but in others, both lungs and kidneys are already involved when the patient is first seen. Frank hematuria is common, and *microscopic hematuria* and *albuminuria* are general and persistent once the kidneys become involved. Patchy involvement of glomeruli can

produce both necrotic and proliferative lesions. Initially focal, these may progress to a diffuse glomerular involvement.

Parenthetically, hypertension is generally absent; this is a point of resemblance to the "microscopic" or small-vessel type of polyarteritis nodosa and, likewise, to Wegener's granulomatosis (see page 167).

Regarding the question of pathogenesis of this disease, the renal lesions appear similar to those seen in other forms of angiitis, and it may not be entirely irrelevant to quote a sentence from Goodpasture's own autopsy findings: "Sections through the hemorrhagic points in the intestine show focal lesions in the wall of arterioles, with fibrinous exudate and a few polymorphonuclears." □

Photomicrographs courtesy of Dr. G. Williams, Department of Pathology, University of Manchester, England, and Dr. G. Berlyne, Central Negev Hospital, Israel.

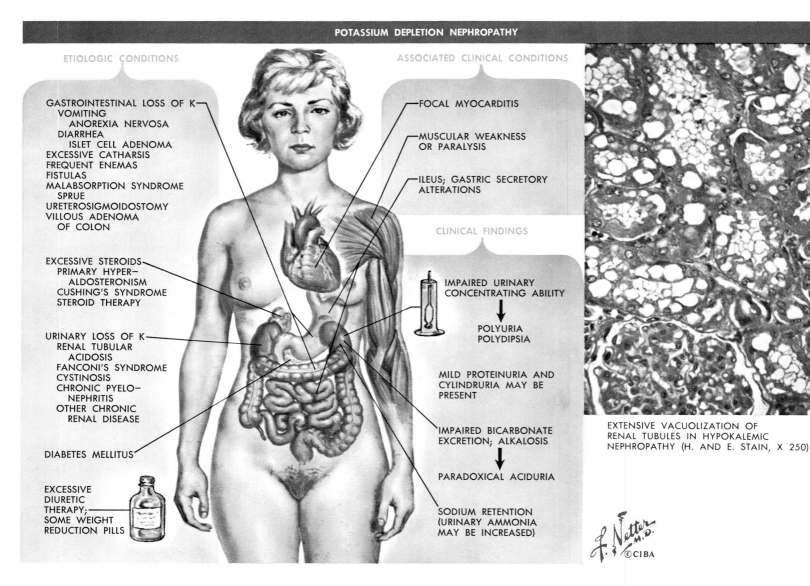

ETIOLOGIC CONDITIONS

GASTROINTESTINAL LOSS OF K
VOMITING
ANOREXIA NERVOSA
DIARRHEA
ISLET CELL ADENOMA
EXCESSIVE CATHARSIS
FREQUENT ENEMAS
FISTULAS
MALABSORPTION SYNDROME
SPRUE
URETEROSIGMOIDOSTOMY
VILLOUS ADENOMA
OF COLON

EXCESSIVE STEROIDS
PRIMARY HYPER–
ALDOSTERONISM
CUSHING'S SYNDROME
STEROID THERAPY

URINARY LOSS OF K
RENAL TUBULAR
ACIDOSIS
FANCONI'S SYNDROME
CYSTINOSIS
CHRONIC PYELO-
NEPHRITIS
OTHER CHRONIC
RENAL DISEASE

DIABETES MELLITUS

EXCESSIVE
DIURETIC
THERAPY;
SOME WEIGHT
REDUCTION PILLS

ASSOCIATED CLINICAL CONDITIONS

FOCAL MYOCARDITIS

MUSCULAR WEAKNESS
OR PARALYSIS

ILEUS; GASTRIC SECRETORY
ALTERATIONS

CLINICAL FINDINGS

IMPAIRED URINARY
CONCENTRATING ABILITY

POLYURIA
POLYDIPSIA

MILD PROTEINURIA AND
CYLINDRURIA MAY BE
PRESENT

IMPAIRED BICARBONATE
EXCRETION; ALKALOSIS

PARADOXICAL ACIDURIA

SODIUM RETENTION
(URINARY AMMONIA
MAY BE INCREASED)

EXTENSIVE VACUOLIZATION OF
RENAL TUBULES IN HYPOKALEMIC
NEPHROPATHY (H. AND E. STAIN, X 250)

Hypokalemic Nephropathy

Conditions associated with the nephropathy of potassium depletion may be divided into four groups:

1. Excessive loss through the gastrointestinal tract from vomiting, diarrhea, excessive catharsis, frequent enemas, fistulas, malabsorption syndrome, ureterosigmoidostomy, villous adenoma of the colon, islet cell adenoma with diarrhea, and anorexia nervosa (see CIBA COLLECTION, Vol. 3/I, 3/II, and 3/III).

2. Excessive loss in the urine including renal tubular acidosis (see page 248), Fanconi's syndrome, cystinosis (see page 247), chronic pyelonephritis (see page 191), and other chronic renal diseases.

3. Excessive steroid levels, especially of aldo-

sterone and hydrocortisone (primary hyperaldosteronism, Cushing's disease, and steroid therapy; see CIBA COLLECTION, Vol. 4).

4. Miscellaneous conditions (use of chlorothiazide, hydrochlorothiazide, and certain weight-reducing medications, and diabetes mellitus).

In addition to nephropathy, potassium deficit may cause muscle weakness or even paralysis, focal myocarditis, ileus, and gastric secretory alterations.

Clinical Findings. It is likely that potassium depletion must exist for a month or so before signs and symptoms occur. Initially, there is an impairment of urine-concentrating ability, not correctable with antidiuretic hormone (ADH). If depletion is severe, diluting ability may also be compromised. Polydipsia, polyuria, and nocturia are noted clinically. Impaired excretion of bicarbonate, producing alkalosis and so-called paradoxical aciduria, may follow. Urinary ammonia may be increased. Retention of sodium to a degree greater than expected from the amount of potassium lost may be seen, apparently caused by replacement of intracellular potassium with sodium and by increased extracellular fluid. Glomerular filtration rate (GFR) may be decreased in some patients, especially if there is dehydration.

Proteinuria, at times slight and intermittent, and cylindruria are observed in many patients. Chronic renal disease may thus be suspected. Occasionally, red cells and leukocytes may be present in the urine.

Histology. The characteristic histologic finding is extreme vacuolization of renal tubular epithelium, more marked in the proximal convoluted tubules than in the distal. The typical vacuole is

clear and does not contain significant fat or glycogen. With electron microscopy, the vacuoles appear to represent widening of the spaces between the infoldings of the basilar cellular membranes. One study reported almost complete separation of adjacent proximal tubule cells with only the integrity of the juxtaluminal tight junctions maintained. Although vacuoles may result from increased extracellular fluid, in at least one patient with severe potassium depletion, large vacuoles appeared to be completely intracellular with no demonstrable connection to basilar infoldings. Thickening of the basement membrane of the tubular epithelium in both cortex and medulla, as well as diffuse mitochondrial swelling, have also been described.

In long-standing cases, either active pyelonephritis or interstitial fibrosis and chronic inflammatory changes may be found. These patients may excrete potassium even in the face of severe depletion. However, it is unsettled as to whether potassium depletion predisposes to chronic pyelonephritis, and it has yet to be shown that renal insufficiency may result from potassium depletion alone.

If the underlying condition is corrected and no complications such as pyelonephritis exist, return to normal function can usually be expected within 6 weeks to 4 months after potassium repletion. Whether or not structural renal changes occur will depend on the duration of the potassium depletion. □

Editor's Note: The effects of renal failure on sodium-potassium metabolism are described on page 116.

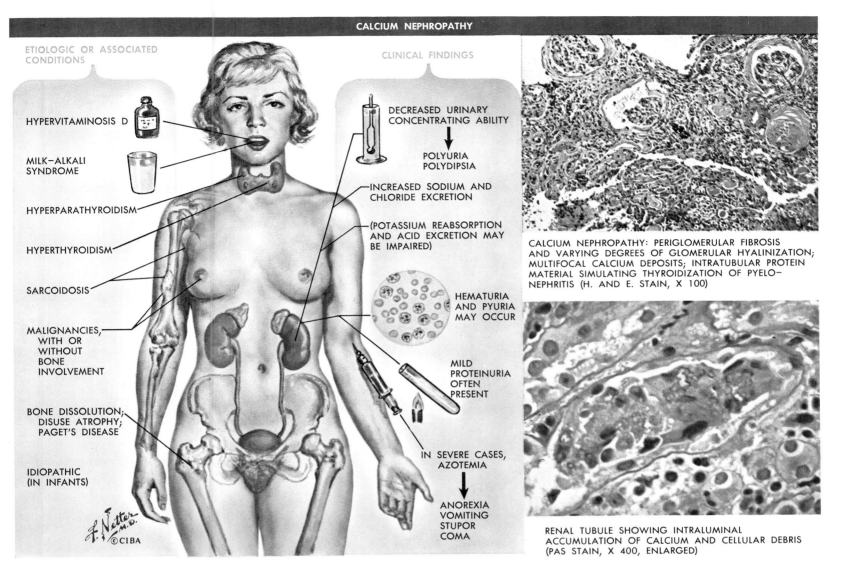

ETIOLOGIC OR ASSOCIATED CONDITIONS

HYPERVITAMINOSIS D

MILK–ALKALI SYNDROME

HYPERPARATHYROIDISM

HYPERTHYROIDISM

SARCOIDOSIS

MALIGNANCIES, WITH OR WITHOUT BONE INVOLVEMENT

BONE DISSOLUTION; DISUSE ATROPHY; PAGET'S DISEASE

IDIOPATHIC (IN INFANTS)

CLINICAL FINDINGS

DECREASED URINARY CONCENTRATING ABILITY → POLYURIA POLYDIPSIA

INCREASED SODIUM AND CHLORIDE EXCRETION

(POTASSIUM REABSORPTION AND ACID EXCRETION MAY BE IMPAIRED)

HEMATURIA AND PYURIA MAY OCCUR

MILD PROTEINURIA OFTEN PRESENT

IN SEVERE CASES, AZOTEMIA → ANOREXIA VOMITING STUPOR COMA

CALCIUM NEPHROPATHY: PERIGLOMERULAR FIBROSIS AND VARYING DEGREES OF GLOMERULAR HYALINIZATION; MULTIFOCAL CALCIUM DEPOSITS; INTRATUBULAR PROTEIN MATERIAL SIMULATING THYROIDIZATION OF PYELO-NEPHRITIS (H. AND E. STAIN, X 100)

RENAL TUBULE SHOWING INTRALUMINAL ACCUMULATION OF CALCIUM AND CELLULAR DEBRIS (PAS STAIN, X 400, ENLARGED)

Calcium Nephropathy

Conditions associated with calcium nephropathy include hyperparathyroidism, sarcoidosis, hypervitaminosis D, milk-alkali syndrome, idiopathic hypercalcemia, hyperthyroidism, malignancies (with and without bony involvement), and conditions such as disuse atrophy and Paget's disease which favor dissolution of bone (see also other CIBA COLLECTION volumes, particularly Vol. 4, pages 179-181, 193, and 194). Regardless of the underlying condition, the resulting abnormalities of renal function and structure are determined largely by the degree and duration of the calcium insult.

Clinical Findings. Initially, there is decreased urine-concentrating ability (resulting in polyuria and polydipsia) which may appear within a few days and without a decrease in glomerular filtration rate (GFR). Reabsorption of solute-free water during osmotic loading is also impaired, and sodium and chloride excretion is increased. These changes appear to be reversible.

Severe acute hypercalcemia may cause rapid development of renal failure and azotemia (the so-called acute hypercalcemia crisis) with anorexia and vomiting, lethargy, stupor, and finally, coma. Distal tubules may be sufficiently damaged to impair the excretion of acid. Hypercalcemia of longer duration may impair the ability to conserve potassium. Chronic or recurrent hypercalcemia can lead to progressive renal failure, often complicated by chronic pyelonephritis, hypertension, and/or nephrolithiasis. Hematuria and pyuria may occur, and mild proteinuria is not uncommon.

If the cause of the hypercalcemia is corrected, there may be a return to normal function, even with residual nephrocalcinosis. However, progressive deterioration may occur in some cases. The eventual outcome is apparently influenced by the amount of calcification and scarring, as well as by the presence of pyelonephritis and/or nephrosclerosis.

Histology. In human biopsy material, multifocal calcification of interstitial tissue, distal convoluted tubules, and collecting ducts may be seen. Calcium may be found in the lumina, in epithelial cells, and in the basement membranes. Glomeruli frequently show partial to complete hyalinization. Variable but usually moderate to marked intertubular and periglomerular fibroses are common. Chronic inflammatory changes are also common but seem to be more marked in hyperparathyroidism and sarcoidosis.

The pathogenesis of this condition has not been demonstrated in humans. Although animal experimental data will be described, it must be

emphasized that comparable human data are not available.

Dogs treated with parathyroid extract develop epithelial degeneration in the distal nephron within 24 hours, followed by necrosis, calcification, and sloughing of cells into the lumen. Here the cells form a nidus for the creation of calcific casts. The resulting obstruction is associated with dilatation of the proximal tubules. These changes tend to be focal, at least in the early stages, and therefore probably do not cause the early renal impairment which frequently occurs.

In rats given vitamin D, there is an apparently increased pinocytotic uptake of calcium by the proximal convoluted tubules within 24 hours, followed by mitochondrial alterations and the accumulation of dense cytoplasmic bodies. Calcium deposits then appear in the cystoplasmic vacuoles, mitochondria, and basement membranes. Simultaneously, there is reduced oxidative phosphorylation in isolated mitochondria. Similar alterations may be produced in rats within 1 hour after the intraperitoneal administration of calcium gluconate. If these changes were to occur in humans, they could explain the early clinical findings.

Persistent hypercalcemia in dogs leads to continued distal tubular obstruction associated with proliferation of epithelial cells. In contrast, proximal tubular epithelium atrophies. Eventually, calcification involves interstitial tissue and is accompanied by fibrosis and the cellular elements of chronic inflammation. □

Editor's Note: The effects of renal failure on calcium-phosphorus metabolism are described on pages 117-119.

Myeloma

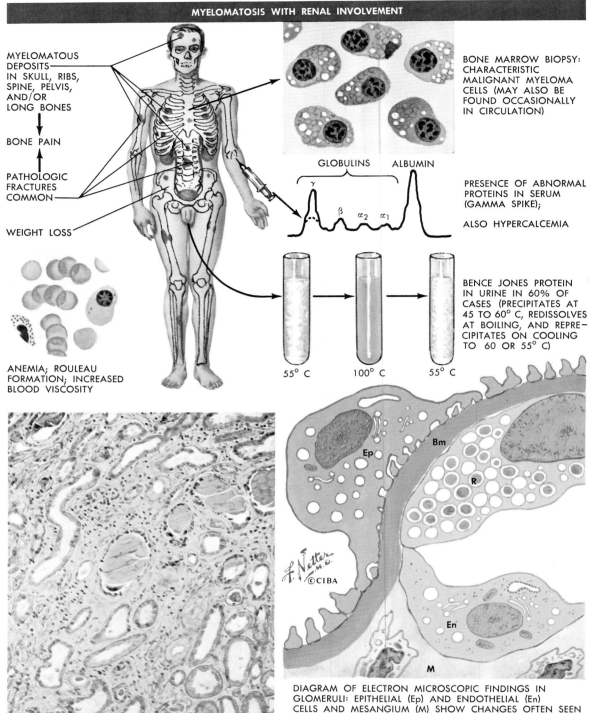

MYELOMATOUS DEPOSITS IN SKULL, RIBS, SPINE, PELVIS, AND/OR LONG BONES

→ BONE PAIN

PATHOLOGIC FRACTURES COMMON

WEIGHT LOSS

ANEMIA; ROULEAU FORMATION; INCREASED BLOOD VISCOSITY

BONE MARROW BIOPSY: CHARACTERISTIC MALIGNANT MYELOMA CELLS (MAY ALSO BE FOUND OCCASIONALLY IN CIRCULATION)

GLOBULINS — ALBUMIN

PRESENCE OF ABNORMAL PROTEINS IN SERUM (GAMMA SPIKE);

ALSO HYPERCALCEMIA

BENCE JONES PROTEIN IN URINE IN 60% OF CASES (PRECIPITATES AT 45 TO 60° C, REDISSOLVES AT BOILING, AND REPRECIPITATES ON COOLING TO 60 OR 55° C)

55° C   100° C   55° C

MYELOMA KIDNEY: MANY DILATED TUBULES CONTAINING EOSINOPHILIC AMORPHOUS CASTS; ATROPHY OF EPITHELIUM; GIANT CELL FORMATION

DIAGRAM OF ELECTRON MICROSCOPIC FINDINGS IN GLOMERULI: EPITHELIAL (Ep) AND ENDOTHELIAL (En) CELLS AND MESANGIUM (M) SHOW CHANGES OFTEN SEEN IN OTHER PROTEINURIC CONDITIONS; FOCAL LOSS OR FUSION OF FOOT PROCESSES; BASEMENT MEMBRANE (Bm) THICKENED BUT FREE OF DEPOSITS; OCCASIONAL CELL ON LUMINAL SIDE SUGGESTIVE OF PLASMA CELL TRANSFORMATION WITH RUSSELL BODIES (R)

Multiple myeloma is now recognized as one type of a clinical spectrum of disorders referred to as paraproteinemias, in which neoplastic plasma cells not only infiltrate bone, lymph nodes, various soft tissues, and rarely, blood, but also elaborate abnormal serum proteins. These proteins may produce a gamma spike on the serum electrophoresis as shown.

Although there have been attempts to relate the ultrastructural appearance of marrow plasma cells to specific serologic types of myeloma, these have been unsuccessful. Furthermore, no correlation between cell types and clinical stages of the disorder (*i.e.,* asymptomatic, incipient, or advanced) has been observed. However, one correlation has been noted: In patients who have plasma cells which contain Russell bodies, Bence Jones proteinuria is absent, and in patients in whom this abnormal urinary protein (light chain) is found, plasma cells which contain Russell bodies are absent. This suggests that Russell bodies may represent an accumulation of light chains which are not being utilized in the biosynthesis of complete globulin molecules.

Approximately 15 percent of individuals with multiple myeloma also exhibit amyloidosis (see page 163), which manifests the tinctorial reactions and a predilection for mesenchymal tissues, both commonly regarded as characteristic of so-called primary amyloidosis.

In addition to the complication of amyloidosis and the sequelae (profound anemia and general debilitation secondary to the neoplastic state) which are experienced by patients with myeloma, renal failure may contribute to death. The structural basis for failure of the kidneys is not entirely clear. Such kidneys frequently reveal a tubular lesion consisting of giant cell transformation of epithelium in association with dense hyaline casts within the tubules; the giant cells frequently penetrate into the interstitium. This transformation has been regarded as a reaction to abnormal urinary proteins, but it is not consistently related to Bence Jones proteinuria. Nevertheless, the presence of giant cell transformation has been considered pathognomonic of multiple myeloma, signifying the so-called myeloma kidney.

Less attention has been directed to the presence of a glomerular defect in kidneys from patients with multiple myeloma. The relatively nonspecific thickening of glomerular capillaries has been observed by light microscopy, and investigations of renal function have disclosed impaired glomerular filtration rate (GFR) and tubular excretory capacity. However, the absence of a consistent fall in GFR tends to minimize its primacy in accounting for the functional renal abnormalities.

Electron microscopic study of glomeruli from the kidneys of patients with multiple myeloma but without overt renal failure has disclosed enlargement and vacuolization of glomerular epithelial cells plus a variable loss of foot processes. Increases in endothelial and mesangial cells are less notable. The lamina densa has been observed at approximately twice its normal thickness but otherwise is unaltered. These glomerular changes are not related to any immunologic type of plasma cell myeloma or the presence or absence of Bence Jones proteinuria. On the other hand, the severity of changes could be correlated with the degree of hyperproteinuria.

The described changes are comparable to those found in man in other proteinuric states of diverse etiology. This information, as well as experimental considerations, is consonant with the view which indicates such ultrastructural abnormalities are the result rather than the cause of proteinuria. This concept applies not only to patients with multiple myeloma but also to patients with other disorders manifested by proteinuria.

Although the glomerular changes do not appear diagnostically specific for multiple myeloma, the occurrence of cells, which resemble plasma cell elements with Russell bodies, probably arising from glomerular endothelium has been noted in several patients. Such an observation represents a unique renal finding. □

Epidemic Hemorrhagic Fever

Epidemic hemorrhagic fever is an acute infectious disease, but the etiologic agent, although filterable, has not yet been identified. Since 1935, the disease has been reported in rural areas of the Amur River basin in Siberia and Manchuria, and in 1951 it appeared in Korea. Subsequently, it has spread westward through the USSR.

The disease is transmitted to man by trombiculid mites that infest the ground vole, a rodent that lives only north of the 38th parallel. The incubation period is usually 14 days but may vary between 9 days and 5 weeks.

The illness varies in severity. The current overall mortality, in patients who receive adequate supportive therapy, is between five and seven percent. In the absence of therapy, mortality may be as high as 20 percent. The majority of deaths occur during the first 10 days, with *shock* as the most common cause. In patients who die later in the course of the disease, acute renal failure, pulmonary edema, and secondary infections contribute to mortality. The basic pathologic changes include capillary dysfunction, necrosis resulting from ischemia, and a mononuclear cellular response. In addition, profound retroperitoneal accumulation of fluid, which has the same protein content as serum, is characteristically found at autopsy in patients who die of shock during the early phases of the disease. This feature is not seen in patients who die in the later two stages (see below). In all patients who die, the kidneys exhibit an extreme degree of congestion localized to the medulla. Necrosis of renal tubules, and sometimes of the renal pyramids, may be present. The right atrium, the anterior pituitary, and the suprarenal medulla also appear hemorrhagic. This hemorrhagic appearance reflects extreme capillary congestion as judged by histologic examination. Congestion of the spleen and gastrointestinal tract also occurs, and petechiae and ecchymoses are common. However, serious hemorrhage from the viscera is rare.

As noted, the disease varies in severity. Many patients exhibit only the signs and symptoms of a moderate febrile illness with heavy proteinuria, an important diagnostic feature. Approximately 25 percent of patients follow a more severe course which can be divided into *five consecutive phases*, each characterized by different pathophysiologic abnormalities.

The initial *febrile phase* of 3 to 8 days is characterized by fever, malaise, flushing of the face and neck, and infection of the eyes and palate. Toward the end of the febrile phase, petechiae appear, platelets decrease, proteinuria develops, and the hematocrit begins to increase.

The *hypotensive phase* develops suddenly and lasts 1 to 3 days. Proteinuria is heavy. The hematocrit may increase greatly and reflects loss of plasma into the retroperitoneal area and other tissues. Nausea and vomiting, abdominal discomfort, and backache may reflect these developments. Despite hypovolemia and shock, the extremities remain warm, and this observation suggests arteriolar dys-

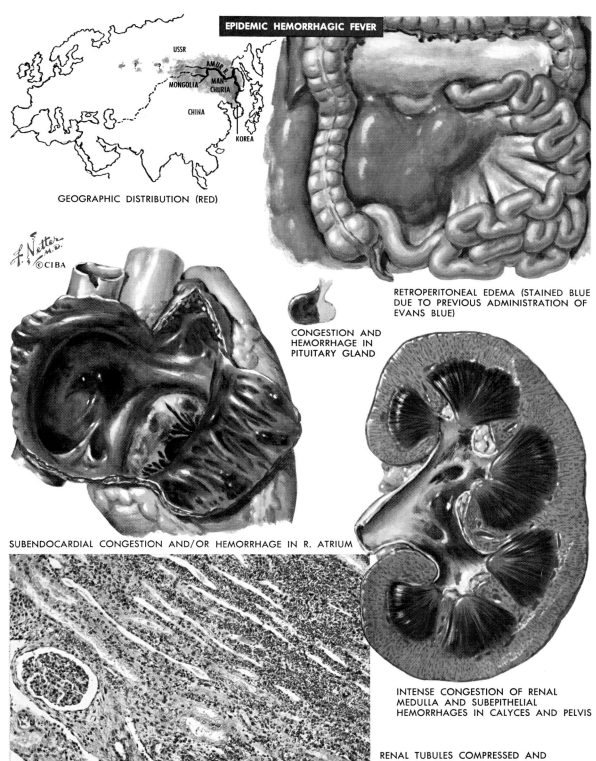

EPIDEMIC HEMORRHAGIC FEVER

GEOGRAPHIC DISTRIBUTION (RED)

RETROPERITONEAL EDEMA (STAINED BLUE DUE TO PREVIOUS ADMINISTRATION OF EVANS BLUE)

CONGESTION AND HEMORRHAGE IN PITUITARY GLAND

SUBENDOCARDIAL CONGESTION AND/OR HEMORRHAGE IN R. ATRIUM

INTENSE CONGESTION OF RENAL MEDULLA AND SUBEPITHELIAL HEMORRHAGES IN CALYCES AND PELVIS

RENAL TUBULES COMPRESSED AND DISTORTED BY MASSES OF RED BLOOD CELLS; ALSO HEMOGLOBIN CASTS

function. Oliguria and renal insufficiency begin during this phase.

The *oliguric phase* begins as sequestered plasma returns to the vascular system. There is increasing renal failure, nitrogen retention, vomiting, and dehydration. Hyperkalemia is common. Despite the disappearance of symptoms which occurred earlier, confusion, restlessness, and hypertension may develop. In some instances these are the result of a relative hypervolemia which will respond to phlebotomy. Hemorrhages in the skin, gastrointestinal tract, lungs, and renal pelves occur but are rarely of dangerous proportions. The oliguric phase usually lasts 3 to 5 days.

The *diuretic phase* initiates clinical recovery and rapid improvement in renal function. However, diuresis with daily formation of up to 8 liters of urine represents a serious hazard since the patients exhibit a brittle fluid and electrolyte homeostasis. There may be rapid

fluctuation between shock and pulmonary edema. Deaths in this phase account for one third of the total deaths and are secondary to the shock of dehydration and to pulmonary infection.

The *convalescent phase* usually requires 3 to 12 weeks. Permanent residual sequelae, even in those who were most severely ill, are extremely rare.

Treatment is entirely supportive. Specific therapy is not available. During the hypotensive phase, the administration of concentrated solutions of human serum albumin, and sometimes of pressor agents, appears to be of benefit. During the oliguric phase, strict control of fluid and food intake must be maintained. Hypervolemia is a serious threat and may require phlebotomy. Also, pulmonary infections are common during the acute phases. In the diuretic phase, adequate and strictly controlled replacement of fluid and electrolytes is necessary. □

Section VI

Diseases of the Urinary System

Frank H. Netter, M.D.

in collaboration with

Thomas Doxiadis, M.D.   *Plate 13*

Paul Kimmelstiel, M.D.   *Plates 5-10*

J. Stauffer Lehman, Jr., M.D., M.P.H.   *Plates 14-15*

J. U. Schlegel, M.D.   *Plates 1-4, 11-12, 16-19, 21-36*

Maurice B. Strauss, M.D.   *Plate 20*

Obstructive Uropathy

Obstruction to the flow of urine causes pathologic changes in the urinary tract referred to as obstructive uropathy and, if uncorrected, will cause obstructive nephropathy. The seriousness of the clinical situation is multiplied enormously if infection is also present. Obstructive uropathy is one of the common causes of the morbidity and mortality associated with renal disease.

A great variety of both congenital and acquired lesions may cause obstructive uropathy (as can be appreciated from Plate 1), and the point or area of obstruction may be anywhere from a renal calyx to the urethral meatus. Depending on the site of obstruction, the condition may be unilateral or bilateral.

The obstruction produces a compensatory hypertrophy of the muscular wall proximal to it. However, when this attempted compensation is insufficient to overcome the obstruction, decompensation and dilatation occur, followed in time by pressure atrophy of renal tissue. Urinary stasis also favors precipitation of dissolved salts, and the resulting calculi may aggravate the destructive process. Nevertheless, the prime danger of obstruction lies not only in the direct effect of altered urodynamics, but also in the consequent increased risk of superimposed infection which can greatly accelerate and amplify the destruction of renal parenchyma.

While *acute* urinary tract obstruction is often manifested clinically by obvious symptoms, *chronic* obstruction can be much more insidious and is often silent. Frequently, the first clinical manifestation of long-standing obstructive uropathy is the onset of infection or the occurrence of acute urinary retention; renal destruction may already be far advanced. This is especially the situation in children, and even if obstructive uropathy is symptomatic in the younger age group, it often produces only vague abdominal discomfort rather than flank pain or urinary complaints. In adults, symptoms may vary from vague, nonspecific complaints to severe, colicky pain associated with acute urinary retention.

At times, advanced azotemia may be present. If the obstructive process involves the lower urinary tract and has produced bilateral kidney damage, there may be elevation of serum creatinine and blood urea nitrogen. However, advanced bilateral hydronephrosis, especially in children, may exist without producing abnormal serum levels of various chemical components.

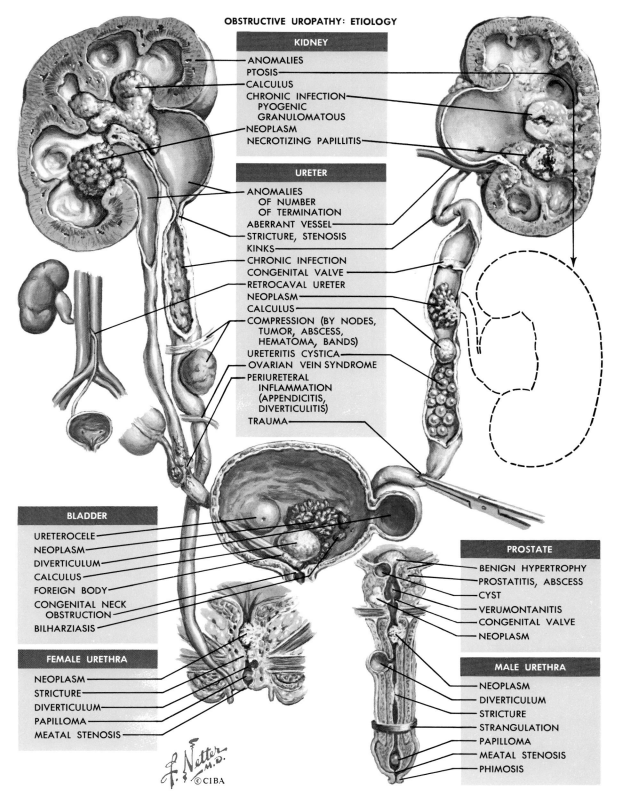

OBSTRUCTIVE UROPATHY: ETIOLOGY

KIDNEY
- ANOMALIES
- PTOSIS
- CALCULUS
- CHRONIC INFECTION
  - PYOGENIC
  - GRANULOMATOUS
- NEOPLASM
- NECROTIZING PAPILLITIS

URETER
- ANOMALIES
  - OF NUMBER
  - OF TERMINATION
- ABERRANT VESSEL
- STRICTURE, STENOSIS
- KINKS
- CHRONIC INFECTION
- CONGENITAL VALVE
- RETROCAVAL URETER
- NEOPLASM
- CALCULUS
- COMPRESSION (BY NODES, TUMOR, ABSCESS, HEMATOMA, BANDS)
- URETERITIS CYSTICA
- OVARIAN VEIN SYNDROME
- PERIURETERAL INFLAMMATION (APPENDICITIS, DIVERTICULITIS)
- TRAUMA

BLADDER
- URETEROCELE
- NEOPLASM
- DIVERTICULUM
- CALCULUS
- FOREIGN BODY
- CONGENITAL NECK OBSTRUCTION
- BILHARZIASIS

FEMALE URETHRA
- NEOPLASM
- STRICTURE
- DIVERTICULUM
- PAPILLOMA
- MEATAL STENOSIS

PROSTATE
- BENIGN HYPERTROPHY
- PROSTATITIS, ABSCESS
- CYST
- VERUMONTANITIS
- CONGENITAL VALVE
- NEOPLASM

MALE URETHRA
- NEOPLASM
- DIVERTICULUM
- STRICTURE
- STRANGULATION
- PAPILLOMA
- MEATAL STENOSIS
- PHIMOSIS

It is thus important to detect even minor indications of obstructive uropathy, such as a decrease in urinary concentrating ability, enuresis, dysuria, polyuria, change in the size and force of the urinary stream, and nocturia. Hematuria and other abnormalities found on examination of the urine also provide diagnostic clues. In addition, since urinary tract infection often indicates more serious underlying pathologic changes, it is always wise to retain a mental picture of Plate 1.

Obstructive uropathy must be diagnosed as early as possible when treatment may still be simple and permanent renal damage preventable. It is a challenge well worth the prize of salvaging renal tissue. For instance, urethral pathology, such as meatal stenosis in children of both sexes and distal urethral stricture in female children, is commonly found and often leads to infectious pyelonephritis (see page 189 and CIBA COLLECTION, Vol. 2, page 30). Such pathology can be recognized readily and is easily corrected.

Since chronic obstructive uropathy is often clinically silent, the diagnostic use of scintillation camera technics (see page 104) may hold the answer to the practice of preventive medicine. It is our opinion that a seemingly healthy population can be adequately screened, using available isotope scanning technics, for the purpose of detecting unsuspected renal or urinary tract disease. If even minor indications suggesting the existence of obstructive uropathy are present, numerous investigative technics are available to assist in making a diagnosis.

Drug treatment of urinary tract infections without correction of any existing obstructive uropathy usually fails to achieve eradication of the infection. Often it only complicates adequate therapy and may, in fact, even endanger the patient's life. *Continued on page 186*

Obstructive Uropathy

Continued from page 185

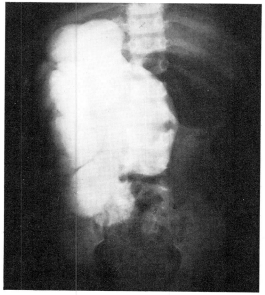

HYDRONEPHROTIC KIDNEY DUE TO URETEROPELVIC STENOSIS

ANTEGRADE PYELOGRAM: 2–YEAR–OLD CHILD WITH LARGE HYDRONEPHROSIS

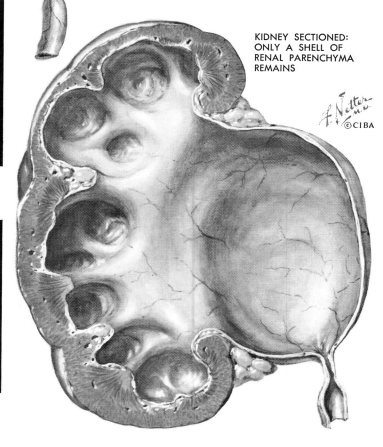

KIDNEY SECTIONED: ONLY A SHELL OF RENAL PARENCHYMA REMAINS

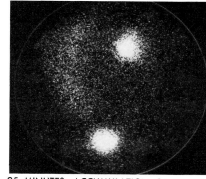

RADIOHIPPURAN SCAN; 2 MINUTES: L. KIDNEY NORMAL; R. KIDNEY SHOWS JUST A RIM OF PARENCHYMA WITH A "COLD" CENTER

25 MINUTES: ACCUMULATION OF RADIO-ACTIVE URINE IN HUGE HYDRONEPHROTIC R. KIDNEY (ALSO IN BLADDER)

Hydronephrosis

Hydronephrosis is a dilatation of the collecting system of the kidney caused by obstruction to the flow of urine. Conversely, however, obstruction does not always result in hydronephrosis. In some patients the obstruction is distal to the bladder which dilates and acts as a buffer zone, thus preventing the occurrence of hydronephrosis. Otherwise, in most instances, obstructive uropathy will sooner or later lead to the development of hydronephrosis. Occasionally, the degree of renal enlargement may reach gigantic proportions, with the collecting system containing several liters of urine.

Almost any type of urinary tract abnormality which leads to obstructive uropathy can eventually result in hydronephrosis; depending on the site of obstruction, the hydronephrosis may be bilateral or unilateral. If no infection is present, the dilatation of the collecting system can be of little or no clinical significance until compression and atrophy of the renal parenchyma occur. However, complete obstruction with gradual dilatation of the collecting system and compression of the renal parenchyma will eventually cause a complete atrophy. This extreme is commonly seen in patients with congenital hydronephrosis (see page 233), which fortunately is often unilateral. Parenthetically, congenital hydronephrosis may give rise to a palpable tumor and present a problem in differential diagnosis (see below).

Asymptomatic or silent hydronephrosis of a lesser degree is often found in adults. Commonly, attention is drawn to this pathology by minor trauma which causes bleeding into the hydronephrotic sac with resulting hematuria. In fact, lesser degrees of hydronephrosis are important primarily because of their susceptibility to trauma and infection which may then create a rather serious clinical situation. Consequently, such kidneys should be approached surgically; either the hydronephrotic kidney should be removed or the obstructive outlet repaired, depending upon, among other things, the degree of compensatory hypertrophy in the contralateral kidney.

Occasionally, when there is a relative ureteropelvic junction obstruction, a high fluid intake results in intermittent hydronephrosis which may be manifested by colicky pain, nausea, and vomiting. This syndrome is named Dietl's crisis.

Differential Diagnosis. As noted before, the finding in a child of a palpable mass in the renal area may lead to a differential diagnosis problem of neoplasm, multicystic disease, or unilateral hydronephrosis. Usu-ally, neoplastic renal disease in an infant is the result of a Wilms' tumor (see page 212). Wilms' tumor produces distortion of the collecting system of the affected kidney, and this can be observed on intravenous urography. It is important to differentiate between a benign lesion such as hydronephrosis and a malignant lesion such as Wilms' tumor, since in patients with the latter, one might employ preoperative radiation prior to surgical exploration.

The differentiation between unilateral multicystic disease (see page 227) and unilateral hydronephrosis can be made by palpation, use of transillumination, and isotope scanning technics (see page 104). It is occasionally possible to make the distinction between multicystic disease and unilateral hydronephrosis by intravenous urography, but this is often not diagnostic, and the final proof lies in exploration and removal of the mass. □

Cystitis

Cystitis, an inflammation of the urinary bladder, can vary in severity from a simple, self-limited disease to a severe condition that may eventually extend to involve the kidney and the upper urinary tract and lead to death in uremia. Fortunately, most cases of cystitis are rather benign.

In the adult female, cystitis, in particular limited to the trigone, often results from an ascending urethritis. Rarely, the infection can progress to a severe, fulminating, ulcerative, or gangrenous cystitis, occasionally with alkaline incrustation. However, it usually follows an uncomplicated course and in most instances responds well to a variety of antibacterial agents.

In the adult male and in children, including female children, the presence of cystitis usually signifies the existence of a precipitating anatomic or physiologic abnormality. It therefore requires a thorough evaluation for diagnosis.

As noted, cystitis generally results from an ascending infection. However, it can also arise from infection in the kidneys, such as tuberculosis (see page 196), schistosomiasis (see page 198), or primary renal infections of other types (see page 189). Usually the organisms causing cystitis are the gram negative enteric bacteria, but staphylococci, and specific organisms such as *Neisseria gonorrhoeae, Treponema pallidum, Trichomonas vaginalis,* and others are occasionally found.

Outlet obstruction is an important precipitating factor in the establishment of cystitis. (The presence of a residual urine provides a medium in which bacteria may grow.) Other pathologic conditions in the bladder which may act as predisposing factors for the establishment of cystitis include the presence of calculi, a neoplasm, and foreign bodies. The resulting cystitis is often difficult to eradicate unless the underlying cause is corrected.

Trauma to the bladder or urethra, either accidental or as a result of instrumentation or surgical procedures, predisposes to the development of cystitis, either directly or indirectly. Therefore, if such clinical conditions exist, it appears justified to use antibacterial agents in order to obtain a urinary concentration of the agent which is sufficient to prevent the establishment of infection. It should be noted, in this connection, that urine which is either very dilute or very concentrated appears to offer a natural barrier against bacterial infections since it does not provide a suitable medium for bacterial growth. However, in diabetic patients this is not the case, and the presence of glucose in the urine actually enhances the possibility of bacterial multiplication. In addition, diabetic patients have lowered tissue resistance to bacterial infections.

The *symptoms* of acute cystitis are annoying and include dysuria, frequency, and occasionally hematuria. There are usually no systemic manifestations, and fever, if present, is low grade. The chief danger of cystitis is the possibility of infection ascending to the kidney.

It is not uncommon to find that a *reflux* of urine from the bladder into the ureters occurs in patients with cystitis. This apparently results from an involvement of

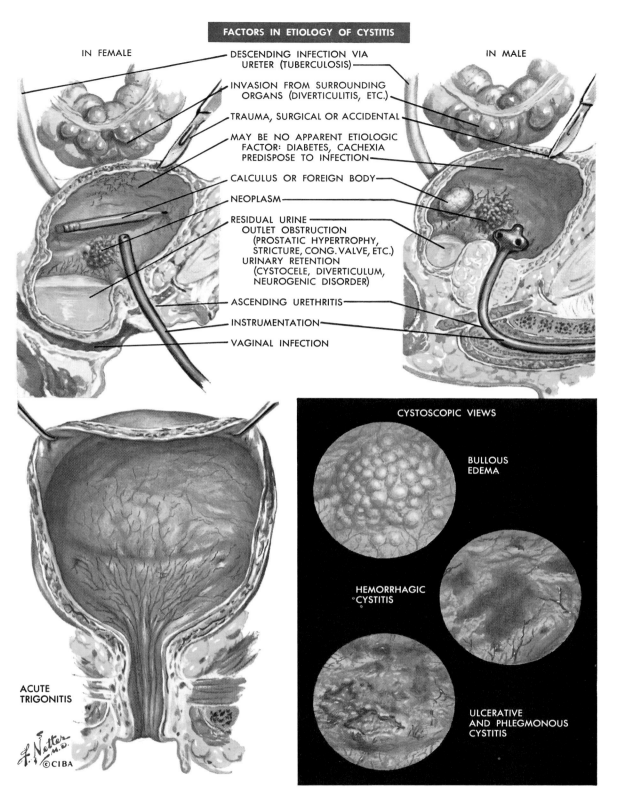

FACTORS IN ETIOLOGY OF CYSTITIS

IN FEMALE

IN MALE

DESCENDING INFECTION VIA URETER (TUBERCULOSIS)

INVASION FROM SURROUNDING ORGANS (DIVERTICULITIS, ETC.)

TRAUMA, SURGICAL OR ACCIDENTAL

MAY BE NO APPARENT ETIOLOGIC FACTOR: DIABETES, CACHEXIA PREDISPOSE TO INFECTION

CALCULUS OR FOREIGN BODY

NEOPLASM

RESIDUAL URINE
OUTLET OBSTRUCTION (PROSTATIC HYPERTROPHY, STRICTURE, CONG. VALVE, ETC.)
URINARY RETENTION (CYSTOCELE, DIVERTICULUM, NEUROGENIC DISORDER)

ASCENDING URETHRITIS

INSTRUMENTATION

VAGINAL INFECTION

ACUTE TRIGONITIS

CYSTOSCOPIC VIEWS

BULLOUS EDEMA

HEMORRHAGIC CYSTITIS

ULCERATIVE AND PHLEGMONOUS CYSTITIS

the intramural portion of the ureters and of the ureteral orifices which is sufficient to interfere with normal physiology. If the bladder urine contains bacteria, it is obvious that infection of the kidney is more or less inevitable. Prompt and long-term antibacterial treatment is imperative in these circumstances. If the reflux is not effectively resolved, surgical procedures involving reimplantation of the ureters may be necessary to prevent recurrent exposure of the kidneys to infected, refluxed urine.

However, it appears that bacteria can reach the kidneys by the ascending route, even in the absence of reflux. This situation is particularly likely if patients are diabetic, or are pregnant, or have preexisting upper urinary tract abnormalities.

Thus, it is important to treat urethritis and trigonitis before a "full-blown" cystitis or pyelonephritis occurs. In the female patient, it is important also to eradicate

any infection of the cervix or vagina which, in conjunction with sexual intercourse, may be the precipitating factor in an ascending urethritis.

Adequate therapy of cystitis with antibacterial agents requires bactericidal concentrations of the drug in the urine. Thus, a urine volume which is too great may defeat this purpose, as will the existence of renal disease which interferes with maximum urinary concentration of solutes, including antibacterial agents.

The actions of various antibacterial agents must be considered, in particular with regard to their method of excretion by the kidney. Proper urinary concentrations must be achieved by means of doses of the drug which are not sufficient to produce toxic serum levels. For instance, if an antibacterial agent is primarily metabolized in the liver to compounds with little or no antibacterial action, and if the parent compound is not excreted by the kidney, *Continued on page 188*

Cystitis

Continued from page 187

this agent would have limited value in the treatment of urinary tract infection. Also, many antibacterial agents work best in either an acid or alkaline medium. Thus, appropriate acidifying or alkalizing drugs administered in conjunction with the bactericidal agent may provide optimum therapeutic effects.

As indicated previously, if any degree of obstructive uropathy is present, or if there are abnormalities in the bladder, such as calculi, foreign bodies, or neoplasm, specific treatment of the underlying condition must be performed before eradication of an existing cystitis is attempted.

Clinical and Pathologic Variations

Inflammation of the bladder mucosa may exhibit considerable variation, depending upon the virulence of the infecting organism and the resistance of the host. The so-called bullous cystitis is one variety of *polypoid cystitis* which results from inflammatory edema that elevates the vesical mucosa. This condition can be either a more severe reaction to an ascending cystitis or the result of infection spreading from a neighboring organ.

The *ulcerative* and *acute hemorrhagic* forms of cystitis are both manifestations of massive infection. They require prompt, adequate therapy.

Often the urine of patients with urethritis and trigonitis is normal on routine examination and sterile when cultured on ordinary media. This situation raises the question whether the urethral and trigonal glands harbor the organisms which classically causes infection, or whether *L-forms, mycoplasma,* or other organisms which do not grow on standard culture media are the cause of the infection. We have cultured L-forms of staphylococci from fresh urine specimens obtained from patients who were suffering from urethritis and cystitis but who also had never received chemotherapy. Whether such L-forms are the etiologic organisms in some instances of urethritis and trigonitis remains to be seen. Nevertheless, female patients with severe symptoms of urethritis and trigonitis, and a sterile urine, frequently have inflammation and edema of the urethra and trigone, as demonstrated by endoscopic examination.

Another type of cystitis, characterized by epithelial proliferation, is called *glandular* or *cystic cystitis.* In this form the lining of the bladder is studded with clear or turbid vesicles. *Cystitis cystica* is a term employed when such lesions are large. The ureter and the pelvis of one or both kidneys, in addition to the bladder, may also be involved. Pyelography may reveal multiple small filling defects which impart a moth-eaten appearance. The cysts often contain coagulated fluid and must be distinguished from *cystitis emphysematosa,* in which the vesicles contain carbon dioxide, a situation usually seen primarily in diabetic patients.

Hunner's ulcer, also named *chronic interstitial cystitis,* is a little understood entity in which no bacteria can be recovered in the urine, and in which there is chronic inflammation of all layers of the bladder wall. On cystoscopic examination, ulcera-

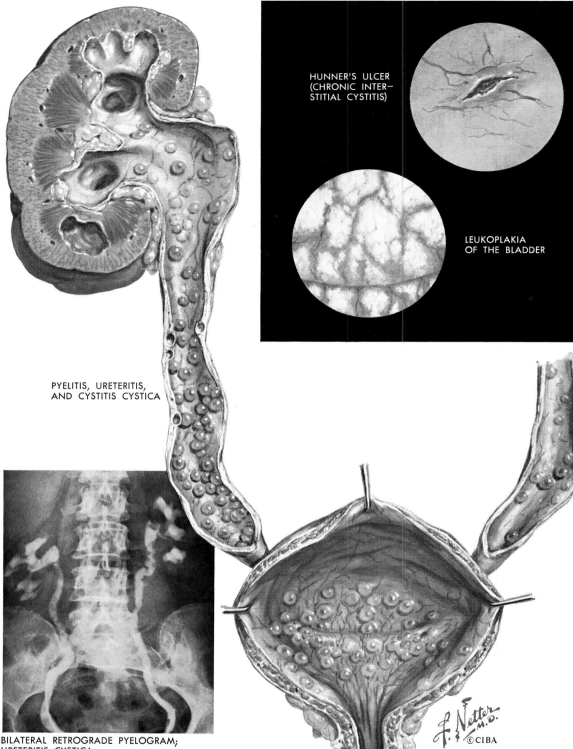

HUNNER'S ULCER (CHRONIC INTERSTITIAL CYSTITIS)

LEUKOPLAKIA OF THE BLADDER

PYELITIS, URETERITIS, AND CYSTITIS CYSTICA

BILATERAL RETROGRADE PYELOGRAM; URETERITIS CYSTICA

tion is evident, especially if the bladder is distended. The condition must be distinguished from leukoplakia which represents an epidermoid transformation of the normal bladder epithelium secondary to chronic inflammation. However, in leukoplakia there is usually evidence of pyuria of long duration and often evidence of mechanical irritation, from either foreign bodies or a residual urine secondary to obstruction.

Hunner's ulcer occurs most frequently in women and, if untreated, leads to a gradual, severe decrease in bladder capacity. Eventually the decrease in bladder size may be incapacitating to the point at which a urinary diversion procedure is necessary. There is no known cure. Dilatation of the bladder under anesthesia may be helpful. (Anesthesia is essential since otherwise this is an extremely painful procedure.) In the author's experience, many cases of early Hunner's ulcer can be treated best by urging the patients not to urinate at their first inclination to do so, but rather to try to retain the urine for as long as possible. This procedure thereby achieves some degree of bladder dilatation and prevents the otherwise inevitable shrinkage in bladder capacity which may eventually become intractable.

Although the incidence of bladder tumors in patients with Hunner's ulcer does not appear to be higher than in the general population, it should be remembered that any patient can develop a bladder tumor (see page 209). We have seen patients in whom bladder tumors were overlooked because, for years, the patients had been treated for interstitial cystitis and additional symptoms were not particularly noticeable. Also, chronic cystitis often precedes the occurrence of a bladder tumor and indeed it may occasionally act as an etiologic agent, as will the existence of residual urine. □

Pyelonephritis

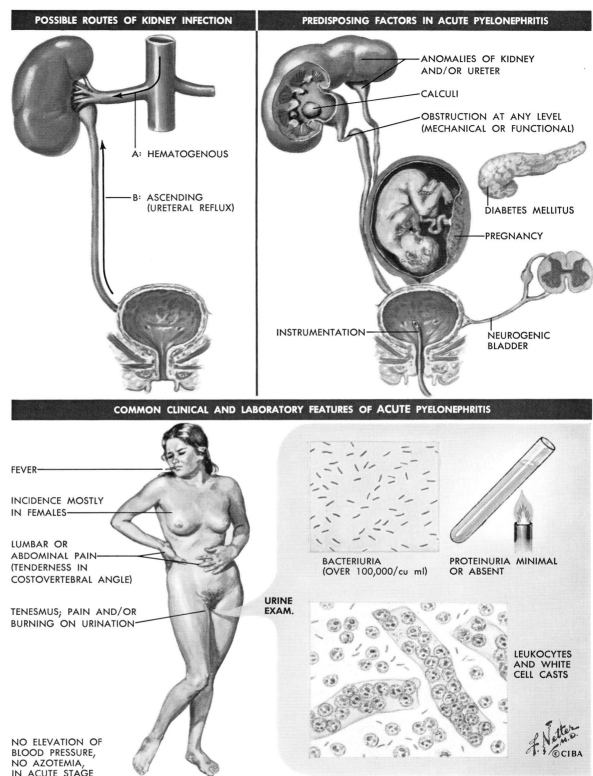

POSSIBLE ROUTES OF KIDNEY INFECTION

A: HEMATOGENOUS

B: ASCENDING (URETERAL REFLUX)

PREDISPOSING FACTORS IN ACUTE PYELONEPHRITIS

ANOMALIES OF KIDNEY AND/OR URETER

CALCULI

OBSTRUCTION AT ANY LEVEL (MECHANICAL OR FUNCTIONAL)

DIABETES MELLITUS

PREGNANCY

INSTRUMENTATION

NEUROGENIC BLADDER

COMMON CLINICAL AND LABORATORY FEATURES OF ACUTE PYELONEPHRITIS

FEVER

INCIDENCE MOSTLY IN FEMALES

LUMBAR OR ABDOMINAL PAIN (TENDERNESS IN COSTOVERTEBRAL ANGLE)

TENESMUS; PAIN AND/OR BURNING ON URINATION

NO ELEVATION OF BLOOD PRESSURE, NO AZOTEMIA, IN ACUTE STAGE

URINE EXAM.

BACTERIURIA (OVER 100,000/cu ml)

PROTEINURIA MINIMAL OR ABSENT

LEUKOCYTES AND WHITE CELL CASTS

Pyelonephritis, defined as an infectious disease of the kidney, is characterized by a primary interstitial inflammation which secondarily involves the tubules and, in later stages, the vessels and glomeruli.

The term implies that the inflammation of the kidney and that of the pelvis are part of the same process. This is the situation in many instances, but the association of pyelitis with infectious interstitial nephritis is often not observed and may, in fact, be absent. However, the absence of pyelitis cannot be used as a criterion to distinguish, pathogenically, nonbacterial interstitial nephritides from the type of interstitial nephritis for which the time-honored term pyelonephritis is retained; nor can the presence of pyelitis be used to establish the diagnosis of pyelonephritis. What really distinguishes pyelonephritis from other, quite similar, interstitial nephritides is that pyelonephritis is caused by invasion of pathogenic organisms and that its initial stage is always purulent. It is customary to distinguish *acute* from *chronic* pyelonephritis.

Acute Pyelonephritis

The clinical manifestations include *fever, leukocytosis, malaise, back pain, tenderness to palpation in the costovertebral area, pyuria,* and *bacteriuria.* In a patient with such a clinical picture, the finding of *leukocyte casts* in the urine strongly suggests the diagnosis of pyelonephritis. The presence of such casts indicates that the polymorphonuclear leukocytes represent inflammation in the kidney rather than in the pelvis or lower urinary tract. Symptoms of dysuria, urgency, and frequency are usually associated with irritation of the lower urinary tract (see page 187) but are not uncommon in patients with acute pyelonephritis. Infants may have no localizing signs and symptoms but merely have general evidence of illness, including vomiting, diarrhea, and fever.

Depending on the extent of involvement of the renal parenchyma, renal function may be considerably reduced. Since interstitial nephritis affects the tubules more than any other anatomic unit, the most important and often the only dysfunction in the acute stage is the inability of the kidney to concentrate the urine.

Acute pyelonephritis may occur in both sexes and at any age, but in the young, it is more common in children and women;

in the older age group, it is most frequent in men with prostatic hyperplasia. Acute pyelonephritis may develop whether or not there is urinary obstruction, but every case should be carefully explored for a possible site of obstruction (see page 185) since treatment cannot be expected to be successful without adequate urinary drainage. In children, congenital malformations frequently are underlying factors (see Section VII), while in adults, calculi, strictures, or space-occupying lesions predominate.

Frequently, acute pyelonephritis is self-limited. However, the disease should not be considered cured unless periodic urine cultures provide assurance of the absence of organisms. Careful follow-up of patients has revealed recurrence of infection with the same or different organisms more often than had been suspected.

In some patients, the disease may progress insidious-

ly, or with episodes of acute exacerbations, into a chronic stage. Intensive antibacterial treatment is indicated, therefore, not only in an attempt to avoid such progression, but also to prevent the dreaded complication of septicemia by gram negative or other types of organisms. The purulent, interstitial inflammation may break through the wall of the intrarenal veins and produce thrombophlebitis, which may serve as a focus of dissemination of organisms into the bloodstream.

Pathology. The gross appearance in acute pyelonephritis is characteristically that of a swollen kidney, with multiple small abscesses on the external surface. On the cut surface, these same abscesses can be found in the cortex, often in continuity with rather poorly defined, linear, yellowish areas radiating from the corticomedullary junction to the surface. If more clearly defined, these lines or streaks continue through the medulla into the papillae. *Continued on page 190*

Pyelonephritis

Continued from page 189

Between the streaks in the involved cortical areas, the parenchyma appears normal. Pyelonephritis is thus a focal disease of the kidney. This feature is important in the differential diagnosis and becomes even more conspicuous in the chronic stage.

Microscopically, there is a heavy interstitial infiltrate, predominantly composed of polymorphonuclear leukocytes. The infiltrate frequently progresses to pus formation with areas of liquefaction necrosis within the cortex corresponding to the grossly visible abscesses. Throughout the cortex and medulla, segments of tubules are destroyed, and dense collections of polymorphonuclear leukocytes appear in the lumina of distal tubules. The leukocytes are held together by a proteinaceous material and are flushed out into the urine as casts. Occasionally, rather discrete areas of tubular and interstitial coagulation necrosis are seen microscopically, and these raise the suspicion that *Proteus mirabilis* is most likely the offending organism.

The infiltrate is patchy in distribution, sparing portions of normal parenchyma, but it may become more confluent with increasing severity of the disease. The preservation of glomeruli and vessels of all calibers, even in the areas of extensive interstitial infiltrate, is remarkable. Only occasionally is a glomerulus destroyed from without by invasion of Bowman's capsule.

Etiology. The most common organisms found in acute pyelonephritis are those of the coliform group, *E. coli* most frequently, followed by *Klebsiella* and paracolon bacilli. Other organisms, such as species of *Proteus,* can be encountered, but they are more often seen after antibiotic treatment of the initial episode, or following instrumentation.

It is of interest to note that protoplasts have been demonstrated in the urine of patients with pyelonephritis. Protoplasts are membrane-free forms of microorganisms which survive in hypertonic media, such as in the renal medulla. It is possible that the conservation of microorganisms in protoplastic forms could account for the continuance of a seemingly sterile inflammation resistant to antibiotic treatment.

Pathogenesis. Microorganisms may reach the kidney by the bloodstream or by ascending within the lower urinary tract. That pyelonephritis can be caused by hematogenous spread can be shown by

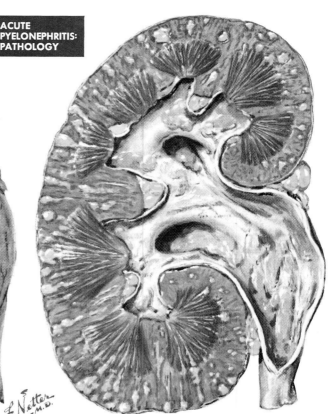

ACUTE PYELONEPHRITIS: PATHOLOGY

SURFACE ASPECT OF KIDNEY: MULTIPLE MINUTE ABSCESSES (SURFACE MAY APPEAR RELATIVELY NORMAL IN SOME CASES)

CUT SECTION: RADIATING YELLOWISH GRAY STREAKS IN PYRAMIDS AND ABSCESSES IN CORTEX; MODERATE HYDRONEPHROSIS WITH INFECTION; BLUNTING OF CALYCES (ASCENDING INFECTION)

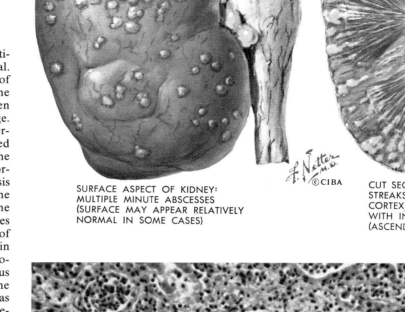
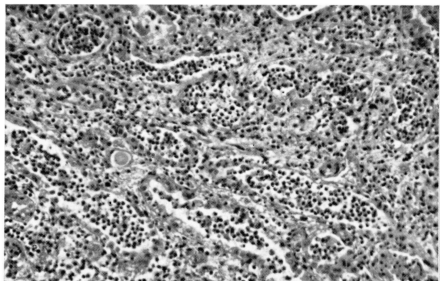

ACUTE PYELONEPHRITIS WITH EXUDATE CHIEFLY OF POLYMORPHONUCLEAR LEUKOCYTES IN INTERSTITIUM AND COLLECTING TUBULES

experiments in which organisms injected intravenously will lodge in the kidney. Here they will produce the characteristic changes of pyelonephritis provided the urine flow is temporarily blocked. The ascending route of infection can be demonstrated experimentally by injecting organisms into the bladder.

However, these experiments do not tell the pathogenesis of pyelonephritis in any given human case. Pyelonephritis is more commonly seen in patients with urinary obstruction, but this observation does not prove that the infection is ascending, for, in any such case of partial obstruction, a fleeting, clinically silent bacteremia may account for hematogenous spread. Clinically, operative procedures on urethral strictures are not infrequently associated with bacteremia, and pyelonephritis may be its sequela.

Catheterization of the urethra, with or without urinary obstruction, particularly with indwelling catheters,

is known to cause cystitis and bacteriuria and may be followed by pyelonephritis. It is not clear, however, which pathways the microorganisms use to reach the kidney. It is reasonable to assume that bacteremia is a result of traumatic catheterization, since this fact has been demonstrated experimentally. However, the literature is conspicuously void of adequate documentation concerning the frequency of bacteremia following catheterization, even though "catheterization fever" is well known to the urologist.

It is equally reasonable to assume that cystitis may compromise the function of the ureteral-vesical valve, causing vesicoureteral reflux and thus jetting infected urine into the renal pelvis. Such vesicoureteral reflux has been shown radiologically to occur in adults, but it is more frequently associated with urinary tract infection in children.

If pyelonephritis arises without obstruction and

Pyelonephritis

Continued

prior to urethral manipulation, additional pathogenetic factors should be considered. Bacteriuria is known to precede pyelonephritis, and it occurs much more commonly in females than in males. This finding may be related to the anatomic features of the female urethra. Organisms normally present in the urethra presumably have ready access to the bladder (*e.g.*, "honeymoon cystitis"). Under such circumstances, one presumes that the resultant pyelonephritis was of ascending pathogenesis. Also, the flow of the urine in the lower urinary tract may be greatly reduced, without mechanical obstruction, by lack of normal ureteral peristalsis. Such instances are regarded as functional obstruction, in contrast to mechanical obstruction.

The role of urinary bacterial inhibitors and of local bladder defense mechanisms (*e.g.*, immunoglobulins) requires more study. In summary, the pathogenesis of pyelonephritis in any individual case is, to a large extent, a matter of inference.

Bacteriuria

Bacteriuria deserves special mention because its significance often has been falsely interpreted. Normal urine is sterile. Bacteria cultured from a midstream specimen under sterile conditions may be derived from the urethral flora (see page 81). A count of colonies grown from such specimens, if less than 1,000 colonies per milliliter, can be assumed to result from contamination. Colony counts between 1,000 and 100,000 are indeterminate, and the procedure must be repeated. More than 100,000 colonies per milliliter is regarded as abnormal and is referred to as significant bacteriuria. If urine is obtained by suprapubic needle puncture of the bladder (see page 71), the presence of any bacteria is regarded as abnormal, but low colony counts may rarely reflect contamination.

Significant bacteriuria is found in nearly all cases of acute pyelonephritis unless a unilateral renal infection is associated with complete obstruction of the respective ureter. However, what is the significance of asymptomatic bacteriuria detected on routine examination? It may mean cystitis, prostatitis, or preexisting pyelonephritis. On the other hand, it may be followed by pyelonephritis, and in this case, it would be reasonable to assume that it is the cause of the subsequent ascending pyelonephritis.

The evaluation of a causative relationship between bacteriuria and pyelonephritis may encounter difficulties in the individual case. In the instance of acute pyelonephritis, the pivotal clinical symptom of pain and tenderness does not occur unless the interstitial nephritis is extensive. In the absence of interstitial nephritis it is virtually impossible either to exclude or to prove the existence of a focal acute pyelonephritis. It should also be remembered that asymptomatic bacteriuria may occur without pyuria, *i.e.*, without evidence of inflammation, and may subside spontaneously. In this case, the significance of bacteriuria may remain obscure.

To prove the existence of pyelonephritis in cases of asymptomatic bacteriuria may require the demonstration of bacteria in urine specimens taken from above the bladder by ureteral catheterization, since percutaneous needle biopsies of the kidney are notoriously unreliable for the diagnosis of pyelonephritis. Nevertheless, clinical judgment often replaces solid proof.

It cannot be sufficiently emphasized that the absence of significant bacteriuria, *i.e.*, less than 100,000 colonies per milliliter, does not rule out an existing pyelonephritis and, conversely, that the presence of bacteriuria does not necessarily indicate pyelonephritis. In addition, the practicing physician should be aware of the fact that a single bacterial colony count is not reliable. At least two counts should be performed.

Chronic Pyelonephritis

Symptoms and signs of acute pyelonephritis can be correlated in most cases with characteristic structural renal lesions. However, this association does not hold for chronic pyelonephritis and the clinical features often are quite vague. In a minority of patients, an adequately documented *Continued on page 192*

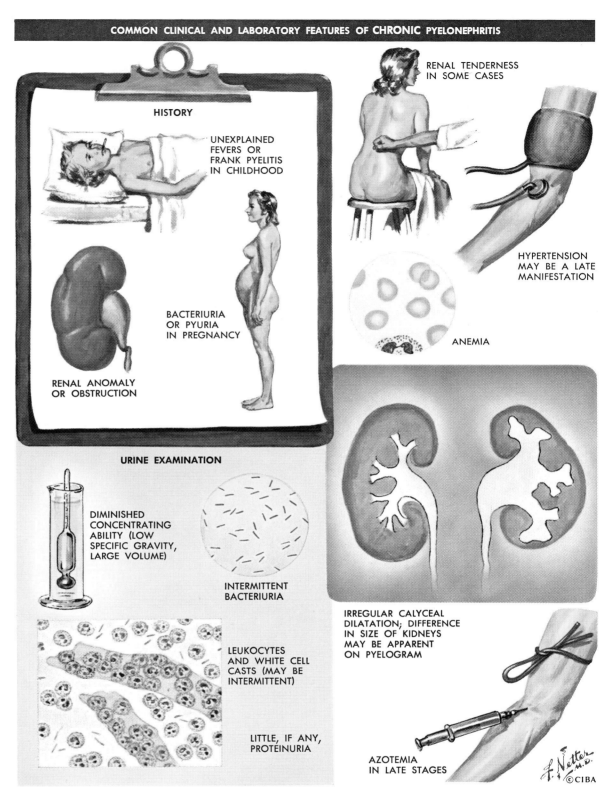

COMMON CLINICAL AND LABORATORY FEATURES OF CHRONIC PYELONEPHRITIS

HISTORY

UNEXPLAINED FEVERS OR FRANK PYELITIS IN CHILDHOOD

BACTERIURIA OR PYURIA IN PREGNANCY

RENAL ANOMALY OR OBSTRUCTION

RENAL TENDERNESS IN SOME CASES

HYPERTENSION MAY BE A LATE MANIFESTATION

ANEMIA

URINE EXAMINATION

DIMINISHED CONCENTRATING ABILITY (LOW SPECIFIC GRAVITY, LARGE VOLUME)

INTERMITTENT BACTERIURIA

LEUKOCYTES AND WHITE CELL CASTS (MAY BE INTERMITTENT)

LITTLE, IF ANY, PROTEINURIA

IRREGULAR CALYCEAL DILATATION; DIFFERENCE IN SIZE OF KIDNEYS MAY BE APPARENT ON PYELOGRAM

AZOTEMIA IN LATE STAGES

Pyelonephritis

Continued from page 191

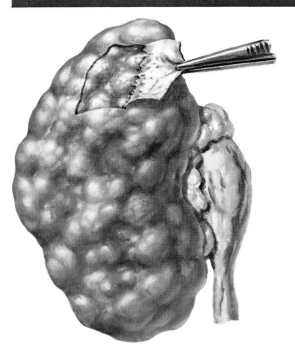

COARSELY GRANULAR CONTRACTED KIDNEY, WITH BLUNT, U–SHAPED DEPRESSIONS SOMETIMES SEEN IN CHRONIC PYELONEPHRITIS; IN MANY INSTANCES THE KIDNEY IS INDISTINGUISHABLE FROM THAT OF NEPHROSCLEROSIS; THICKENED CAPSULE IS ADHERENT

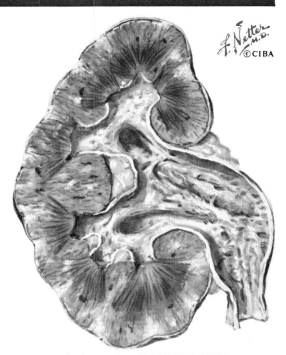

THINNING OF RENAL PARENCHYMA WITH WEDGE–SHAPED SUBCAPSULAR SCARS; BLURRING OF CORTICOMEDULLARY JUNCTION; DILATED, FIBROSED PELVIS AND CALYCES SEEN IN MANY BUT NOT ALL CASES OF CHRONIC PYELONEPHRITIS

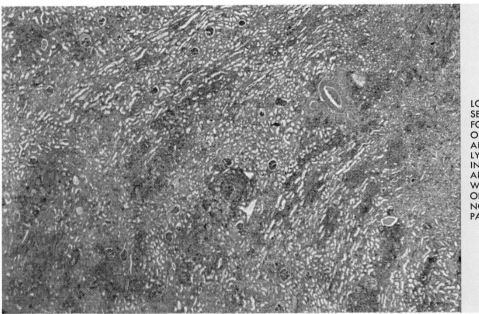

LOW–POWER SECTION SHOWING FOCAL NATURE OF INVOLVEMENT: AREAS OF LYMPHOCYTIC INFILTRATION ALTERNATING WITH AREAS OF RELATIVELY NORMAL PARENCHYMA

acute onset may be followed by repeated episodes of exacerbations between months or years of good health. In such cases, renal failure may become apparent only in the late stage when the loss of renal parenchyma by scarring overbalances the compensation of the remaining intact kidney tissue. Of course, this decompensation may never occur in the not infrequent instances of unilateral pyelonephritis.

Whether episodes of renal infection precede the chronic stage, or the latter begins entirely insidiously, the clinical manifestations of late-stage pyelonephritis include azotemia and late onset of hypertension. As may be expected from our knowledge of the renal structural damage, a diminution of urine-concentrating power precedes and is disproportionately greater than a reduction in glomerular filtration rate.

Chronic pyelonephritis is often associated with obstruction. Bacteriuria and pyuria may be present but are not necessarily of renal origin. They are frequently absent in patients who are diagnosed as having chronic pyelonephritis on purely morphologic grounds, by radiologic findings, at nephrectomy, or at autopsy.

Proteinuria is often present in patients with chronic pyelonephritis. However, in the differential diagnosis, if the amount exceeds 3.5 gm/day, it indicates the nephrotic syndrome and must be taken as evidence against the diagnosis of chronic pyelonephritis (see page 123). Moreover, the nephrotic syndrome and pyelonephritis are associated infrequently.

Pathology. In documented chronic pyelonephritis, structural changes are quite characteristic. They consist of widespread focal interstitial infiltration by lymphocytes, plasma cells, histiocytes, and variable numbers of polymorphonuclear leukocytes. Many tubules are destroyed, and within the affected areas, those remaining are dilated, lined by flattened epithelial cells, and filled with homogeneous, proteinaceous material, reminiscent of thyroid alveoli. Arteriosclerosis is almost always prominent, but arteriolosclerosis is not conspicuous. Many glomeruli show a thickening of Bowman's capsule, *i.e.,* periglomerular fibrosis. Other glomeruli show a peculiar intracapsular deposit of an acid mucopolysaccharide which compresses the glomerular tuft into an ec-

centric ball of collapsed and thick-walled capillaries.

The histologic changes correspond to the gross features of an extremely irregular contraction of one or both kidneys. The kidney surface is uneven and bumpy, and wide, flat scars are apparent.

The gross changes are radiologically demonstrable. The contraction of the renal parenchyma and retraction of papillae also cause a widening of the calyces and "blunting" of papillae. These are characteristic radiologic features observed in retrograde pyelograms (see page 96). Among the various acquired renal diseases resulting in marked diminution of size, chronic pyelonephritis may lead to the smallest kidneys.

Pathogenesis. It is generally accepted that acute pyelonephritis, after subsidence, may progress insidiously without demonstrable presence of pathogenic organisms. However, this process is not understood. As stated previously, bacteria may change into proto-

plasts, which can be recognized by means of a modification of growth technics, but systematic studies disclosing protoplasts in abacterial chronic pyelonephritis are not available.

There is also controversy as to whether the perpetuation of interstitial nephritis is a result of a continuation of an antigen-antibody reaction. Isolated reports have suggested this pathogenesis, and an experimental pyelonephritis has been produced by injection of dead bacilli into the pelvis, or its wall, of previously sensitized animals. Nevertheless, the immunogenic evolution of chronic pyelonephritis is still hypothetical.

Severe sclerosis of the interlobar, arcuate, and interlobular arteries is the rule in chronic pyelonephritis and may play an important role in the pathogenesis of hypertension. Yet, the frequent occurrence of severe arteriosclerosis accompanying chronic pyelonephritis is difficult to understand. It has been assumed that

Pyelonephritis

Continued

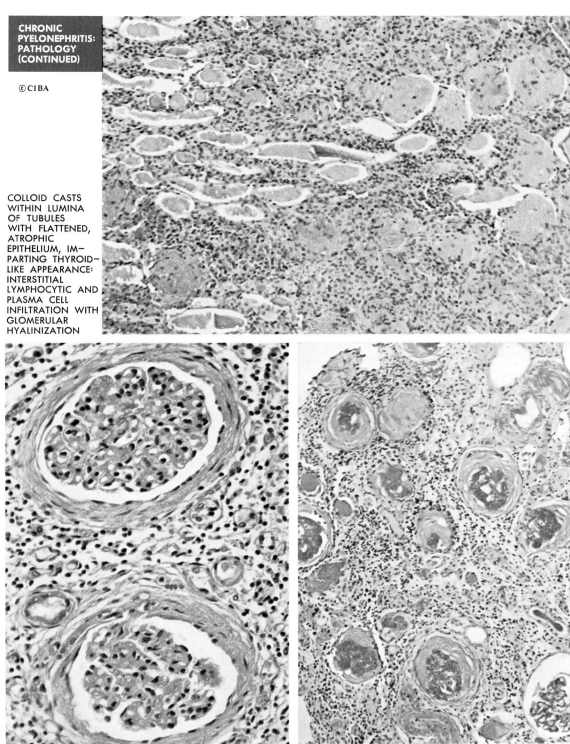

CHRONIC PYELONEPHRITIS: PATHOLOGY (CONTINUED)

COLLOID CASTS WITHIN LUMINA OF TUBULES WITH FLATTENED, ATROPHIC EPITHELIUM, IMPARTING THYROID−LIKE APPEARANCE: INTERSTITIAL LYMPHOCYTIC AND PLASMA CELL INFILTRATION WITH GLOMERULAR HYALINIZATION

PERICAPSULAR GLOMERULAR FIBROSIS WITH TUBULAR ATROPHY AND INTERSTITIAL INFLAMMATION

INTRACAPSULAR HYALINIZING GLOMERULAR FIBROSIS: PAS−POSITIVE MATERIAL IN BOWMAN'S SPACE WITH COMPRESSED CAPILLARY TUFT

the lesion is a sequela of arterial inflammation during the acute stage of pyelonephritis, but in the experiences of other investigators, the occurrence of an arteritis is as uncommon as "invasive glomerulitis."

Many cases of chronic pyelonephritis are diagnosed at autopsy by the criteria mentioned above as characteristic for the late stage of the disease. These criteria, however, are not pathognomonic, as will be discussed subsequently, and extreme variations in assessing the prevalence of chronic pyelonephritis have thus resulted. It can be safely stated that chronic pyelonephritis has often been overdiagnosed.

Chronic pyelonephritis has often been considered as a condition superimposed on other renal diseases. However, an interstitial nephritis with tubular atrophy, even with "thyroidization," has a manifold pathogenesis and should not be identified as pyelonephritis, unless known to be infectious in origin.

Differential Diagnosis of Chronic Pyelonephritis

Two major groups of diseases are to be distinguished from chronic pyelonephritis—primary glomerular and primary vascular diseases. Both of these may lead to azotemia, hypertension, and extreme destruction of renal parenchyma. The onset and duration of azotemia may be so insidious as to be of little assistance in the differential diagnosis. However, if the onset of hypertension precedes that of significant azotemia by a considerable period of time, it weighs heavily against chronic pyelonephritis, since hypertension is a late manifestation of this disease.

As mentioned before, the earliest functional deficiency in pyelonephritis, in contrast to primary glomerular or vascular diseases, is the inability to concentrate the glomerular filtrate. This fact may help to establish the diagnosis. However, in late stages of chronic pyelonephritis, particularly if obstruction is absent and documentation of preceding episodes of renal infection is lacking, the diagnosis rests on radiologic findings which indicate the focal nature of the renal disease, *i.e.,* the gross irregularity of the scarring.

When we attempt to distinguish chronic pyelonephritis on purely morphologic grounds from primary glomerular and vascular diseases, we must take into consideration that all the changes occurring in the kidneys in documented cases of chronic pyelonephritis are also seen in kidneys affected by chronic glomerulonephritis and ischemia. The effect on the renal parenchyma of gradually increasing ischemia, such as occurs with arteriosclerosis, is primarily that of atrophy and destruction of the vulnerable structures, specifically the tubules, with preservation of the glomeruli, and an accumulation of an interstitial infiltrate dominated by lymphocytes. These renal structural changes secondary to ischemia are essentially the same as those seen in chronic pyelonephritis, except for the nature of the interstitial infiltrate which is most pleomorphic in chronic pyelonephritis. Indeed, how much of the interstitial infiltration, "thyroidization," glomerular changes, and tubular damage in documented cases of chronic pyelonephritis is secondary to the original infection and how much is the result of the always present arteriosclerosis, can be assessed

only by inference and not on morphologic grounds.

In "end-stage kidneys," chronic glomerulonephritis may be diagnosed if the great majority of nonhyalinized glomeruli show evidence of active inflammation, partial hyalinization, or at least multiple synechiae. In primary arterio- and arteriolosclerosis there is much less, if any, involvement of residual glomeruli. Nevertheless, as noted, the most persuasive criterion for the diagnosis of pyelonephritis is the nature of the interstitial infiltrate, which contains more plasma cells than in other diseases. The infiltrate becomes suggestive of chronic pyelonephritis if there are aggregates of polymorphonuclear leukocytes.

Generally, purely morphologic changes should be regarded as suggestive, rather than pathognomonic, of chronic pyelonephritis. The final diagnosis must depend on the documentation of renal infection, past or present. □

Papillary Necrosis

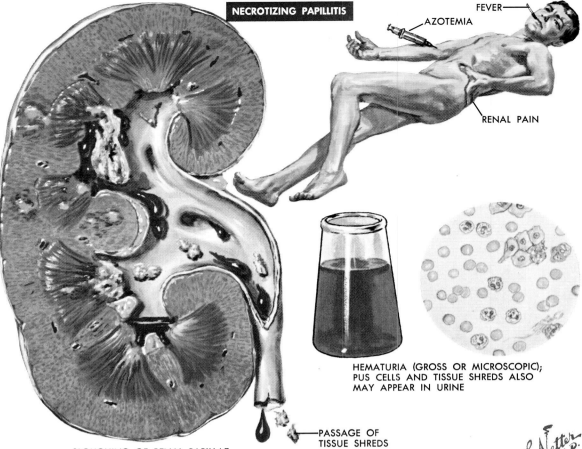

NECROTIZING PAPILLITIS

FEVER

AZOTEMIA

RENAL PAIN

HEMATURIA (GROSS OR MICROSCOPIC); PUS CELLS AND TISSUE SHREDS ALSO MAY APPEAR IN URINE

SLOUGHING OF RENAL PAPILLAE

PASSAGE OF TISSUE SHREDS

The papillae and portions of the medulla may undergo coagulation necrosis and, if sloughed into the renal pelvis, may be passed with dramatic clinical consequences. The patient may become critically ill with fever, renal colic, oliguria, and azotemia and may even die in uremia. In the light of such a clinical picture, hematuria is an important sign which should alert the clinician to suspect the possibility of a sloughed papilla.

In some patients, particularly those with long-standing azotemia, sloughing of the papillae can be observed to occur over a prolonged period of time without episodes of acute renal failure. In these patients, the prognosis depends on the severity of the associated renal disease. A definitive clinical diagnosis can be made by pyelography and by finding fragments of necrotic papillae in urine strained through cloth.

Papillary necrosis has been recognized for many years. It is more frequent in older people and in patients with diabetes or pyelonephritis, particularly those with lower urinary tract obstruction.

Grossly, the necrotic papilla is friable, yellowish in color, and sharply demarcated from adjacent tissue. A portion of the medulla may also be sloughed. Necrosis may occur in one or more papillae. When the necrotic tissue sloughs, the concave inner border of the medulla remains and may gradually be covered by epithelium. This defect produces a characteristic ring shadow on retrograde pyelography.

Microscopically, the papillary tissue is most often completely necrotic, but if the necrosis is incomplete, the epithelial lining of the collecting ducts of Bellini may be preserved. At the zone of demarcation, a heavy infiltration of polymorphonuclear leukocytes may be found. Under certain circumstances, no inflammatory response occurs, yet the demarcation is sharp.

Etiology. The cause of papillary necrosis is poorly understood. It was once thought to be caused by pyelonephritis,

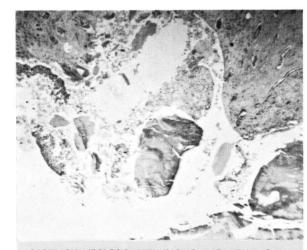

PAPILLARY NECROSIS WITH SLOUGHING, LEAVING A CONCAVE INNER BORDER OF THE MEDULLA. DETACHED DEAD FRAGMENTS CAN BE FOUND IN THE URINE

PAPILLARY NECROSIS WITHOUT INFLAMMATORY REACTION: BELIEVED BY SOME TO BE CHARACTERISTIC OF ANALGESIC PAPILLARY NECROSIS

but more recent evidence indicates that papillary necrosis may be found in patients who do not have pyelonephritis. Thus, the role that pyelonephritis plays in the pathogenesis is uncertain. Moreover, the assumption that papillary necrosis is the result of ischemia has never been substantiated adequately.

In recent years, our concept of the pathogenesis of papillary necrosis has changed significantly. Whereas papillary necrosis had once been observed in only about 0.2 percent of routine autopsies, its frequency has risen sharply in Scandinavia, Switzerland, and Australia and now ranges from one to three percent. Indirect evidence suggests that this increase may be related to an abuse of analgesic drugs. Interstitial nephritis, which is frequently but not always associated with papillary necrosis, was originally thought to be caused by phenacetin. However, more recently it was proposed that analgesics (other than phenacetin) have

a primary necrotizing effect on the papillae (where these drugs are found in high concentration), and that interstitial fibrosis and inflammation in the cortex are sequelae to papillary necrosis. Under these circumstances, an infiltration by polymorphonuclear leukocytes at the zone of demarcation may be absent.

The hypothesis that analgesic drugs—if taken excessively—act primarily on the papillae is attractive. It can be shown experimentally that injections of certain chemical compounds (*e.g.*, 2-bromoethylamine hydrobromide) in optimal doses produce a noninflammatory necrosis of the papillae without any demonstrable effect on the remainder of the kidney or any other organ. However, additional confirmatory data are needed to show whether the chronic interstitial nephritis or pyelonephritis, described as a characteristic manifestation of analgesic abuse, is a sequela of papillary necrosis. □

Renal Carbuncle and Perirenal Abscess

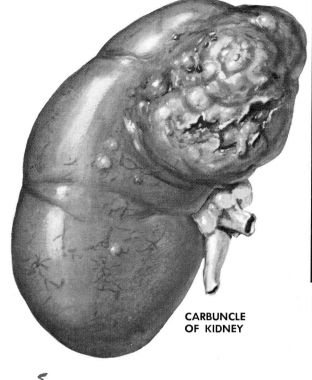

CARBUNCLE OF KIDNEY

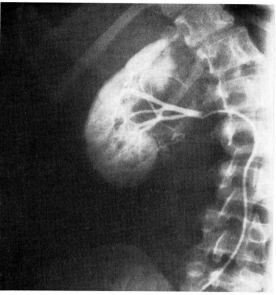

ARTERIOGRAM: NUMEROUS VESSELS AROUND MASS SURROUNDED BY HOMOGENEOUS BLUSH IN UPPER POLE OF KIDNEY, SUGGESTIVE OF INFLAMMATORY PROCESS (CARBUNCLE); ALSO MARKED LUMBAR SCOLIOSIS

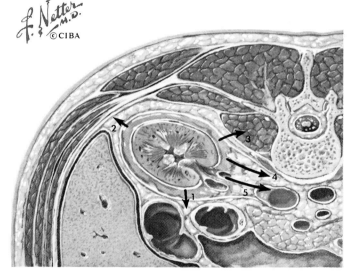

PERIRENAL ABSCESS

ROUTES OF SPREAD:

1 = THROUGH RENAL FASCIA (OF GEROTA) TO RETROPERITONEAL TISSUES; 2 = TO FLANK; 3 = TO PSOAS MUSCLE; 4 = TO MIDLINE (PREVERTEBRAL); 5 = TO INFERIOR VENA CAVA; 6 = TO RETROHEPATIC AND SUBPHRENIC AREAS; 7 = THROUGH DIAPHRAGM TO PLEURAL CAVITY; 8 = TO PELVIC RETROPERITONEAL TISSUES

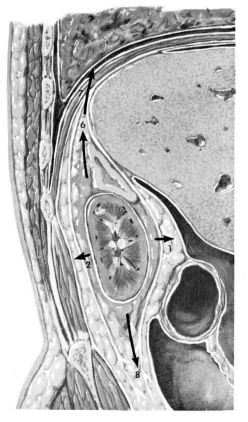

Both renal carbuncle and perirenal abscess are septic conditions which clinically produce unilateral flank pain, chills and fever, and pointed tenderness in the costovertebral angle. Both conditions are often caused by the staphylococcus which reaches the renal or perirenal tissue by either hematogenous or lymphogenous spread. The *primary lesion* is usually a skin furuncle, or some other type of skin infection, the importance of which is not recognized by the patient. It may have appeared months before the onset of the renal or perirenal infection.

A *renal carbuncle* is an abscess in the renal cortex and usually results from the union of several smaller abscesses. The carbuncle may occasionally rupture into the collecting system or it may rupture through the capsule and so cause a perirenal abscess.

A *perirenal abscess* may, as mentioned, arise as a result of rupture of a renal carbuncle, but more often it does not involve the kidney. Instead it is a primary abscess in the perirenal fat inside Gerota's fascia.

Radiologic Findings. In patients who have a perirenal abscess, fluoroscopic examination often shows that the diaphragm is elevated and fixed on the affected side. Also, a roentgenogram may

show that the psoas muscle is obliterated, a feature not found in patients with renal carbuncle. In addition, the X-ray examination will often reveal a scoliosis with the concavity of the curvature toward the affected side. In some patients the presence of a soft tissue mass will suggest the location of the abscess.

Intravenous pyelography, as well as retrograde pyelography, may be important in distinguishing between the two conditions. However, sometimes a cortical abscess will be demonstrated on IVP as an elongation of a major calyx and thus be confused with a neoplasm (see page 205). If a cortical abscess has ruptured, there may be an extravasation of the radiopaque medium. In such a case, the degree of perinephritis can be judged by the lack of ptosis of the involved kidney. In addition, the normal movement of the kidney caused by respiration or a change from the recumbent to the upright position may be decreased or completely absent. These

findings indicate an inflammatory condition in the perinephric fat, especially if there has been extension through Gerota's fascia.

Laboratory Findings. Both renal carbuncle and perirenal abscess usually produce a very high blood leukocyte count. Microscopically, the urine is within normal limits in the majority of patients in whom the infection is secondary to hematogenous spread. However, a renal abscess may originate in a pyelonephritic kidney and this may also spread to form a perinephric abscess; in these patients, especially if there are renal calculi causing partial obstruction, the urine will be infected.

Treatment. Drainage of an abscess at the earliest possible time is indicated. If external drainage is not established, rupture of the abscess may occur with spread of the infectious material in several directions, as shown in the illustration. □

Tuberculosis of the Urinary Tract

Tuberculosis of the urinary tract occurs more frequently in males and has a peak incidence between ages 30 and 50. In countries where bovine tuberculosis has been adequately controlled, renal tuberculosis is usually a complication of the pulmonary form. The tubercle bacilli are hematogenously disseminated throughout the body and frequently lodge in the kidney, a fact which is not surprising since the kidneys receive approximately 25 percent of the cardiac output.

It follows that the disease usually affects both kidneys, although the degree of involvement may be greater on one side. However, the reason why tuberculous lesions commonly develop in the upper pole of a kidney is less well understood.

Involvement of the urinary tract, including the prostate, seminal vesicle, vas deferens, epididymis, and testis, is almost always secondary to tuberculous infection of the kidney.

The renal manifestations of tuberculosis vary enormously, depending upon the virulence of the infecting organism and the defense mechanism of the host. As previously indicated, the infecting organism is usually the human type in countries where milk and dairy controls are strict, but the bovine type is prevalent in many other parts of the world. Regardless of whether the infection is bovine or human, the renal lesions appear to be identical and may be predominantly nodular, fibrotic with severe scarring, or caseous and cavernous like those in the lung. Calcification is not uncommonly found in older lesions. As the disease progresses, irregular cavities may appear in the renal tissue. In addition, hydronephrosis or perirenal abscess may be encountered.

If the bacilli dislodge into the urinary collecting system, the ureters and bladder are exposed and may become secondarily involved. Tuberculous ureteritis causes fibrosis and scarring which produce a shortening of the ureter. This shortening causes retraction of the ureteral orifice, and the so-called golf hole appearance may be recognized on cystoscopic examination. Involvement of the bladder results in ulceration and fibrosis of the wall and decreases the capacity of the bladder.

Clinical Findings. Renal tuberculosis often produces only vague symptoms. If there is involvement of the urinary tract, particularly the bladder, the first symptoms noted by the patient may be urgency, burning, and tenesmus. Often, however, urinary tract tuberculosis first becomes manifest years after the appearance of a primary renal lesion. Nevertheless, it is important to search for possible renal involvement whenever tuberculosis is diagnosed in any organ in the body. In fact, in patients with miliary tuberculosis, a large number will have urine cultures positive for tubercle bacilli. Many male patients

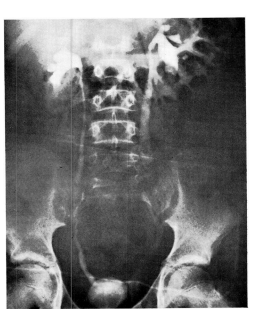

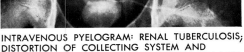

INTRAVENOUS PYELOGRAM: RENAL TUBERCULOSIS; DISTORTION OF COLLECTING SYSTEM AND DILATATION OF URETER, MOST MARKED ON LEFT

TUBERCULOSIS OF KIDNEY INVOLVING PELVIS AND URETER

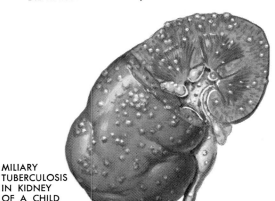

MILIARY TUBERCULOSIS IN KIDNEY OF A CHILD

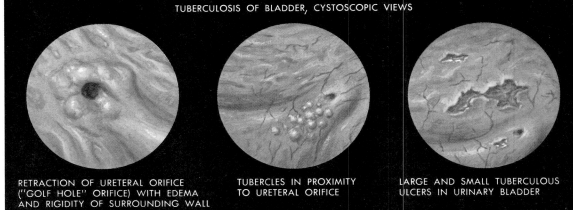

TUBERCULOSIS OF BLADDER, CYSTOSCOPIC VIEWS

RETRACTION OF URETERAL ORIFICE ("GOLF HOLE" ORIFICE) WITH EDEMA AND RIGIDITY OF SURROUNDING WALL

TUBERCLES IN PROXIMITY TO URETERAL ORIFICE

LARGE AND SMALL TUBERCULOUS ULCERS IN URINARY BLADDER

with urinary tract tuberculosis present with complaints referable to tuberculous epididymitis (see CIBA COLLECTION, Vol. 2, pages 50 and 83).

Hematuria is common and deserves special mention. Whenever hematuria and pyuria are found on standard microscopic examination and there is no evidence of bacteriuria, one should have a high degree of suspicion that urinary tract tuberculosis is present. A diligent search should then be made for acid-fast bacteria in the urine. However, urinary tract infection caused by the usual urinary pathogens is also common in patients with urinary tract tuberculosis, especially in advanced cases. The gram negative organisms appear as secondary invaders and are difficult to eradicate unless the primary disease is corrected. Therefore, hematuria, whether occurring as a silent symptom or associated with dysuria, should always be considered an indication for thorough urologic evaluation. Before

one can consider hematuria a harmless coincidence, the existence of urinary tract tuberculosis or neoplastic disease (see page 206) or other serious renal or urinary tract abnormality should be excluded (see page 73).

In the investigation of patients with urinary tract tuberculosis, calcification within the kidney may be observed on X-ray. Intravenous urography or retrograde pyelography often shows a loss of cupping of the calyces, especially of the upper ones, and a typical "moth-eaten" appearance. In advanced cases, radiologic findings of hydronephrosis (see page 186) or perirenal abscess (see page 195) may also be found.

Since chemotherapy is highly effective, surgery is rarely indicated today in the treatment of urinary tract tuberculosis. Nevertheless, certain advanced cases, particularly those with secondary infections, may need surgical intervention. □

Echinococcus Disease

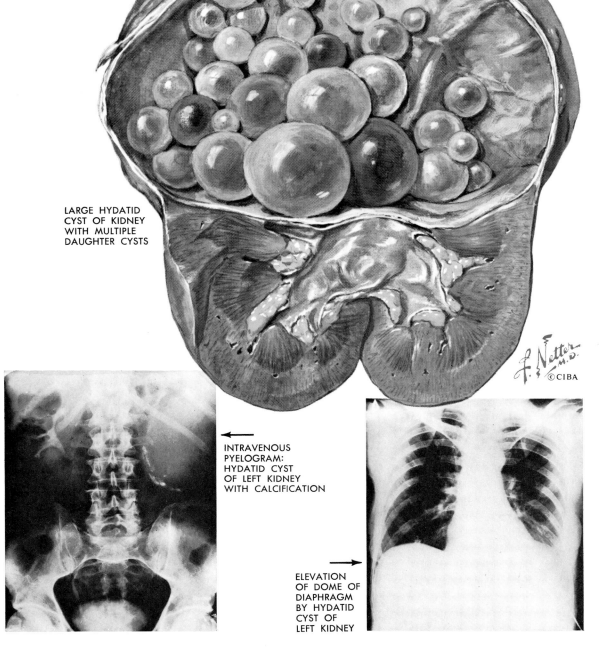

LARGE HYDATID CYST OF KIDNEY WITH MULTIPLE DAUGHTER CYSTS

INTRAVENOUS PYELOGRAM: HYDATID CYST OF LEFT KIDNEY WITH CALCIFICATION

ELEVATION OF DOME OF DIAPHRAGM BY HYDATID CYST OF LEFT KIDNEY

The *Taenia echinococcus,* or *Echinococcus granulosus,* is a tapeworm. However, it is of small size, reaching only 3 to 5 mm in length in the adult stage. It lives in the small intestines of dogs and other canines which become infected either by eating the scolices-containing viscera of other animals, mainly sheep, or by drinking contaminated water.

In the canine intestine, the scolices develop into adult taeniae. Each tapeworm consists of a head, a short neck, and only a few segments, of which the terminal (third) proglottis contains as many as 500 ova. These are excreted in the feces and are subsequently ingested by the *larval* or *intermediate host.* Sheep, cattle, hogs, and man thus become infected.

In the intestine of an intermediate host, the larvae hatch from the ova and migrate to the liver. The liver is the most frequently infected organ, but some larvae pass through it and infect other organs, including those of the genitourinary system. The kidney is involved in about two percent of infections.

When a larva reaches an organ, it develops into a *hydatid cyst* consisting of an outer dense fibrous shell (the result of an inflammatory reaction in the host organ), a middle layer composed mainly of elastic tissue, and an inner germinal layer. The middle layer is a membrane which serves the purpose of protecting and nourishing the scolices within the cyst, and thus this tissue is foreign to the host. The germinal layer gives rise to the embryonal scolices, either directly or after formation of invaginations (brood capsules) which eventually become *endogenous daughter cysts.* Following continuous invagination and development of successive generations of daughter cysts, the original cyst is filled with hundreds of daughter cysts of various sizes.

Daughter cysts may also be seen as outpouchings of the wall of the main cyst or in the surrounding tissues. Occasionally, they are implanted in the peritoneal lining of the mesentery or, at other times, on the calyx or renal pelvis. This latter implantation occurs chiefly in adults, probably only after the disease is contracted in childhood.

Echinococcus infection occurs most frequently in sheep-raising countries, without regard for climatic conditions. In the United States, dogs are rarely infected, and the disease is seen primarily in previously infected immigrants.

Clinically, the symptoms produced by echinococcus disease of the kidney are related to the size of the cyst or to the occurrence of infection or rupture. As the cyst enlarges in the renal area, a dull ache or mild pain and a sense of abdominal fullness may be experienced in the flank or lumbar region of the affected side. If the cyst is large enough to compress other organs, clinical symptoms related to compromised function in these organs may appear. Continued enlargement of the hydatid cyst in the kidney compresses the adjacent renal tissue and eventually erodes the wall of a calyx or the renal pelvis itself. Rupture is then likely and, once this occurs, will produce a fistula between the cyst and the urinary passage. A sharp, stabbing pain in the flank, accompanied by hematuria, usually signals such rupture and is followed by colicky pain as the scolices and cellular debris pass down the ureter.

The continued presence of a fistula between the urinary passage and the cyst will eventually lead to infection of the cyst which may then progress to a renal abscess. At this point, surgical removal is imperative, for otherwise the prognosis is grave.

Diagnostically, the finding of hydatid material in the urine establishes the presence of the disease. In the absence of such findings, however, the radiologic signs are quite important, but these will vary with the size of the cyst and the presence or absence of a fistula between the cyst and the calyces or pelvis. It is not always possible to differentiate a hydatid cyst from other cystic conditions or new growths within the renal tissue. Intradermal and complement fixation tests may be helpful diagnostically.

Surgical removal of the infected kidney is the accepted treatment, since, if untouched, hydatid cysts will practically destroy the whole kidney. The surgical procedure may be tedious, and great care must be taken to prevent spilling the contents of the cyst into the open wound. Following removal of the cyst, the complement fixation test eventually becomes negative. If it is negative 1 year following surgery, the patient may be considered cured. □

Urinary Schistosomiasis

LIFE CYCLE OF SCHISTOSOMA HAEMATOBIUM

SCHISTOSOMULA DEVELOP INTO MALE AND FEMALE ADULT WORMS IN PORTAL AND MESENTERIC VEINS

SCHISTOSOMULA MIGRATE VIA HEART TO PORTAL VEIN

WORMS COPULATE AND MIGRATE TO VESICAL VEINS; EGGS ARE DEPOSITED HERE IN GREAT NUMBERS AND ARE EXTRUDED THROUGH BLADDER MUCOSA

MIRACIDIA ENTER SNAILS AND UNDERGO CYCLE

EGGS HATCH, RELEASING MIRACIDIA IN WATER

EGGS PASSED IN URINE

CERCARIAE PENETRATE UNBROKEN SKIN OR MUCOUS MEMBRANES BY MEANS OF ENZYMATIC SECRETIONS OF CEPHALIC GLANDS

CERCARIAE EMERGE FROM SNAILS

GEOGRAPHIC DISTRIBUTION OF SCHISTOSOMIASIS

SCHISTOSOMA HAEMATOBIUM

SCHISTOSOMA MANSONI

SCHISTOSOMA HAEMATOBIUM AND MANSONI

SCHISTOSOMA JAPONICUM

Urinary schistosomiasis results from infection by the blood fluke *Schistosoma haematobium*. Other human parasites of this genus of trematodes include *S. mansoni* and *S. japonicum*, which cause intestinal schistosomiasis.

S. haematobium is found throughout much of Africa and the Middle East and on Madagascar and Mauritius. It is probable that the species referred to as *S. haematobium* is, in fact, a composite of several morphologically similar forms. *S. mansoni* occurs in parts of Africa and the Middle East, on some Caribbean islands, and throughout much of the northern and eastern areas of South America. *S. japonicum* is distributed in areas of China and on the islands of Japan, the Philippines, and the Celebes.

The life cycles of the schistosomes are generally similar, requiring *waterborne* transmission of infection between man and snail. An infected man contaminates freshwater canals and streams with egg-laden urine *(S. haematobium)* or feces *(S. mansoni* or *S. japonicum)*. Eggs hatch immediately to release *miracidia,* free-swimming *larval forms* which, within 16 to 32 hours, must locate and penetrate appropriate snail hosts.

Inside the snail, each miracidium transforms into a *sporocyst stage,* within which *cercariae* develop over a 6-week period. One miracidium may give rise asexually to many thousands of cercariae, which emigrate from the snail host into water and have about 3 days in which to find a human host.

The cercariae penetrate normal human skin or mucous membrane by both mechanical action and enzymatic secretions of the cephalic glands. Migration of these *schistosomula* (developmental stage) takes place through the lymphatic and circulatory systems, via the heart, to the portal vein, where they mature into adult and female worms. These then mate and travel to the vesical *(S. haematobium)* or mesenteric *(S. mansoni* and *S. japonicum)* veins, to commence egg laying. Eggs first appear in urine or stools at 4 to 9 weeks after initial infection.

Nature of Infection. The infection is chronic, as the worms have been known to live for 20 or 30 years. Repeated reinfection is common in areas in which water sources are heavily infested. Disease in the human host is produced by the presence of the eggs, not of the worms. Female worms, residing in venules, extrude eggs through vessel walls and mucosa into the bladder or intestinal lumen. Eggs cause irritation and microhemorrhage of the mucosa during extrusion. However, the more important process results from eggs

remaining in tissues or embolizing to liver and lungs. Local egg deposition is the more important pathologic process in *S. haematobium* infection and results in urinary tract abnormalities. However, in *S. mansoni* and *S. japonicum* infections, the major morbidity arises because eggs impact in the portal tracts, causing liver disease.

Initially, granulomatous reactions take place around schistosome eggs, producing *pseudotubercles.* The eggs of *S. haematobium* have a remarkable tendency to calcify, leading, at times, to calcification of the entire bladder. The progression of all lesions is toward a later fibrotic stage, which is frequently associated with anatomic distortion of the genitourinary tract.

The consequences of *S. haematobium* infection are probably a result of the described pathologic progression. Granulomatous and fibrotic changes lead to ureteral stenosis, incompetence of the ureterovesical

Urinary Schistosomiasis

Continued

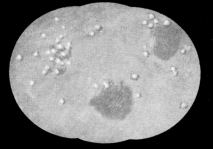

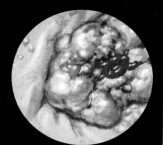

SCHISTOSOMIASIS OF THE URINARY BLADDER

SCHISTOSOMAL TUBERCLES AND NONSPECIFIC PATCHES OF EDEMA AND CONGESTION

SCHISTOSOMAL PAPILLOMAS AND TUBERCLES

NODULAR CARCINOMA IN A SCHISTOSOMAL BLADDER

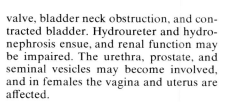

"END-STAGE" SCHISTOSOMAL BLADDER: FIBROSIS AND CALCIFICATION OF THE BLADDER WALL, NUMEROUS PAPILLOMAS AND NODULES, SANDY PATCHES WITH PALE YELLOW AVASCULAR APPEARANCE, CHRONIC ULCERS, ENCRUSTATION, BLADDER NECK AND LEFT URETERAL ORIFICE OBSTRUCTED

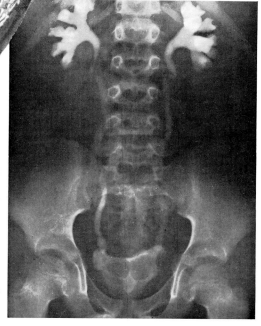

PLAIN FILM DEMONSTRATING CALCIFICATION OF THE BLADDER

INTRAVENOUS PYELOGRAM: BLADDER FILLING DEFECTS, HYDROURETER, AND HYDRONEPHROSIS

valve, bladder neck obstruction, and contracted bladder. Hydroureter and hydronephrosis ensue, and renal function may be impaired. The urethra, prostate, and seminal vesicles may become involved, and in females the vagina and uterus are affected.

Diagnosis is made by finding terminally spined eggs of *S. haematobium* in urine, or observing typical abnormalities by cystoscopy or intravenous urography. Early lesions of the bladder include mucosal hyperemia and edema, tubercles, nodules, and polyps and may be seen through the cystoscope. Chronic changes frequently observed are mucosal pallor and granularity, sandy patches, chronic ulcers, and bladder neck contracture. Typical urographic abnormalities include bladder calcification, filling defects of the bladder, ureteral stenosis, hydroureter, and hydronephrosis.

Clinically, the infection can be divided into acute and chronic phases. Local skin erythema and itching may follow cercarial penetration. From 4 to 6 weeks later, febrile and toxic illness may occur, accompanied by eosinophilia and other allergic phenomena. This phase tends to resolve spontaneously, although egg laying by the adult worms continues.

The chronic illness appears after months or years and is chiefly a result of lesions caused by the eggs. It is marked by intermittent terminal hematuria and dysuria. Bladder or renal colic is common. However, symptoms are not incapacitating, and the disease may progress rather silently to bilateral obstructive uropathy with abnormalities of renal function and eventually uremia and death.

Tubular function, particularly maximal urinary concentrating ability, is affected first. Glomerular function remains normal until late in the course of the disease. Superimposed bacterial urinary tract infection probably plays a significant role in the production of advanced impairment of renal function.

In several countries of North Africa and the Middle East, particularly Egypt, it is claimed that squamous cell carcinoma of the bladder is associated with vesical schistosomiasis. In fact, a high prevalence of bladder cancer is noted in certain of these countries.

The most serious manifestations of urinary schistosomiasis are seen in Egypt, where the disease is endemic and the intensity of infection is probably great. Many other parts of Africa and the Mediterranean area have endemic foci, and perhaps 200 million people are infected. In some areas, young patients are as frequently and as severely affected as adults.

It is probable that considerable morbidity and mortality are a result of urinary schistosomiasis in certain developing countries, but good public health data are lacking. Frequently, patients in such countries are malnourished and are infected concomitantly with other helminths and protozoa which cause further difficulty in estimating the significance of urinary schistosomiasis.

Treatment generally employs trivalent antimony compounds, of which intravenous potassium antimony tartrate (tartar emetic) is the most successful. The use of such drugs is time-consuming, and drug reactions are frequent. Experience with the nonmetallic, oral drug niridazole promises good results in young patients with urinary schistosomiasis.

Problems of education, sanitation, and snail eradication have not yet been solved but are crucial to the control of schistosomiasis. □

Urinary Tract Calculi

Urinary calculi have plagued mankind for at least six or seven thousand years. There is a recorded case of a urinary tract calculus found in a mummy in Egypt which dated to 4800 B.C. Analysis of this stone disclosed that it had a nucleus of uric acid with layers of calcium phosphate, calcium carbonate, and magnesium ammonium phosphate.

Even today, in spite of sophisticated research technics and an expanded understanding of disease processes, urinary calculi are a major problem. In recent years, an average of one in every 1,000 residents in the United States has been hospitalized for urinary stones. Some authorities have recorded the incidence of renal stones at autopsy as slightly more than one percent. Other authors claim a figure as high as five percent, but this figure includes small, insignificant calculi. In only about 0.4 percent of cases were renal calculi responsible for death, either directly or indirectly.

No age group is spared, and calculi can be found in children. Nevertheless, the prime age group in which calculi occur is between 20 and 55 years of age.

Etiology

A clearly defined etiology for urinary calculi has not yet been established. So-called geographic "stone belts" have been described, and unquestionably there are areas in the world where the incidence of urinary calculi is high. Apart from such "stone belts," hot climates also favor stone formation. This is especially true in people who are exposed for the first time to an environment in which insensible water loss is high. If fluid intake is not adequate in these circumstances, urine output is apt to be curtailed; the urine is thus more concentrated, and precipitation of dissolved salts is more likely.

Most stones originate in the kidney and are composed of a framework of an organic matrix which, in the majority of cases, contains variable mixtures of calcium oxalate, calcium phosphate, or magnesium ammonium phosphate. Occasionally stones contain uric acid or cystine. Calculi may also have a uric acid or cystine core around which there are layers of calcium oxalate. At other times, there is a central core of calcium phosphate surrounded by layers of magnesium ammonium phosphate.

Certain metabolic diseases are associated with the formation of particular types of calculi. Thus, in patients with cystinuria there is impaired renal tubular absorption of the amino acids cystine, lysine, arginine, ornithine, and homocystine. Since cystine is relatively insoluble, it tends to precipitate in the urinary tract and form calculi. Similarly, in the hereditary disease *glycinuria,* glycine stones may be formed.

In the rare condition *hyperoxaluria,* calcium oxalate stones may occur, but it must be pointed out that most patients

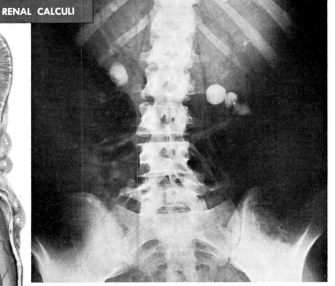

PLAIN FILM: MULTIPLE RENAL CALCULI

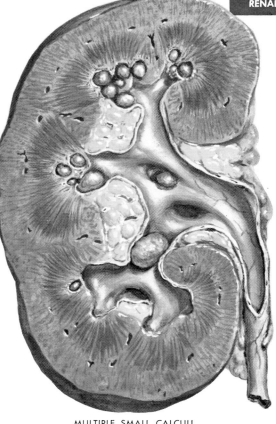

MULTIPLE SMALL CALCULI

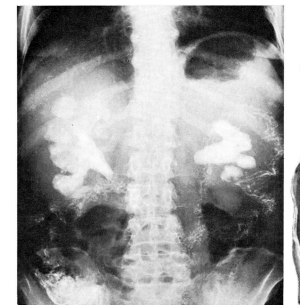

BILATERAL STAGHORN CALCULI

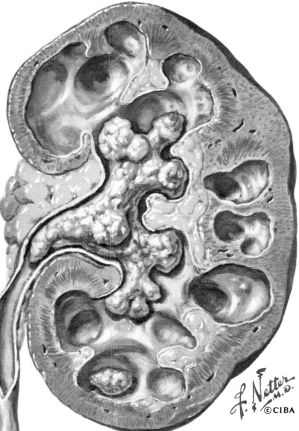

STAGHORN CALCULUS PLUS SMALLER STONE

who form calcium oxalate stones do not excrete excessive amounts of oxalate.

The formation of radiolucent uric acid stones in an acid urine in patients who have gout is well known; gouty patients often pass so-called urinary "gravel" or "sand" consisting of multiple small uric acid stones. Nevertheless, most patients with urate calculi do not have hyperuricemia or increased urinary excretion of uric acid. Instead, for some unknown reason, these patients who form uric acid calculi have an increased tendency to excrete an extremely acid urine; from this acid urine the uric acid, which is present in normal concentration, readily precipitates.

In many patients who form calcium stones, there is an increased urinary excretion of calcium. This may result from a variety of causes such as hyperparathyroidism, milk-alkali syndrome, excessive vitamin D intake, and certain bone diseases. In other patients, an abnormally high urinary excretion of calcium exists for no known reason. Nevertheless, in most patients who have recurrent formation of calculi, urinary excretion of calcium and phosphorus is normal.

The presence of urinary tract infection is undoubtedly a factor in the formation of calculi, especially if the infection is caused by urea-splitting organisms. If urinary stasis and hydronephrosis are also present, the chances of calculi formation are increased. Conversely, a calculus may produce obstruction and urinary stasis which thus predispose to infection (see page 185).

Irrespective that the presence of certain conditions as described above provides the rational explanation for the occurrence of stones in some patients, it is important to remember that not all people with these conditions form stones. Moreover, in approximately half the patients who develop calculi, no predisposing factor can be found. It is therefore logical to ask why this

Urinary Tract Calculi
Continued

is the case. At the present time no answer is forthcoming. Obviously an interdisciplinary approach may be required before the etiology can be established.

There is agreement that whatever the basic pathologic condition which leads to the formation of calculi, a high urine volume will dilute any substances apt to be precipitated and so will decrease the likelihood of calculi formation.

Renal Calculi

Renal calculi may be solitary or multiple and may either remain in the pelvis of the kidney or pass down the ureter. A calculus which remains in the kidney may grow to a large size and eventually form a cast of the entire calyceal and pelvic collecting system — the so-called staghorn calculus.

Damage to the renal parenchyma may occur because either the size of the calculus creates pressure necrosis or the location of the calculus produces obstruction with resulting hydronephrosis. As noted before, infection is more likely to occur if there is urinary stasis, and this in turn may accelerate destruction of the renal parenchyma. At the same time, urinary tract obstruction, either with or without infection, is a factor in the further development of the calculus. Thus, the removal of a stone which is producing obstruction and urinary stasis is most important.

Clinically, symptoms may be entirely absent. Unless there is obstruction of the ureteropelvic junction, pain is rarely a symptom of a renal calculus. However, vague abdominal or flank pain may be complained of chronically. If the calculus is radiopaque, it may be discovered during the course of radiographic examination of the abdomen for unrelated reasons. Sometimes, the patient will present with symptoms related to obstruction or infection. At other times, passage of the calculus into the ureter may cause symptoms typical of renal colic (see below). Hematuria, either gross or microscopic, is a common accompaniment of renal calculi. If obstruction and infection are present, pyuria may also be observed.

Treatment. It should be emphasized that the general therapeutic rule of achieving a dilute urine by means of adequate hydration applies in the prevention of all urinary calculi regardless of etiology (see below). Small calculi formed of either uric acid or cystine, which are precipitated in an acid urine, may be dissolved by alkalizing the urine. Additionally, the use of allopurinol may be of value in decreasing both serum and urinary uric acid levels. Similarly, the use of *d*-penicillamine appears to be promising in increasing the solubility of cystine by forming a cystine-penicillamine disulfide which is more soluble than cystine alone.

If infection is present, as either a primary or a secondary factor, appropriate therapy is of the greatest importance, and the infecting organism should be eradi-

STONE REMOVED VIA INCISION IN LATERAL MARGIN OF KIDNEY POLE; RENAL VASCULAR PEDICLE COMPRESSED BY BULLDOG CLAMP TO CONTROL BLEEDING

KIDNEY SPLIT AND WIDELY LAID OPEN FOR REMOVAL OF MULTIPLE STONES

STONE REMOVED VIA INCISION IN RENAL PELVIS

cated. However, bacteriologic cure usually cannot be expected to occur without the removal of the calculus.

Surgical treatment is required for stones which are too large to pass spontaneously and which cannot be reduced in size. Such calculi are usually composed of calcium oxalate, calcium phosphate, or magnesium ammonium phosphate mixed with calcium oxalate, but they also incorporate matrix calculi.

If removal through the pelvis and renal hilus is not feasible, incisions into the renal parenchyma may be required to remove large renal calculi and staghorn calculi. However, if stones are primarily located in one pole of a kidney, removal of this portion of the organ, together with the calculus or calculi, is often the more desirable approach. If a stone is trapped in a calyx, it can often be removed by a nephrotomy in which the calyx is exposed. This is a preferable method for removal of the calculus, since attempted removal via the

renal pelvis will often injure the infundibulum and lead to scarring and postoperative obstruction. A calculus present in the renal pelvis may be removed by a pyelotomy incision. If calculi are present in the calyces as well as in the renal pelvis, a combination of the described maneuvers is usually performed.

Ureteral Calculi

Occasionally, calculi are formed in the ureter, usually as a result of urinary stasis secondary to conditions such as ureterocele, diverticula, or other congenital or acquired abnormalities. More often, however, a ureteral calculus is formed in the kidney and moves into the ureter, where it may cause obstruction or may pass to the bladder, depending on its size and surface texture. If a ureteral calculus causes obstruction, severe colicky pain usually results. In fact, as noted previously, this is often the method by *Continued on page 202*

Urinary Tract Calculi

Continued from page 201

which a renal calculus becomes clinically manifest. However, if renal function is depressed so that the urinary pressure proximal to the calculus is inadequate and little or no distention of the ureter occurs, colicky pain will not be a feature. Thus, it is important to recognize that even bilateral obstruction secondary to ureteral calculi may occur with little or no pain in patients with bilateral chronic renal disease. The occurrence of anuria without pain may thus indicate bilateral obstruction or obstruction to the outflow from a solitary kidney. In such patients, it is important to rule out obstruction by a carefully taken history and possibly by the use of radiologic examinations or retrograde catheterization.

In the patient with normal renal function, ureteral and renal colic can be extremely severe. The pain is felt in the renal and ureteral area of the affected side and comes in waves. With upper urinary tract calculi, nausea and vomiting may also be present. If the calculus is in the lower two thirds of the ureter, the pain may radiate into the scrotum (or labial region) and along the inner aspect of the thigh, as illustrated. Gross or microscopic hematuria may be observed, and if infection is also present, there usually will be pyuria. Urgency and frequency often occur concomitantly, particularly if there is associated infection or if the stone is near the ureterovesical junction.

On radiologic examination, a radiopaque calculus can usually be detected on a plain film of the abdomen, but an intravenous pyelogram with delayed films and oblique views is necessary to locate the exact area of obstruction. If such examinations fail to reveal the exact site of either a calculus or obstruction in patients presenting with symptoms of ureteral colic, a retrograde pyelogram can provide additional information.

With pure uric acid stones, which are radiolucent, it may be possible to locate the point of obstruction but impossible to tell the cause of the obstruction. In such instances, the passage of a ureteral catheter, the tip of which has been dipped in wax, can be very helpful. When the ureteral catheter is withdrawn, examination with a hand lens will often show a telltale scratch made in the wax by a calculus.

A partial or completely obstructing calculus does not represent an emergency unless infection is present proximal to the site of obstruction, or unless the obstruction occurs in a solitary functioning kidney. Generally, a smooth-surfaced stone with a diameter less than 6 mm will pass spontaneously with no permanent damage to an uninfected kidney or ureter, even if complete obstruction continues for as long as 5 to 10 days. However, if the stone has a rough surface, or is larger than considered feasible for spontaneous passage, or is associated with infection proximal to the obstruction, or is obstructing

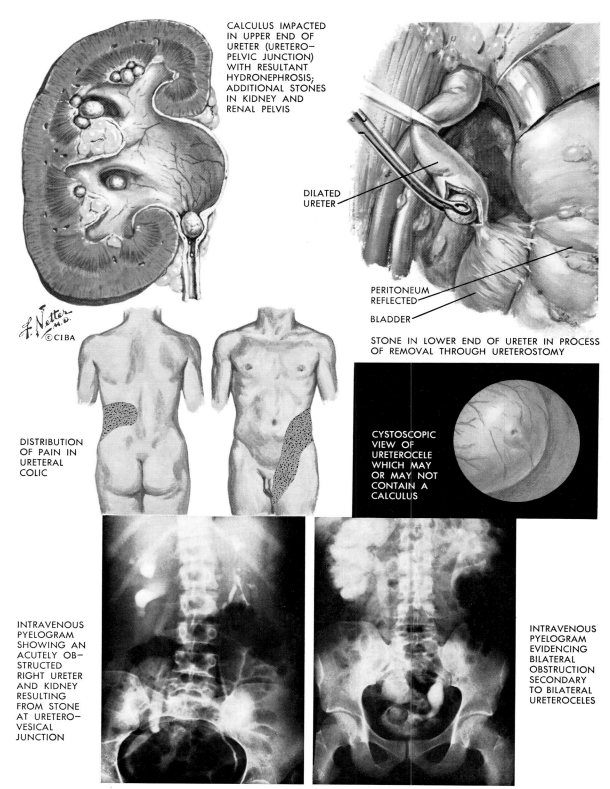

CALCULUS IMPACTED IN UPPER END OF URETER (URETERO–PELVIC JUNCTION) WITH RESULTANT HYDRONEPHROSIS; ADDITIONAL STONES IN KIDNEY AND RENAL PELVIS

DILATED URETER

PERITONEUM REFLECTED

BLADDER

STONE IN LOWER END OF URETER IN PROCESS OF REMOVAL THROUGH URETEROSTOMY

DISTRIBUTION OF PAIN IN URETERAL COLIC

CYSTOSCOPIC VIEW OF URETEROCELE WHICH MAY OR MAY NOT CONTAIN A CALCULUS

INTRAVENOUS PYELOGRAM SHOWING AN ACUTELY OB–STRUCTED RIGHT URETER AND KIDNEY RESULTING FROM STONE AT URETERO–VESICAL JUNCTION

INTRAVENOUS PYELOGRAM EVIDENCING BILATERAL OBSTRUCTION SECONDARY TO BILATERAL URETEROCELES

the outflow from a solitary kidney, surgical removal as soon as possible is indicated.

Not infrequently in patients with renal papillary necrosis (see page 194), a renal papilla is passed and occasionally causes ureteral obstruction with symptoms indistinguishable from those of a ureteral calculus. Since the very nature of renal papillary necrosis most often is a fulminating infection, it is extremely important that the obstruction be released promptly. (A renal papilla obstructing a ureter will have the exact same effect as a stone obstructing the ureter of an infected kidney.) It may be sufficient to pass a ureteral catheter and bypass the obstruction. Vigorous therapy of the accompanying pyelonephritis should be instituted simultaneously. If upon removal of the ureteral catheter 4 or 5 days later the sloughed papilla is not passed and obstruction still persists, surgical removal is necessary. Most often, however, a necrotic papilla will

pass into the bladder and can often be ultimately recovered in the urine.

Vesical Calculi

Most bladder calculi represent stones which are formed in the kidney and passed to the bladder but which are not excreted during micturition. Frequently, there is also lower urinary tract obstruction, caused by conditions such as benign prostatic hypertrophy or urethral stricture, which aids in the retention of the stones in the bladder. However, bladder stones may also form in diverticula (see page 218) and around foreign bodies (see page 219). The calculi may be solitary or multiple and occasionally may become quite large.

Today, in the western world, bladder calculi are relatively uncommon, found primarily in the elderly male. However, in Europe just over 100 years ago,

Urinary Tract Calculi

Continued

stones in the bladder were extremely frequent. Bladder calculi still afflict a large percentage of the population in India and China, and in these countries bladder calculi are frequently found in children in association with renal calculi.

The symptoms associated with vesical calculi depend to a great extent upon the degree of the accompanying cystitis as well as the physical characteristics of the stone, *i.e.,* whether it is rough or smooth surfaced. In most instances symptoms are those of an accompanying cystitis (see page 187), and hematuria is frequently observed.

Diagnosis of bladder calculi may be made by radiologic examination. Most calculi will be detected provided they are large enough and are not composed primarily of uric acid which would make them radiolucent. Confirmation of the diagnosis should be made by cystoscopic examination.

Surgical removal is essential since treatment of the accompanying cystitis is useless unless the bladder calculi are first removed. Removal may be carried out endoscopically or through a suprapubic incision as illustrated. The calculus can be crushed with a lithotrite provided that it is not too large and the bladder capacity is ample enough. Otherwise, injury to the bladder wall and perforation may occur.

Prevention and Treatment

The importance of adequate hydration in the prevention of urinary calculi, regardless of etiology, has been mentioned before (see page 200) but cannot be overemphasized. Yet, many patients with calculi who have been instructed to maintain a high fluid intake are found to have a urine which is concentrated. Apparently it is difficult for patients to understand what is meant by such nonspecific instructions. Particularly in hot climates where insensible water loss is high despite seemingly adequate fluid intake, an inadequate urine volume often occurs. As a result, urine solutes such as calcium, uric acid, or cystine fail to remain in solution.

It is more practical to insist that a patient have a high urine volume, since it is easier for the patient to check urine output than it is to check fluid intake. Importantly, it is wise to remember that during the night, urine concentration is usually greatest. From a therapeutic point of view, the patient should drink extra fluids late at night. If nocturia results (once or twice per night), it is a good sign that fluid intake is adequate. A patient should also be instructed to have water at the bedside. This water can be taken at the time the patient arises to urinate. Thus, an adequate volume of dilute urine is assured for the remainder of the night. A high urine volume means at least 2 and preferably 3 or 4 liters per 24 hours.

Beyond achieving a high urine volume to dilute whatever solute is apt to be pre-

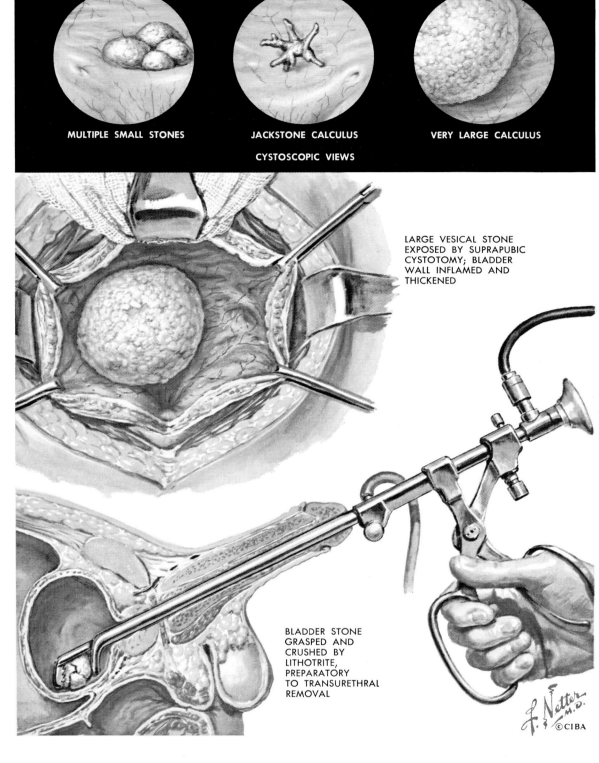

MULTIPLE SMALL STONES **JACKSTONE CALCULUS** **VERY LARGE CALCULUS**

CYSTOSCOPIC VIEWS

LARGE VESICAL STONE EXPOSED BY SUPRAPUBIC CYSTOTOMY; BLADDER WALL INFLAMED AND THICKENED

BLADDER STONE GRASPED AND CRUSHED BY LITHOTRITE, PREPARATORY TO TRANSURETHRAL REMOVAL

cipitated, prevention of recurring urinary calculi centers around a knowledge of the chemical composition of the stones. Using this knowledge, one can attempt to achieve a urinary pH which will provide the highest degree of solubility for the particular substance. In addition, any metabolic defects should be corrected if at all possible. Removal of existing stones which act as nidi for further calculi formation is also important.

Indwelling Catheters. Special mention should be made of patients who are required to have indwelling catheters for even short periods of time. These patients are prone to infection with urea-splitting organisms and to the development of calculi secondary to incrustations on the indwelling catheter. Such incrustations can be prevented if proper and adequate nursing care procedures are instituted. A high urine volume must be maintained, and the catheter should

be changed relatively frequently. In addition, regular bladder irrigation with a buffered acid solution in order to dissolve small calcium-containing plaques is important.

It can be readily appreciated that calcified plaques dislodged from an indwelling catheter may act as foreign bodies within the bladder. Just as importantly, retained pieces of rubber from a ruptured balloon of a catheter may act as nidi for the formation of calculi. Thus, if an indwelling Foley or similar type catheter is inadvertently expelled because of a collapse of the balloon, it must be inspected to ensure that no pieces are missing.

In many male patients, a more satisfactory way to maintain long-term drainage of the bladder is the use of a suprapubic tube. However, the cautions and statements which apply to indwelling catheters apply also to suprapubic tubes. □

Sponge Kidney

Sponge kidney was first described more than 60 years ago as an incidental finding in four patients who had died of nonrenal causes. In the last 30 years, several hundred additional cases have been reported, mostly as a result of urologic radiography. Fewer than 10 percent of the diagnoses were verified histologically.

As far as can be ascertained, *sponge kidney* is entirely asymptomatic unless accompanied by the passage of stones or the presence of obstruction or infection. Renal function in uncomplicated cases is generally normal, although inability to acidify the urine maximally has been reported, as have both defective ammonium excretion and hypercalciuria. Of the reported cases, about two thirds were in the 30- to 60-year age range with no apparent racial, familial, or sexual preponderance.

Moderate enlargement of one or both kidneys occurs in about one third of patients. In most cases, *radiopaque calculi*, varying in size from being barely visible to a diameter of 5 mm or more, and in number from a solitary stone to hundreds, are seen on plain films. On intravenous urography, *cavities* are the first structures filled with contrast medium and appear more distinct if pressure is applied to the ureter. The cavities may appear as greatly dilated collecting tubules and may be rounded, oval, triangular, or irregularly shaped and contain calculi.

The cavities are invariably confined to the pyramids, mainly in the papillary portion and practically never extending to the corticomedullary junction. There may be involvement of only a single pyramid of one kidney or of every pyramid of both kidneys. The involved pyramids and corresponding calyces are commonly enlarged. The lesions generally remain unaltered over long periods, but the number and size of calculi increase.

Retrograde pyelography seldom reveals as many cavities as intravenous urography. However, when calculi have eroded into a calyx, cysts may be demonstrated on retrograde studies. Cavities not visible on urography may be seen on retrograde study, suggesting that they open into a calyx but are no longer connected to functioning nephrons.

Ekström and his associates have reported on 44 patients, the largest single series, many studied for a prolonged period of time. Silent hematuria, either gross or microscopic, occurred in eight patients and acute renal colic in 25. Seven patients presented with urinary tract infection and four were asymptomatic, diagnosis being made incidentally.

The gross and microscopic appearance of the kidney in uncomplicated cases is characteristic. The pyramids, to which the lesions are limited, are paler than normal and irregularly demarcated. The papillary region contains varying numbers of cavities ranging from barely visible to 7 to 8 mm in diameter. These contain material which may be clear to opaque, and liquid, jellylike, or grumous. Frequently, there are also smoothly surfaced, pale yellow to black calculi in the cavities. In the absence of secondary infection, the pelvic and calyceal mucosae are normal.

Microscopically, both dilatation of col-

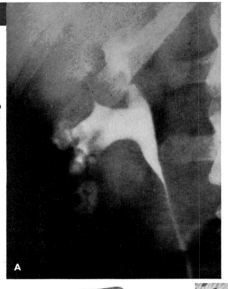

A: INTRAVENOUS PYELOGRAM SHOWING OPACIFIED AREAS OF VARIOUS SHAPES AND SIZES ADJACENT TO CALYCES; PLAIN FILM HAD REVEALED A NUMBER OF CALCULI IN THESE AREAS

B: RETROGRADE PYELOGRAM: MOST OF THE SPACES SHOWN IN "A" ARE NOT FILLED

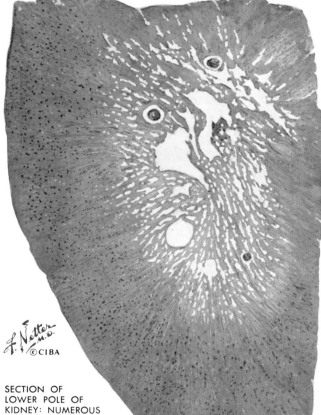

SECTION OF LOWER POLE OF KIDNEY: NUMEROUS CYSTS AND CLEFTLIKE DILATATIONS OF TUBULES IN THE PYRAMIDS; CALCULI IN SOME OF THE CYSTS; THE CORTEX APPEARS RELATIVELY NORMAL

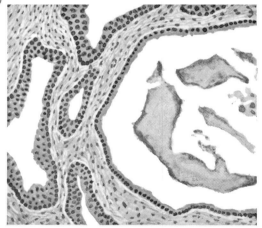

COLLECTING TUBULE LINED BY COLUMNAR EPITHELIUM THREE OR MORE LAYERS DEEP; PROLIFERATION OF INTERSTITIAL TISSUE

CYST CONTAINING BLUISH STAINED MATERIAL (CALCIUM?) LINED BY SINGLE LAYER OF CUBOIDAL EPITHELIUM AND DILATED TUBULES WITH MULTILAYERED EPITHELIUM

lecting ducts and rounded or irregularly shaped cysts are seen. In some instances, connection with tubules or calyces is obvious, but in others, the cysts appear to be isolated. The cysts may contain desquamated cells, precipitated calcium salts, or solid calculi. The dilated tubules may be lined with more or less normal appearing cells or with several layers of cuboidal or columnar epithelium of transitional type.

The cortex ordinarily shows no abnormalities unless there has been concomitant infection. However, the interstitial tissue in the affected areas is infiltrated with round cells and occasionally with eosinophils, even in the absence of infection.

Most of the difficulties encountered by patients with sponge kidney are secondary to calculus formation, but there is no known way to prevent this. The treatment of impacted stones and of urinary tract infection does not differ from the therapy of these conditions in the

absence of sponge kidney. Occasionally, in patients who recurrently pass stones and in whom the condition is limited to one pole or to one kidney, surgical excision of one pole or one kidney has been employed. If massive hematuria occurs, blood transfusion may be required but nephrectomy has not been necessary.

In contrast to the situation in patients with the uremic form of medullary cystic disease (see page 229), the prognosis is good. In 21 of 44 patients followed by Ekström *et al.* from 5 to 15 years, there were no deaths from renal failure. In five patients, recurring stone passage, hydronephrosis from obstruction, and recurring pyelonephritis led to renal functional impairment.

Four patients, subjected to unilateral nephrectomy, developed serious disease in the remaining kidney. Thus conservatism and the avoidance of unnecessary instrumentation would appear to be the watchwords of treatment. □

Benign Renal Tumors

Benign tumors of the kidney are important clinically because they may mimic malignant tumors or present a problem in the differential diagnosis of a renal cyst (see pages 227 and 228), but otherwise they are of little or no consequence. They may arise from the renal parenchyma, the capsule, or the renal pelvis. The latter will be considered separately (see page 208).

Renal adenomas are usually small nodules which cause no symptoms but are found incidentally at autopsy. They occur in older patients, and not infrequently the kidneys in which they arise show evidence of chronic pyelonephritis or arteriosclerosis. Occasionally, a large, single adenoma may be found.

These tumors often grow within small cysts and are usually papillomatous structures. They may also be tubular or alveolar in structure, and different structural types can be found within the same tumor or in different areas in the same kidney. The growth pattern is regular, and anaplasia is absent.

The cells of adenomas are usually cuboidal and show well-differentiated morphologic features. Vacuoles are frequent and these apparently contain either lipids or cholesterol. The alveolar type of adenoma may be difficult to distinguish from a renal adenocarcinoma, and indeed, both tumors may be present in the same kidney. Also, the alveolar type of adenoma is suspected of a tendency to degenerate into adenocarcinoma and probably should be considered premalignant if large enough to diagnose by radiologic means.

The papillary type of renal adenoma is usually considered benign, but if it is incised, the contents will often spill into the wound and thus give a false impression of a malignant tumor. Papillary cyst adenomas are usually small but may occasionally become large enough to produce clinical symptoms.

Connective tissue tumors which arise in the kidney include fibroma, lipoma, myoma, and hemangioma. The small tumor found most often in the medulla is a *fibroma*. However, this tumor may also originate in the peripheral areas of the cortex. It rarely attains a large size. *Lipomas* rarely occur in the renal parenchyma. However, renal sinus lipomatosis, which represents an excessive accumulation of adipose tissue within the renal sinus, may be confused with either polycystic disease (see page 227) or neoplasm on intravenous urography. *Myomas* are also rare tumors usually first discovered at autopsy. They may be difficult to distinguish from fibromas. However, myomas have a tendency to undergo malignant change.

Hemangioma may occur surrounding the base of a pyramid or at the apex of a pyramid, immediately deep to the mu-

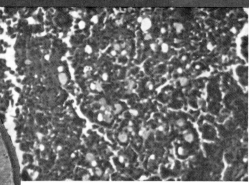

ADENOMA OF KIDNEY

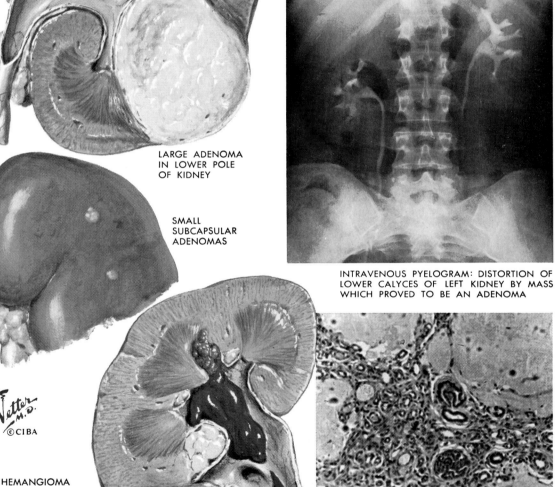

LARGE ADENOMA IN LOWER POLE OF KIDNEY

SMALL SUBCAPSULAR ADENOMAS

INTRAVENOUS PYELOGRAM: DISTORTION OF LOWER CALYCES OF LEFT KIDNEY BY MASS WHICH PROVED TO BE AN ADENOMA

HEMANGIOMA WITH HEMORRHAGE (CLOT) IN CALYCES AND PELVIS

HAMARTOMA OF KIDNEY

cous membrane of a calyx. This tumor is usually solitary but occasionally may be multiple. The clinical importance of a hemangioma results from the common occurrence of gross hematuria, which may be severe enough to necessitate nephrectomy. It is questionable if a hemangioma represents a true tumor or instead is a conglomeration of small, thin-walled blood vessels which have formed secondary to tissue repair because of trauma or infection. Regardless of their true origin, however, hemangiomas are difficult to diagnose because they are often too small to produce visible changes on either intravenous urograms or angiograms. Therefore, in any patient with hematuria which cannot be otherwise explained, it is wise to rule out various nonrenal causes for hematuria (such as sickle cell disease or bleeding abnormalities) before the diagnosis of hemangioma is made and before surgery is performed (see page 75).

Angiomyolipoma (hamartoma) is a mesenchymal tumor composed of blood vessels, fat, and muscles. (The term hamartoma implies a tumorlike overdevelopment of various tissue elements normally found at a particular site, but in abnormal proportions and without evidence of active growth.) This tumor is important because of its tendency to bleed. If it is large enough, massive retroperitoneal hemorrhage may occur. Hamartomas are often associated with the rare congenital disorder called *tuberous sclerosis,* and about 50 percent of patients with this condition have kidney hamartomas.

Renal capsule tumors are similar to the tumors of the same cell type which arise from the parenchyma. Thus, it is often difficult to tell whether a fibroma or myoma arose from the renal capsule or from the renal parenchyma. These types of tumors are of no particular pathologic importance. □

Malignant Tumors of the Kidney

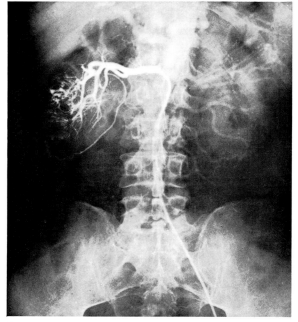

SELECTIVE RIGHT RENAL ARTERIOGRAM SHOWING TYPICAL TUMOR VESSEL PATTERN CHARACTERISTIC OF ADENOCARCINOMA (HYPERNEPHROMA)

ADENOCARCINOMA OF UPPER POLE OF KIDNEY WITH DISTORTION OF COLLECTING SYSTEM

EXTENSIVE ADENO—CARCINOMA OF KIDNEY INVADING RENAL VEIN AND INFERIOR VENA CAVA

Malignant tumors of the kidney may arise from the parenchyma, the pelvis, or the capsule, or they may be metastatic. The latter include lymphoma, leukemia, myeloma, Hodgkin's disease, reticulum cell sarcoma, and primary malignancies of the lungs, breasts, or stomach. Usually, metastatic tumors affect both kidneys, but if only one kidney is involved, metastatic lesions may be mistaken for primary renal neoplasms.

Fibrosarcoma, myosarcoma, liposarcoma, and angioendothelioma are rare tumors which may originate in the renal capsule or the renal parenchyma. Malignant tumors of the renal collecting system and ureters, and nephroblastoma (Wilms' tumor) require special mention (see pages 208 and 212).

Renal Adenocarcinoma

The most common renal neoplasm, representing about three fourths of all renal malignancies, is *adenocarcinoma*. This tumor is known by a variety of names such as hypernephroma, granular cell carcinoma, clear cell carcinoma, renal cell carcinoma, and alveolar cell carcinoma. The term adenocarcinoma thus includes all malignant epithelial renal tumors of parenchymal origin.

Adenocarcinoma most commonly occurs after the age of 50 and is only very rarely encountered in children. It affects males twice as often as females. This tumor may be bilateral but more often is unilateral and solitary; it may arise from either pole or from the central area of the kidney.

The neoplasm is usually encapsulated, firm, and solid. Occasionally it may undergo necrosis—an occurrence which may make diagnosis difficult. The cells may be granular, clear, or anaplastic. Occasionally various cell types are intermixed in any one tumor, while in other tumors only one cell type predominates. (The similarity of the cells of a clear cell carcinoma to the cells in the suprarenal cortex is the reason for the original name given to this tumor—hypernephroma.)

Clinically, there are few, if any, early symptoms. Often complaints referable to metastases first bring the patient to the physician. A *mass* in the flank may be palpable but usually not until late in the course of the disease. *Microscopic* or *gross hematuria* may signal invasion into the collecting system and is an early sign in over half the patients. Pain is uncommon unless secondary to ureteral obstruction caused by blood clots. However, there may be a dull ache in the flank. *Fever,* the cause of which has not been explained, is usually a bad prognostic sign and does not necessarily result from necrosis of the tumor. *Weight loss* is usually a rather late manifestation and often indicates distant metastases.

In two to three percent of patients with carcinoma of the kidney, polycythemia may occur. It may also be found *after removal* of a primary renal tumor and in this latter situation is apparently secondary to erythropoietin production by metastatic lesions.

Radiologically, a renal tumor is usually readily detectable on intravenous urogram. Apart from the appearance of a mass, distortion of the collecting system commonly occurs. In addition, the presence of a tumor is usually readily detectable on a renal scan utilizing either ^{197}Hg- or ^{203}Hg-labeled chlormerodrin or ^{131}I-

Malignant Tumors of the Kidney
Continued

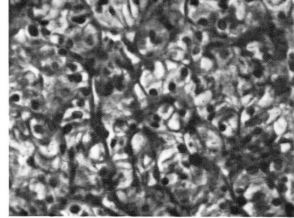

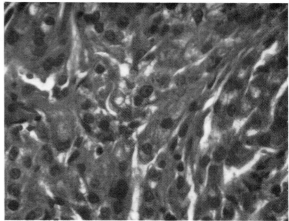

CLEAR CELL ADENOCARCINOMA OF KIDNEY (H. & E.), THIS TYPE OCCASIONALLY REFERRED TO AS "HYPERNEPHROMA"

ADENOCARCINOMA OF KIDNEY COMPOSED OF GRANULAR CELLS RESEMBLING CELLS OF DISTAL TUBULE (H. & E.)

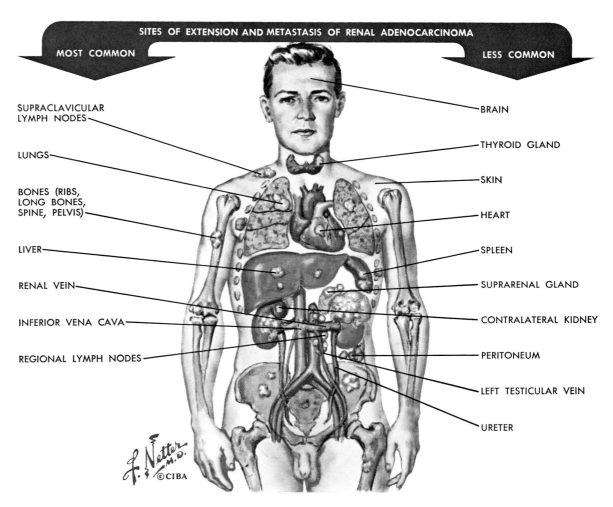

SITES OF EXTENSION AND METASTASIS OF RENAL ADENOCARCINOMA

MOST COMMON

- SUPRACLAVICULAR LYMPH NODES
- LUNGS
- BONES (RIBS, LONG BONES, SPINE, PELVIS)
- LIVER
- RENAL VEIN
- INFERIOR VENA CAVA
- REGIONAL LYMPH NODES

LESS COMMON

- BRAIN
- THYROID GLAND
- SKIN
- HEART
- SPLEEN
- SUPRARENAL GLAND
- CONTRALATERAL KIDNEY
- PERITONEUM
- LEFT TESTICULAR VEIN
- URETER

labeled sodium iodohippurate. The latter isotope requires the use of a scintillation camera (see pages 103-106). On renal scan, a mass in the kidney may show as a "cold" area. An additional technetium scan utilizing a scintillation camera will help differentiate a benign cyst from an adenocarcinoma. If adenocarcinoma is present, there will be prompt appearance of the technetium unless the tumor is necrotic. If the mass is a cyst, the area of lack of filling with technetium will coincide with the demonstrated "cold" spot on the radiohippurate or ^{203}Hg- or ^{197}Hg-labeled chlormerodrin scan.

Additional diagnostic procedures include retrograde pyelography (if complete delineation of the collecting system has not been feasible by intravenous urography), angiography, and nephrotomography. As noted previously (see page 100), angiography, and especially selective angiography, may show the typical appearance of a vascularized tumor with the contrast medium showing the so-called tumor stains caused by pooling in the abnormal vessels of the tumor. The injection of vasoconstrictors provides an additional refinement of angiography by causing vasoconstriction of the normal renal arteries but not the tumor vessels. Thus the diagnostic value of the angiogram is enhanced.

Nephrotomography (see page 98) will often yield valuable information, inasmuch as a cyst will appear as a radiolucent mass while a neoplasm will usually give a dense shadow, often slightly more opacified than the adjacent normal renal parenchyma.

While it is recommended by most urologists that a patient with a renal mass should be surgically explored even though the mass is probably a cyst, in poor-risk patients every effort should be made to improve the preoperative diagnostic accuracy. Unfortunately, the occasional occurrence of a small, solid carcinoma in the wall of a cyst complicates the problem. Nevertheless, the diagnostic accuracy can be improved by percutaneous puncture of a cyst (see page 102) with drainage and collection of fluid. (Such fluid must be subjected to cytologic examination—see page 79.) Contrast material may be injected directly into the cyst to provide additional information. Thus, with good diagnostic workup it should be possible to make an accurate diagnosis in 95 to 98 percent of patients.

Percutaneous biopsy (see page 107) is sometimes suggested but may lead to spread of the tumor into the needle tract. Therefore, the procedure is used infrequently. In contrast, the danger of spreading the tumor by percutaneous kidney puncture with a small, sharp needle is probably of no consequence.

Adenocarcinoma of the kidney often metastasizes via the bloodstream, but lymphatic spread also occurs. (Plate 23 shows the sites at which metastases may occur.) If there is no indication of distant metastases, surgical exploration (with preparation of the patient for radical nephrectomy) should be performed once the diagnosis of a renal cell carcinoma has been established or is considered most likely. However, it is not uncommon to find invasion either of the main renal vein or of its branches. Thus, at the time of surgery it is of utmost importance to open the renal vein and be sure that possible tumor emboli are removed. □

Tumors of the Pelvis and Ureter

Comprising about seven to eight percent of all renal tumors, epithelial neoplasms of the renal collecting system are the most important renal tumors. Histologically, most of these tumors are transitional cell papillomas or transitional cell carcinomas. In rare instances, metastatic tumors may be found. The squamous cell carcinoma is less common, and adenocarcinoma is encountered quite rarely. Transitional cell papilloma is histologically a benign tumor (whether it occurs in the renal pelvis, ureter, or bladder) but must be considered potentially malignant.

Transitional cell tumors of the renal pelvis occur primarily in patients in the older age group, although there are a few cases recorded in children. The incidence is much higher in males, as is also true for ureteral and bladder tumors.

In the majority of cases, transitional cell tumors are papillomatous in structure, may be single or multiple, and are usually unilateral. However, bilateral occurrence has been reported. The tumor may originate in a calyx, the infundibulum, or the pelvis and may seed into the ureter and bladder, often surrounding the ipsilateral ureteral orifice. The tumor may also arise as a primary growth in the ureter, and such a carcinoma usually metastasizes quite early, probably because the wall of the ureter is thin and has an abundant lymphatic supply.

The squamous cell (epidermoid) carcinoma usually appears as a flat, firm lesion which is often ulcerated. It tends to metastasize early and not infrequently invades the renal parenchyma. For this reason it is often considered more malignant than transitional cell tumors. In many cases squamous cell carcinoma is also associated with renal calculi and infection.

Clinical Manifestations. In patients with tumors of the calyx, pelvis, or ureter, symptoms are surprisingly few in the early stages. Pain is not a prominent feature and usually occurs secondary to obstruction and hydronephrosis or may be produced by blood clots passing down the ureter. However, pain occurs more frequently in patients with ureteral tumors since partial obstruction by the tumor is more likely to take place.

Hematuria happens frequently and may be microscopic or gross; at times it may even be profuse. It is usually intermittent and may be associated with renal colic. Since hematuria is such a common symptom of pelvic and ureteral malignancy, its occurrence should always precipitate a thorough investigation to exclude neoplasm anywhere in the urinary tract.

If a patient is suspected of having a urinary tract malignancy, an intravenous pyelogram must be done. However, it is extremely important that complete visualization of the entire collecting system be obtained, since otherwise a small papillary tumor may be missed. A frequent mistake made in failure to diagnose transitional cell carcinoma of the kidney is to misinterpret the intravenous pyelogram

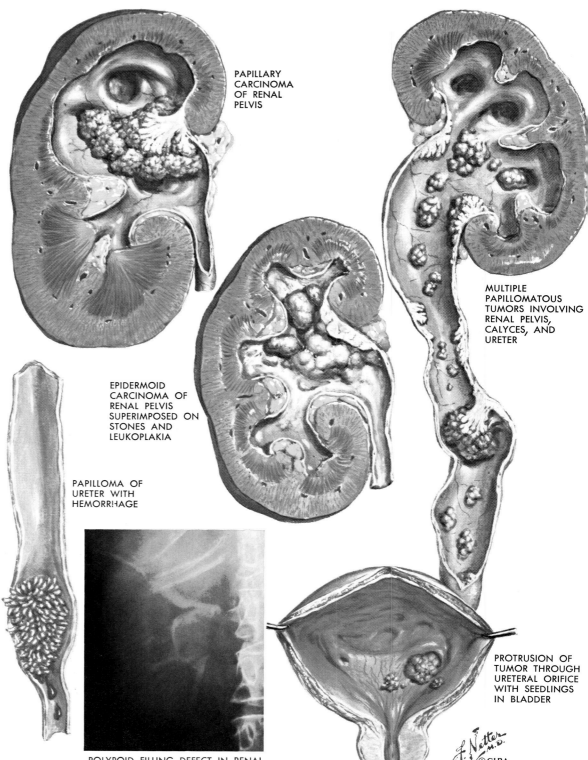

PAPILLARY CARCINOMA OF RENAL PELVIS

MULTIPLE PAPILLOMATOUS TUMORS INVOLVING RENAL PELVIS, CALYCES, AND URETER

EPIDERMOID CARCINOMA OF RENAL PELVIS SUPERIMPOSED ON STONES AND LEUKOPLAKIA

PAPILLOMA OF URETER WITH HEMORRHAGE

PROTRUSION OF TUMOR THROUGH URETERAL ORIFICE WITH SEEDLINGS IN BLADDER

POLYPOID FILLING DEFECT IN RENAL PELVIS DUE TO CARCINOMA

as normal when the procedure was not diagnostically accurate. An intravenous pyelogram should never be considered normal simply because one cannot see any pathologic disfigurations. Rather, the term normal should be applied only to a urogram in which all portions of the collecting system are well outlined and are indeed normal. The use of ureteral compression and the infusion of larger amounts of contrast medium (see page 91) greatly enhance the diagnostic qualities of a pyelogram and should be used whenever any suspicion exists of a renal transitional cell carcinoma. Of course, the intravenous pyelogram should also completely outline each ureter in its entirety in order to rule out the presence of a ureteral tumor.

If complete delineation of the collecting system and ureter cannot be accomplished by intravenous urography, retrograde pyelography should be performed. Since it is mandatory to perform cystoscopy in a pa-

tient with hematuria, retrograde pyelography can be performed at the same time. Also, when the ureteral catheter is in place in the renal pelvis of the suspect kidney, urine can be readily collected and examined for neoplastic cells by the use of the Papanicolaou stain (see page 79). Of course, if tumor cells are discovered in the urine, the procedure will have been invaluable in establishing a positive diagnosis.

Urinary tract carcinomas metastasize to both regional and distant lymph nodes and via the bloodstream to lungs, liver, and bone. Nevertheless, there is no reason to believe that an early carcinoma cannot be cured. However, it is extremely important to make the diagnosis early, particularly with tumors of the ureter, which tend to metastasize even earlier than calyceal or pelvic neoplasms. Prompt, radical surgery should be performed, as soon as possible, providing there is no evidence of metastatic lesions. □

Tumors of the Bladder

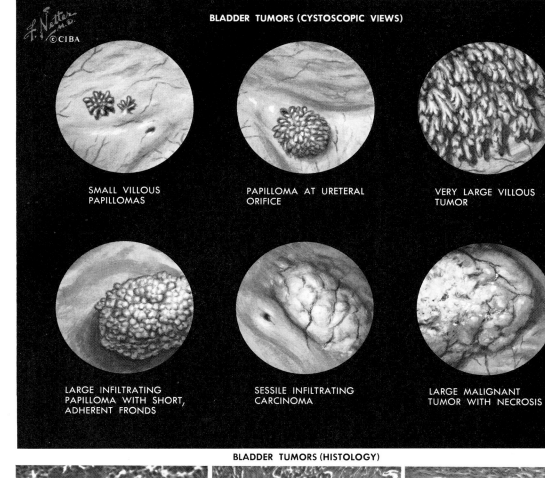

BLADDER TUMORS (CYSTOSCOPIC VIEWS)

SMALL VILLOUS PAPILLOMAS

PAPILLOMA AT URETERAL ORIFICE

VERY LARGE VILLOUS TUMOR

LARGE INFILTRATING PAPILLOMA WITH SHORT, ADHERENT FRONDS

SESSILE INFILTRATING CARCINOMA

LARGE MALIGNANT TUMOR WITH NECROSIS

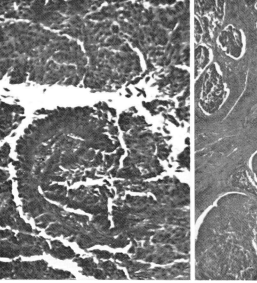

BLADDER TUMORS (HISTOLOGY)

PAPILLARY CARCINOMA

INFILTRATING CARCINOMA

SQUAMOUS CELL CARCINOMA

Most bladder tumors arise from the mucous membrane and, with few exceptions, are of transitional cell type. Benign papillomas (which must be considered premalignant), malignant papillomas (papillary carcinomas), noninvasive sessile carcinomas, and undifferentiated carcinomas may all occur. Squamous cell (epidermoid) carcinomas are occasionally found in areas of leukoplakia. Adenocarcinoma, which occurs rarely, may be mucus-producing. Epithelial mesenchymal tumors are found even more rarely.

As with tumors in the collecting system and ureters, bladder neoplasms occur principally in older adults; males are affected more frequently than females. In 25 percent of cases the lesions are multiple.

Etiology. Vesical neoplasms are of worldwide importance and offer an important research field in the area of the etiology of cancer. It is known, for instance, that certain chemical agents produce bladder tumors, both experimentally in animals and clinically in man; there are well-recognized industrial carcinogens. Similarly, the incidence of bladder carcinoma is higher in areas infected with schistosomiasis, and in the Balkan countries it appears that urinary tract carcinoma is considerably more frequent in patients afflicted with Balkan nephritis (see page 145). Also, cigarette smokers seem to have a higher incidence than non-smokers. In bladder exstrophy (see page 243), adenocarcinoma may occur in conjunction with cystitis glandularis.

An observation which warrants further study is the fact that tumors of the collecting system, ureters, and bladder occur more often in males. This finding may or may not be related to the more frequent occurrence of obstructive uropathy secondary to prostatic disease in the male, or alternatively, it may be related to hormonal factors.

In 1895, Rehn suggested that bladder tumors which occurred in employees of an aniline-manufacturing plant were caused by aniline vapors. This was the first suspected association between a carcinogen and a tumor. It has since been proven, however, that aniline is not the primary carcinogen, but that the true agent is β-naphthylamine. This compound has proven to be carcinogenic in man and certain animals, especially the dog. Workers in the aniline dye industry are excessively exposed.

Since Rehn's original observations, other chemicals have been implicated as the cause of bladder tumors in people who are exposed to them. These exogenous chemicals ultimately appear in the urine as ortho-amino-phenolic compounds. Quite commonly, such carcinogens are conjugated in the liver with sulfuric acid or glucuronic acid, and it has been suggested that liberation of the free carcinogens may take place in the urine as a result of enzymes such as sulfatase and glucuronidase. Furthermore, it has been suggested that such liberation of the free ortho-amino-phenols in the urine will be facilitated if there is a residual urine. Under such circumstances, the exposure time of the conjugant to the enzymes which produce deconjugation would be prolonged.

Several metabolites of the essential amino acid tryptophan are excreted in the urine as ortho-amino-phenolic compounds. Consequently, it has been suggested by Price and others that these metabolites may be responsible for at least some of the spontaneously occurring bladder carcinomas in man. These workers have found that approximately 50 percent of patients with bladder carcinoma excreted increased amounts of ortho-amino-phenolic metabolites after a loading dose of tryptophan was given by mouth.

Recently, the author has suggested that the urinary content of antioxidants may be an important factor in prevention of carcinogenesis. The carcinogens known to produce bladder tumors are inactive if oxygen is not available. Thus, if ascorbic acid is administered in amounts great enough to produce *Continued on page 210*

Tumors of the Bladder

Continued from page 209

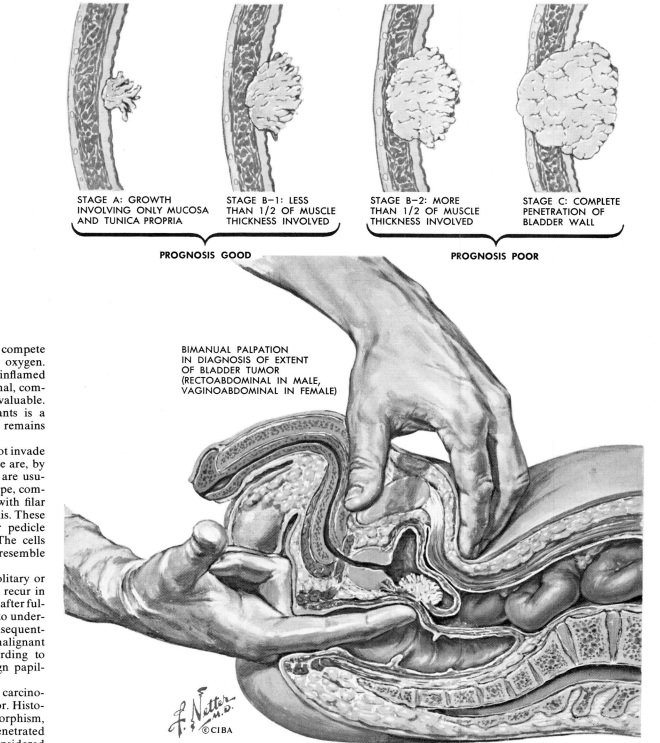

STAGE A: GROWTH INVOLVING ONLY MUCOSA AND TUNICA PROPRIA

STAGE B-1: LESS THAN 1/2 OF MUSCLE THICKNESS INVOLVED

STAGE B-2: MORE THAN 1/2 OF MUSCLE THICKNESS INVOLVED

STAGE C: COMPLETE PENETRATION OF BLADDER WALL

PROGNOSIS GOOD

PROGNOSIS POOR

BIMANUAL PALPATION IN DIAGNOSIS OF EXTENT OF BLADDER TUMOR (RECTOABDOMINAL IN MALE, VAGINOABDOMINAL IN FEMALE)

its excretion in the urine, it will compete with potential carcinogens for oxygen. If oxygen influx through an inflamed bladder wall is in excess of normal, competition for oxygen may be valuable. However, the use of antioxidants is a theoretical consideration which remains unproven.

Pathology. Tumors which do not invade the delicate basement membrane are, by definition, noninfiltrating. They are usually the benign papillomatous type, composed of a central villous tuft with filar projections from the primary axis. These tumors usually have a slender pedicle which may be long or short. The cells coating the villi histologically resemble normal bladder epithelium.

Benign papillomas may be solitary or may occur in clusters and often recur in different locations of the bladder after fulguration. They have a tendency to undergo malignant change and consequently should be considered as premalignant or potentially malignant. According to Jewett's classification, the benign papillomas are considered Stage 0.

The earliest form of bladder carcinoma is a noninvasive, sessile tumor. Histologically, the cells show pleomorphism, but because the tumor has not penetrated the basement membrane, it is considered *carcinoma in situ.* However, once the tumor has penetrated the basement membrane, it must be considered infiltrating regardless of how superficial the degree of penetration.

In Jewett's classification, Stage A indicates an infiltrating tumor which has penetrated into the submucosa but not into the muscle. Stage B-1 indicates superficial muscle invasion and B-2 deep muscle invasion. Stage C denotes penetration through the bladder wall into the perivesical tissues and lymphatics. Stage D is sometimes used to indicate a tumor that has involved regional lymph nodes.

The staging of a tumor is an evaluation based on information derived from the histologic picture as obtained by biopsy, physical examination, intravenous urography to assess possible ureterovesical

junction obstruction, and bimanual examination, illustrated in Plate 26. Staging determines to a great extent the choice of therapy and the prognosis, but tumor grading must also be considered. Grading depends principally on Broders' classification of the degree of malignancy. This is a histologic assessment as to the extent to which the tumor cells have changed from the normal epithelium of the vesical mucosa — the more undifferentiated the cells of the tumor, the more malignant the tumor.

Clinical Features. Most patients who have bladder tumors have gross hematuria, usually lasting throughout all of the period of urination. However, papillary bladder tumors which are situated around the bladder neck will often produce hematuria only at the end of micturition as the bladder contracts to near its smallest size. Symptoms of bladder irritability may be present in some patients, but usually the hematuria is

unaccompanied by either pain or discomfort.

A bladder tumor usually produces a filling defect in a cystogram and intravenous urogram. Nevertheless, cystoscopy, which provides direct visual examination of the bladder mucosa, is mandatory in all patients with hematuria. Even though many women suffer from recurrent cystitis and occasionally from hemorrhagic cystitis, complacency in the evaluation of a patient with hematuria is not justified, and cystoscopic examination should be mandatory. If the index of suspicion about the presence of a bladder tumor is high enough, cystoscopy should be performed under anesthesia since a bimanual examination is an essential part of the evaluation. Moreover, a biopsy can be more readily performed under these circumstances. In performing the biopsy it is important to obtain a section of tissue which includes enough of the bladder wall to assess the possible infiltrating nature of a neo-

Tumors of the Bladder

Continued

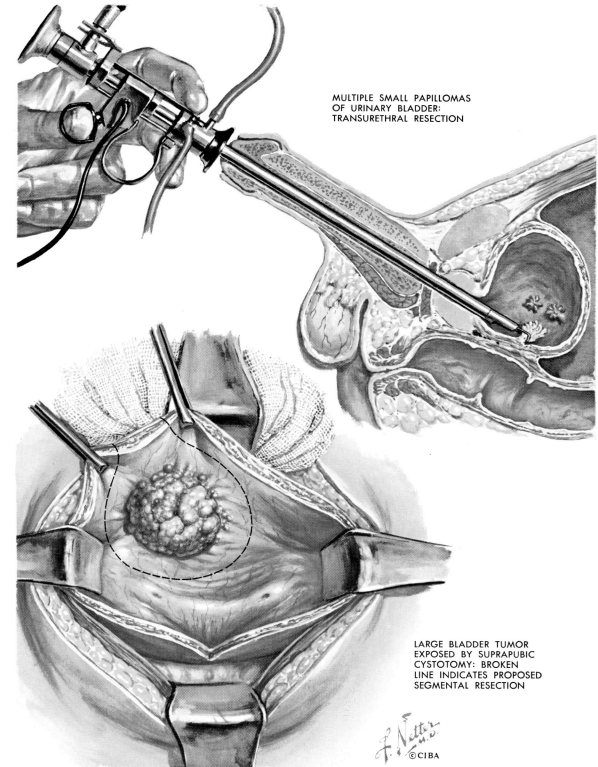

MULTIPLE SMALL PAPILLOMAS
OF URINARY BLADDER:
TRANSURETHRAL RESECTION

LARGE BLADDER TUMOR
EXPOSED BY SUPRAPUBIC
CYSTOTOMY: BROKEN
LINE INDICATES PROPOSED
SEGMENTAL RESECTION

plasm. Also, it should be recognized that many bladder tumors will show a histologic pattern on the surface different from the one that exists deep within the tumor.

Cystoscopic Findings. On cystoscopic examination, a histologically benign papilloma usually appears as a fine villous structure attached to the bladder by a thin, long pedicle. Within this pedicle there is a central core of blood vessels. On the other hand, a papillary carcinoma is usually a denser tumor and has a cauliflower type of appearance. The pedicle is usually short and thick. If the tumor is infiltrating, the surrounding bladder mucosa may look edematous, and in more advanced cases, necrosis with possible incrustation on the surface can be clearly visualized.

The sessile bladder carcinoma usually appears as a brownish, fleshy mass with thick, rounded margins projecting into the bladder. Necrosis of the tumor usually produces a crater in the central portion and calcification may be present in this area. If the tumor has been present for a long period and has diffusely infiltrated the wall, there is decreased bladder capacity. However, if there is also inflammation, the decrease in bladder capacity may be a result of inflammatory changes. In such a situation, the value of anesthesia for cystoscopic examination becomes apparent. Ordinarily, if bladder capacity is decreased because of acute cystitis, it will increase under anesthesia, but if the capacity has been decreased secondary to tumor infiltration, no change will occur with anesthesia.

If the orifice of a ureter is invaded by tumor, with resulting obstruction, the prognosis is bad since there is generally deep infiltration. Moreover, it should be recalled that transitional cell tumors arising in the ureter or upper urinary tract may seed into the bladder, often surrounding the ureteral orifice. Thus, it is important to determine if a bladder tumor has arisen from the upper urinary tract.

Treatment. The treatment of a patient found to have a bladder tumor depends upon the cystoscopic appearance, the histologic grading, the clinical staging as judged by bimanual examination and biopsy, the findings of a metastatic survey, and the patient's general clinical condition.

Noninfiltrating tumors of low grade malignancy can usually be removed adequately by electrocoagulation alone. However, it is important that the patient be checked frequently since recurrence of this type of tumor is the rule.

Infiltrating tumors are usually treated more aggressively depending upon their location. Either a segmental resection of the bladder or total cystectomy with urinary diversion should be employed. In addition, in many medical centers it has become customary to treat infiltrating bladder tumors with cobalt or supervoltage radiation prior to surgery. However, at this time it is too early to judge whether presurgical radiation will improve the prognosis. It is generally agreed that radiation alone, whether external or local, should be re-served as the sole therapy for patients who constitute a poor surgical risk because of their general condition. In some patients such therapy can be curative.

Although information about the possible *prevention* of bladder tumors is inadequate, a number of points are worth considering. Exposure to the known carcinogens should obviously be minimal or eliminated altogether. In addition, obstructive uropathy distal to the bladder neck should be corrected since it will cause a residual urine which appears to be a factor predisposing to bladder tumor formation. (The desirability of treating obstructive uropathy from the point of view of infection and decompensation of the urinary bladder and upper tract has been discussed elsewhere; see page 186.) The value of oral administration of high doses of ascorbic acid in order to achieve a high ascorbic acid concentration in the urine, because of the antioxidant effect, is at present unproven. □

Nephroblastoma (Wilms' Tumor)

A malignant tumor in childhood presenting as a mass in the upper abdomen is usually either a neuroblastoma (see CIBA COLLECTION, Vol. 4, page 231) or a nephroblastoma (Wilms' tumor). Conversely, an upper abdominal mass in an infant or child statistically is more likely to be a benign condition such as ureteropelvic junction obstruction, with or without associated pyelonephritis (see page 233), or multicystic kidney (see page 227).

Neuroblastoma most often originates in the suprarenal medulla but may displace the kidney by its rapid growth and distort the calyces and ureter. Thus, neuroblastoma may be difficult to distinguish from a Wilms' tumor. *Nephroblastoma* contains both epithelial and connective tissue elements with various degrees of cellular differentiation and is thought to arise from the metanephrogenic blastema (see page 30). Comprising six to eight percent of all renal tumors, Wilms' tumor is found primarily in infancy and childhood and occasionally in adults. It is usually unilateral.

Clinical Findings. Often the presence of an abdominal mass is the first indication of disease in the child or infant. However, general malaise, weakness, and failure to gain weight may have been noted, and the older child may complain of pain in the loin or abdomen. In advanced cases, fever, weight loss, anemia, and hypertension may be present. Hematuria is uncommon.

When an upper abdominal mass is found in an infant or child, it becomes a matter of urgency to establish the diagnosis as soon as possible. Even though statistically the mass is probably a benign condition, it should be suspected of being malignant until proven otherwise. Once a diagnosis of Wilms' tumor is considered likely, it is important not to subject the child to further physical examination since palpation of the tumor makes the likelihood of spread of tumor cells by the hematogenous route a real possibility.

Differential Diagnosis. One must differentiate between hydronephrosis (such as occurs in ureteropelvic junction obstruction), multicystic kidney, and nephroblastoma or neuroblastoma. Multicystic kidney does not function and thus does not appear either on a radiohippurate scan or on an intravenous urogram. Palpation of a multicystic kidney often reveals a large, hard mass with an uneven surface. The organ does not transilluminate. A hydronephrotic kidney secondary to ureteropelvic junction obstruction may occasionally show delayed function but usually does not. On palpation it is usually hard, smooth, and, like a Wilms' tumor, ballottable. It may be transilluminated with a strong light source, a feature usually diagnostic of a hydronephrotic kidney.

In contrast to the situation in patients with multicystic kidney or hydronephrotic kidney, malignant tumors such as Wilms' tumor and neuroblastoma do not generally cause complete destruction of the renal parenchyma. However, distortion of the collecting system is common. Thus, intravenous urogram will show a functioning kidney with distortion of the calyceal system, and radiohippurate scan

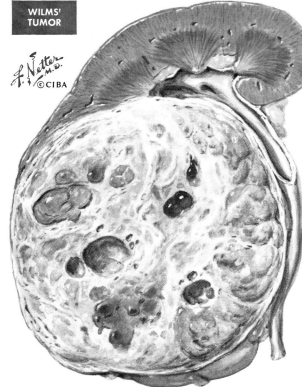

WILMS' TUMOR WITH PSEUDOCAPSULE AND CHARACTERISTIC VARIEGATED STRUCTURE

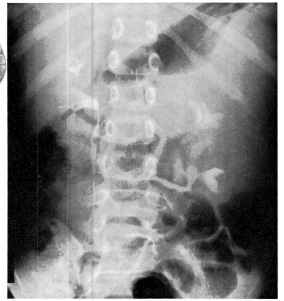

INTRAVENOUS PYELOGRAM: DISTORTION OF COLLECTING SYSTEM OF LEFT KIDNEY BY WILMS' TUMOR IN AN INFANT

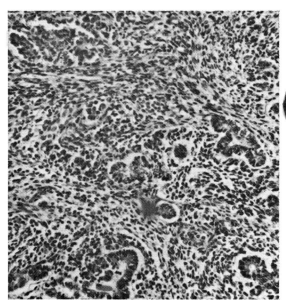

STROMA OF SARCOMALIKE SPINDLE CELLS WITH ISLANDS OF MALIGNANT COLUMNAR CELLS IN IRREGULAR TUBULAR ARRANGEMENTS TYPICAL OF WILMS' TUMOR

CLINICAL FEATURES OF WILMS' TUMOR

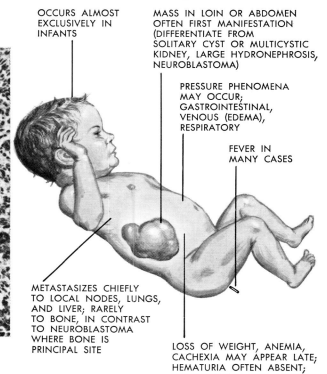

OCCURS ALMOST EXCLUSIVELY IN INFANTS

MASS IN LOIN OR ABDOMEN OFTEN FIRST MANIFESTATION (DIFFERENTIATE FROM SOLITARY CYST OR MULTICYSTIC KIDNEY, LARGE HYDRONEPHROSIS, NEUROBLASTOMA)

PRESSURE PHENOMENA MAY OCCUR; GASTROINTESTINAL, VENOUS (EDEMA), RESPIRATORY

FEVER IN MANY CASES

METASTASIZES CHIEFLY TO LOCAL NODES, LUNGS, AND LIVER; RARELY TO BONE, IN CONTRAST TO NEUROBLASTOMA WHERE BONE IS PRINCIPAL SITE

LOSS OF WEIGHT, ANEMIA, CACHEXIA MAY APPEAR LATE; HEMATURIA OFTEN ABSENT; HYPERTENSION MAY APPEAR

will show a nonradioactive mass replacing a portion of the kidney — findings highly suggestive of a Wilms' tumor. In a few patients, a retrograde pyelogram is necessary to complete the investigation before the presumptive diagnosis of malignancy is made.

Treatment. Since the tumor metastasizes primarily to lungs, liver, and lymph nodes, and less frequently to bones, early treatment of a Wilms' tumor is important. The accepted treatment of the tumor is radical surgical removal at the earliest possible time. However, the need for early treatment does not mean surgical removal of the tumor as an emergency procedure without adequate preoperative diagnostic workup, as is occasionally advocated. This is not acceptable since adequate diagnostic studies are essential before surgery. When one considers that preoperative radiation is sometimes advocated to improve the prognosis of a patient with Wilms' tumor, it is obviously important to establish a proper diagnosis; otherwise, one may radiate a child with a benign lesion such as unilateral hydronephrosis or multicystic kidney.

It is pertinent to mention that the author has developed a technic whereby a radiohippurate scan of even small infants is simplified. The procedure requires an intramuscular injection of radiohippurate mixed with hyaluronidase.

The question of preoperative radiation of Wilms' tumor is as yet unresolved. In general, the prognosis in a patient with nephroblastoma is usually poor, especially if the tumor is found after the age of 2 years, but it remains to be seen whether preoperative radiation will improve the prognosis. For now the accepted treatment is nephrectomy at the earliest possible time followed immediately by radiation and possibly the use of actinomycin D and vincristine intravenously. □

Renal Trauma

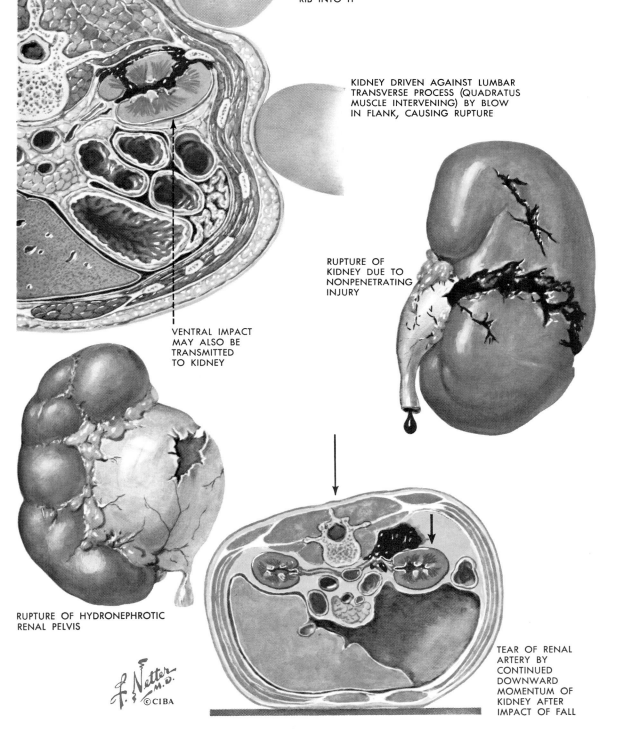

DORSOLATERAL BLUNT IMPACT, RUPTURING KIDNEY BY DRIVING 12th RIB INTO IT

KIDNEY DRIVEN AGAINST LUMBAR TRANSVERSE PROCESS (QUADRATUS MUSCLE INTERVENING) BY BLOW IN FLANK, CAUSING RUPTURE

RUPTURE OF KIDNEY DUE TO NONPENETRATING INJURY

VENTRAL IMPACT MAY ALSO BE TRANSMITTED TO KIDNEY

RUPTURE OF HYDRONEPHROTIC RENAL PELVIS

TEAR OF RENAL ARTERY BY CONTINUED DOWNWARD MOMENTUM OF KIDNEY AFTER IMPACT OF FALL

It is fortunate that the majority of renal injuries are minor bruises which usually heal without sequelae. Depending on the manner in which they occur, renal injuries are classified as either nonpenetrating or penetrating.

Nonpenetrating injuries of the kidney are most often the result of direct injury to the back, the flank, or the abdomen.

A less common but extremely important cause is a fall in which, after the patient has landed, one or both kidneys continue to descend, stretching the renal artery or arteries and sometimes causing an avulsion of a blood vessel.

While a *severe avulsion of the renal artery* leads to the rapid accumulation of a large hematoma and may be fatal in short order, a *less serious avulsion with a resultant thrombosis* can be most subtle in its symptoms, and may, in fact, be recognized only when the kidney's lack of function becomes apparent, often too late to salvage the organ. Early use of angiography is therefore of utmost importance in patients in whom the type of injury suggests renal trauma, if the kidney is to be saved. *Injuries short of avulsion* may also lead to renal artery thrombosis as a result of an intimal tear followed by formation of a subintimal hematoma—a type of injury whose frequency is becoming more appreciated with the increase in early use of angiography.

Fortunately, most renal artery lesions of the stretching-avulsion type are unilateral. (The author has seen only one case of bilateral renal artery thrombosis.) Thus, the less severe forms of the injury are not necessarily life-threatening if eventually recognized.

The majority of renal injuries caused by blunt trauma are compounded by multiple injuries to other organs, a situation quite frequently seen following traffic accidents. The most common type of renal trauma in such cases results from the kidney's being forcibly pushed against a transverse process or being punctured by a fractured twelfth or, occasionally, eleventh rib. The type of laceration encountered can vary from a simple bruising without rupture of the renal capsule to a complete shattering of the renal parenchyma. Renal lacerations most commonly radiate from the hilus, and a complete transection, as shown, is not an unusual finding in severe blunt trauma. Also, since an abnormal kidney, especially a hydronephrotic one, is very susceptible to trauma, it is not uncommon for patients with unsuspected hydronephrosis to sustain a rupture of the renal pelvis as a result of even minor injury to the kidney.

Because renal trauma may or may not involve the urinary collecting system, lack of hematuria does not necessarily assure that kidney injury has not occurred. Also, it should be remembered that a blood clot obstructing the ureter can obscure renal bleeding, and lack of hematuria would not rule out a kidney injury.

With more severe lacerations of the kidney, serious hemorrhage may occur which can cause a state of shock requiring immediate blood transfusion. In such instances, a flank mass is usually present, although a concurrent rupture of the peritoneum may prevent its formation by allowing the blood to leak into the peritoneal cavity.

Penetrating wounds of the kidney are usually caused by knives, bullets, or shrapnel. Since such injuries often involve simultaneous damage to intestines, liver, spleen, or other vital organs, surgical exploration is often essential—especially if there are indications of sustained blood loss or penetrating injury to the intestines. Continued on page 214

Renal Trauma

Continued from page 213

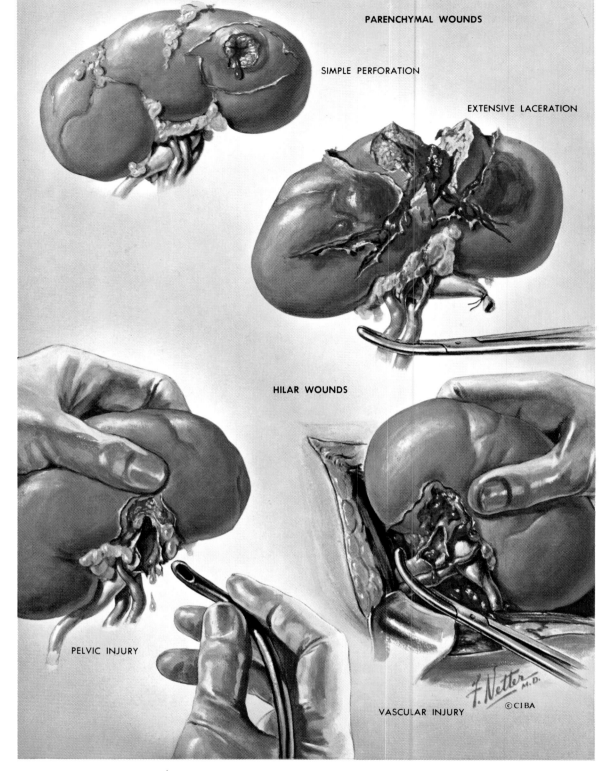

PARENCHYMAL WOUNDS

SIMPLE PERFORATION

EXTENSIVE LACERATION

HILAR WOUNDS

PELVIC INJURY

VASCULAR INJURY

When the patient is in shock, the need for surgical exploration assumes emergency proportions. Nonetheless, an intravenous urogram to evaluate the status of the unaffected kidney should be performed *before* surgical intervention. Such evaluation can prevent decisions leading to procedures that might render a patient anephric.

Evaluation and Management of the Patient. Whenever renal injury is suspected, either by the nature of the trauma and/or by the presence of hematuria, an investigation of the extent and type of kidney injury should be made as early as possible.

If the patient is in shock, vital signs should preferably be stabilized before an evaluation of renal function is made, since reduced kidney function may otherwise merely reflect decreased renal blood flow secondary to shock (see page 111).

If there are no externally obvious injuries and the overriding concern is for intraabdominal lesions, it is probably wise to obtain diagnostic urograms to ascertain the functional status of both kidneys. It should be remembered, however, that a normal intravenous pyelogram does not necessarily rule out lacerations of the renal parenchyma. Conversely, lack of function does not always indicate severe renal injury but certainly constitutes an indication for obtaining an angiogram to clarify underlying pathology.

Scanning procedures, utilizing [197]Hg- or [203]Hg-labeled chlormerodrin or ^{131}I-labeled iodohippurate, are excellent tools for the initial evaluation, and a technetium scan may add further information concerning possible renal artery lesions (see page 104). If such scans are normal, there is little reason to proceed to other diagnostic measures. If they are abnor-

mal, however, intravenous urography, angiography, and possibly even retrograde pyelography are indicated, depending on the patient's general condition.

The major concern in treating penetrating or nonpenetrating trauma of the kidney is first to ascertain whether the patient has two functioning kidneys so that a unilateral nephrectomy can be performed if necessary without endangering the patient's life.

The next consideration is to preserve salvageable kidney function to the greatest extent possible, while at the same time considering possible long-term consequences, especially in regard to hypertension. Secondary scarring which results when the kidney heals itself has been implicated as a not infrequent cause of renal hypertension which may develop at a later date. A conservative surgical approach may prevent such sequelae and lower the morbidity. However, in these cases, it is probably a misconcept to consider "conser-

vative" identical with a "wait-and-see" attitude. "Conservative" should be used to mean whatever approach is considered the one that will preserve the most nephrons without resulting in disease entities such as hypertension which may arise secondary to the trauma.

The arguments concerning indications for surgery will not be discussed here at any length. Even severe renal trauma does not necessarily constitute an indication for surgery, unless lack of stability of vital signs suggests continuous bleeding. However, since angiography, especially in the nephrogram stage (see page 100), can give clear evidence of the degree of parenchymal involvement, the surgeon can, if necessary, promptly remove devitalized portions of the kidney and approximate viable tissue in a primary repair. This course of action will often lead to a decrease in morbidity, a shorter hospital stay, and better return of renal function. □

Ureteral Injuries

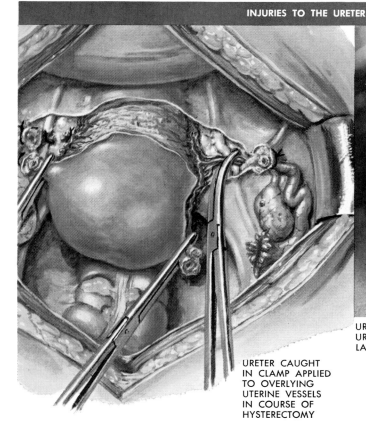

URETER CAUGHT IN CLAMP APPLIED TO OVERLYING UTERINE VESSELS IN COURSE OF HYSTERECTOMY

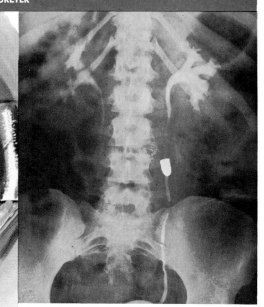

URETERAL INJURY BY GUNSHOT WOUND: IVP; URINARY EXTRAVASATION ABOVE AND LATERAL TO BULLET

IVP; DELAYED FILM: URINARY EXTRAVASATION FROM LEFT URETER INJURED BY CATHETERIZATION

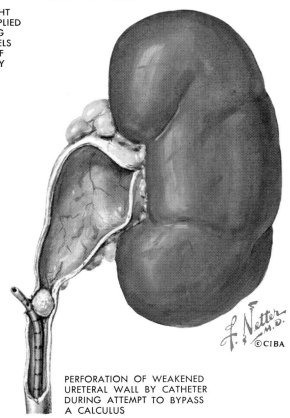

PERFORATION OF WEAKENED URETERAL WALL BY CATHETER DURING ATTEMPT TO BYPASS A CALCULUS

Ureteral injury is most commonly the result of surgery, although it may also be caused by penetrating wounds from knives or firearms.

Surgical injury to the ureter can occur as a result of ureteral catheterization, especially if the ureter is the site of pathologic changes secondary to a stone or neoplasm. Injury can also occur during open surgical procedures, especially in patients who have carcinoma in whom it may be difficult to identify the ureter properly and thus protect this structure from injury. In many major surgical procedures, especially for cancer of the uterus or sigmoid, the anatomic landmarks are so grossly distorted or the ureter so encased in neoplastic mass that injury is virtually unavoidable. (In such complicated surgical cases it may be necessary to pass a ureteral catheter prior to surgery to make the ureter easier to identify. This maneuver will not only help prevent injury but will also assure that, should injury occur, it will be readily recognized.) Ureteral injury can also result from attempted stone removal with baskets or loops.

The most important aspect of treating surgical injury to the ureter is to recognize it *early* so that proper corrective measures can be instituted quickly enough to avoid severe complications. In fact, it is often desirable to perform intravenous urography on patients prior to any abdominal surgery that carries a risk of ureteral injury. Thus, an immediate comparison between postoperative and preoperative status should permit prompt detection of any ureteral injury.

Surgical trauma to the ureter usually results in some degree of obstruction and therefore is easily detectable by intravenous urography, especially with delayed films. The site of obstruction as well as any possible extravasation should be clearly revealed.

Injuries to the ureter caused by a ureteral catheter are usually readily recognized at the time they occur, since adequate X-ray studies are generally part of procedures in which such catheterization is performed.

External Trauma to the Ureter. What has been mentioned in regard to ureteral injury caused by surgical trauma applies equally to ureteral injury resulting from *external trauma*, except that complete transection of the ureter may not result in obstruction. Diagnosis is especially complicated in these latter cases since extravasation of contrast material is likely to be retroperitoneal and difficult to recognize. Delayed films are usually somewhat more successful in revealing the extravasation, especially if larger than normal amounts of radiopaque media are injected.

As with most other aspects of trauma to the urinary tract, it is important to have an adequate awareness of the possible occurrence and possible consequences of ureteral injuries, whether as a result of penetrating trauma or surgical procedures. Because of the difficulty in recognizing the anatomic structures in certain surgical situations, the assistance of available up-to-date technology becomes invaluable in facilitating the surgeon's task and in improving the patient's chances for an uncomplicated surgical procedure. Should ureteral injury occur despite all precautions, however, early recognition followed by prompt corrective measures constitutes the best chance for returning the urinary tract function to normal. □

Trauma to the Bladder

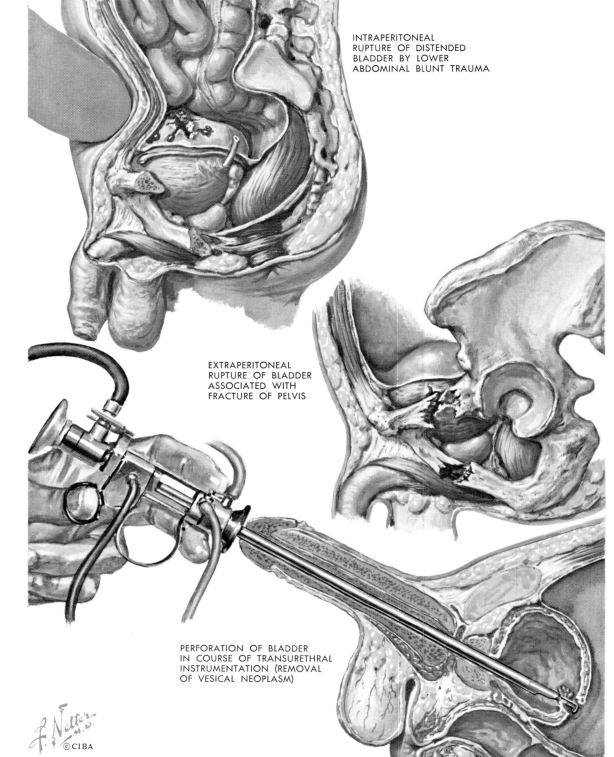

INTRAPERITONEAL
RUPTURE OF DISTENDED
BLADDER BY LOWER
ABDOMINAL BLUNT TRAUMA

EXTRAPERITONEAL
RUPTURE OF BLADDER
ASSOCIATED WITH
FRACTURE OF PELVIS

PERFORATION OF BLADDER
IN COURSE OF TRANSURETHRAL
INSTRUMENTATION (REMOVAL
OF VESICAL NEOPLASM)

Bladder trauma rarely presents any significant problem unless there is actual rupture of the bladder wall with subsequent leakage of urine.

Iatrogenic ruptures of the bladder wall constitute a calculated risk in certain surgical procedures. They can ordinarily be successfully managed if recognized at the time, whether the procedure involves open surgical intervention in the area of the bladder or endoscopic manipulations.

For example, perforation of the bladder wall by resectoscope loop, especially when one is resecting a bladder tumor, is often unavoidable. Nevertheless, unless intraperitoneal leakage of urine results, such injury requires nothing more than to maintain adequate urinary drainage (see below). If the perforation is through the peritoneum-covered portion of the bladder wall, however, and results in leakage of urine into the peritoneal cavity, open suturing of the ruptured bladder wall is necessary in conjunction with evacuation of the extravasated urine from the peritoneal cavity. Then, adequate urinary drainage must be established (see below).

Another potentially dangerous situation, which also lends itself to iatrogenic injury of the bladder wall with possible leakage of infected urine either retroperitoneally or intraperitoneally, is the crushing of stones with a lithotrite in a bladder with a small capacity. Stone crushing should never be undertaken if the bladder capacity is insufficient to allow enough room to operate the instrument easily, for otherwise the risk of injuring the bladder wall is considerable.

Blunt trauma to the lower abdominal area can lead to a rupture of the bladder wall. Even *mild* degrees of trauma will readily rupture a bladder which is dis-

tended. *Severe* trauma may cause rupture of the undistended bladder if the bony pelvis is fractured. Such injury may affect not only the bladder but also the urethra; especially in the male, complete or partial transection of the urethra, usually at the apex of the prostate, in the area of the membranous urethra, may occur.

Penetrating trauma caused by firearms, knives, splinters, or other sharp objects can also rupture the bladder wall. As in injury by blunt trauma, the bladder is much more liable to rupture if it is partially or fully distended than when it is empty and hidden below the bony pelvis.

Whenever bladder injury is suspected, either by history or by physical findings such as shock and hemorrhage, lower abdominal pain, hematuria, or the inability to void following trauma, it is necessary to act without delay. The diagnosis must be estab-

Trauma to the Bladder

Continued

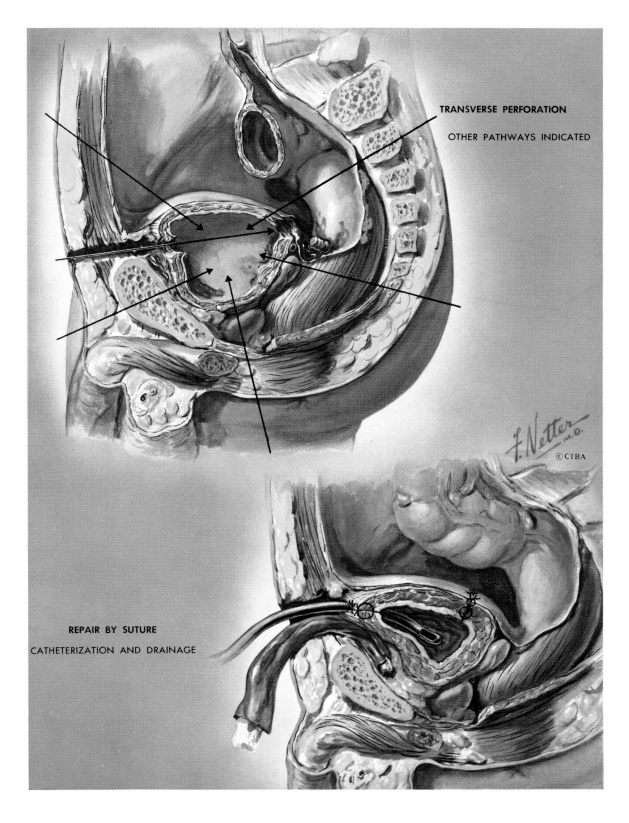

TRANSVERSE PERFORATION

OTHER PATHWAYS INDICATED

REPAIR BY SUTURE

CATHETERIZATION AND DRAINAGE

lished, and corrective measures taken.

An intravenous urogram is always advisable in such cases. It may promptly reveal the correct diagnosis; even if it does not, it will inform the physician about the status of the upper urinary tract.

A urethral catheter should be passed, if possible, to obtain a cystogram. This should clearly demonstrate if extravasation of urine is present and, if it is, should further allow the physician to distinguish between intraperitoneal and retroperitoneal extravasation.

Intraperitoneal extravasation, especially of infected urine, is usually fatal if not dealt with immediately by open surgical exploration, evacuation of urine from the peritoneal cavity, and meticulous closure of the bladder rupture. Adequate urinary drainage is essential. In the male, it is probably wise to drain the urine through a suprapubic cystotomy tube, although in the female, a urethral catheter may serve equally well. If, however, there is any contraindication for the use of a suprapubic tube in a male patient, urethral drainage may be substituted, as long as urinary drainage from the bladder is adequate to keep the bladder empty and so give the repaired bladder a chance to heal.

Retroperitoneal extravasation of urine is not as potentially dangerous as intraperitoneal extravasation, and drainage of the extravasated urine followed by adequate urinary drainage, as described above, may constitute sufficient treatment. When possible, however, it is generally desirable to repair the bladder lesion surgically since this operation will definitely speed up the healing process and decrease the period of time that the patient needs to be incapacitated.

Rupture of the membranous urethra in the male requires primary anastomosis, if possible. If, for any reason, this repair cannot be done, the application of tension to an indwelling catheter may assure approximation of the severed portions of the urethra. Late strictures are very common sequelae to this type of injury and repair, and the patients should be followed carefully for such a possibility.

The prognosis of a patient with a rupture of the bladder wall, whether from iatrogenic sources or from blunt or penetrating trauma, is dependent not only on the type of treatment he or she receives but also on the speed with which it is instituted. If a ruptured bladder is recognized immediately and correctly handled, it usually constitutes a minor problem. If it is not recognized and dealt with properly, however, it may be a fatal disorder. □

Diverticula of the Bladder

Diverticula of the bladder are described separately, even though in most if not all cases they could logically be included in the discussion on obstructive uropathy (see page 185). However, bladder diverticula are of striking appearance on intravenous urograms and are also of diagnostic significance in evaluating the importance of symptoms of lower urinary tract infection. Furthermore, their very presence often constitutes a problem in itself, even after the causative pathology has been corrected. An analogy may be made to urinary tract calculi (see page 201) which are also commonly the result of another disease process such as urinary tract obstruction or infection.

Bladder diverticula start as cellules—small pouches which grow between hypertrophied muscle bundles as a result of bladder outlet obstruction. As obstruction progresses, this beginning decompensation of the detrusor muscle (the external muscle layer of the bladder—see page 22) gradually forms one or more true diverticula of various sizes, occasionally with a diameter larger than that of the bladder itself.

The diverticulum *opening* is usually narrow, the *lumen* covered with uroepithelium, and the *wall* constructed primarily of connective tissue with moderately thin strands of muscle fibers.

Although *congenital diverticula* have been described as separate entities, it is probable that all diverticula are secondary to obstruction, and the congenital aspect is primarily concerned with the fact that the formation of a diverticulum usually occurs in congenitally weak areas of the bladder.

The incidence of bladder diverticula is far greater in men than in women and is usually associated with bladder outlet obstruction resulting from prostatic enlargement.

Cystoscopic examination will not necessarily reveal the presence of a diverticulum since the opening may be so small that it is missed. Thus, in patients with uropathy secondary to bladder outlet obstruction, the performance first of cystography to determine if diverticula are present is mandatory. Retrograde cystography is the best technic for demonstrating bladder diverticula.

If diverticula are present, it is necessary to determine whether or not they retain urine and cause urinary stasis, a

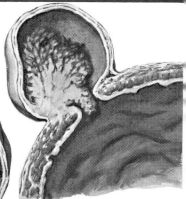

PAPILLARY NEOPLASM
WITHIN A DIVERTICULUM

MULTIPLE DIVERTICULA
OF THE BLADDER, ONE
CONTAINING CALCULI;
PROSTATIC HYPERTROPHY
AND TRABECULATION OF
THE BLADDER WITH
CELLULE FORMATION

CYSTOSCOPIC VIEW:
OPENING OF
DIVERTICULUM
CLOSE TO URETERAL
ORIFICE

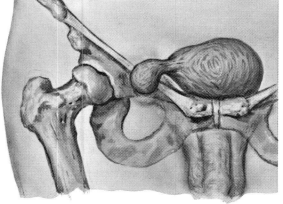

BLADDER DIVERTICULUM IN AN INGUINAL HERNIA

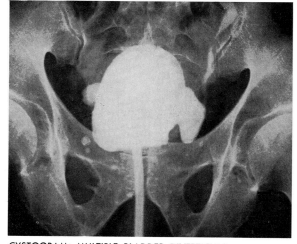

CYSTOGRAM: MULTIPLE BLADDER DIVERTICULA

A VERY LARGE AND SEVERAL SMALLER DIVERTICULA

condition which can lead to stone formation and/or infection and even, on occasion, be associated with a neoplasm. Bladder tumors formed in diverticula are particularly malignant because of the ease with which they can spread through the thin wall and invade a neighboring structure.

Occasionally, a bladder diverticulum may protrude, with a hernia sac, through the abdominal wall; both conditions result from bladder outlet obstruction.

It is of prime importance to *relieve the obstruction* which caused the formation of the diverticula. In some cases, it is necessary to *remove the diverticula* as well, in order to clear a persistent infection.

Large diverticula which often originate in the posterior or lateral walls of the bladder can be difficult to remove surgically. However, since they may significantly add to the morbidity of a patient suffering from relatively long-term urinary tract obstruction, it

becomes especially important in such a patient to evaluate the need for resection and removal of the diverticula. Since diverticula are usually seen in the male with obstructive uropathy resulting from an enlarged prostate, adequate evaluation of the need for their surgical removal will also play a role in deciding the type of prostatectomy advisable.

Whether or not to remove bladder diverticula surgically can best be decided by draining the bladder with a catheter and then observing whether contrast material injected in retrograde fashion is retained in the diverticula. If it is, surgical removal is usually indicated.

When surgery is performed, one should always be mindful that the wall of a diverticulum may contain a ureter, and that, at times, a ureter may even terminate in a diverticulum. Thus, care is required to prevent accidental sectioning of a ureter. □

Foreign Bodies in the Bladder

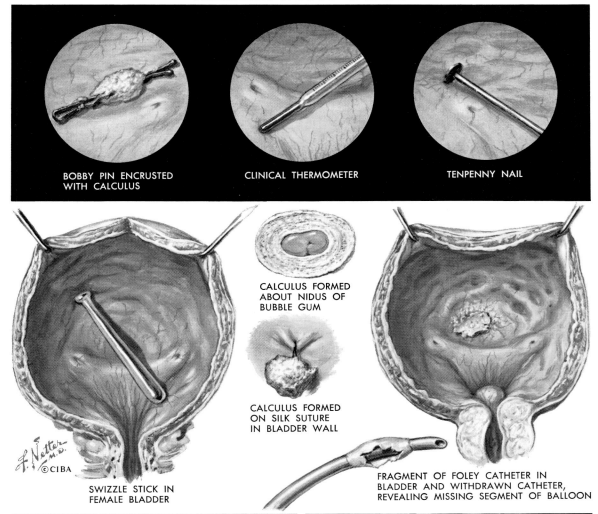

BOBBY PIN ENCRUSTED WITH CALCULUS

CLINICAL THERMOMETER

TENPENNY NAIL

CALCULUS FORMED ABOUT NIDUS OF BUBBLE GUM

CALCULUS FORMED ON SILK SUTURE IN BLADDER WALL

SWIZZLE STICK IN FEMALE BLADDER

FRAGMENT OF FOLEY CATHETER IN BLADDER AND WITHDRAWN CATHETER, REVEALING MISSING SEGMENT OF BALLOON

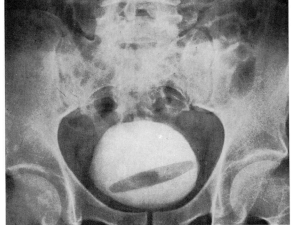

CYSTOGRAM: FISHING CORK IN BLADDER

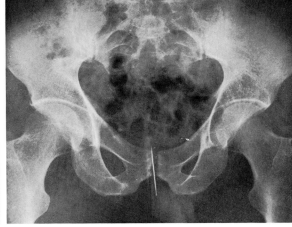

PLAIN FILM: NEEDLE IN URETHRA

Foreign bodies in the bladder cause virtually the same symptoms as bladder calculi (see page 203) and, indeed, often become so covered with and embedded in calcium deposits that the foreign-body nucleus is not even recognized unless the calculus is carefully examined. Accompanying infection is the rule, often with urea-splitting bacteria, a situation which further increases the incrustation with calcium salts.

Foreign bodies in the bladder (other than renal calculi) usually result from retrograde passage of an object mistakenly inserted into the urethra by a patient. The accompanying illustration gives some idea of the incredible variety of objects that have been recovered from bladders.

In the female, foreign bodies in the bladder are usually the result of an attempt to cope with a urethral itch—the object slips from the patient's fingers and passes upward in the urethra. Occasionally, the objects are inserted to induce abortion, with the patient mistaking the urethral for the vaginal opening. Rarely do foreign bodies in the female bladder represent misguided sexual impulses, as is commonly the situation with foreign bodies in the male bladder.

In the male, it is not uncommon that the patient or his partner, under the influence of alcohol, may introduce foreign bodies into the urethra which eventually migrate to the bladder. Understandably, such patients often feel reluctant to reveal what, under more sober conditions, they may consider embarrassing, and thus it is not unusual to see foreign bodies that have been in the bladder for a consider-

able period of time. Often these patients have intractable cystitis.

Although the object may originally have been composed of radiolucent material, by the time the patient sees the physician, it is often sufficiently covered with calcium deposits to be detected on X-ray. The ultimate diagnosis, however, particularly if there is intractable cystitis, is made by cystoscopy. It should be remembered, though, that materials lighter than water will float and thus may occasionally be difficult to find because of constantly changing positions.

It has been previously mentioned that indwelling Foley catheters can fall out if the balloon ruptures, leaving behind a piece of rubber which will form a nidus for stone formation (see page 203). It is also not unusual to find a male patient with an indwelling Foley catheter who, prompted by urethral irritation, has cut the catheter at the urethral meatus; unfortu-

nately, the most proximal part of the catheter will then have slipped back into the bladder and will require endoscopic or suprapubic removal.

Filiform catheters may accidentally break off in the bladder. However, this event should be recognized when it occurs, and endoscopic removal is usually possible at the time.

On rare occasions, a sponge or other object may inadvertently be left behind during an open and unusually bloody surgical procedure. Also, because remaining suture material will form a nucleus for stone formation, it is important that only absorbable sutures be used in bladder surgery.

Finally, foreign bodies may occasionally enter the bladder from other nearby organs such as the bowel. Bone fragments from fractures of the pelvis or migrating bone fragments that are sometimes seen secondary to osteomyelitis may also enter the bladder. □

Neurogenic Bladder

The serious problem of neurologic impairment of bladder function can stem from a broad variety of conditions as shown in the accompanying illustration. While interruption of either *motor* or *sensory nerves* can lead to interference with the normal ability to empty the bladder, it is the *site* of the injury or disease which determines the type of abnormality—the innervation of different parts of the bladder arises from distinct segments of the nervous system.

Motor nerves to the detrusor muscle (external muscle layer—see page 22) are part of the parasympathetic nervous system and arise from preganglionic cells located in the second to fourth sacral segments (S2 to S4) of the spinal cord. The trigonal area is innervated by sympathetic motor fibers from the upper two lumbar segments (L1, 2) and perhaps the lowest two thoracic segments (T11, 12) of the spinal cord. The external sphincter and perineal muscles are supplied by somatic fibers of the pudendal nerves also arising from spinal segments S2 to S4 (see pages 27–29).

Sensory afferent nerve fibers from the bladder accompany parasympathetic and somatic nerves and enter the cord at segments S2 to S4 and, as well, accompany sympathetic nerves to the upper lumbar and perhaps lower thoracic spinal cord segments. The afferent and efferent fibers of the sacral portions of the cord form a spinal voiding reflex (see pages 27–29).

Upper motor neuron lesions usually result in a spastic bladder which, on cystograms, gives a characteristic "Christmas tree" appearance with heavy trabeculation and numerous small diverticula. However, it should be remembered that spinal shock from lesions of the cord less severe than complete interruption (spinal concussion) may be temporary; spinal cord function, including bladder function, may return completely or almost completely.

Lower motor neuron lesions, on the other hand, result in a flaccid bladder, with an increased capacity and a tendency to retain large amounts of residual urine.

Complications of Neurogenic Bladder. The primary consideration in patients with neurogenic bladder is the prevention of eventual damage to the upper urinary tract from *infection, urolithiasis,* and *obstruction.*

Infection is the almost inevitable result of the common use of indwelling catheters (see page 187). In the male, there is the additional danger of the development

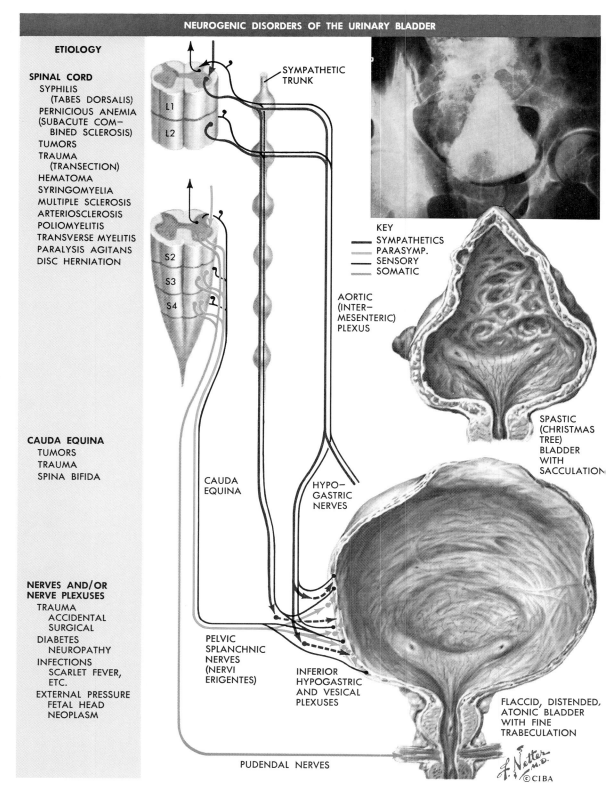

NEUROGENIC DISORDERS OF THE URINARY BLADDER

ETIOLOGY

SPINAL CORD
SYPHILIS
  (TABES DORSALIS)
PERNICIOUS ANEMIA
  (SUBACUTE COM-
    BINED SCLEROSIS)
TUMORS
TRAUMA
  (TRANSECTION)
HEMATOMA
SYRINGOMYELIA
MULTIPLE SCLEROSIS
ARTERIOSCLEROSIS
POLIOMYELITIS
TRANSVERSE MYELITIS
PARALYSIS AGITANS
DISC HERNIATION

CAUDA EQUINA
TUMORS
TRAUMA
SPINA BIFIDA

**NERVES AND/OR
NERVE PLEXUSES**
TRAUMA
  ACCIDENTAL
  SURGICAL
DIABETES
  NEUROPATHY
INFECTIONS
  SCARLET FEVER,
  ETC.
EXTERNAL PRESSURE
  FETAL HEAD
  NEOPLASM

SYMPATHETIC TRUNK

L1
L2

S2
S3
S4

KEY
— SYMPATHETICS
— PARASYMP.
— SENSORY
— SOMATIC

AORTIC
(INTER-
MESENTERIC)
PLEXUS

CAUDA
EQUINA

HYPO-
GASTRIC
NERVES

PELVIC
SPLANCHNIC
NERVES
(NERVI
ERIGENTES)

INFERIOR
HYPOGASTRIC
AND VESICAL
PLEXUSES

PUDENDAL NERVES

SPASTIC
(CHRISTMAS
TREE)
BLADDER
WITH
SACCULATION

FLACCID, DISTENDED,
ATONIC BLADDER
WITH FINE
TRABECULATION

F. Netter ©CIBA

of urethritis (see CIBA COLLECTION, Vol. 2, page 37), which can follow the use of a catheter too large to allow adequate drainage of secretions from the urethral glands that surround the catheter.

Urolithiasis occurs more frequently because of the increased calcium excretion in the urine which is associated with immobilization of the patient (see page 200).

Obviously, in dealing with these virtually unavoidable factors, measures to decrease the bacterial count and the calcium concentration in the urine must be pursued with vigor. Otherwise the stage will be set for *chronic urinary infection* with *secondary stone formation* leading to *deterioration of kidney function* so that even if the underlying disease is dealt with adequately, the patient may still succumb to *uremia.*

It is therefore of utmost importance that the physician keep in mind the inherent potential dangers of the

neurogenic bladder in trying to maintain normal renal function while attempting to rehabilitate the patient. This awareness is particularly important when neurogenic bladder is secondary to spinal shock with only temporary paralysis; vesical drainage should be instituted immediately and maintained in such a way as to prevent infection or urolithiasis.

In any patient with neurogenic bladder, certain simple but important measures which will help avoid these problems include: (1) use of small catheters, especially in the male, (2) maintenance of high urine volume by adequate hydration, (3) bladder irrigation with a solution which will dissolve calcium salts, and (4) administration of antibacterial agents. Furthermore, because of the danger of urethritis in male patients, it is sometimes advisable to use a suprapubic tube, instead of an indwelling catheter, when prolonged catheterization is necessary. □

Section VII

Congenital and Hereditary Disorders

Frank H. Netter, M.D.

in collaboration with

J. U. Schlegel, M.D.   *Plates 5-6*

Maurice B. Strauss, M.D.   *Plate 7*

Howard G. Worthen, M.D., Ph.D.   *Plates 1-4, 8-27*

Anomalies in Number

Anomalies considered here are bilateral or unilateral renal agenesis and supernumerary kidney. Each of these conditions is more common in males than in females.

Bilateral Renal Agenesis. Complete absence of the kidneys and ureters is associated with a definite clinical picture characterized by a peculiar facial appearance, pulmonary abnormalities, and often, a single umbilical artery. The facial appearance, termed "Potter facies," is identified by low-set (elfin) ears, hypertelorism, prominent epicanthal folds, a flat, broad nose, and a receding chin. Skeletal, gastrointestinal, and cardiovascular anomalies are also frequently present. Renal agenesis may often be diagnosed in the delivery room since the absence of urine during gestation results in severe oligohydramnios.

Agenesis may be caused by a failure of formation of either the ureteric bud or the nephrogenic blastema, both of which are necessary for normal development of the kidney (see page 30). Other possible causes are an interruption of the blood supply to these tissues or some unknown adverse event occurring at a critical period in gestation.

The connection between renal agenesis and other anomalies of the Potter syndrome is unknown. The altered facial features and pulmonary hypoplasia may be secondary to oligohydramnios since similar changes have been found in newborns who have had intrauterine anuria from other causes.

Renal agenesis is incompatible with life; most infants do not survive long enough to develop uremia. Many are stillborn while others die from either pulmonary hypoplasia or pneumothorax within a few minutes of birth.

Unilateral Renal Agenesis. Absence of one kidney and ureter occurs more frequently than bilateral agenesis. If the solitary kidney and other organs are intact, a normal life span is possible. Unfortunately, a significant number of patients also have anomalies elsewhere in the genitourinary system, in the gastrointestinal tract, or in the cardiopulmonary system. In males, an undescended testicle on the same side as the agenesis is fairly common and may be the only external evidence of the condition.

The ureter and hemitrigone are absent on the affected side in 90 percent of the patients. In the remainder, a rudimentary, blind-ending ureter is found. Thus the presence of a ureteral orifice cannot be used as evidence to exclude the diagnosis of renal agenesis on that side. In this situation, it is extremely difficult clinically to distinguish agenesis from *primary atrophy* such as renal dysplasia or severe hypoplasia (see page 224). On the other hand, *secondary atrophy* with nonfunction can usually be diagnosed by retrograde pyelography.

If the solitary kidney is normal, compensatory hypertrophy will maintain re-

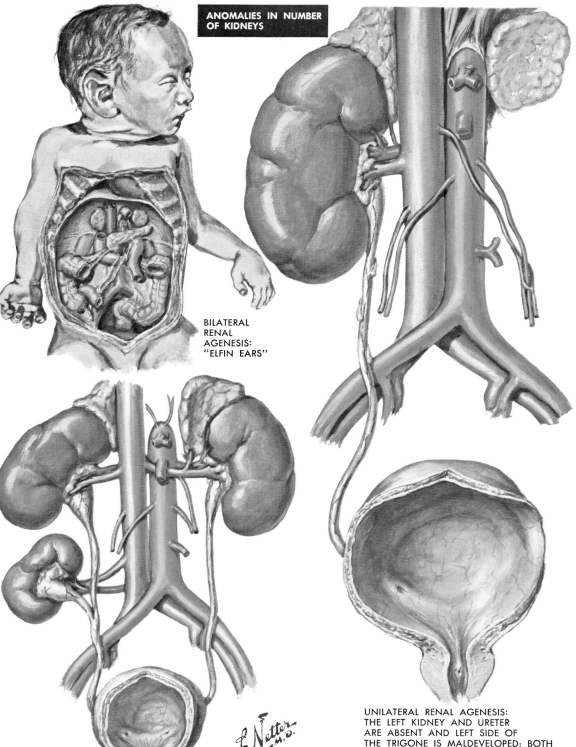

ANOMALIES IN NUMBER OF KIDNEYS

BILATERAL RENAL AGENESIS: "ELFIN EARS"

SUPERNUMERARY RIGHT KIDNEY

UNILATERAL RENAL AGENESIS: THE LEFT KIDNEY AND URETER ARE ABSENT AND LEFT SIDE OF THE TRIGONE IS MALDEVELOPED; BOTH SUPRARENAL GLANDS PRESENT IN NORMAL POSITION

nal function at a normal level. Unilateral agenesis is thus an incidental finding. However, as many as one half of the patients with unilateral renal agenesis have serious renal disease in the remaining kidney.

It is important to diagnose unilateral renal agenesis in order to obviate the possibility that nephrectomy of the solitary organ (which may be performed for a variety of reasons) would result in the removal of all functioning renal tissue. For instance, a large solitary kidney, particularly if mobile, may simulate an abdominal mass. Various acute abdominal symptoms might then be ascribed to this mass, and emergency surgery could result in removal of the enlarged kidney. Adequate preoperative evaluation would avoid such a catastrophe.

Supernumerary kidney is a rare condition in which there is complete duplication of the kidney, pelvis, and ureter, presumably caused by a splitting of the neph-

rogenic blastema before, or at the time of, union with the ureteric bud. The condition occurs with equal frequency on either side and may also be bilateral. The supernumerary kidney is generally smaller than, and situated inferior to, the regular kidney of the same side. The ureter of the supernumerary kidney usually joins the ureter of the upper kidney so that there is a common ureteral opening into the bladder on the affected side. Occasionally, however, the ureter of the supernumerary kidney has a separate bladder orifice.

Unlike the situation with partial duplication, the capsule and blood supply of the supernumerary kidney are entirely separate from those of the regular kidney of the same side. The diagnosis of supernumerary kidney may be made by intravenous pyelography (see page 91), but often the accessory kidney functions poorly and retrograde pyelograms may be necessary to demonstrate its presence. □

Renal Hypoplasia

The classification of hypoplastic kidneys remains in controversy, but the majority of authors now use the term to describe the pure form of the disease. This may be defined as a congenitally small kidney which contains a small number of well-formed nephrons, and in which renal function is normal in proportion to the mass of the kidney. As so defined, renal hypoplasia is an exceedingly rare disease.

In the vast majority of congenitally small kidneys, the morphology is abnormal, and changes resembling dysplasia, or evidence of scarring and cellular infiltration may be found. The presence of the latter changes makes it difficult to decide whether the kidney was indeed congenitally small or whether it has shrunk from the effects of postnatal disease. As a result, the term renal hypoplasia is occasionally used to describe any small kidney, providing there is evidence that the decrease in size dates from early life. However, two apparently specific varieties of renal hypoplasia are considered separately—oligonephronic hypoplasia and the Ask-Upmark kidney.

Like renal agenesis, hypoplasia is believed to result from a failure of normal development of the metanephric blastema, the duct, or the blood supply to these areas (see page 31). However, the defective development is only partial since the formation of the kidney proceeds to a limited degree.

Unilateral Hypoplasia. Many patients with unilateral hypoplasia are asymptomatic, and the condition is discovered as an incidental clinical finding or at autopsy. Other patients have persistent or recurrent lumbar pain on the side of the hypoplastic kidney, but the exact cause of this pain is unknown. In still other patients, the condition is discovered because of investigation for either urinary tract infection or hypertension.

Excretory urography (see page 91) may show a small renal outline, a small, often simplified pelvis, and a reduced number of calyces. However, retrograde pyelography (see page 96) may be required if function in the hypoplastic kidney is poor. This will demonstrate the small collecting system and uniformly narrowed ureter without evidence of obstruction or scarring. Aortography (see page 100) may demonstrate an artery of uniformly narrowed caliber, commensurate in size to the small kidney. The uniformly small blood vessels and ureter help to distinguish hypoplasia from acquired disease, especially pyelonephritis, in which the narrowing of these structures is not uniform.

Morphologically, the diagnosis is established by the finding of a reduced number of renal lobules (reniculi) and a relatively normal microscopic appearance.

Hypertension secondary to unilateral hypoplasia has been reported, and removal of the affected kidney has resulted in either complete cure or marked amelioration of the hypertension. Therefore routine removal of the hypoplastic kid-

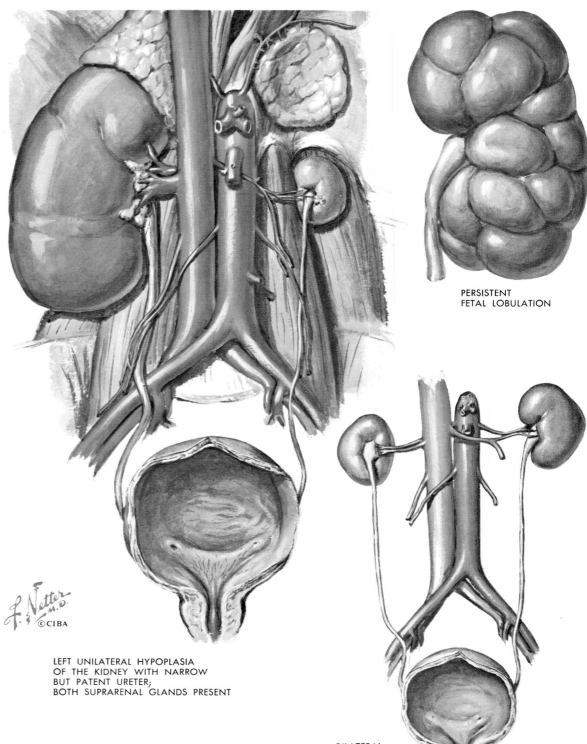

PERSISTENT
FETAL LOBULATION

LEFT UNILATERAL HYPOPLASIA
OF THE KIDNEY WITH NARROW
BUT PATENT URETER;
BOTH SUPRARENAL GLANDS PRESENT

BILATERAL
RENAL HYPOPLASIA

ney has been advocated on the assumption that it is more susceptible to infection or more likely to produce hypertension. However, unless there is evidence that the hypoplastic kidney is producing symptoms, surgery is not generally recommended.

Bilateral hypoplasia presumably has the same origin as the unilateral variety, but the clinical consequences are much more severe. Usually patients with bilateral hypoplasia have evidence of renal insufficiency such as defective urine concentration and acidification, and eventually renal osteodystrophy occurs. Patients may survive only a few weeks or as long as a few years, and uremia often develops.

Intravenous pyelography may fail to demonstrate the calyces and pelves because of diminished concentration of contrast material by the hypoplastic kidneys, and retrograde pyelography may be required.

The criteria for diagnosis of bilateral hypoplasia are the uniform narrowing of the blood vessels and ureters, the simplification of the pelves, and the absence of pyelonephritic scars. However, differentiation from acquired parenchymal renal diseases, such as chronic glomerulonephritis or chronic pyelonephritis, is often difficult and usually requires microscopic examination of renal tissue.

Persistent Fetal Lobulation. Normally, lobulation is present until 4 or 5 years of age and if it persists beyond this time is considered an inconsequential anatomic variant. Although some authors believe that persistent fetal lobulation represents a relative immaturity of renal development, all renal function studies indicate normal maturation. Occasionally an erroneous diagnosis of cystic disease is made—for instance, if the lobulations are palpated on clinical examination or if the abnormal shape of the kidney is observed on X-ray. □

Renal Dysplasia

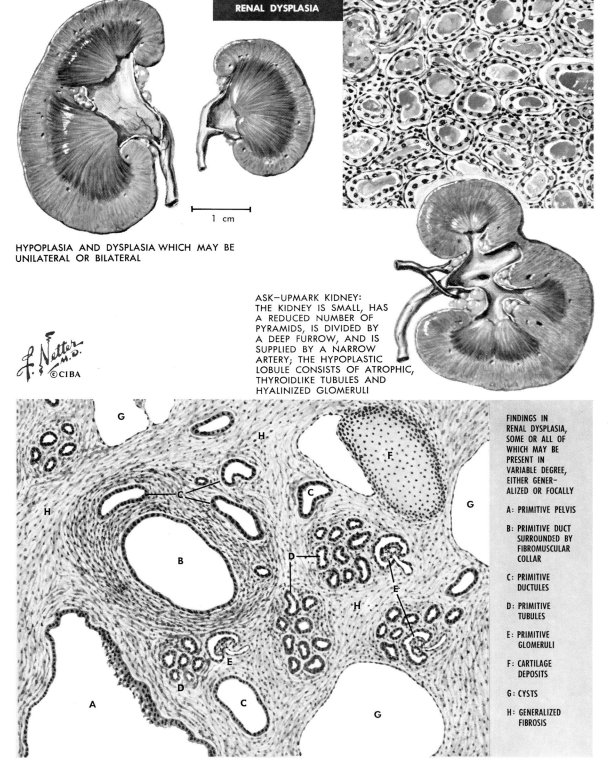

RENAL DYSPLASIA

HYPOPLASIA AND DYSPLASIA WHICH MAY BE UNILATERAL OR BILATERAL

ASK–UPMARK KIDNEY: THE KIDNEY IS SMALL, HAS A REDUCED NUMBER OF PYRAMIDS, IS DIVIDED BY A DEEP FURROW, AND IS SUPPLIED BY A NARROW ARTERY; THE HYPOPLASTIC LOBULE CONSISTS OF ATROPHIC, THYROIDLIKE TUBULES AND HYALINIZED GLOMERULI

FINDINGS IN RENAL DYSPLASIA, SOME OR ALL OF WHICH MAY BE PRESENT IN VARIABLE DEGREE, EITHER GENERALIZED OR FOCALLY

A: PRIMITIVE PELVIS

B: PRIMITIVE DUCT SURROUNDED BY FIBROMUSCULAR COLLAR

C: PRIMITIVE DUCTULES

D: PRIMITIVE TUBULES

E: PRIMITIVE GLOMERULI

F: CARTILAGE DEPOSITS

G: CYSTS

H: GENERALIZED FIBROSIS

Renal dysplasia, as noted on page 224, is frequently confused with renal hypoplasia. The term dysplasia should be reserved for those kidneys which, in addition to being smaller than normal, have certain microscopic abnormalities believed to be characteristic.

Histologically, primitive ducts and ductules consisting of tall, columnar epithelium surrounded by a fibromuscular collar have been described. In addition, there are poorly formed, primitive glomeruli covered by cuboidal epithelium and associated with primitive tubules. The primitive tubules, embedded in a fibrous matrix, are devoid of features which permit normal differentiation of the various segments of the mature tubule. Diversely sized cysts, most of which are believed to represent portions of dilated tubules, and metaplastic cartilage in the kidney complete the picture.

If all such pathologic findings are present, and if evidence of postnatal inflammation is absent, the distinction between dysplasia and postnatal disease of the kidney is not difficult. Unfortunately, primitive tubules, glomeruli, and cysts can occur in acquired renal diseases so that in some cases the distinction between dysplasia and acquired disease may not be possible unless one can find evidence of cartilage or primitive ducts.

The exact cause of renal dysplasia is obscure. The microscopic abnormalities are believed to result from either a failure of differentiation of the metanephros or a persistence of mesonephric remnants (see pages 30–31). In most patients, dysplasia is associated with obstruction of the urinary tract, and this suggests that obstruction may, in some way, interfere with normal maturation of the kidney. In fact, many of the features of dysplasia have been produced by experimental obstruction. However, obstruction is not invariably found in association with dysplasia, and thus it appears probable that other factors acting on the kidney during embryogenesis also contribute to the dysplasia.

The small, malformed dysplastic kidney usually functions poorly, if at all. Consequently, when the disorder is bilateral, it is clearly incompatible with survival of the infant. However, less severe degrees of bilateral dysplasia may permit survival for variable periods. In contrast, unilateral dysplasia is often an incidental finding since the opposite, normal kidney can adequately sustain life. Infection, though, is frequently superimposed on dysplasia, particularly if there is obstruction. Also, hypertension is sometimes observed in association with either the dysplasia or the superimposed pyelonephritis.

Oligonephronic hypoplasia, a distinctive form of bilateral renal hypoplasia, is characterized by a reduction in the number of nephrons and hypertrophy of those that remain. The kidneys are extremely small and have a reduced number of pyramids.

Early in the course of the disease, the glomeruli are very large, often two to three times normal size. The tubules are also markedly hypertrophied and hyperplastic. In children who die later in the course of the disease, interstitial fibrosis, cellular infiltration, hyalinized glomeruli, and tubular atrophy may be found. These later changes could represent superimposed pyelonephritis, but similar changes have been observed late in the course of experimental disease in which a large part of functioning renal tissue has been removed. Thus, they may result from an excessive load placed on the residual functional renal tissue over a long period of time.

Clinically, oligonephronic hypoplasia is distinguished by the appearance of *Continued on page 226*

Renal Dysplasia

Continued from page 225

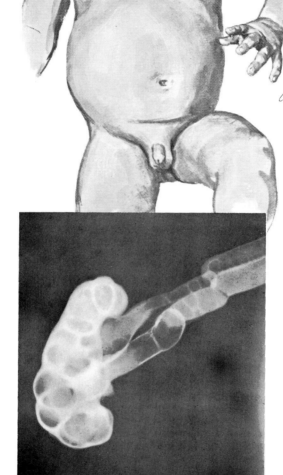

UNILATERAL MULTICYSTIC KIDNEY

PALPABLE MASS IN ABDOMEN AND FLANK: TO BE DIFFERENTIATED FROM HYDRONEPHROSIS, NEUROBLASTOMA, AND WILMS' TUMOR

MULTICYSTIC KIDNEY IN SITU: NARROW, CORDLIKE URETER

MULTICYSTIC KIDNEY WITH DUPLICATION OF URETER

CYSTIC MASS SECTIONED: LOOSELY AGGLOMERATED LARGE CYSTS

insidious renal insufficiency early in life, usually early in childhood; polyuria, polydipsia, proteinuria, and acidosis may be observed. Patients may survive for long periods, even after the onset of uremia, with little evidence of progression of the renal insufficiency. Children who survive long enough eventually develop renal dwarfism (see CIBA COLLECTION, Vol. 4, pages 228-230) and renal osteodystrophy (see page 117). Ultimately the deterioration of renal function progresses to the point where uremia is fatal.

The disorder can be explained by an interruption of bilateral nephrogenesis in embryonic life (see page 31). Consequently too few nephrons are formed. When the disease is bilateral, the load placed on the remaining nephrons leads to marked hypertrophy and ultimately to renal damage. In unilateral hypoplasia, the presence of a normal kidney eliminates the excessive load upon the few hypoplastic and residual nephrons, so that, in the absence of such stimulation, nephron hypertrophy does not occur.

Ask-Upmark kidney is a peculiar form of hypoplasia or dysplasia which is almost always unilateral. It is characterized by a groove on the surface of the kidney which marks the plane of separation between a relatively normal portion and the hypoplastic area. Within the hypoplastic area, there are atrophic "thyroidlike" tubules and a few hyalinized glomeruli.

The usual way the disorder is found is during the evaluation of hypertensive patients. However, in some patients the condition is discovered as an incidental finding or in association with other urinary tract symptoms. In a few hypertensive patients, nephrectomy has been followed by a return of blood pressure to normal, while in other patients the blood pressure has remained elevated, possibly because of changes in the other kidney.

The unilateral multicystic kidney represents an extreme form of cystic renal dysplasia. Most of the renal tissue is replaced by cysts connected by fibrous tissue. Often, the cysts are quite large, and the volume of the kidney is increased, sometimes forming a large abdominal mass.

Characteristically, the condition is unilateral, although bilateral multicystic kidneys have been described (see page 227). When one kidney is normal, the prognosis is excellent, but cases have been described in which a unilateral multicystic kidney has been associated with dysplasia or hydronephrosis in the other organ.

Usually, the renal pelvis of the affected kidney is absent, and the ureter either is completely absent or shows atresia. As with other forms of dysplasia, the multicystic, dysplastic kidney is assumed to be the result of obstruction early in embryonic life. However,

the mechanism by which the massive cysts form in the absence of recognizable glomeruli remains unknown. Secretion by the epithelium of the cysts is perhaps responsible.

Clinically, multicystic kidney generally presents as an abdominal mass in a newborn infant. Palpation may reveal the lobulated nature of this mass and could help distinguish it from hydronephrosis, neuroblastoma, or Wilms' tumor (see pages 186 and 212). The mass generally transilluminates well, and even when palpation does not reveal lobulation, it can almost always be determined, prior to surgery, that the mass is cystic.

The prognosis in patients found to have multicystic kidney depends entirely on the condition of the opposite kidney since the affected cystic kidney is not functional. If the opposite kidney is normal, surgery should be curative. □

Renal Cystic Diseases

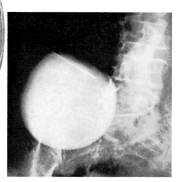

RENAL CYST INJECTED WITH
CONTRAST MEDIUM BY
PERCUTANEOUS NEEDLE
PUNCTURE

LARGE THIN—WALLED
CYST OF MIDPORTION
OF RIGHT KIDNEY

THICK—WALLED
CYST WITH
CALCIFICATION

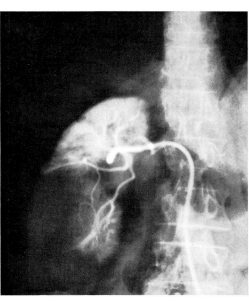

RENAL ANGIOGRAM REVEALING EVIDENCE OF
SOLITARY CYST IN LOWER POLE OF KIDNEY

Several important types of cystic diseases of the kidneys can be distinguished from the point of view of diagnosis, therapy, and prognosis. However, from a pathologic point of view all renal cystic disease can be classified as forms of renal dysplasia (see page 225).

The important entities are: (1) polycystic disease of the kidney (adult type), (2) polycystic disease of the kidney (infantile type), (3) unilateral multicystic disease (some pathologists prefer the term unilateral renal dysplasia), (4) simple cysts (single, multiple, and multilocular), and, to complete the list, (5) various cysts of lesser clinical importance (which will not be described in detail), such as retention or inflammatory cysts, parapelvic and peripelvic cysts, and cysts secondary to hematoma, echinococcus infection (see page 197), pyelonephritis (see page 189), and other specific disease entities.

Polycystic Disease of the Kidney

The incidence of this disease entity is not high and is estimated at less than one per 1,000 people by the age of 80. However, because of the hereditary characteristics, polycystic disease is an important condition. There appears to be a distinct difference between the polycystic disease in adults and that in infants (see page 225), inasmuch as the disease in adults shows a regular autosomal *dominant* heredity, while in infants it appears to be an autosomal *recessive* characteristic. The

presence of polycystic disease in adults is thus an important factor in advising patients in regard to the likelihood that the condition will be transmitted to their children. Since the dominant gene has a high penetration, the risk is considerable.

It is estimated that if an individual lives to the age of 80 carrying the dominant gene, there is a 100 percent chance of affliction. In the adult type, it appears that the disease process may have been latent for many years and becomes manifest in renal tissue which previously had functioned and developed normally. However, even though the dominant gene has an extraordinarily high penetration, the variation in the time of onset of the disease makes it difficult to predict the prognosis before symptoms become manifest.

The infantile form of polycystic disease is much rarer than the adult form and usually leads to a very early death of the infant (see page 226). Of course,

patients afflicted with the infantile form who die in the first month of life have not transmitted their genetic inheritance. This is an important difference between the infantile and adult forms of renal polycystic disease.

Since polycystic disease is often a slowly progressive condition which may develop over a number of years, it is often initially asymptomatic. In the more advanced stages, destruction of renal tissue results in azotemia and physical discomfort from the sheer size of the large cystic masses. These cysts are not necessarily of identical size. Not infrequently there are complicating infections which produce local and possibly systemic manifestations. Thus, symptoms of urinary tract infection are common. Hypertension occurs frequently. Albuminuria is found in approximately 50 percent of patients afflicted with either associated hypertension or urinary tract infection. *Continued on page 228*

Renal Cystic Diseases

Continued from page 227

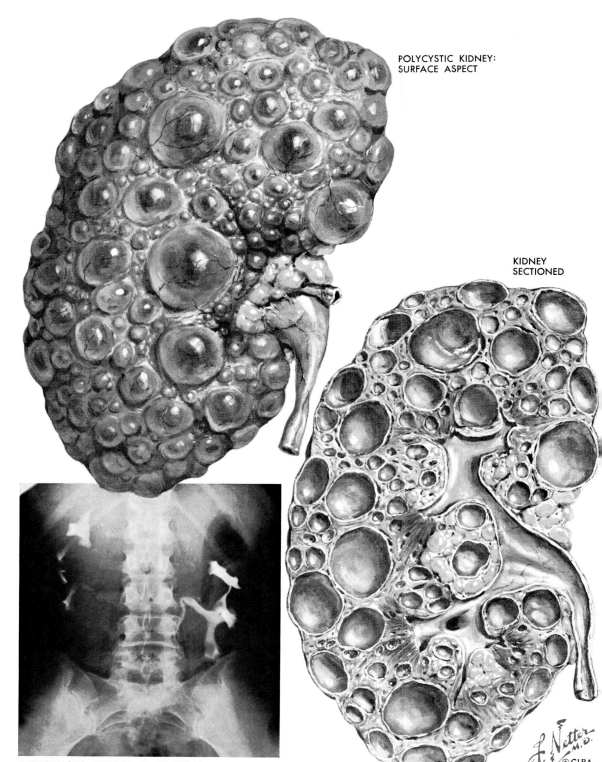

POLYCYSTIC KIDNEY:
SURFACE ASPECT

KIDNEY
SECTIONED

INTRAVENOUS PYELOGRAM: BILATERAL
POLYCYSTIC DISEASE

Unfortunately, there is no specific therapy for polycystic disease. Unless infected cysts necessitate surgical exploration and drainage, good supportive medical care with treatment of individual symptoms as they appear is the only recourse. Occasionally, surgery may be indicated if a polycystic kidney, because of its size, handicaps the individual's activity. Not only pain and discomfort, but sometimes the increased risk of trauma, may impose limitations. In such patients, unroofing of as many cysts as possible may temporarily alleviate the patient's discomfort (Rovsing procedure). However, it appears that such an attempt has no beneficial effect upon kidney function which is already severely depressed in these patients.

Unilateral Multicystic Disease

In children, unilateral multicystic disease is the most common childhood renal cystic disease. It is an important clinical entity because it often presents a problem in differential diagnosis. The child with a large mass in the flank, which is also palpable through the abdomen, is more likely to have unilateral multicystic disease than Wilms' tumor (see page 212), neuroblastoma, or unilateral hydronephrosis (see page 186).

Intravenous urograms typically demonstrate lack of renal function on the same side as the mass, and a normal kidney on the contralateral side. Not infrequently

it is possible to palpate the uneven surface of the mass. Nephrectomy should be performed since normal renal parenchyma is completely missing.

Simple Cysts

Simple cysts may be solitary or multiple, thin walled or thick walled. They may be trabeculated and also may be multilocular. The fluid within the cyst or cysts may be clear, straw colored, or hemorrhagic. Occasionally, the walls of the cyst contain calcium. In two to three percent of cases, adenocarcinoma of the wall may occur.

Simple cysts are usually cortical and bulge through the renal capsule. Sometimes, however, simple cysts occur deep within the cortex and even in the medulla. Such cysts may infrequently cause partial obstruction of the collecting system. Atrophy of the renal parenchyma may result because of the size of the cyst.

Differential Diagnosis. Renal cysts are extremely common, and it is felt that at least half of all people beyond the age of 50 have one or more cysts in their kidneys. However, such cysts are of little or no consequence unless carcinoma is present in the wall or unless the cysts interfere with renal function because of pressure on the parenchyma or the collecting system. The main problem lies in differentiating a simple cyst from adenocarcinoma, and this problem is especially pertinent in distinguishing simple cysts from an adenocarcinoma which has developed a necrotic center.

The use of various scanning procedures and radiologic technics (see pages 103 and 98) can increase the accuracy of diagnosis of renal cysts to the 95 to 98 percent range. Nevertheless, if a patient is a good surgical risk, it is advisable to explore the patient surgically to confirm the diagnosis. □

Cystic Disease of Renal Medulla

Medullary cystic disease, first clearly delineated in 1945, occurs predominantly in young people of either sex. Most of the first reported cases of medullary cystic disease occurred sporadically. In Switzerland and Scandinavia the disorder was labeled familial juvenile nephronophthisis, and initially the two conditions were not recognized as being clinically and pathologically identical.

Autosomal recessive inheritance has been suggested for some of the familial cases, but the data are relatively scant. Nevertheless, in several families extensively studied, it is very clear that autosomal dominant transmission is probable. The failure to observe male-to-male transmission suggests either sex linkage or preferential segregation of an abnormal autosome. Many cases occur sporadically, and patients have been observed to develop the disorder as late in life as the sixth decade. For this reason the term medullary cystic disease seems preferable to the designation familial juvenile nephronophthisis.

Clinical and Laboratory Findings. Symptoms produced by a normocytic and normochromic anemia of insidious onset are often the presenting manifestations and, in turn, lead to the discovery of a coexisting azotemia. Polyuria and nocturia frequently have been present for so long that patients do not consider them abnormal. Except for the occurrence of pallor, physical examination is generally unremarkable. Bone changes are rarely manifested clinically and are observed only in children, who also may suffer retarded growth.

Laboratory findings, as illustrated, are those which would be expected in patients with chronic renal insufficiency. Urine concentrating ability is lost, but the ability to dilute the urine is not. Hyposthenuria accounts in part for the minimal or absent proteinuria found on qualitative testing of randomly collected urine specimens and the sparsity of formed elements in the sediment. Serum bicarbonate concentration is almost always reduced, but symptoms of acidosis are unusual. Serum alkaline phosphatase is generally elevated in the young patient.

Urinary wasting of sodium is observed frequently, and commonly it is severe enough to require a sodium intake of several hundred milliequivalents daily in order to maintain balance. In the past, such wasting of sodium often led to a diagnosis of adrenocortical insufficiency, when in fact secondary suprarenal hyperplasia is common.

Radiographic examination of the urinary system has seldom been revealing except for demonstration of small kidneys.

The clinical course of this disorder has been quite variable and depends on how advanced the renal insufficiency is at the time the patients are first seen. Inexorable progression appears to be the rule, but a number of patients have survived for some years.

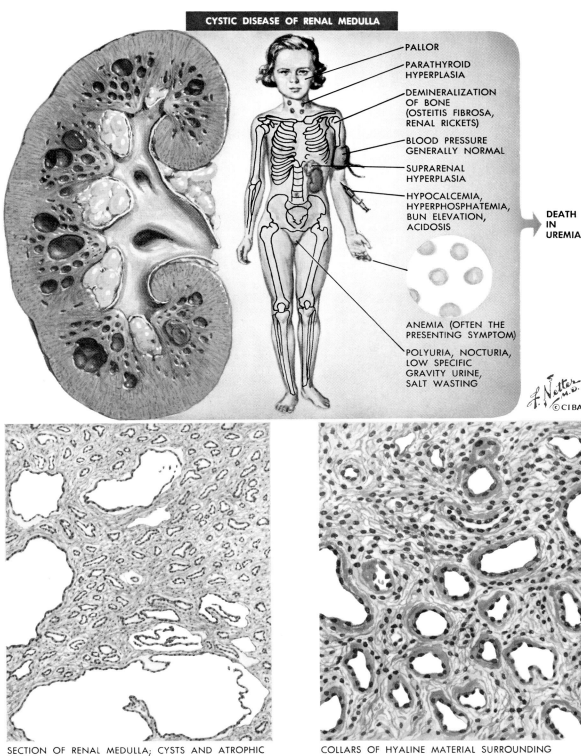

CYSTIC DISEASE OF RENAL MEDULLA

PALLOR

PARATHYROID HYPERPLASIA

DEMINERALIZATION OF BONE (OSTEITIS FIBROSA, RENAL RICKETS)

BLOOD PRESSURE GENERALLY NORMAL

SUPRARENAL HYPERPLASIA

HYPOCALCEMIA, HYPERPHOSPHATEMIA, BUN ELEVATION, ACIDOSIS

DEATH IN UREMIA

ANEMIA (OFTEN THE PRESENTING SYMPTOM)

POLYURIA, NOCTURIA, LOW SPECIFIC GRAVITY URINE, SALT WASTING

SECTION OF RENAL MEDULLA; CYSTS AND ATROPHIC AND DILATED TUBULES SURROUNDED BY RELATIVELY ACELLULAR CONNECTIVE TISSUE

COLLARS OF HYALINE MATERIAL SURROUNDING TUBULES IN SUBCORTICAL AREA

The treatment is that of chronic renal insufficiency in general. Particular attention must be paid to an adequate intake of sodium (as both the chloride and the bicarbonate) in patients with the severe salt-wasting form of the disorder. This is especially important in the later stages when too little salt rapidly leads to hypovolemia and a small excess of salt leads to salt retention, edema, and a rise in blood pressure.

Pathologic Findings. The *kidneys* generally are equally reduced in size, and the calyceal and pelvic mucosae are smooth and not thickened. Cysts vary in size from less than 1 mm to more than 5 cm in diameter and are usually located just beneath the cortex.

Microscopically, the cortex is thin and poorly demarcated, and a majority of the glomeruli are partially or completely hyalinized. Some glomeruli are abnormally small while others show no abnormality except for occasional hypertrophy. Periglomerular fibrosis may be seen. Practically all the cortical tubules, except for a few proximal convolutions, have an atrophic or unspecialized epithelium and are engulfed in fibrous tissue. Many tubules evidently have disappeared. Collecting ducts are distorted and, near the papilla, are sometimes extremely narrow or obliterated, with concentrically thickened PAS-positive basement membranes. The interstitial tissue, aside from extensive diffuse fibrosis, contains lymphocytes, macrophages, and occasional plasma cells.

The *parathyroid glands* are often markedly enlarged and extremely hyperplastic. Renal osteodystrophy, often both renal rickets and osteitis fibrosa, is observed. The bone marrow is hypoplastic and may have areas of fibrosis. The *suprarenal glands* are enlarged in those patients who have marked wasting of sodium, and the zona glomerulosa is moderately prominent. □

Anomalies in Rotation

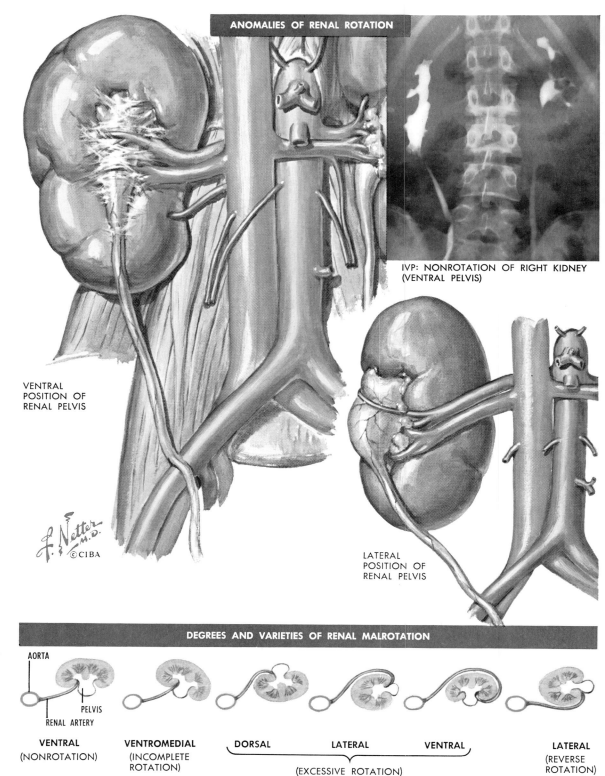

IVP: NONROTATION OF RIGHT KIDNEY
(VENTRAL PELVIS)

VENTRAL
POSITION OF
RENAL PELVIS

LATERAL
POSITION OF
RENAL PELVIS

DEGREES AND VARIETIES OF RENAL MALROTATION

AORTA

PELVIS

RENAL ARTERY

VENTRAL (NONROTATION)	VENTROMEDIAL (INCOMPLETE ROTATION)	DORSAL	LATERAL	VENTRAL	LATERAL (REVERSE ROTATION)
			(EXCESSIVE ROTATION)		

During its embryonic ascent from pelvis to abdomen, the kidney normally rotates medially so that the hilus, which originally faced ventrally, ultimately occupies a medial position in adult life (see page 35). Abnormalities of this normal rotational process may thus occur in one of three ways: (1) The kidney may fail to rotate; (2) it may rotate excessively; or (3) it may rotate laterally rather than medially.

The most common anomaly of rotation is nonrotation or incomplete rotation. In this condition, the kidney hilus remains facing in a ventral or ventromedial position.

Excessive rotation usually results in a dorsal or lateral placement of the hilus of the kidney. Occasionally, however, the kidney may rotate completely, through 360 degrees, so that the hilus is ventrally located as in incomplete rotation or nonrotation, but the renal vessels and the ureter, on leaving the hilus, pass lateral and posterior to the kidney before emerging on the medial aspect.

Reverse rotation results in a laterally placed renal pelvis, but in this condition, the ureter and renal vessels, on leaving the hilus, pass medially and cross anterior to the kidney.

Malrotation of any type is frequently accompanied by failure of the kidney to ascend to its normal midlumbar position. This, in turn, is responsible for the frequent association of ectopic kidney with the condition of malrotation. In fact, in about 50 percent of malrotated kidneys, the organ is displaced far enough caudally to be classified as ectopic.

Unilateral malrotation occurs more often than the bilateral variety. The condition occurs with approximately equal frequency on the two sides and somewhat more commonly in males than in females.

Malrotation is considered to be an incidental finding except when obstruction of the pelvis or ureter has occurred. This may result from compression of the ureter or pelvis by the kidney. Alternatively, associated anomalies, such as high insertion of the ureter into the pelvis, or anomalous blood vessels, may cause compression. Massive hydronephrosis (see page 186) is not common in patients with malrotation, but moderate degrees of obstruction with urinary stasis are. This predisposes to urinary tract infection, the most common complication of malrotation.

The diagnosis of malrotation can usually be established without difficulty by intravenous urography (see page 91). The narrow pelvis with obscured calyces, or calyces viewed in their short dimensions, is usually characteristic. Another useful pyelographic finding is lateral displacement of the ureter in its course to the bladder. The aortographic finding (see page 100) of elongated and sometimes curved vessels is another indication that the hilus is further removed from the midline than normal. Aortography may also reveal vascular anomalies that will complicate subsequent surgery. Occasionally, even though the investigation has been adequate, a malrotation may mimic compression of the pelvis by a renal tumor (see page 206) or pelvicalyceal distortion from pyelonephritis (see page 189). Thus, the physician must be alert to the possibility of malrotation in order to prevent unnecessary surgery. □

Ectopia of the Kidney

Ectopia results from a failure of the normal embryonic process of ascent of the kidney from its original low, pelvic position to a position opposite the second lumbar vertebra. Thus, the kidney may fail to ascend *(pelvic ectopic kidney),* it may ascend excessively *(thoracic kidney),* or it may cross to the other side *(crossed ectopia of the kidney).*

Ectopic kidney occurs more often in males than in females and is two to three times more frequent on the left side than on the right. In approximately 10 to 20 percent of cases the condition is bilateral, while in a relatively low but significant percentage of patients, the ectopic kidney is a solitary organ.

Ectopic kidney is also frequently associated with abnormalities of the spine, particularly myelomeningocele. In addition, anorectal anomalies may be found to occur concomitantly, and ectopic kidney is a frequent incidental finding in patients who have imperforate anus.

Pelvic Kidney. The most common variety of ectopia is pelvic. This presumably results from persistence of the early fetal vascular connections which prevent the kidney from ascending normally. Thus, the arterial supply of the pelvic kidney may arise from the lower aorta or from the iliac vessels. The ureter is short, and malrotation with a ventrally placed renal pelvis is usual.

Clinically, the pelvic kidney may produce symptoms referable to the lower abdomen because of pressure on blood vessels, nerves, or adjacent organs. It may also produce constipation by displacement of or pressure on the colon, and it may cause dystocia by similar effects on the uterus.

Often, the pelvic kidney is easily palpable and thus may be mistaken for a solid pelvic tumor. The diagnosis, however, is usually made by urography. This shows the abnormally low, often malrotated pelvis, a short ureter, and frequently a filling defect in the bladder from impingement by the low-lying kidney.

Pelvic kidney must be distinguished from ptosis of the kidney. The finding on excretory urography of a ureter of normal length, but with redundancy, indicates nephroptosis. In addition, aortography will demonstrate the normal origin of the blood supply to the kidney in the case of ptosis, whereas in the case of pelvic ectopia, the abnormal source of the arterial supply will be apparent. (Aortography is also a useful preoperative procedure since it serves to alert the surgeon to anomalies of the vasculature which may affect the outcome of the surgery.)

Ectopia may be complicated by obstruction and stones which occur more commonly than in normally placed kidneys (see page 200). The resulting infection is a common presenting complaint of patients with pelvic ectopic kidneys.

If a pelvic ectopic kidney is found as an incidental finding, no therapy is required. Nephropexy is usually difficult because of the short ureter and the anomalous blood supply. Thus, if a normal kidney is present on the contralateral side, ne-

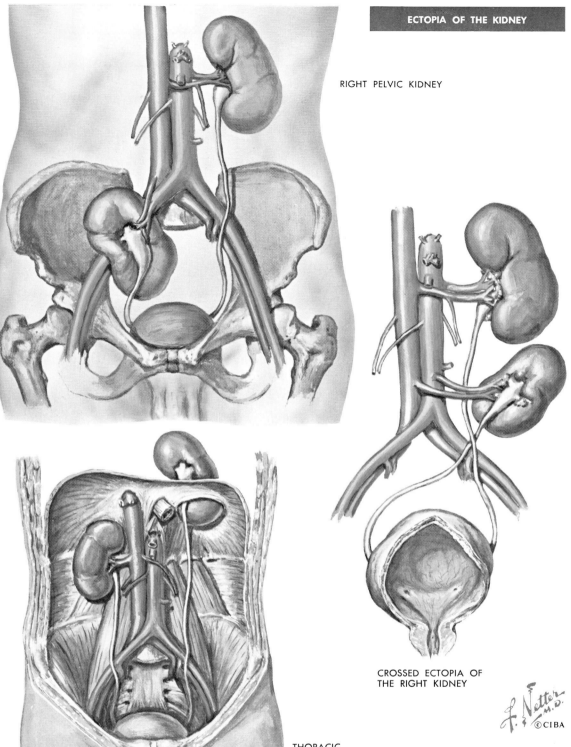

RIGHT PELVIC KIDNEY

CROSSED ECTOPIA OF
THE RIGHT KIDNEY

THORACIC
KIDNEY

phrectomy may be indicated if the pelvic kidney produces symptoms which are severe enough to warrant a surgical procedure.

Thoracic Kidney. Excessive ascent of the kidney during embryonic life results in thoracic kidney. The arteries to the ectopic kidney usually arise from a point on the aorta which is higher than normal. The ureter is excessively long.

Symptoms of diaphragmatic hernia may be present, or the kidney may plug the opening in the diaphragm and prevent development of symptoms. Thoracic symptoms may be produced if the ectopic kidney becomes infected or obstructed.

Crossed ectopia without fusion is an uncommon condition. Both kidneys are located on one side of the body, and the crossed kidney is usually inferior to and smaller than the normal kidney. The vessels to the ectopic crossed kidney may arise normally and cross to the opposite side of the body with the kidney. Alternatively, the blood supply may arise on the contralateral side so that both renal arteries arise from the same side of the aorta and both renal veins enter the inferior vena cava on the same side. The ureter of the ectopic kidney usually enters the bladder at the normal site. As in other forms of ectopia, malrotation is common, and the usual abnormality is a ventrally placed renal pelvis.

The abnormally long and tortuous course of the blood vessels and ureter of the ectopic crossed kidney makes obstruction and infection more likely. In addition, the ureter from the normally placed kidney may become obstructed.

The diagnosis of crossed ectopia is made with the aid of intravenous pyelography. However, the distinction from the much more common crossed ectopia with fusion may be difficult to make preoperatively. □

Renal Fusion

Renal fusion is a commonly occurring abnormality of the kidneys and is named according to either the shape or location. The most frequently encountered form is the *horseshoe kidney* which, like most renal anomalies, occurs more frequently in males than females, in a ratio of about 2:1. The predominant theory of the mechanism by which fusion occurs is that nephrogenic blastemas unite early in the course of their ascent into the abdomen.

Horseshoe kidney occurs when the kidneys, situated on their respective sides of the abdomen, are connected across the midline by an isthmus which generally runs anterior to the aorta and vena cava. The isthmus may be simply a cord or fibrous band; more often it consists of functional renal tissue and occasionally is drained by a separate pelvis and ureter. Fusion of the lower poles is the most common form, but fusion of the middle of the kidneys or upper poles may also occur.

Because of the fusion, the kidneys are closer than normal to the midline and are usually lower than normal. The arterial supply often arises from the inferior end of the aorta or from the iliac artery. In addition, there may be multiple renal arteries which may present serious problems during surgery.

Since renal fusion prevents the normal rotation of the kidneys, malrotation almost invariably accompanies horseshoe kidney as well as the other types of fusion. Moreover, the combination of malrotation and the location of the ureters anterior to the isthmus is primarily responsible for the associated obstruction which may occur in one or both sides of the horseshoe kidney.

Clinically, patients with horseshoe kidneys may be asymptomatic or may present with symptoms secondary to the common complications of hydronephrosis, infection, and calculi. Recurrent periumbilical pain is said to be characteristic of horseshoe kidney but, unfortunately, is of little value in establishing a diagnosis.

Intravenous pyelography may show the pelves close together and abnormal in appearance because of malrotation. If the inferior poles are fused, they will be closer to the midline than the upper poles, in contrast to normal, when the lower poles are further from the midline than the upper poles. Compression of the ureter by the isthmus occurs frequently and causes obstruction. Stones may be seen in one or both pelves on the initial scout film.

Aortography or renal arteriography may reveal the anomalous vasculature present in most patients and help in establishing the diagnosis.

No therapy is required for uncomplicated horseshoe kidney. However, if obstruction occurs, either pyeloplasty or division of the isthmus may be required.

Crossed ectopia with fusion is the second most frequently occurring form of renal

RENAL FUSION

SIMPLE CROSSED ECTOPIA WITH FUSION

S-SHAPED OR SIGMOID KIDNEY

PELVIC CAKE OR LUMP KIDNEY

HORSESHOE KIDNEY

fusion. It differs from horseshoe kidney in that the renal mass is located entirely on one side of the abdominal cavity. Generally, the ectopic kidney is inferior and medial to the normal kidney.

The clinical picture is similar to that described for horseshoe kidney. The diagnosis is suspected when pyelography reveals two pelves close together on one side of the abdomen, with a ureter going to each side of the bladder. Distinction from crossed ectopia without fusion, however, may not be possible prior to surgery. Generally speaking, no treatment is required for the primary condition. As with horseshoe kidney, obstruction, infection, and stone formation are frequent complications and may require therapy.

Cake or lump kidney is a variant of horseshoe kidney in which the medial surfaces of the two organs are fused along their entire border. Thus malrotation and failure of ascent are invariably associated.

The signs and symptoms are similar to those of horseshoe kidney except that the mass of renal tissue in the lower abdomen or pelvis is often easily palpated and may be mistaken for a pelvic or lower abdominal tumor. Pyelography may establish the diagnosis and frequently shows the malrotated pelves close together in the lower abdomen or pelvis. Because of the severe malrotation and the frequency of anomalous vessels, obstruction is more likely than in other forms of renal fusion. As with other forms of renal fusion, therapy depends on complicating abnormalities.

The sigmoid kidney (S-shaped) is another variant of horseshoe kidney. The upper pole of one kidney is fused with the lower pole of the other across the midline. Alternatively, the entire mass of the sigmoid kidney may be on one side of the abdomen. As with the other variants, there are malrotation (the pelves usually facing ventrally) and an anomalous vasculature. □

Anomalies of Renal Pelvis and Calyces

A number of anomalies of the renal pelvis and calyces may occur in otherwise normal kidneys and are of no clinical consequence. Among these, the most commonly found abnormality is the *bifid* or *duplicated renal pelvis* which rarely produces symptoms. However, if one of the pelves becomes stenotic, obstruction will result and may produce symptoms.

The spider-shaped kidney is an anomaly in which the calyces are spread and elongated in an unusual configuration. Consequently, the condition may be confused on radiologic examination with a tumor or other space-occupying lesion. Adequate preoperative evaluation, including renal arteriography (see page 100), should assist in establishing the correct diagnosis.

Extrarenal pelvis appears to be more susceptible to obstruction and stasis than the normally situated pelvis, presumably because the lack of protection normally offered by the renal parenchyma makes the anomalous pelvis more susceptible to extrinsic obstruction. In addition, a high ureteropelvic junction and various anomalies of the kidney are more commonly associated with the extrarenal pelvis than with the normal intrarenal pelvis.

Congenital calyceal diverticulum (calyceal cyst) is an infrequent anomaly. There is a marked dilatation of one calyx, and the resulting cyst is usually smooth and round, and lined with normal urothelium. There is no obstruction distal to the cyst.

Many such calyceal diverticula are incidental findings and do not appear to predispose to infection or to become progressively worse. These observations plus the frequent association with anomalous vertebrae suggest congenital rather than acquired lesions.

Clinically, calyceal cyst may be difficult to distinguish from stenosis of a calyx or obstruction in a single or duplicated pelvis. However, communication of the cyst directly with the remainder of the renal pelvis and the absence of stenosis usually help distinguish calyceal cyst.

Ureteropelvic junction (UPJ) obstruction is the most important and most common abnormality of the renal pelvis. Formerly, anomalous vessels were thought to kink the ureter or lower end of the pelvis and so cause UPJ obstruction. However, the frequency with which UPJ obstruction occurs in association with normal vessels and the frequency with which anomalous vessels occur without UPJ obstruction suggest that the obstruction is a result of other factors. For instance, bands or adhesions which kink the ureter and an unusual angle or location of the insertion of the ureter into the pelvis may be at fault. However, in many cases, the cause of UPJ obstruction is not related to stenosis, aberrant vessels, or other extrinsic factors, and it is assumed that a functional defect prevents normal emptying of the renal pelvis.

Some authors believe UPJ obstruction can be acquired by patients who have persistent long-standing vesicoureteral reflux. Whether UPJ obstruction is secondary to reflux, or whether the two conditions represent coincidental congenital

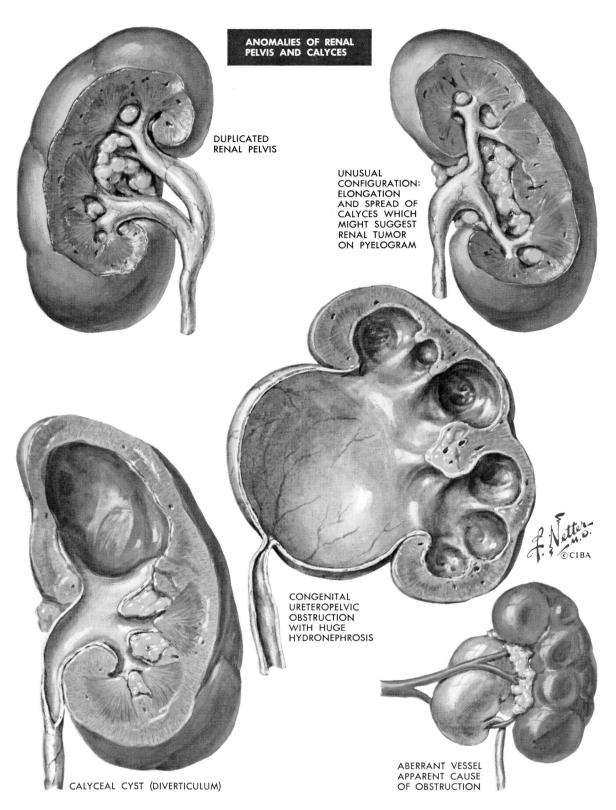

ANOMALIES OF RENAL PELVIS AND CALYCES

DUPLICATED RENAL PELVIS

UNUSUAL CONFIGURATION: ELONGATION AND SPREAD OF CALYCES WHICH MIGHT SUGGEST RENAL TUMOR ON PYELOGRAM

CONGENITAL URETEROPELVIC OBSTRUCTION WITH HUGE HYDRONEPHROSIS

CALYCEAL CYST (DIVERTICULUM)

ABERRANT VESSEL APPARENT CAUSE OF OBSTRUCTION

events, the physician must be alert to the possibility of UPJ obstruction in such patients.

Frequently, extrarenal pelvis is associated with UPJ obstruction, and although the extrarenal pelvis may have contributed to the obstruction, the distensibility of the pelvis acts as a safety valve and delays the onset of calyceal distention and hydronephrosis.

UPJ obstruction is bilateral in many patients, particularly those in whom symptoms develop early in life. When it is unilateral, UPJ obstruction is often associated with other anomalies in the contralateral kidney.

Clinically, UPJ obstruction with marked hydronephrosis commonly presents in infants as an abdominal mass, usually unilateral but occasionally bilateral. In patients who have no mass, the diagnosis may be delayed for some time since other symptoms are nonspecific: feeding problems, failure to thrive, and unexplained fever. In many patients, a search for the cause

of urinary tract infection leads to detection of the UPJ obstruction. Urinary tract infection or pain localized to the side of the lesion are the most common identifiable symptoms in older patients. Hematuria, particularly following mild trauma, is a common occurrence in hydronephrosis from any cause and may be observed in patients with UPJ obstruction. If the obstruction is bilateral or if it occurs in a single kidney, the patient may present with signs of renal failure including polyuria and hypertension.

Prolonged obstruction may produce marked calyceal dilatation and renal parenchymal compression. Nevertheless, even though the kidney looks nearly destroyed and renal function is markedly depressed, a considerable return of function is possible following relief of obstruction. Thus, many surgeons are conservative about recommending nephrectomy for UPJ obstruction, particularly in young children. □

Ureteral Duplication and Ectopic Ureter

Ureteropelvic duplication is the most common anomaly of the upper collecting system. The duplication is *complete* when there are two separate pelves, each with a complete ureter and separate ureteral orifice. In contrast, duplication is *incomplete* when the ureters join prior to entry into the bladder so that a single ureteral orifice is present.

Complete duplication is less common than incomplete duplication, but is more commonly associated with obstruction, infection, and anomalies of insertion. Thus, a relatively large percentage of patients who have symptomatic urinary tract disease caused by a ureteral duplication will have the complete form.

Ureteropelvic duplication is believed to arise from either the formation of two ureteral buds or the division of a single ureteral bud during embryogenesis. During normal development, the insertions of the ureters into the bladder migrate superiorly and laterally to occupy the positions normally occurring in the newborn infant. If ureteral duplication develops, the ureter from the lower pole of the kidney migrates in a relatively normal pattern, whereas that from the upper pole does not. Therefore, the bladder orifice of the ureter from the lower pole of the kidney generally is found in the normal position, and the bladder orifice of the ureter from the upper pole is located more medially and inferiorly. In a fairly large percentage of cases, the bladder orifice of the ureter from the upper pole is so far inferior to that from the lower pole as to be considered an ectopic orifice. As a corollary, in the vast majority of cases, an ectopic ureteral orifice associated with duplication belongs to the ureter which drains the upper pole of the kidney.

Complete Ureteral Duplication

Clinically, whether or not patients with complete duplication have symptoms depends primarily on the sites of the ureteral orifices and the competence of the ureterovesical junctions. When the ureters end close to the normal position at the trigone, the ureter from the lower pole generally penetrates the bladder wall in a more perpendicular direction and so has a shorter intramural course. For this reason, reflux into the lower pole ureter is common. Thus, parenchymal damage to the lower renal pole may occur because of obstruction and infection. Paradoxically, when the upper pole ureter enters the bladder far distal to the orifice of the lower pole ureter, damage to the parenchyma of the upper renal pole occurs. Obstruction, reflux, or both are frequent. Also, dysplasia of the upper pole is commonly associated.

In patients who have duplication without ectopic ureteral orifices, recurrent or persistent urinary tract infection, presumably caused by reflux into, and/or obstruction of, one of the anomalous ureters, may occur, or the duplication may be discovered incidentally.

On intravenous pyelogram, duplication of the pelvis and ureter may be seen unless the renal tissue drained by a du-

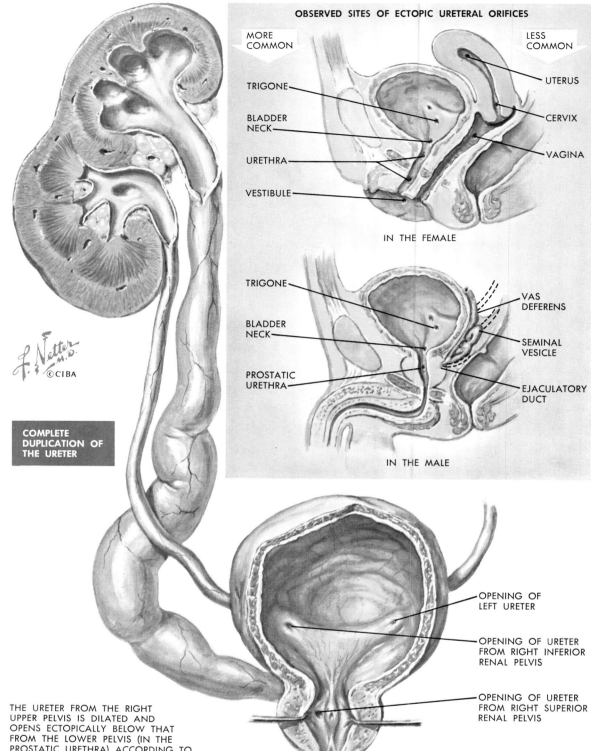

OBSERVED SITES OF ECTOPIC URETERAL ORIFICES

MORE COMMON — LESS COMMON

TRIGONE / BLADDER NECK / URETHRA / VESTIBULE / UTERUS / CERVIX / VAGINA

IN THE FEMALE

TRIGONE / BLADDER NECK / PROSTATIC URETHRA / VAS DEFERENS / SEMINAL VESICLE / EJACULATORY DUCT

IN THE MALE

COMPLETE DUPLICATION OF THE URETER

THE URETER FROM THE RIGHT UPPER PELVIS IS DILATED AND OPENS ECTOPICALLY BELOW THAT FROM THE LOWER PELVIS (IN THE PROSTATIC URETHRA) ACCORDING TO THE WEIGERT—MEYER LAW

OPENING OF LEFT URETER

OPENING OF URETER FROM RIGHT INFERIOR RENAL PELVIS

OPENING OF URETER FROM RIGHT SUPERIOR RENAL PELVIS

plicated ureter is nonfunctional. In that case, the pelvis of the visualized segment will be smaller than that of the opposite, normal side, with a reduced number of calyces. Generally, the nonvisualized pelvis also causes flattening of the upper part of the visualized pelvis. Voiding cystourethrogram may show reflux into the nonfunctioning system and cystoscopic examination may reveal the two ureteral orifices. Retrograde pyelography will confirm the diagnosis.

Incomplete Ureteral Duplication

Incomplete duplication is more common than the complete form but is less frequently associated with reflux or ectopic ureteral orifices. Thus, such duplication is less likely to cause symptoms and is more often found incidentally. However, a kidney drained by a partially duplicated ureter is still more likely to show anomalies than one drained by a single ureter.

The extent of duplication of the ureter varies from a simple bifid pelvis with a single ureter to a duplication that is complete except for the last few millimeters where the ureters join together in the bladder wall. In all cases of incomplete duplication there is a common ureteral orifice so that the incidence of reflux is much lower than with complete duplication. Also, there is an infrequent association of ectopic ureteral orifices.

Clinically, most of the problems presented by patients with incomplete duplication are caused by obstructions in the distal ureter, or by uretero-ureteral reflux. In this type of reflux the urine from one limb of the Y-shaped ureter refluxes into the other limb with consequent stasis and resulting infection. Some authorities believe that defective peristalsis at the site where the ureters join is the principal cause of this type of reflux.

In most patients, incomplete duplication is detected as an incidental finding during the course of investigation for infection or other renal problems. In a small percentage of patients, the incomplete duplication produces symptoms. If both urinary tract infection and partial duplication are present, however, it may be difficult to determine whether the duplication has contributed to the infection or is an incidental finding. In these patients, catheterization of both ureteral orifices is necessary to obtain urine for examination and culture. The presence of infection bilaterally suggests that the duplication may not be a contributing factor, whereas infection only on the side of the duplication suggests that ureteroureteral reflux may play a causal role.

Less common forms of duplication include those in which either the superior or the inferior end of the duplicated ureter is atretic. If the atresia occurs proximally while the ureter is patent distally, urine may reflux into this blind-ending ureter and produce dilatation, stasis, and infection. Functionally, this partial duplication behaves the same as a diverticulum of the ureter. Also, if urine-producing renal tissue is present superior to the area of atresia, sufficient urine may be produced to create a large cystic mass which may be mistaken for a tumor.

Rarely, the distal ureters are not duplicated at the proximal, renal end. In this situation two ureteral orifices are present, one of which communicates with the kidney while the other ends blindly, with or without an atretic cord continuing to the kidney. The blind-ending ureter functionally resembles a diverticulum of the bladder (see page 218) and may produce symptoms if it becomes infected or dilated. Clinically, diagnosis of the duplicated lower urinary tract may be made by cystoscopy or by the voiding cystourethrogram if reflux into the blind-ending ureter occurs.

Ectopic Ureter

It will be recalled that in the embryo the metanephric duct or primitive ureter arises as a bud from the mesonephric or wolffian duct (see page 31). As the embryo develops, the metanephric duct and the mesonephric duct acquire their own orifices into the cloaca. After the development of the vesicoureteral canal, the metanephric duct begins shifting, and eventually the opening of the metanephric duct, now called the ureter, is superior to the orifice of the wolffian duct. Thus, failure of the ureteric bud to ascend normally will result in an anomalous or ectopic orifice. The ectopic orifice may be located in the bladder neck or the urethra, or occasionally in the wolffian duct remnants in the male or the müllerian duct derivatives in the female (see page 34).

In female patients, ectopic ureter is nearly always associated with duplication of the upper urinary tract, and in nearly every patient, the ectopic ureter comes from the upper pole of the kidney. The ectopic ureteral orifice very often opens distal to the urethral sphincter, and this insertion is responsible for one of the characteristic symptoms of the disorder—dribbling incontinence.

On the other hand, in male patients

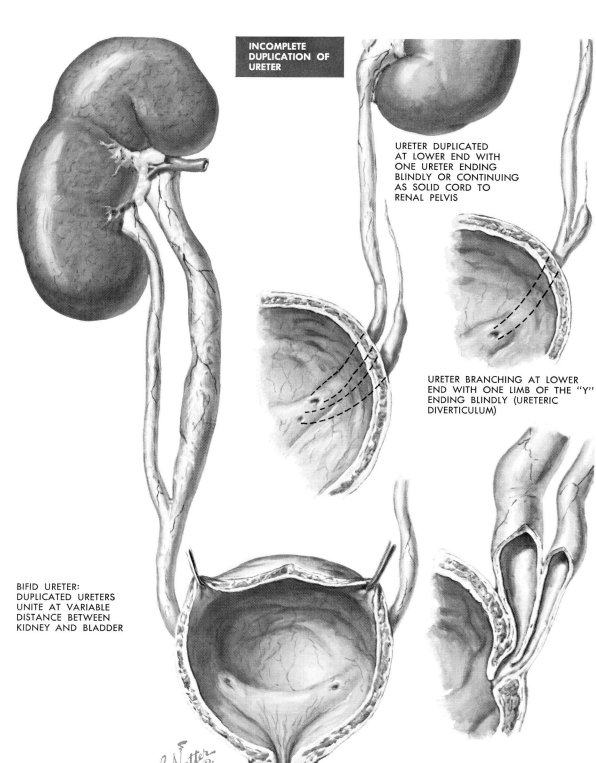

BIFID URETER: DUPLICATED URETERS UNITE AT VARIABLE DISTANCE BETWEEN KIDNEY AND BLADDER

INCOMPLETE DUPLICATION OF URETER

URETER DUPLICATED AT LOWER END WITH ONE URETER ENDING BLINDLY OR CONTINUING AS SOLID CORD TO RENAL PELVIS

URETER BRANCHING AT LOWER END WITH ONE LIMB OF THE "Y" ENDING BLINDLY (URETERIC DIVERTICULUM)

DUPLICATED URETERS UNITING IN BLADDER WALL TO ENTER BLADDER BY A COMMON ORIFICE

an ectopic ureter is less likely to be associated with duplication of the ureters, and the ectopic ureter nearly always terminates proximal to the external sphincter. Thus, incontinence occurs much less commonly in males with ectopic ureters.

Clinically, in a female patient the diagnosis may be suspected because of the occurrence of relatively constant urinary dribbling despite normal voiding patterns. If the ureter opens into the vagina or uterus, signs of vaginitis may be present. In the majority of male patients and in female patients in whom dribbling is absent, symptoms of urinary tract infection may be the first clinical manifestation.

The diagnosis of ectopic ureter may be difficult to establish if there is no history of dribbling. However, cystoscopy, urethroscopy, or vaginoscopy may reveal the ectopic orifice, or on a voiding cystourethrogram the orifice may be discovered to fill.

Treatment

Uncomplicated duplication requires no treatment. However, if complications such as infection occur, duplication with or without ectopic ureter is nearly always managed surgically. If the condition is discovered before serious renal damage has occurred and before there is massive ureteral dilatation, reimplantation of the ureter may be feasible. In patients with duplication without ectopia, the ureters are usually contained within a single sheet, and reimplantation of the ureters as a single unit is the best procedure.

If, however, significant renal damage has occurred in one or the other of the duplicated segments, heminephrectomy with ureterectomy is usually the treatment of choice. When both poles of the kidney are badly damaged and a normal kidney is present on the other side, nephroureterectomy may be preferred. □

Ureterocele

BILATERAL URETEROCELES: ORIFICE OF
RIGHT URETEROCELE NOT VISIBLE BECAUSE
IT IS ON UNDERSURFACE OF THE CYST

BLADDER
MUCOSA

URETERAL
MUCOSA

URETER

ORIFICE

BLADDER
WALL

A ureterocele is a cystic ballooning of the intramural portion of the ureter. It is believed to be caused by a stricture of the tip of the ureter which raises intraureteral hydrostatic pressure sufficiently to balloon the ureter into the bladder. However, why the dilatation involves only the intravesicular portion of the ureter, rather than the entire structure, is not known. In any case, as the ureter protrudes inward, it carries with it the adjacent bladder wall. The wall of the ureterocele thus consists of a covering of bladder mucosa, an attenuated connective tissue and muscle layer, and a lining of ureteral mucosa.

Ureteroceles may be unilateral or bilateral, may occur in duplicated, ectopic, or otherwise normal ureters, and may or may not cause obstruction of the bladder outlet. In children, a ureterocele is commonly associated with duplication of the ureter and usually involves the orifice of an ectopic ureter draining the upper renal pole. An ectopic ureterocele is much more common in girls and is likely to cause obstruction of the bladder neck, of the ureter draining the lower pole of the duplicated system, or even of the contralateral ureter. In older children and adults, the more common forms of ureterocele arise in either normally placed single ureters or duplicated ureters without ectopia and, again, may be unilateral or bilateral. Also, this condition is usually accompanied by an obstruction of the ureter associated with the ureterocele. Occasionally, obstruction of the contralateral ureter is observed. If the ureterocele involves a duplicated urinary tract, reflux into the nonaffected ureter on the ipsilateral side is frequent.

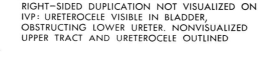

RIGHT-SIDED DUPLICATION NOT VISUALIZED ON
IVP: URETEROCELE VISIBLE IN BLADDER,
OBSTRUCTING LOWER URETER. NONVISUALIZED
UPPER TRACT AND URETEROCELE OUTLINED

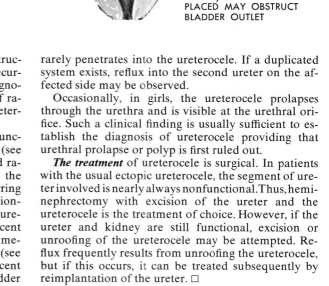

URETEROCELE AT ECTOPIC
ORIFICE OF A DUPLICATED
URETER; URETEROCELE SO
PLACED MAY OBSTRUCT
BLADDER OUTLET

Clinically, ureteroceles of all types produce obstruction, and the common presenting symptom is recurrent or persistent urinary tract infection. The diagnosis of ureterocele is usually made with the aid of radiologic and cystoscopic studies employed to determine the cause of such infection.

If the ureter affected by the ureterocele drains functional renal tissue, the intravenous pyelogram (see page 91) often pictures the ureterocele as a round radiopacity with a radiolucent rim projecting into the bladder. However, in the more commonly occurring situation in which the ureter drains a poorly functioning kidney (observed particularly in ectopic ureterocele), the ureterocele appears as a radiolucent area in a bladder otherwise filled with contrast medium. Similarly, the voiding cystourethrogram (see page 97) also shows the ureterocele as a radiolucent shadow since the radiopaque medium in the bladder

rarely penetrates into the ureterocele. If a duplicated system exists, reflux into the second ureter on the affected side may be observed.

Occasionally, in girls, the ureterocele prolapses through the urethra and is visible at the urethral orifice. Such a clinical finding is usually sufficient to establish the diagnosis of ureterocele providing that urethral prolapse or polyp is first ruled out.

The treatment of ureterocele is surgical. In patients with the usual ectopic ureterocele, the segment of ureter involved is nearly always nonfunctional. Thus, heminephrectomy with excision of the ureter and the ureterocele is the treatment of choice. However, if the ureter and kidney are still functional, excision or unroofing of the ureterocele may be attempted. Reflux frequently results from unroofing the ureterocele, but if this occurs, it can be treated subsequently by reimplantation of the ureter. □

Retrocaval Ureter

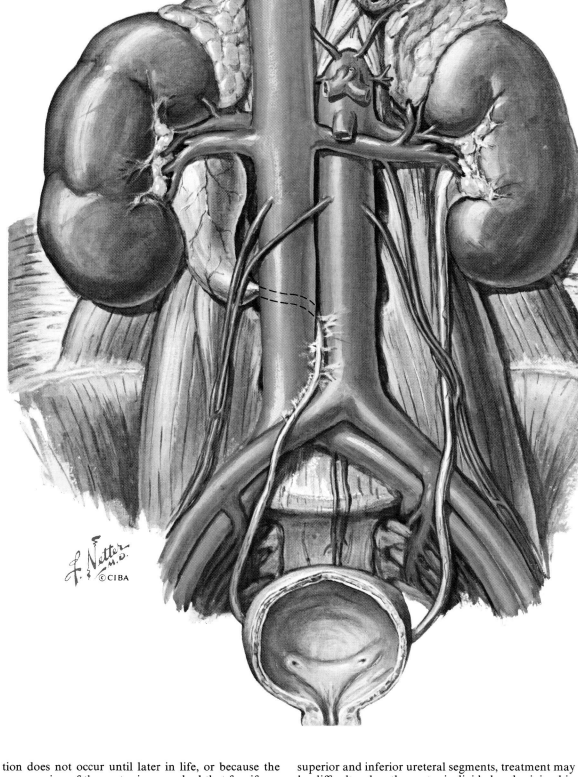

Retrocaval ureter is a relatively uncommon condition in which the *right ureter* passes *posterior* to, rather than anterior to, the *inferior vena cava* before reaching the bladder.

The displaced position of the ureter is actually caused by an anomaly of the abdominal venous system. During normal development of the embryo, the definitive inferior vena cava arises from a persistence of the right subcardinal vein caudal to the kidney (see page 17 and CIBA COLLECTION, Vol. 5, pages 129-133). However, if the posterior cardinal vein persists to form the infrarenal portion of the inferior vena cava, the right ureter becomes trapped posterior to the inferior vena cava.

The right posterior cardinal vein is initially dorsal and lateral to the subcardinal vein. As the metanephros ascends, the right posterior cardinal vein eventually crosses anterior to the metanephros. At the same time, the portion of the subcardinal vein which normally would form the infrarenal portion of the inferior vena cava lies posterior to both the ureter and metanephros. Thus, if the right posterior cardinal vein (instead of the subcardinal vein) forms the infrarenal part of the inferior vena cava, the ureter takes a circular route posterior, medial, and then anterior to the vein before reaching the bladder.

If sufficient space remains between the inferior vena cava and the lumbar vertebral column, the abnormal course of the right ureter causes no difficulty. However, when the ureter is compressed between the vena cava and the spine, the resulting obstruction will lead to right-sided hydroureter and hydronephrosis. The ureter often becomes fibrotic and stenosed in the compressed area.

Clinically, right flank pain, recurrent urinary tract infection, renal calculi, and hematuria occasionally develop in early childhood. Usually, however, the first symptoms do not appear until the third or fourth decade, either because obstruc-

tion does not occur until later in life, or because the compression of the ureter is so gradual that few if any symptoms are produced. In adults, intermittent or persistent right flank pain and recurrent urinary tract infections which are resistant to therapy may be present.

Diagnosis and Treatment. Intravenous or retrograde urography will usually demonstrate a marked discrepancy between the sizes of the superior and inferior sections of the right ureter. A spiraling of the narrowed ureter around the inferior vena cava can usually be detected, but sometimes this is recognized only because the ureter is displaced medially. Occasionally, a patient may have a radiologic examination because of symptoms which predate obstruction. In this situation, a medial displacement and spiraling course of the ureter without a discrepancy in size may be the only findings on which to base the diagnosis.

Because of the marked differences in sizes of the

superior and inferior ureteral segments, treatment may be difficult unless the ureter is divided and rejoined in the dilated segment at a point where postoperative stricture seems less likely to occur. If there is stenosis of the retrocaval portion of the ureter or if the ureter adheres to the vena cava, it may be necessary to excise the stenotic or adherent portion of the ureter and then to anastomose the narrowed distal segment with the dilated proximal segment.

It should be noted that compression of the ureter may also be produced by anomalous arteries, most of which obstruct the distal portion rather than the mid-portion of the ureter. Obstructions have been produced by the umbilical branch of the hypogastric artery, the obturator artery, or the iliac artery. These conditions are similar to retrocaval ureter; treatment consists of resection and anastomosis of the ureter or reimplantation into the bladder. □

"Prune-Belly" Syndrome

Congenital absence of the abdominal musculature, the "prune-belly" syndrome, is a rare disorder which affects males almost exclusively. Most of the medial and inferior musculature of the abdominal wall either is entirely absent or has been replaced by a homogeneous ground substance without recognizable muscle tissue. The musculature of the ureters and bladder appears to be affected by a similar process, with attenuation of the muscle fibers and replacement by fibrous tissue. Often there are associated urinary tract anomalies and undescended testes. The cause is unknown.

Although the abnormality of the abdominal wall musculature is prominent, it causes surprisingly little difficulty except for pulmonary disorders attributable to poor abdominal support, and a weak cough. Also, if there is urethral obstruction (see below), severe oligohydramnios may result and be associated with pulmonary hypoplasia and talipes equinovarus. Just as importantly, gastrointestinal and cardiac anomalies are frequently associated with the syndrome. Nevertheless, survival of children with "prune-belly" syndrome depends primarily on the severity of the renal and urinary tract anomalies.

Urinary Tract Abnormalities. The urinary tract is diffusely affected. The bladder is markedly dilated and contracts poorly; the ureters are dilated, and peristalsis is either absent or markedly diminished; hydronephrosis is present bilaterally. In many patients, the kidneys are dysplastic, presumably as a result of obstruction during gestation.

The dilatation of the bladder, ureters, and renal pelves can be explained in some patients by an obstruction in the lower urinary tract. Other patients have no detectable obstruction, and the dilatation is assumed to be caused by the intrinsic defect in the musculature of the urinary tract. However, in some patients, the presence of defective urinary tract musculature may be difficult to establish since the histology of the bladder is normal.

Clinical Findings. The discovery of a lax, protuberant, thin abdominal wall with multiple creases usually leads to the diagnosis of "prune-belly" syndrome at the time of birth. The absence of muscular tissue in the abdominal wall may be established by palpation of the abdomen, particularly when the infant is crying. Almost invariably, the presence of bilateral cryptorchidism further supports the diagnosis. Since the inferior abdominal muscles are more severely affected than the superior musculature, attempted contraction of the abdominal muscles

produces an upward movement of the umbilicus.

Radiologically, the usual finding in patients with "prune-belly" syndrome is the presence of a grossly dilated urinary tract often associated with poor renal function as judged by the intravenous pyelogram. Bilateral reflux is frequently seen in the voiding cystourethrogram. The ureters are tortuous and may show segmental or saccular dilatation with delayed emptying times. The bladder is usually large, and the apex of the bladder extends to, and is often attached to, the umbilicus.

The only disorder likely to be confused with the "prune-belly" syndrome is congenital urethral valves with massive hydronephrosis (see CIBA COLLECTION, Vol. 2, page 30). In the latter condition, prolonged distention of the abdomen *in utero* leads to a flabby musculature which, when combined with uremia and generalized dilatation of the urinary tract, closely simu-

lates "prune-belly" syndrome. Generally, when the infant is a male with undescended testes and complete absence, rather than attenuation, of abdominal musculature, the diagnosis of "prune-belly" syndrome is indicated. However, in the exceptional instance, it may be necessary to exclude the possibility of posterior urethral valves before the diagnosis can be considered established.

Prognosis. Whether children with this syndrome survive depends primarily on the severity of the renal and urinary tract anomalies. Generally, the early mortality rate is high; 20 percent of the patients die within the first month of life, and 50 percent within 2 years. The cause of death is uremia or urinary tract infection. Those patients without marked urinary tract anomalies may live reasonably normal lives, and as they grow older, the abdominal wall defect becomes less obvious. □

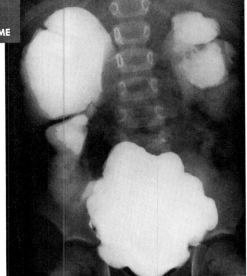

VOIDING CYSTOGRAM: REFLUX INTO MASSIVELY DILATED URINARY TRACT AND ABNORMALITY OF BLADDER MUSCULATURE

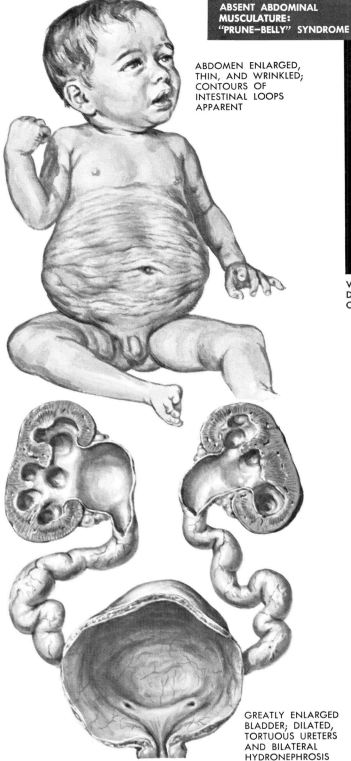

ABSENT ABDOMINAL MUSCULATURE: "PRUNE-BELLY" SYNDROME

ABDOMEN ENLARGED, THIN, AND WRINKLED; CONTOURS OF INTESTINAL LOOPS APPARENT

GREATLY ENLARGED BLADDER; DILATED, TORTUOUS URETERS AND BILATERAL HYDRONEPHROSIS

ABDOMINAL LAXITY BECOMES LESS APPARENT WITH AGE

Anomalies of the Urachus

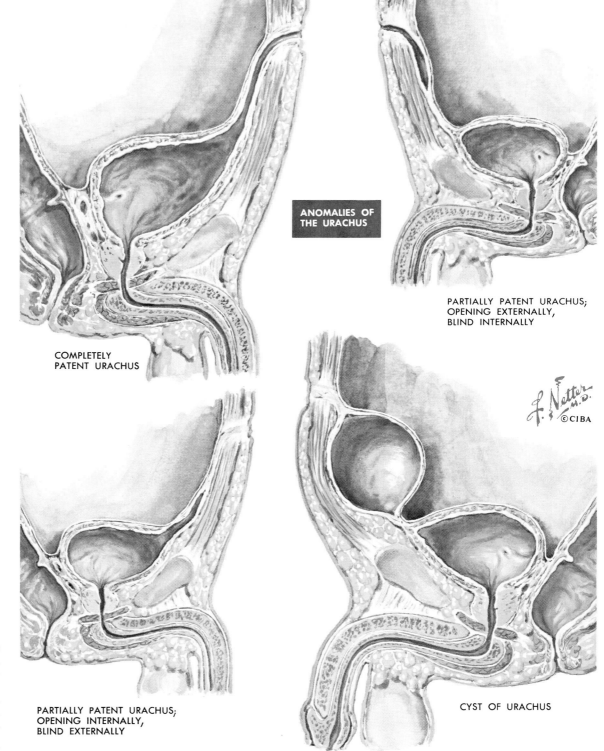

ANOMALIES OF
THE URACHUS

COMPLETELY
PATENT URACHUS

PARTIALLY PATENT URACHUS;
OPENING EXTERNALLY,
BLIND INTERNALLY

PARTIALLY PATENT URACHUS;
OPENING INTERNALLY,
BLIND EXTERNALLY

CYST OF URACHUS

In the human embryo, the bladder develops from that portion of the cloaca at which the allantois joins the urogenital sinus (see page 34). By late fetal life, the allantois has narrowed to form the urachal canal which closes at birth, or soon afterward, to form the middle umbilical ligament. Urachal anomalies include a failure of the urachal canal to close, either partially or completely. A patent urachus may lead to formation of a sinus or cyst, which may in turn produce clinical symptoms.

Completely patent urachus is caused by a failure of obliteration of the urachal canal. Often, an accompanying obstruction distal to the bladder prevents normal bladder emptying. Urine forced through the urachus to drain externally from the umbilicus thus maintains urachal patency. Also, because of the attachment to the umbilicus, the bladder usually is located high in the abdomen.

Clinically, a completely patent urachus is usually indicated by a profuse watery discharge from the umbilicus which increases during voiding. The diagnosis may be confirmed by cystography in which the dye can be seen to pass through the fistulous tract and externally through

the umbilicus. Injection of radiopaque dye directly into the fistula will also demonstrate a connection between the urachal canal and the bladder. Either cystoscopy or voiding cystourethrography may be used to demonstrate obstruction distal to the bladder. A patent urachus is treated by removal of any obstruction and excision of the urachal tract.

Partially patent urachus may persist as a diverticulum superior to the bladder. In this instance, the urachal tract is patent at the vesical end but is closed toward the umbilicus. The condition is usually asymptomatic unless urinary infection or calculi develop. Urachal diverticula produce symptoms similar to those of other bladder diverticula (see page 218).

Umbilical Sinus. If the urachal canal is obliterated at the bladder end but remains patent near the umbilicus, an umbilical sinus is formed. Providing there is sufficient secretion into the urachal canal, persis-

tent drainage from the umbilicus will occur. Most of the blind-ending tracts located at the umbilicus will close spontaneously. However, occasionally, excision may be required if secretion persists.

Urachal Cyst. When the urachal canal is obliterated at both ends but remains patent in the central portion, a cyst of the urachus may develop if there is continued exudation of fluid from the urachal epithelial lining. Most urachal cysts are small and without clinical significance. Occasionally, a cyst will become large enough to produce symptoms of an abdominal mass and, if infection supervenes, may simulate an intra-abdominal abscess. Such an infected urachal cyst may rupture into the abdominal cavity or into the bladder. Diagnosis of a urachal cyst is often very difficult and is usually made following an exploratory laparotomy. If the cyst is not infected, it should be excised; if the cyst is infected, marsupialization is indicated.□

Megacystis Syndrome

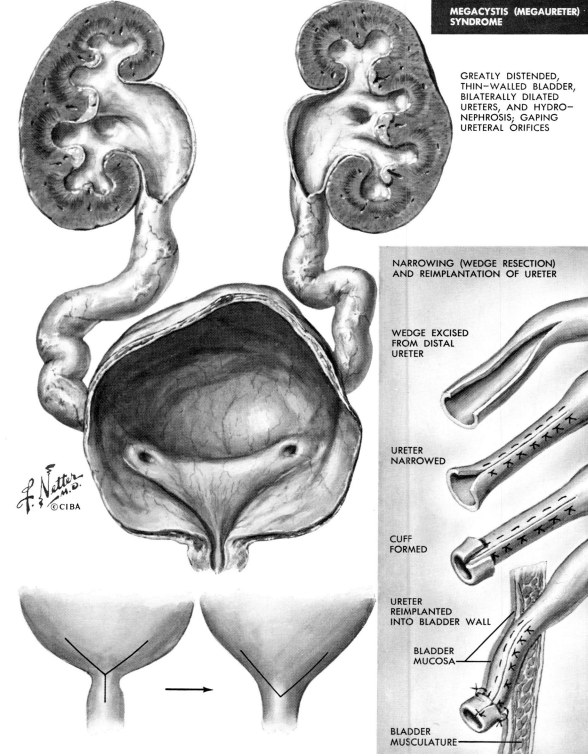

GREATLY DISTENDED, THIN-WALLED BLADDER, BILATERALLY DILATED URETERS, AND HYDRO-NEPHROSIS; GAPING URETERAL ORIFICES

NARROWING (WEDGE RESECTION) AND REIMPLANTATION OF URETER

WEDGE EXCISED FROM DISTAL URETER

URETER NARROWED

CUFF FORMED

URETER REIMPLANTED INTO BLADDER WALL

BLADDER MUCOSA

BLADDER MUSCULATURE

PRINCIPLE OF ANTERIOR Y-V PLASTY OF BLADDER NECK

The megacystis-megaureter syndrome is an ill-defined condition in which there is massive dilatation of the bladder and ureters, bilateral reflux, but no evidence of obstruction distal to the bladder to explain the massive dilatation.

The symptoms of this syndrome are difficult to define because few values are available for normal bladder capacity and voiding pressure in children. Nevertheless, it is generally assumed that a child's bladder capacity should not exceed 200 to 300 ml, and a capacity greater than 500 ml must be considered abnormal. It is also difficult to determine definitively the presence or absence of infravesical obstruction by radiologic or endoscopic procedures currently available.

Megacystis is nonetheless defined as a condition in which the bladder has a large capacity (at least 500 ml), a smooth rather than a trabeculated wall, and the capability of emptying itself completely with a relatively normal intravesical pressure. The trigone is also enlarged, and the ureteral orifices are far apart, each with a rounded rather than a crescentic shape which is usually described as "patulous." Whether the large trigone is a primary defect leading to reflux, or whether it enlarges along with the rest of the bladder as a secondary effect of the megacystis is unknown.

Free reflux occurs into both ureters, which are usually markedly dilated and often longer and more tortuous than normal. The kidneys are frequently hydronephrotic with marked dilatation of the calyces and pelves as well as thinning of the parenchyma. Dysplastic areas are also seen.

Most authorities have discarded the possibility that obstruction of the bladder outlet might explain the megacystis and refluxing megaureters. The normal voiding pressures, the lack of trabeculation, and the failure to find any detectable lesion by cystoscopy all suggest that organic obstruction cannot account for this syndrome.

The possibility that abnormal innervation of the bladder and ureters might cause the massive dilatation, in a manner analogous to the causation of Hirschsprung's disease, has been considered. However, an apparent deficit of ganglion cells originally thought to be pathologic has since been shown to be normal.

Another possibility is that the megacystis represents a functional defect caused by persistent reflux of a large portion of the bladder contents into the ureters during voiding. After voiding, rapid refilling of the bladder occurs as the ureters discharge not only the refluxed but also the newly formed urine. Thus, the bladder is kept in an almost constant state of distention which leads to the persistent dilatation seen in this syndrome. The functional defect could therefore be similar to that seen in infants with neonatal diabetes insipidus (see page 246), in whom the ureters and bladder become persistently dilated because of the large volume of urine passed.

Because the greatest danger in megacystis is kidney damage from ureteral reflux, reimplantation of the ureters into the bladder in such a way as to prevent future reflux appears to be the treatment of choice. In simple vesicoureteral reflux, in which the ureters have not yet become dilated, the Leadbetter-Politano procedure is generally used. However, when the ureter is massively dilated, the extravesical approach of Paquin, as illustrated above, is preferred.

Although obstruction distal to the bladder is not considered a causative factor in megacystis, some surgeons believe a Y-V plasty at the bladder neck is helpful in decreasing voiding pressure and thus in minimizing the chance of reflux. The Y-V plasty increases the effective aperture of the bladder neck and, because of the conversion of a longitudinal incision into a transverse one (see illustration), effectively shortens the urethra. □

Congenital Bladder Outlet Obstruction

In the past, congenital obstruction of the bladder outlet was considered to be a condition commonly responsible, in childhood, for many cases of hydroureter and hydronephrosis, as well as for recurrent urinary tract infections with or without reflux. Recently, however, objections have been raised to the belief that bladder outlet obstruction is of major importance in causing upper tract pathology in children.

In particular, the concept of *bladder neck obstruction* has been questioned. The lack of definitive endoscopic, radiographic, or cystometric criteria for this type of obstruction makes it especially difficult to evaluate the significance of such a lesion in causing obstruction to the bladder outlet.

The changes in the bladder neck seen on the voiding cystourethrogram or endoscopy are now considered by many to be variants or alterations within the normal range. Furthermore, many patients in whom bladder neck revision had been performed to relieve recurrent cystitis or ureteral reflux had shown no objective evidence of obstruction at the bladder neck. For this reason, bladder neck revision has fallen into disrepute among many urologists. The use of such surgery, therefore, remains controversial, with some centers reporting not one bladder neck revision in over 5 years, and others still performing many plastic procedures or transurethral resections for bladder neck obstruction.

The lesion first described by Bodian as *fibroelastosis of the prostate* has recently met with the same skepticism as has bladder neck obstruction. Ironically, Bodian originally used the possibility of fibroelastosis to cast doubt on bladder neck obstruction. He pointed out a distal lesion that might cause hypertrophy of the bladder neck. However, most urologists have been unable to confirm the existence of this lesion and therefore cast doubt on both bladder neck obstruction and fibroelastosis of the prostatic urethra as causes of bladder outlet obstruction.

The only congenital obstructive lesion of the posterior urethra which has not been seriously questioned is *congenital posterior urethral valves.* In this condition, the normal ridges which run from the lower portion of the verumontanum to the lateral urethral wall characteristically are sufficiently hyperplastic to form folds of mucous membrane. These folds act as a valvular obstruction to the outflow of urine. As a result, the posterior urethra becomes dilated, and the bladder musculature becomes markedly hypertrophied, forming the typical trabeculated bladder detected by cystography or cystoscopy.

In all but the mildest cases of posterior urethral valves, the ureters become markedly dilated, and hydronephrosis is produced by the severe obstruction. In addition to the renal damage produced by obstruction, dysplasia of the kidneys is frequently found.

In the most severe cases, the findings

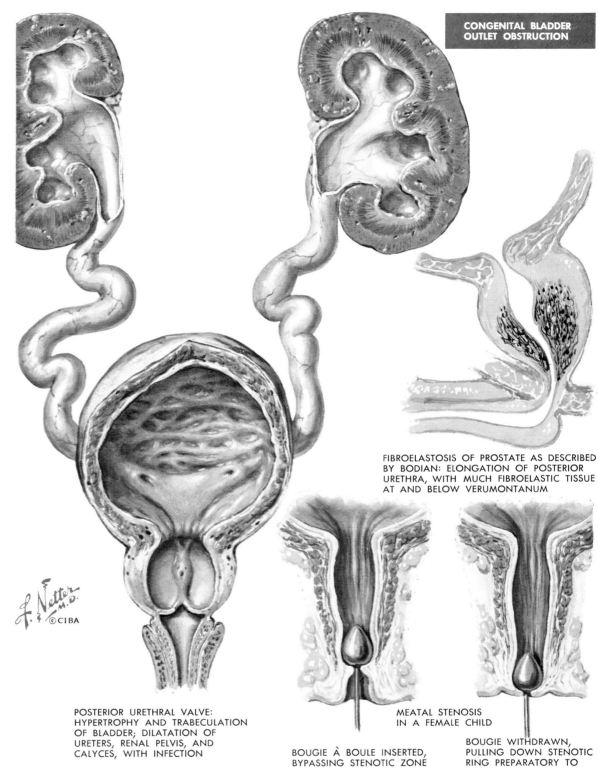

FIBROELASTOSIS OF PROSTATE AS DESCRIBED BY BODIAN: ELONGATION OF POSTERIOR URETHRA, WITH MUCH FIBROELASTIC TISSUE AT AND BELOW VERUMONTANUM

POSTERIOR URETHRAL VALVE: HYPERTROPHY AND TRABECULATION OF BLADDER; DILATATION OF URETERS, RENAL PELVIS, AND CALYCES, WITH INFECTION

MEATAL STENOSIS IN A FEMALE CHILD

BOUGIE À BOULE INSERTED, BYPASSING STENOTIC ZONE

BOUGIE WITHDRAWN, PULLING DOWN STENOTIC RING PREPARATORY TO RUPTURE OR INCISION

are those of prolonged obstruction: anuria or dribbling incontinence, distention of the abdomen, vomiting or weight loss, and the chemical findings of renal insufficiency. When the obstruction is less severe, the child may simply develop urinary tract infection at a later age.

The diagnosis is usually made by the characteristic findings on voiding cystourethrogram, the most prominent of which is a bulging dilatation of the posterior urethra with a sudden transition to a very narrowed distal urethra. The valves themselves may or may not be observed. Massive reflux into both ureters is seen. Other common findings are a dilated, trabeculated bladder and dilated ureters, pelves, and calyces.

The first aim in therapy is to remove the obstructing valves, using an infant resectoscope. In many instances, this procedure alone is adequate to permit gradual restoration of the urinary tract. However, in

some patients, secondary changes at the ureteropelvic junction continue to cause persistent obstruction or reflux even after removal of valves. In these cases, reimplantation of the ureters or urinary diversion is required.

Meatal stenosis is a common obstructive lesion in males, but the presence of meatal or distal urethral stenosis in females is much rarer. Such a lesion is frequently implicated by some urologists as a cause of infection. It is presumed to consist of a collagenous ring in the distal part of the urethra.

Although the diagnosis of distal urethral stenosis may be suggested by the voiding cystourethrogram or by the character of the urinary stream, calibration with the *bougie à boule* is the definitive method. The *bougie à boule* is also used in treating the lesion by withdrawing the stenosed ring prior to rupture or incision as illustrated. □

Duplication and Septa of the Bladder

Complete duplication of the bladder presumably results from a sagittal splitting of the anlage of the bladder during embryogenesis. Usually the rest of the lower genitourinary tract is also duplicated, each bladder being drained by a separate urethra which, in the male, passes through a separate penis. Since each bladder drains an individual ureter and since the musculature of each bladder is relatively normal, the duplication itself is compatible with normal urinary tract function. However, the duplication is frequently associated with anomalies elsewhere, in particular duplication of the large bowel, with consequent problems from intestinal obstruction and rectourethral fistulae. Other anomalies are common and frequently lead to obstruction of one or both urethras or bladders.

The treatment of complete duplication usually requires a plastic procedure for restoration of normal appearance. The usual method consists of removing one of the duplicated bladders along with its urethra and reimplantation of the respective ureter into the remaining bladder.

Incomplete duplication of the bladder is a less serious anomaly which consists of partial duplication of the upper portion of the bladder without duplication of the trigone or urethra. The division of the two portions of the bladder is usually sagittal, but frontal duplication has also been noted. Other anomalies, particularly bowel abnormalities, are much less common than with complete duplication, a fact which is reflected in the much better prognosis of the incomplete form. The only condition likely to be confused clinically with incomplete duplication is a vesical diverticulum into which a ureter empties (see page 218). However, a diverticulum usually lacks a complete muscular coat and is more frequently associated with obstruction. Thus, the differentiation of these two conditions should not be difficult.

Incomplete duplication requires no therapy unless obstruction, infection, or stones occur. In such cases, it may be necessary to remove the obstructing segment of bladder and reimplant the ureter. However, if severe damage to the kidney drained by that segment has occurred, nephrectomy and ureterectomy may be required.

The "hourglass" bladder is usually considered to be a variety of incomplete duplication. Because of its distinctive appearance, however, it is sometimes thought of as a separate entity, even though it results from an incomplete duplication of the bladder in a horizontal plane. When the ureters enter the upper portion of the hourglass bladder, little

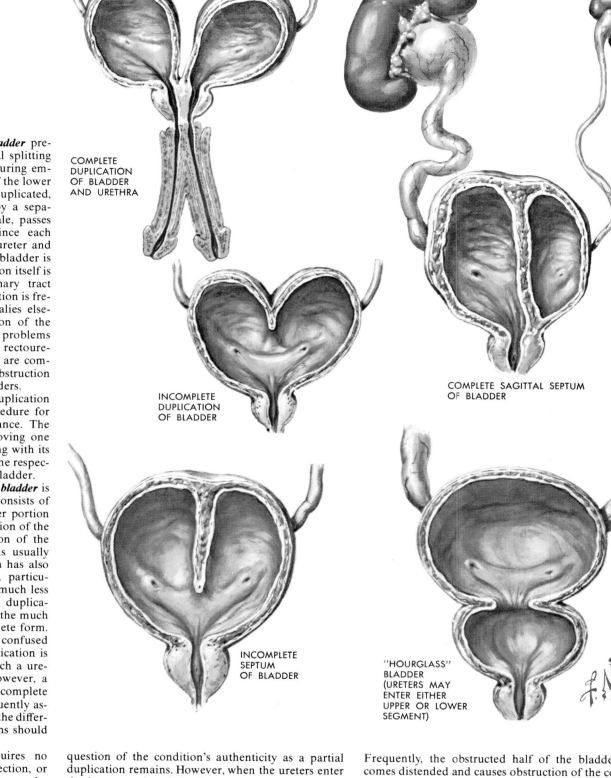

COMPLETE DUPLICATION OF BLADDER AND URETHRA

INCOMPLETE DUPLICATION OF BLADDER

COMPLETE SAGITTAL SEPTUM OF BLADDER

INCOMPLETE SEPTUM OF BLADDER

"HOURGLASS" BLADDER (URETERS MAY ENTER EITHER UPPER OR LOWER SEGMENT)

question of the condition's authenticity as a partial duplication remains. However, when the ureters enter the lower portion, it is difficult to be certain that a true hourglass bladder is present since a urachal diverticulum may mimic the hourglass bladder and confuse the diagnosis (see page 239).

Treatment for hourglass bladder is dependent on the presence of obstruction and the efficiency with which the bladder empties.

Septa of the bladder are analogous to duplication except that the external appearance of the bladder is normal. The septum may be *complete* or *incomplete*. Complete sagittal septum is the most serious anomaly of this group because it impairs urinary tract function. Since only a single urethra is present, the septum nearly always causes complete obstruction to the drainage of one kidney and ureter with resultant atrophy and/or dysplasia of the kidney on that side.

Frequently, the obstructed half of the bladder becomes distended and causes obstruction of the contralateral ureter, leading to renal damage from hydronephrosis on that side.

The treatment for complete septum of the bladder is the removal of the septum, with or without nephroureterectomy on the side that was originally completely obstructed.

Incomplete septum of the bladder is the least serious of these anomalies since obstruction is rather infrequent. This anomaly may be discovered only incidentally during urologic study or autopsy. Since it is frequently associated with other anomalies, its discovery during routine urologic tests may be an indication to search for abnormalities elsewhere, particularly in the colon. In an occasional patient, obstruction is found with resultant infection and renal damage. Then, surgical removal of the septum may be required. □

Exstrophy of the Bladder

Exstrophy of the bladder is a serious genitourinary anomaly in which both the lower portion of the anterior abdominal wall and the anterior wall of the bladder are missing. In addition, the posterior wall of the bladder is everted and fused laterally with the remaining abdominal wall.

Complete exstrophy of the bladder, the most common form, is accompanied by wide separation of the pubic bones and by epispadias with a rudimentary broad penis in boys or a cleft clitoris in girls. In both sexes, the urethra is a short, flat strip of mucosa, and the bladder neck is rudimentary or nonexistent.

In addition to these nearly constant features of exstrophy, the frequency of other anomalies, particularly skeletal and intestinal malformations, is high.

The diagnosis of complete exstrophy of the bladder is made by inspection, but the detection of associated anomalies and the evaluation of the functional state of the upper urinary tract require further study. An intravenous pyelogram is the most useful tool for detection of the presence of ureteral duplication and uretero-vesical junction obstruction, two of the urinary tract abnormalities which commonly accompany exstrophy (see pages 233 and 234).

The exact embryologic mechanism of exstrophy is unknown. One theory is that nonregression of the cloacal membrane early in gestation prevents both meso-dermal ingrowth into the anterior abdominal wall and closure of the bladder itself, and holds apart the ischiopubic bones. This theory would also explain the epispadias and bifid phallus which accompany exstrophy. Experimentally, exstrophy has been produced in animals by a procedure which mimics nonregression of the cloacal membrane.

In the patient with uncorrected exstrophy, the persistent urinary incontinence produces excoriation and ulceration of the bladder and surrounding skin. The inflamed vesical mucosa becomes hyperplastic and polypoid, and malignant change is frequent if the patient survives to adult life (see page 209).

Other notable findings are the waddling gait resulting from external rotation of the acetabula, rectal prolapse, and umbilical and inguinal hernias. Urinary tract infection is a constant danger, and although the exact incidence of infection in these patients is unknown, pyelonephritis is reported to be the most common cause of death. Prior to the availability of antibiotics, two thirds of the patients with uncorrected exstrophy died in the first decade of life. Most of the deaths were caused by infection, and few patients survived to adulthood.

The therapy for exstrophy is difficult at best, always time-consuming, and frequently disappointing. In a few patients, it has been possible to reconstruct the

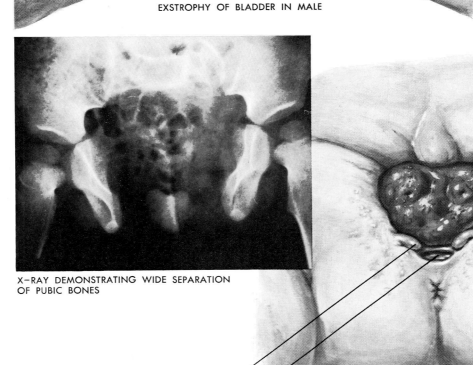

EXSTROPHY OF BLADDER IN MALE

UMBILICAL HERNIA
BLADDER MUCOSA
URETERAL ORIFICES
GLANS PENIS
CRYPTORCHIDISM
SCROTUM

X-RAY DEMONSTRATING WIDE SEPARATION OF PUBIC BONES

DIVIDED CLITORIS
VAGINA

EXSTROPHY OF BLADDER IN FEMALE

bladder and the urethra, to draw the pubic bones together, and to construct a relatively normal phallus, resulting in a patient who is continent, free of infection, and capable of normal sexual activities later in life. However, the number of cases in which such therapy is successful is very small, only five to 10 percent, even in very competent hands. The majority of patients are left with a bladder which is too small, and they continue to suffer incontinence, reflux, and recurrent urinary tract infections. Therefore, most patients ultimately have some form of urinary diversion with removal of the bladder. If the rectum is otherwise normal, ureterosigmoidostomy appears to be the procedure of choice. Even when the anus and rectum appear normal, however, a number of patients have persistent urinary incontinence. In addition, ascending infection from the sigmoid is a constant threat. Therefore, many surgeons prefer to construct an iso-

lated ileal conduit, using the Bricker procedure, even though this means that an external appliance must be worn.

Variants of exstrophy which are milder or more severe than the classic form described above may occur. *Incomplete exstrophy* is a much less common condition in which the pubis is intact and the genitalia are normal, with defects only in the abdominal wall and bladder to indicate the presence of exstrophy. In this relatively mild condition, plastic closure of the bladder and abdominal wall may be all that is required to produce complete rehabilitation.

Exstrophy of the cloaca, on the other hand, is a more serious problem than complete exstrophy of the bladder, for in addition to the bladder, the bowel and other abdominal organs are eventrated. Surgery for such a condition is generally considered by most authorities to be extremely difficult, if not impossible. □

Hereditary Glomerulonephritis

Hereditary glomerulonephritis is a separate clinical and pathologic entity which has been distinguished from other renal diseases by studies done in recent years on a number of affected families. Although more than one variety of hereditary nephritis exists, all are grouped under the term hereditary glomerulonephritis, since the hereditary nature of the renal disease appears to be the most characteristic feature of all cases.

The differences among the various forms of the disease lie chiefly in the *nonrenal abnormalities* which accompany the nephritis. For example, in Alport's syndrome, the nephritis is accompanied by *nerve deafness*, in hyperprolinemia by *elevated plasma proline*, and in other variants by *ocular abnormalities* and *mental retardation*. In other cases, *anatomic renal anomalies* have been observed. These abnormalities may appear alone or in varying combinations associated with the nephritis. Hereditary nephritis may also occur without any of the abnormalities mentioned above.

The best-described and apparently the most frequently occurring form of hereditary glomerulonephritis is Alport's syndrome—hereditary nephritis with nerve deafness. It appears to be transmitted as either a sex-linked partial dominant or an autosomal dominant with preferential attachment to the X chromosome. Males are affected less often than females but contract a more severe case of the disease. The genetic transmission from females to males and the virtual absence of genetic male-to-male transmission favor the probability of a sex-linked mode.

Clinically, the disorder usually appears in males as recurrent gross hematuria with or without hypertension. Edema is common, but oliguria and azotemia are variable. The patient is often thought to have acute glomerulonephritis until the frequent recurrences or family history indicate more serious disease.

The disease in males tends to be progressive, terminating in uremia between the second and fourth decades of life. During the late stages of the disease, symptoms of renal failure are found, with malaise, weakness, headache, edema, vomiting, and polyuria. By that time, azotemia, anemia, and isosthenuria are present (see pages 113-122).

In females, the course is less severe and often is characterized by pyuria and symptoms of urinary tract infection rather than by nephritis. A history of recurrent gross hematuria is infrequent, and asymptomatic disease is more common than in males. Also, the disease progresses at a much slower rate than in males, and uremia, if it occurs, is often delayed until the sixth decade.

The laboratory findings are virtually the same as those in nephritis of any cause and, in the absence of a family history, are not usually distinctive enough to separate these patients from those with sporadic nephritis (see pages 134-137). Persistent hematuria and proteinuria, either

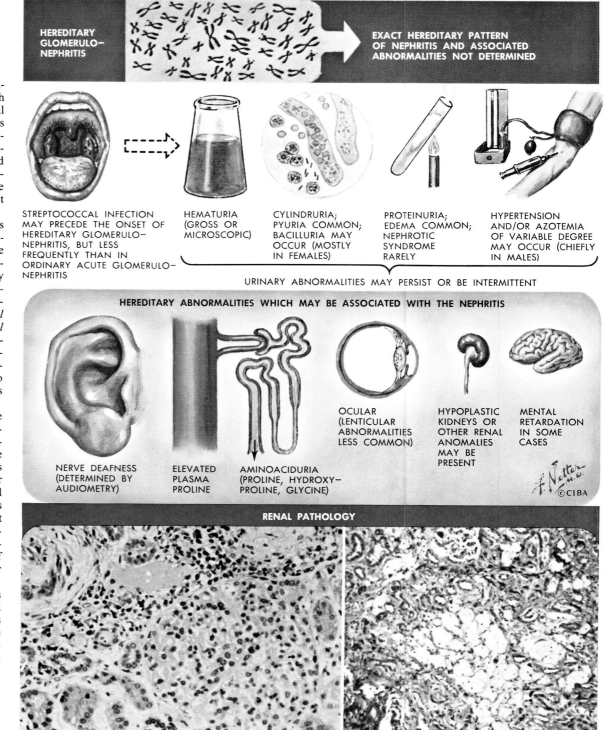

HEREDITARY GLOMERULO-NEPHRITIS → EXACT HEREDITARY PATTERN OF NEPHRITIS AND ASSOCIATED ABNORMALITIES NOT DETERMINED

STREPTOCOCCAL INFECTION MAY PRECEDE THE ONSET OF HEREDITARY GLOMERULO-NEPHRITIS, BUT LESS FREQUENTLY THAN IN ORDINARY ACUTE GLOMERULO-NEPHRITIS

HEMATURIA (GROSS OR MICROSCOPIC)

CYLINDRURIA; PYURIA COMMON; BACILLURIA MAY OCCUR (MOSTLY IN FEMALES)

PROTEINURIA; EDEMA COMMON; NEPHROTIC SYNDROME RARELY

HYPERTENSION AND/OR AZOTEMIA OF VARIABLE DEGREE MAY OCCUR (CHIEFLY IN MALES)

URINARY ABNORMALITIES MAY PERSIST OR BE INTERMITTENT

HEREDITARY ABNORMALITIES WHICH MAY BE ASSOCIATED WITH THE NEPHRITIS

NERVE DEAFNESS (DETERMINED BY AUDIOMETRY)

ELEVATED PLASMA PROLINE

AMINOACIDURIA (PROLINE, HYDROXY-PROLINE, GLYCINE)

OCULAR (LENTICULAR ABNORMALITIES LESS COMMON)

HYPOPLASTIC KIDNEYS OR OTHER RENAL ANOMALIES MAY BE PRESENT

MENTAL RETARDATION IN SOME CASES

RENAL PATHOLOGY

GLOMERULAR HYPERCELLULARITY; THICKENING OF VESSEL WALL

FOAM CELLS IN KIDNEY (BIOPSY, AZAN STAIN)

following an acute exacerbation or as an original finding in an otherwise asymptomatic individual, are common in male patients with hereditary nephritis. The diagnosis has been made by urinalysis of a specimen from an infant with a positive family history.

Usually, the diagnosis is confirmed either by the discovery of the patient's (or another family member's) high-tone nerve deafness or by the presence of renal disease in other family members. Audiometry may be necessary to detect hearing loss early in life but is unnecessary later when overt deafness is present.

Pathologically, the presence of *foam cells* in the kidney constitutes the most important finding in this disease, along with the usual changes seen in the kidneys of patients with nephritis. The exact nature and the cause of the foam cells which characterize hereditary nephritis are unknown. Staining by fat stains indicates that they are composed of lipids, but beyond that, lit-

tle is known of their content. Furthermore, no abnormality of plasma lipids or any other blood constituent has been found that could explain the presence of the foam cells. Although these cells occur in other forms of renal disease, their occurrence in hereditary nephritis is frequent enough to suggest this disease in a previously unsuspected case.

Glomerular changes are dominated by *hypercellularity* and *mesangial sclerosis* early in the course of the disease and an increasing number of hyalinized glomeruli as the disease progresses. *The tubules* usually show few early changes, but progressive tubular atrophy does occur in the late stages of the disease. An *interstitial infiltrate* may be present early and, in female patients, often dominates the microscopic picture. When the disorder is far advanced, interstitial fibrosis is found, accompanied by periglomerular fibrosis and generalized shrinkage of the kidney. □

Infantile Nephrosis

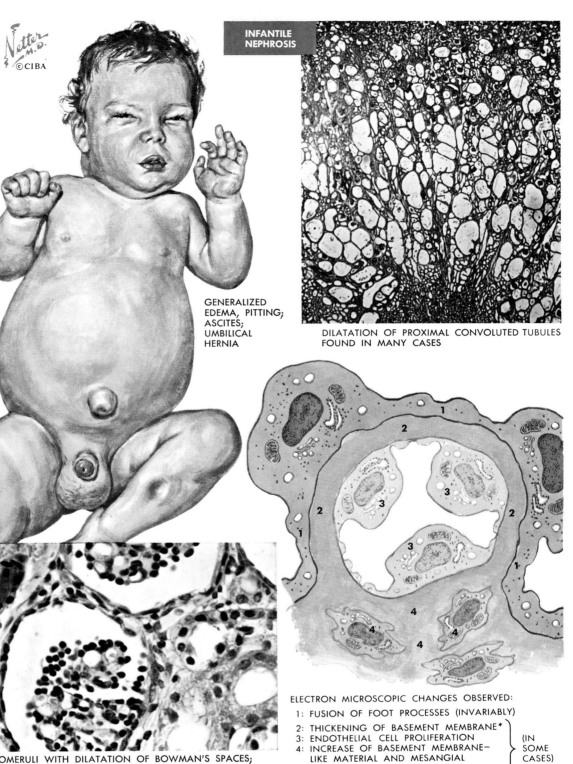

GENERALIZED EDEMA, PITTING; ASCITES; UMBILICAL HERNIA

INFANTILE NEPHROSIS

DILATATION OF PROXIMAL CONVOLUTED TUBULES FOUND IN MANY CASES

GLOMERULI WITH DILATATION OF BOWMAN'S SPACES; LOBULATION AND MODERATE MEMBRANOUS AND PROLIFERATIVE CHANGES FOUND IN SOME CASES

ELECTRON MICROSCOPIC CHANGES OBSERVED:
1: FUSION OF FOOT PROCESSES (INVARIABLY)
2: THICKENING OF BASEMENT MEMBRANE*
3: ENDOTHELIAL CELL PROLIFERATION
4: INCREASE OF BASEMENT MEMBRANE—LIKE MATERIAL AND MESANGIAL CELLS IN GLOMERULAR TUFT
    *SEE TEXT
(IN SOME CASES)

Childhood nephrosis (childhood nephrotic syndrome) is a relatively benign disorder which occurs most frequently between the ages of 2 and 5 years. On rare occasions, however, the nephrotic syndrome develops during *infancy*, at some time from the neonatal period through the first year of life. Although certain aspects of this early-onset form appear identical to those of the disease in older children, there are differences which clearly separate the infantile from the childhood form of this disease.

For example, patients with infantile nephrosis (infantile nephrotic syndrome) may have proteinuria, hypoproteinemia, edema, and hypercholesterolemia; these findings are also observed in patients with childhood nephrosis. However, the two forms differ in *familial incidence, pathologic findings*, and *prognosis*.

The familial incidence of infantile nephrosis is much higher than that of childhood nephrosis. In approximately 25 percent of cases of early-onset disease, another sibling in the family also has the disease. Although some sort of adverse *in utero* factor might explain the familial incidence, the occurrence of the condition in succeeding generations of siblings without the disease suggests the possibility that the disease is hereditary, with an autosomal recessive pattern of inheritance.

The renal pathologic changes in a small percentage of the infants are so different from those seen in any other patients with nephrosis that an entirely different disease is suggested. Such changes include a striking dilatation of the tubules (which may be great enough to give the appearance of cysts) and, in some patients, a dilatation of Bowman's spaces. Because of these appearances, the name "microcystic disease of the kidneys" is sometimes used.

Histologic sections of the kidneys of most patients with infantile nephrosis, however, look normal by light microscopy. In other patients, particularly if the disease is of long standing, the kidneys show membranous or proliferative lesions similar to those seen in older patients with severe nephrotic syndrome. Nevertheless, even when kidneys seem otherwise normal, Bowman's spaces are often dilated. This dilatation suggests that

there may be a connection with the microcystic form.

Electron microscopy of the glomerulus early in the course of infantile nephrosis reveals in all patients a characteristic picture: The basement membrane is extremely thin, and the epithelial cell foot processes are replaced by a continuous layer of epithelial cytoplasm spread over the basement membrane. With advancing time and increasingly severe disease, mesangial proliferation and sclerosis occur and the basement membrane becomes thicker in most patients.

The pathogenesis of infantile nephrosis is, at present, completely unknown, but there are a number of hypotheses. An autoimmune mechanism similar to that suggested for childhood nephrosis has been proposed, although most of the studies to date have failed to give any direct support to this theory. Another thesis is that during gestation the mother produces a substance which damages the infant's kidney.

A third theory is that a metabolic disorder in the infant, possibly inherited as an autosomal recessive trait, causes the production of a substance which is toxic to the kidney.

The prognosis in infantile nephrosis is much less favorable than in the childhood form of the disease. One of the most characteristic and discouraging features of the early-onset form is its almost total lack of response to adrenocorticosteroid therapy. An exceptional patient responds to treatment and recovers from the disease. Such favorable response has occurred only in patients with nephrotic syndrome secondary to a known toxin, or in patients whose disease started late in the first year of life. Thus, the mortality is exceedingly high, close to 100 percent. The life span varies from a few weeks in those children who die of electrolyte imbalance or sepsis, to 8 or 9 years in those who die of progressive uremia. □

Nephrogenic Diabetes Insipidus

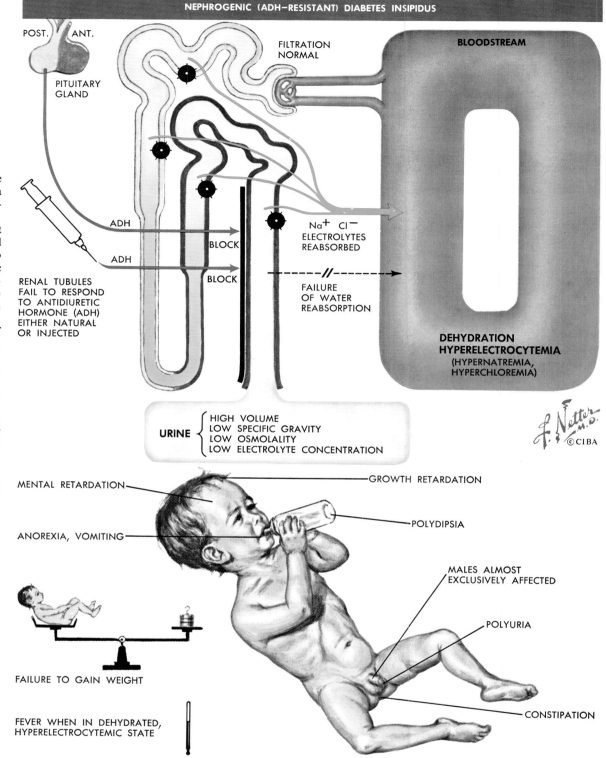

POST. ANT.

PITUITARY GLAND

FILTRATION NORMAL

BLOODSTREAM

ADH

ADH

BLOCK

BLOCK

RENAL TUBULES FAIL TO RESPOND TO ANTIDIURETIC HORMONE (ADH) EITHER NATURAL OR INJECTED

Na⁺ Cl⁻ ELECTROLYTES REABSORBED

FAILURE OF WATER REABSORPTION

DEHYDRATION HYPERELECTROCYTEMIA (HYPERNATREMIA, HYPERCHLOREMIA)

URINE { HIGH VOLUME / LOW SPECIFIC GRAVITY / LOW OSMOLALITY / LOW ELECTROLYTE CONCENTRATION }

MENTAL RETARDATION

ANOREXIA, VOMITING

FAILURE TO GAIN WEIGHT

FEVER WHEN IN DEHYDRATED, HYPERELECTROCYTEMIC STATE

GROWTH RETARDATION

POLYDIPSIA

MALES ALMOST EXCLUSIVELY AFFECTED

POLYURIA

CONSTIPATION

Nephrogenic diabetes insipidus is a rare hereditary disorder with severe polyuria and hyposthenuria which are not responsive to antidiuretic hormone (ADH).

Because the disorder occurs almost exclusively in males and is transmitted by females, it originally was thought to be inherited as a recessive characteristic linked to the X chromosome. Subsequently, however, female carriers have been discovered who have mild defects in urinary concentrating ability, and, in some families, mothers and sisters of affected males have equally severe forms of the disease. These observations suggest the current theory of an X-linked dominant inheritance with variable penetrance in the hemizygous females. Apparent examples of the male-to-male genetic transmission of this disease, which would indicate an autosomal form of transmission, have been questioned by most authorities, the majority of whom favor a sex-linked dominance.

The disorder clearly seems to result from an inability of the distal portion of the nephron, particularly the collecting duct, to respond to endogenously produced or exogenously administered ADH. (Adequate levels of endogenous ADH are present in the serum, and normal amounts are found in the urine.) The urinary excretion of a larger than normal fraction of administered ADH suggests that the basic defect may be a failure of the collecting duct to bind this hormone. No evidence of any ADH-inhibiting agent has been found.

Shortly after birth the infant develops symptoms and signs such as episodic irritability, fever of unknown origin, vomiting, constipation, and excessive intake of water, if offered. If the parents (or physician) are alerted by the presence of the disease in other family members, the disorder may be recognized early. Otherwise, the diagnosis may be delayed until irreparable brain damage has occurred.

Infants who will take an almost unlimited amount of water, who even when they are dehydrated have excessively wet diapers, and most importantly, who have hypotonic urine despite clinical dehydration are exhibiting symptoms of this disease. Hypernatremia and hyperchloremia are also useful indications of excessive water loss, and every infant with hypertonic dehydration should be evaluated for the possibility of nephrogenic diabetes insipidus.

Older children may show signs of irritability and fatigue from lack of sleep because of frequent nocturia. Physical retardation is common because of diminished food intake secondary to the excessive water ingestion. In an unfortunately

high percentage of children, mental retardation occurs as a result of hypertonic dehydration.

Other disorders which may mimic nephrogenic diabetes insipidus include renal tubular acidosis (see page 248), hyperaldosteronism or hypokalemia from other causes, sickle cell disease, chronic renal failure (see page 113), and obstructive uropathy (see page 185).

The diagnosis of diabetes insipidus is made by demonstrating that the urine remains hypotonic (usually less than l00 mOsm/kg) despite prolonged water deprivation. The diagnosis of *nephrogenic* diabetes insipidus is made by demonstrating that ADH administration does not correct the hyposthenuria. The ADH-response test is performed initially by administering aqueous ADH in a dose of 0.5 unit/m² and measuring the urine concentration for a period of 4 to 6 hours. If no response occurs, a second test is performed using up to 2 units/m² to demonstrate that, despite the

blanching of the skin produced by the larger dose, no increase in the urine concentration results.

The treatment of patients with nephrogenic diabetes insipidus consists of ensuring adequate water intake by making water freely available. A simultaneous reduction of solute intake will help decrease the large urine volume.

Some patients with nephrogenic diabetes insipidus respond to chlorothiazide and other diuretics by a reduction in urine volume and an increase in urine concentration. The reason for this paradoxical effect of diuretics is not certain, but it is probably caused by sodium depletion which decreases filtration of sodium (and possibly water). Proximal tubular reabsorption of filtered sodium results in the entrance of a smaller volume of fluid into the distal nephron, so that enough fluid can be reabsorbed to decrease urine volume and raise urine concentration. □

Cystinosis

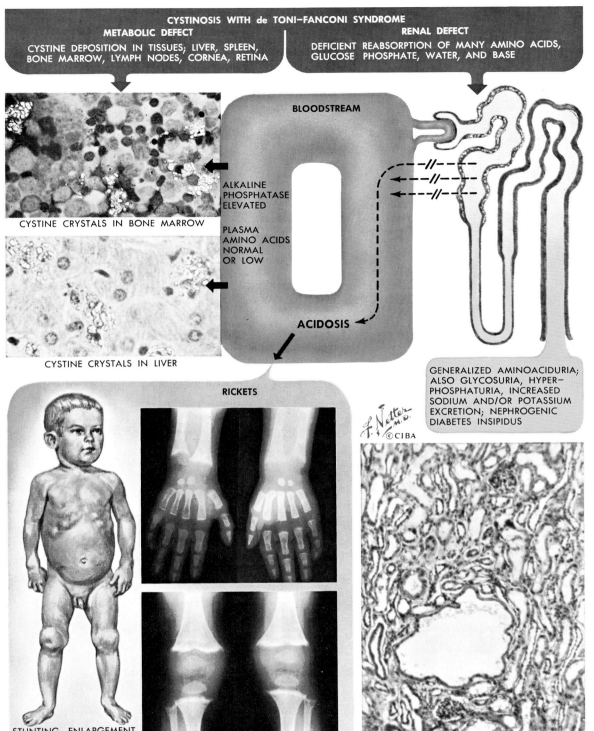

CYSTINOSIS WITH de TONI-FANCONI SYNDROME

METABOLIC DEFECT
CYSTINE DEPOSITION IN TISSUES; LIVER, SPLEEN, BONE MARROW, LYMPH NODES, CORNEA, RETINA

RENAL DEFECT
DEFICIENT REABSORPTION OF MANY AMINO ACIDS, GLUCOSE PHOSPHATE, WATER, AND BASE

BLOODSTREAM

CYSTINE CRYSTALS IN BONE MARROW

ALKALINE PHOSPHATASE ELEVATED

PLASMA AMINO ACIDS NORMAL OR LOW

CYSTINE CRYSTALS IN LIVER

ACIDOSIS

GENERALIZED AMINOACIDURIA; ALSO GLYCOSURIA, HYPER-PHOSPHATURIA, INCREASED SODIUM AND/OR POTASSIUM EXCRETION; NEPHROGENIC DIABETES INSIPIDUS

RICKETS

STUNTING, ENLARGEMENT OF WRISTS AND KNEES; COSTOCHONDRAL BEADING; WADDLING GAIT

X-RAY EVIDENCE OF RICKETS

RENAL CORTEX: DILATATION AND DEGENERATION OF PROXIMAL TUBULES

Cystinosis is a rare inborn error of metabolism transmitted by an autosomal recessive gene and manifested by the deposition of crystals of cystine throughout the body. Accompanying the cystinosis in all children reported to date has been the Fanconi syndrome of proximal tubular malfunction. This syndrome produces glycosuria, aminoaciduria, hyperphosphaturia, and renal tubular acidosis and leads to rickets and growth failure early in life. Renal damage from accumulated cystine causes gradual deterioration of glomerular function, which, in turn, inevitably leads to renal insufficiency in the first or early in the second decade of life.

The cause of the accumulation of cystine is unknown. However, cystine is an extremely insoluble amino acid and could be expected to precipitate even if its concentration within the cell or in the total body fluids were only slightly increased. Most of the cystine accumulates in phagocytes of the liver, spleen, bone marrow, and lymph nodes. This fact led to the assumption that such accumulation of cystine resulted in its deposition by precipitation. However, recent studies have shown little or no increase in circulating blood cystine levels. This observation has led to the hypothesis that the deposition of cystine is caused by an abnormal compartmentalization of the amino acid within cell organelles, presumably the lysosomes. This theory also suggests that cystine accumulates in those cells in which it is produced in excess.

The early accumulation of cystine in the proximal tubular cells, the presumed cause of the Fanconi syndrome, would be compatible with either of these concepts. Still to be explained by the more recent theory, however, is the preferential accumulation of cystine in phagocytes and in the nearly acellular cornea.

Whatever the cause, the most harmful effects of cystine accumulation are produced on the kidney; the Fanconi syndrome is produced by an inhibition of the enzymes or transport systems of the proximal convoluted tubule. Later, interstitial fibrosis and glomerular hyalinization appear and lead to progressive renal insufficiency.

The clinical consequences of cystine accumulation in the kidney are striking. Symptoms usually appear in the first year of life and include growth retardation, anorexia, polyuria and polydipsia, constipation, and heat intolerance. Rickets can usually be detected radiologically

during the first 2 years of life. A retarded bone age is also often obvious.

If a careful slit-lamp examination is performed, cystine crystals may be detected in the cornea by 6 months of age. Later in life, when the amount of cystine is greater, crystals can be seen with the aid of an ophthalmoscope.

Both fair hair and skin, which are often much lighter than those of parents or siblings, may be present. A "cherubic facies" has been described in many patients.

Glycosuria without hyperglycemia, aminoaciduria without elevation of the blood amino acids, systemic acidosis with an alkaline urine, hypokalemia, hypophosphatemia, and an elevated alkaline phosphatase are nearly constant findings in patients with cystinosis and the Fanconi syndrome. Renal function studies usually show diminished glomerular filtration rate as measured by inulin or creatinine clearance, and a marked

reduction in the PAH clearance and in the Tm_{PAH}.

No specific treatment of the cystine accumulation is available; therapy is directed at the secondary consequences which constitute the Fanconi syndrome. Sodium and potassium citrate are given to combat the acidosis and hypokalemia. Vitamin D in large doses and extra calcium are given to combat rickets (see pages 113-122). With this therapy, the patient may be asymptomatic until the uremic stage of the disorder, although growth failure may persist. Renal transplant has been performed occasionally and appears to be potentially useful for patients with cystinosis.

Death from electrolyte imbalance, particularly acidosis and hypokalemia, poses a constant threat in early life. Children who survive the early period of life face the certainty of gradually reduced renal function and death from uremia, unless chronic dialysis or a kidney transplant is possible. □

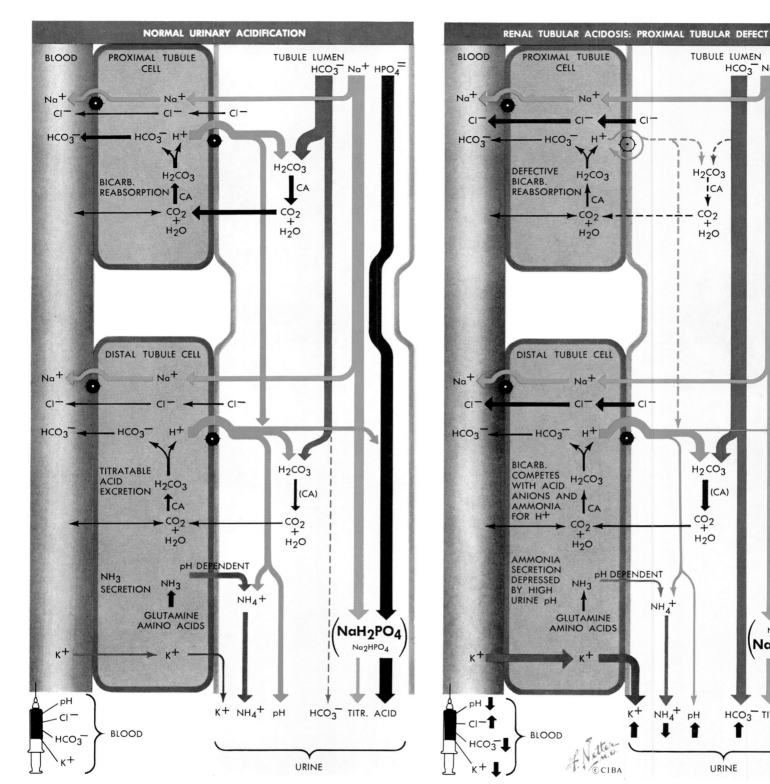

NORMAL URINARY ACIDIFICATION

RENAL TUBULAR ACIDOSIS: PROXIMAL TUBULAR DEFECT

Renal Tubular Acidosis

In renal tubular acidosis (RTA) the renal mechanisms for acid excretion are insufficient to guard the integrity of the acid-base balance of the body so that systemic acidosis develops.

(The role of the kidney in maintaining the pH of body fluids has been discussed in detail on pages 61 through 64. To understand renal tubular acidosis, one should first review those pages, particularly in conjunction with the portion of Plate 26 showing normal urinary acidification.)

Two forms of renal tubular acidosis have been described which are distinguished by the presumed site of the metabolic defect. Whether such a distinction is valid or not is uncertain, but the distinction forms a convenient basis for explaining biochemical variations in patients with RTA.

Proximal renal tubular acidosis is thought to be caused by a deficiency in the proximal tubular mechanism for bicarbonate reabsorption. The failure of bicarbonate reabsorption in the proximal tubule is assumed to allow an excess of bicarbonate to enter the distal tubule. This flooding of the distal tubular acidification mechanism with bicarbonate not only causes bicarbonate to be excreted in the urine but also allows it to compete with distal tubular mechanisms for acidification. Such competition effectively prevents the formation of titratable acid from phosphate and other urinary buffers, as well as the formation of ammonium ion from ammonia. Thus, increased excretion of bicarbonate, decreased excretion of titratable acid and ammonium, and elevated urine pH occur. In addition, excretion of potassium is markedly augmented.

Distal renal tubular acidosis is believed to be a deficiency of those reactions which normally take

place in the distal tubule. Thus, proximal tubular bicarbonate reabsorption is assumed to be normal. Instead, the ability to acidify the urinary buffers is impaired, possibly because the distal tubule is unable to secrete hydrogen ions against an unfavorable concentration gradient. (Distal RTA is sometimes called gradient RTA; see page 115.) The urinary phosphate thus remains in the dibasic ($HPO_4^=$) form rather than being converted to the monobasic ($H_2PO_4^-$) form. Other buffers remain in combination with cations besides hydrogen, so that ammonium (NH_4^+) secretion, which requires the trapping of ammonia (NH_3) by the hydrogen ion, is effectively prevented. As in proximal RTA, the secretion of potassium is markedly increased, excretion of bicarbonate is increased, excretion of titratable acid and ammonium is decreased, and urine pH is elevated. One physiologic and apparently reliable difference between the two forms is that bicarbonate Tm

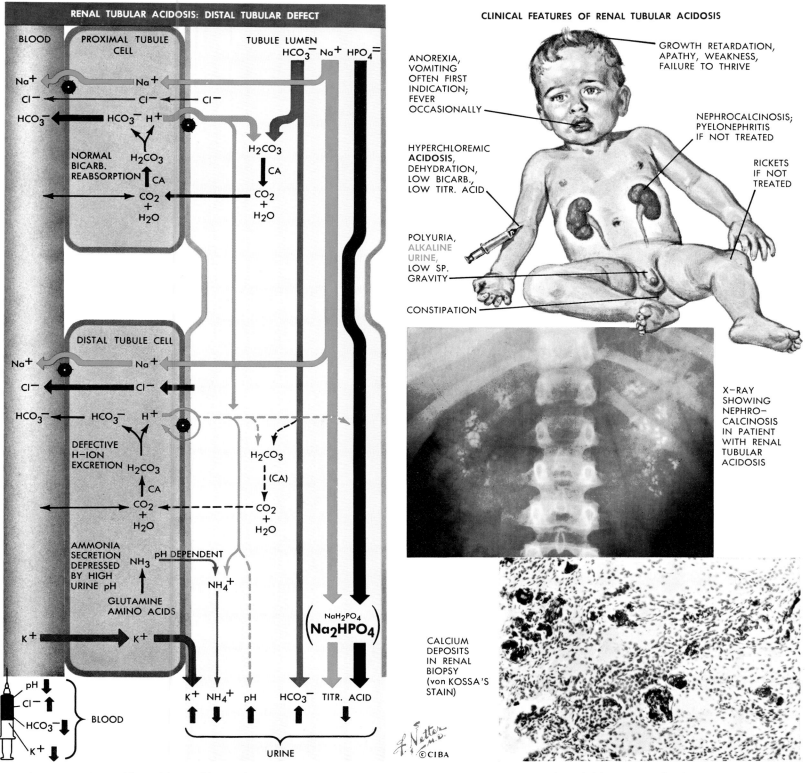

CLINICAL FEATURES OF RENAL TUBULAR ACIDOSIS

BLOOD | **PROXIMAL TUBULE CELL** | **TUBULE LUMEN**

HCO_3^- Na^+ $HPO_4^=$

Na^+ — Na^+

Cl^- — Cl^- — Cl^-

HCO_3^- — HCO_3^- H^+

NORMAL BICARB. REABSORPTION

H_2CO_3 — CA

H_2CO_3 — CA

$CO_2 + H_2O$ — $CO_2 + H_2O$

ANOREXIA, VOMITING OFTEN FIRST INDICATION; FEVER OCCASIONALLY

GROWTH RETARDATION, APATHY, WEAKNESS, FAILURE TO THRIVE

NEPHROCALCINOSIS; PYELONEPHRITIS IF NOT TREATED

RICKETS IF NOT TREATED

HYPERCHLOREMIC **ACIDOSIS**, DEHYDRATION, LOW BICARB., LOW TITR. ACID

POLYURIA, ALKALINE URINE, LOW SP. GRAVITY

CONSTIPATION

DISTAL TUBULE CELL

Na^+ — Na^+

Cl^- — Cl^-

HCO_3^- — HCO_3^- H^+

DEFECTIVE H−ION EXCRETION

H_2CO_3 — CA

H_2CO_3 — (CA)

$CO_2 + H_2O$ — $CO_2 + H_2O$

AMMONIA SECRETION DEPRESSED BY HIGH URINE pH

NH_3 — pH DEPENDENT

NH_4^+

GLUTAMINE AMINO ACIDS

K^+ — K^+

(NaH_2PO_4) (Na_2HPO_4)

X−RAY SHOWING NEPHRO−CALCINOSIS IN PATIENT WITH RENAL TUBULAR ACIDOSIS

pH ↓
Cl^- ↑
HCO_3^- ↓
K^+ ↓

BLOOD

K^+ NH_4^+ pH HCO_3^- TITR. ACID

CALCIUM DEPOSITS IN RENAL BIOPSY (von KOSSA'S STAIN)

URINE

F. Netter M.D.
©CIBA

and bicarbonate threshold are decreased in proximal RTA but normal in distal RTA.

Rickets and nephrocalcinosis occur in RTA as a result of systemic acidosis and secondary hyperparathyroidism. (The disturbances in metabolism of calcium-phosphorus are described on pages 117-120. It is sufficient to note here that rickets and nephrocalcinosis with nephrolithiasis may occur.)

Clinically, when renal tubular acidosis becomes manifest in infancy, common initial symptoms are vomiting, anorexia, fever, polyuria, and dehydration. Within a few months, growth failure may be evident, together with increasing apathy, weakness, and tissue wasting. In succeeding months, nephrocalcinosis and rickets occur.

If the disease does not appear until later in childhood, growth failure and signs of rickets, and urinary tract infection are common initial findings, but some patients may complain of weakness or even paralysis from hypokalemia.

The most common chemical changes in the blood are depressed serum bicarbonate and pH and elevated serum chloride. Hypokalemia is frequently present, as are chemical findings associated with rickets, such as normal serum calcium, low serum phosphorus, and elevated alkaline phosphatase.

The usual finding in the urine is a relatively alkaline pH associated with low titratable acidity and ammonium content. Occasionally, a patient with proximal tubular acidosis may have a low urine pH while the systemic acidosis is exceptionally severe. However, even in such a patient, the urine usually becomes alkaline with only partial correction of the acidosis, while the serum bicarbonate and pH remain depressed. Polyuria and decreased urinary concentrating ability are frequent.

The therapy for renal tubular acidosis is usually not difficult, unless nephrocalcinosis and pyelonephritis are complicating factors. The correction of acidosis with sodium citrate or other sodium salts, and the provision of sufficient potassium to correct the hypokalemia will usually maintain a patient in adequate balance and allow normal growth and development. (Patients with proximal RTA may require larger doses of citrate than patients with distal RTA.) Vitamin D in large doses may be required to correct rickets. However, after correction of rickets and acidosis, the dose of vitamin D may be reduced to a level sufficient to prevent recurrence.

In some patients with nephrocalcinosis, the calcium deposits are reabsorbed after prolonged alkali therapy; in other patients, the nephrocalcinosis seems to be permanent. The prognosis depends, ultimately, on the extent of renal damage prior to treatment and the degree of reversibility of renal damage which is possible with alkali therapy. □

Section VIII

Therapeutics

Frank H. Netter, M.D.

in collaboration with

G. M. Berlyne, M.D., F.R.C.P.   *Plate 5*

Paul J. Cannon, M.D.   *Plates 1-4*

Michael E. DeBakey, M.D.   *Plates 16-17*

John P. Merrill, M.D.   *Plates 12-15*

J. U. Schlegel, M.D.   *Plates 18-19*

George E. Schreiner, M.D.   *Plates 6-11*

Diuretics

The development of drugs which promote diuresis by interfering with sodium reabsorption in renal tubular cells has been a major advance in the therapy of patients who have cardiac failure, cirrhosis with ascites, or the nephrotic syndrome.

Each of the several classes of diuretics specifically affects the transport processes located in different regions of the nephron. Each drug may be expected to produce characteristic effects on the electrolyte and acid-base balances of the patient. Thus, many of the electrolyte and acid-base imbalances that result from diuresis may be anticipated and forestalled. Also, consideration of the *sites* of action may facilitate the choice of diuretic combinations for patients with edema resistant to a single agent.

Mercurial Diuretics

Mercurial diuretics, used since early in this century, are usually administered by intramuscular injection. They produce a substantial diuresis which is sustained for 12 to 24 hours. Mercurial diuretics do not influence the glomerular filtration rate (GFR) but inhibit the tubular reabsorption of sodium and chloride which, in turn, results in diminished reabsorption of water.

Although the exact site of action of the mercurial diuretics in the nephron is uncertain, sites in the ascending limb of the loop of Henle and distal tubule have been suggested by recent micropuncture experiments and by the ability of many of the organic mercurials to promote an isotonic diuresis. On the other hand, certain preparations of organic mercurials, such as meralluride, are formulated with theophylline and may induce a hypotonic diuresis. Such preparations are especially useful in treating edematous patients with renal retention of water (dilutional hyposmolality).

Mercurial diuretics partially inhibit distal tubular reabsorption of sodium chloride and the exchange of sodium in luminal fluid for potassium, but they do not interfere with distal sodium-hydrogen exchange. Nevertheless, since the inhibition of sodium and chloride reabsorption in the proximal tubule and loop of Henle results in the delivery of greater amounts of sodium to the distal nephron during diuresis, both urinary potassium excretion and urinary hydrogen excretion (sum of urinary ammonium and titratable acid minus urinary bicarbonate) may rise.

These mercurial diuretics may induce potassium depletion and hypokalemia, as well as a hypochloremic metabolic alkalosis. The alkalosis causes mercurial diuretics to lose their effectiveness in promoting additional sodium excretion. Diuretic responsiveness may be restored by the administration of ammonium chloride or acetazolamide which induces hyperchloremia and metabolic acidosis.

Occasionally, patients exhibit hypersensitivity to mercurial compounds which is manifested by stomatitis, fever, or rashes. Small doses are therefore advisable when therapy is initiated. Also, because acute tubular nephrosis has been associated with the administration of mercurial diuretics in patients who have

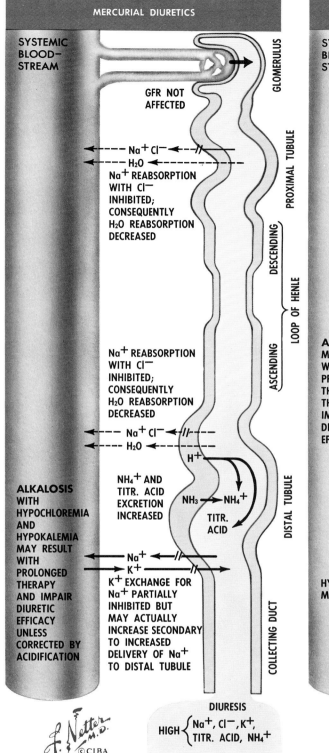

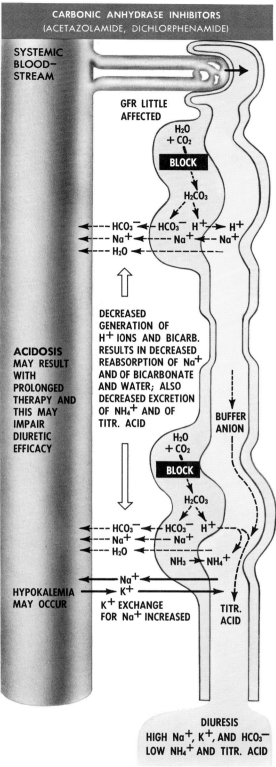

severe degrees of oliguria or who have extensive renal parenchymal disease, larger doses should not be given to patients with such conditions.

Carbonic Anhydrase Inhibitors

The demonstration, in 1949, that sulfanilamide, one of the sulfonamide antibiotics, produced diuresis in patients who had congestive heart failure followed earlier observations that the antibiotic also produced acidosis by inhibition of carbonic anhydrase. Subsequently, the diuretic action of sulfanilamide was also related to inhibition of carbonic anhydrase, and this observation led to the introduction of sulfonamide inhibitors of the enzyme as the first oral diuretic agents.

Carbonic anhydrase inhibitors, which have little effect on GFR, decrease the generation of carbonic acid from carbon dioxide and water by the proximal and distal renal tubular cells. These agents reduce the

amount of hydrogen ion available for secretion into the tubular lumen so that sodium-hydrogen exchange is decreased. Reabsorption of filtered sodium and bicarbonate in the proximal tubules is thus inhibited, promoting diuresis (see pages 61-64).

Because the sodium which was not reabsorbed in the proximal tubules is selectively reabsorbed in the ascending limb of the loop of Henle and in the distal tubules, the urine is hypotonic but contains both sodium and bicarbonate. There is little change in urinary chloride excretion, but as a consequence of diminished sodium-hydrogen exchange, urinary titratable acid and ammonium are reduced. Increased distal tubular sodium reabsorption in exchange for potassium may result in hypokalemia.

Since peak natriuresis is less than two percent of filtered sodium, carbonic anhydrase inhibitors are mild diuretics and are now rarely *Continued on page 254*

Diuretics

Continued from page 253

used as primary therapy for edema. However, a larger increment of sodium excretion can be achieved if these diuretics are administered intermittently to patients with elevated plasma bicarbonate concentrations, as in metabolic alkalosis or cor pulmonale.

Because of reduced urinary hydrogen ion excretion, patients may develop hyperchloremic metabolic acidosis after about 48 hours of administration of carbonic anhydrase inhibitors. In this case these agents are no longer natriuretic.

Carbonic anhydrase inhibitors reduce the diuresis produced by mercurial diuretics but add to or potentiate that induced by drugs whose major sites of action are beyond the proximal tubules.

Thiazides (Chloruretic Sulfonamides)

Chlorothiazide, the first of the chloruretic sulfonamides, was introduced in 1958. It is one of a class of diuretics called the benzothiadiazides, or, more simply, the thiazides. They are among the most effective and widely used oral diuretics for the treatment of both edema and diastolic hypertension. The duration of action of chlorothiazide is 6 to 12 hours, but some derivatives promote diuresis lasting 12 to 72 hours.

These drugs are potent inhibitors of the tubular reabsorption of sodium and chloride. However, because they inhibit selective sodium reabsorption in those portions of the nephron where tubular fluid is rendered hypotonic (the ascending limb of the loop of Henle and the distal tubule; see pages 51–59), these agents may contribute to the development of dilutional hyponatremia in edematous patients whose water intake is large. Nevertheless, urinary concentrating ability is not impeded by the thiazides.

Sodium-potassium exchange in the distal tubule is increased during thiazide-induced diuresis with resulting potassium depletion and hypokalemia. In the digitalized patient, the risk of digitalis intoxication would thus increase. This complication can be prevented by intermittent administration of the diuretic drug together with either increased oral intake of potassium or the simultaneous administration of a potassium-retaining agent.

Unlike carbonic anhydrase inhibitors, thiazides do not induce acidosis but may cause mild metabolic alkalosis with hypokalemia. Possibly because of a slight degree of carbonic anhydrase inhibition, net hydrogen ion excretion does not rise appreciably during the first few days of therapy. Also, these drugs may depress GFR and so induce reversible azotemia in some patients.

In low oral doses, thiazides promote urate reabsorption and thus may induce hyperuricemia and precipitate attacks of gouty arthritis. On the other hand, large intravenous doses of the thiazides are uricosuric.

Potassium-Retaining Diuretics

The suprarenal mineralocorticoid aldosterone produces a slight increase in sodium and chloride reabsorption in water-impermeable sites in the distal nephron and also accelerates reabsorption of sodi-

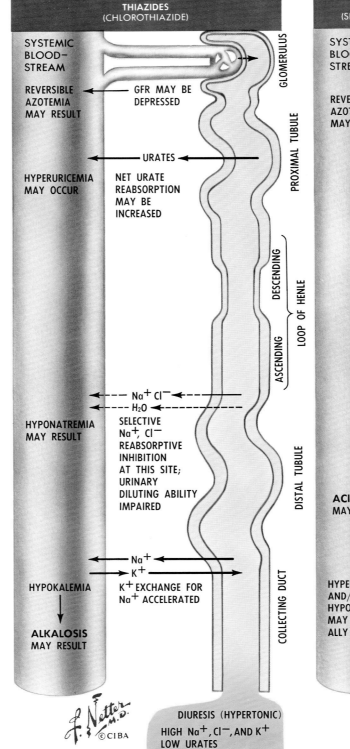

um, in exchange for potassium and hydrogen, in the distal tubule and collecting duct. As a result, urinary excretion of potassium, titratable acid, and ammonium rises.

Two types of compounds have been introduced which antagonize the actions of aldosterone or have similar overall effects on electrolyte excretion. Spironolactone, a compound of the first type, is a competitive inhibitor of aldosterone at the renal sites of action but does not affect the electrolyte excretion pattern of individuals with nonfunctioning suprarenal tissue. The second type of compound is typified by triamterene and amiloride. These drugs directly inhibit renal tubular reabsorption of sodium and chloride in the distal nephron and also impair distal secretion of potassium and hydrogen ions. Both produce natriuresis, potassium retention, and diminished hydrogen excretion, even in the absence of suprarenal glands.

Spironolactone has little effect on renal hemodynamics, but triamterene and amiloride may reduce GFR. All three drugs impede urinary dilution and reduce potassium and hydrogen ion excretion.

Although natriuretic effects of these drugs are slight, cumulative diuretic effects after prolonged administration may be substantial, particularly in patients with marked hypersecretion of aldosterone which may occur in cirrhosis with ascites or the nephrotic syndrome. These diuretic compounds, which affect the distal nephron, are especially effective when administered with other diuretics which inhibit sodium reabsorption more proximally. For instance, when the potassium-retaining agents are combined with mercurial diuretics, thiazides, ethacrynic acid, or furosemide, potassium is conserved and sodium excretion is increased.

These drugs, particularly triamterene and amilo-

Diuretics

Continued

ride, may cause reversible azotemia because of reduced GFR. Hyperkalemia, especially in patients with kidney disease, and metabolic acidosis, in patients with hepatic or renal failure, may occur. Hyponatremia may also develop because of reduced sodium transport in water-impermeable portions of the distal nephron.

Ethacrynic Acid and Furosemide

Ethacrynic acid and furosemide are two potent diuretic compounds which may be administered orally or parenterally in the treatment of edema. Both drugs are effective even when edema is accompanied by electrolyte or acid-base disturbances or azotemia. Intravenous administration of either agent is useful in the treatment of pulmonary edema.

Although ethacrynic acid is derived from aryloxyacetic acid and furosemide from anthranilic acid, they are remarkably similar in pharmacologic properties. Oral administration produces a peak diuresis in 2 hours which lasts 6 to 12 hours; intravenous injection causes diuresis almost immediately, with a peak effect in 30 minutes to 1 hour.

In usual doses, neither drug significantly affects GFR, but in high doses, both may produce dilatation of the renal vasculature which may be useful in the therapy of oliguria and/or renal parenchymal disease.

These drugs produce a marked rise in urinary excretion of sodium and chloride and a lesser but significant increase in potassium excretion. Both agents reduce renal diluting and concentrating ability and thus are thought to promote natriuresis primarily by inhibiting chloride and sodium reabsorption in the ascending limb of Henle's loop. Micropuncture studies also indicate a lesser effect on proximal tubular sodium reabsorption.

During the diuresis produced by either drug in patients with cardiac, cirrhotic, or nephrotic edema, up to 30 percent of the filtered sodium may be excreted. Since increased sodium is delivered to the distal nephron, sodium-potassium and sodium-hydrogen ion exchanges are also accelerated. The consequent urinary losses of potassium and hydrogen may cause potassium depletion and metabolic alkalosis.

The magnitude of potassium depletion during diuresis with ethacrynic acid and furosemide appears to be related to the aldosterone secretion rate of the patient. Greater potassium losses for a given degree of natriuresis occur in patients who have higher circulating levels of aldosterone. Thus, either of the loop diuretics used with an aldosterone antagonist or other potassium-retaining diuretic not only augments sodium excretion but also may significantly reduce potassium losses.

Metabolic alkalosis caused by increased net acid excretion in the urine is slightly less likely to occur with furosemide than with ethacrynic acid because of a mild carbonic anhydrase-inhibiting activity of furosemide. Other factors which may contribute to the induction of metabolic alkalosis in edematous patients who receive these compounds are potassium depletion and disproportionate losses of urinary chloride. The latter

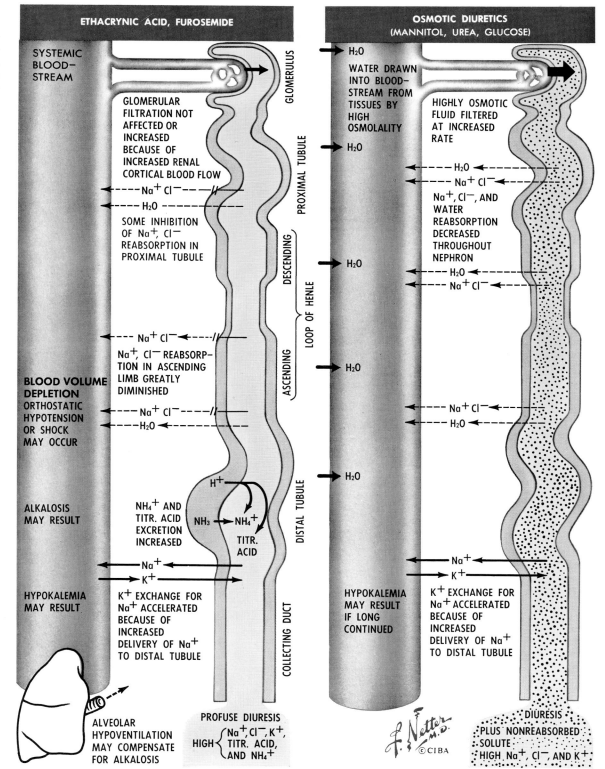

event causes the chloride-bicarbonate ratio in urine to exceed that normally present in extracellular fluid.

Intravenous administration of furosemide or ethacrynic acid increases urate excretion, but prolonged oral use causes urate retention and hyperuricemia.

Both drugs may cause ototoxicity when administered in high doses to patients with renal disease. Increased hyperglycemia has been observed in diabetic patients after treatment with furosemide.

Because orthostatic hypotension and shock may be produced by an excessively rapid and large diuresis, therapy with ethacrynic acid or furosemide should be initiated cautiously by determining sensitivity to a single dose before protracted treatment is begun.

Osmotic Diuretics

The osmotic diuretics, urea and mannitol, are administered intravenously in the treatment of patients

with oliguria, edema, or increased intracranial pressure caused by cerebral edema, and for certain drug intoxications. When these agents are present in hypertonic concentrations within the blood, interstitial fluid enters the circulation; when they are present in hypertonic concentrations in interstitial fluid, fluid leaves the cells and enters the interstitial fluid.

The ability of osmotic diuretics to maintain urinary volume is useful in the treatment of oliguria, while their capacity to initiate and sustain diuresis is useful in the treatment of drug intoxications. However, because administration of these substances may increase blood volume, they must be used with caution, if at all, in the treatment of cardiac failure.

Although the osmotic diuretics may increase renal blood flow in ischemic kidney tissue by preventing the swelling of vascular and other cells because of anoxia, these diuretics also act to maintain *Continued on page 256*

DRUG →	MERCURIALS (e.g., MERALLURIDE, CHLORMERODRIN)	CARBONIC ANHYDRASE INHIBITORS (e.g., ACETAZOLAMIDE, DICHLORPHENAMIDE)	THIAZIDES (e.g., CHLOROTHIAZIDE)	POTASSIUM–RETAINING DIURETICS (e.g., SPIRONOLACTONE, TRIAMTERENE, AMILORIDE)	ETHACRYNIC ACID FUROSEMIDE	OSMOTIC DIURETICS (e.g., MANNITOL)
ROUTE OF ADMINISTRATION	INTRAMUSCULAR	ORAL	ORAL	ORAL	ORAL OR PARENTERAL	INTRAVENOUS
MAJOR SITES OF ACTION	PROXIMAL AND/OR DISTAL TUBULES AND LOOP OF HENLE	PROXIMAL TUBULES	LOOP OF HENLE AND DISTAL TUBULE WITHIN RENAL CORTEX	DISTAL TUBULES, COLLECTING DUCTS	ASCENDING LIMB OF HENLE'S LOOP	PROXIMAL TUBULES, ASCENDING LIMB OF HENLE'S LOOP
MAJOR EFFECT ON SODIUM REABSORPTION	BLOCK ISOSMOTIC Na^+, Cl^- REABSORPTION	REDUCE SECRETION OF H^+ AND NET Na^+, HCO_3^- REABSORPTION BY INHIBITION OF CARBONIC ANHYDRASE	INHIBIT SELECTIVE Na^+, Cl^- REABSORPTION AT DISTAL DILUTING SEGMENT (URINARY DILUTION IMPAIRED)	SPIRONOLACTONE: COMPETITIVE ANTAGONIST OF ALDOSTERONE–STIMULATED REABSORPTION OF Na^+ WITH Cl^- AND OF Na^+ REABSORPTION IN EXCHANGE FOR H^+ AND K^+ TRIAMTERENE AND AMILORIDE: DIRECTLY INHIBIT DISTAL Na^+, Cl^- REABSORPTION AND DISTAL Na^+ EXCHANGE FOR H^+ AND K^+	BLOCK SELECTIVE Cl^- AND Na^+ REABSORPTION, INHIBITING ABILITY OF KIDNEY TO DILUTE OR TO CONCENTRATE URINE	PRESENCE OF OSMOTIC PARTICLES WITHIN NEPHRON RETARDS H_2O REABSORPTION AND REDUCES NET Na^+, Cl^- TRANSPORT
RELATIVE DIURETIC POTENCY	+ + + +	+ +	+ + +	+	+ + + + +	VARIABLE: RELATED TO DOSE
EFFECT ON POTASSIUM	PARTIAL INHIBITION OF DISTAL K^+ SECRETION BUT HYPOKALEMIA MAY OCCUR	K^+ SECRETION INCREASED	K^+ SECRETION INCREASED	SPIRONOLACTONE: RETARDS K^+ SECRETION STIMULATED BY ALDOSTERONE TRIAMTERENE AND AMILORIDE: DEPRESS K^+ EXCRETION	K^+ SECRETION INCREASED	K^+ SECRETION SLIGHTLY INCREASED
EFFECT ON ACID EXCRETION	H^+ SECRETION INCREASED	H^+ EXCRETION DIMINISHED (BICARBONATE DIURESIS)	LITTLE EFFECT ON NET ACID BASE	SPIRONOLACTONE: RETARDS ALDOS–TERONE–STIMULATED H^+ EXCRETION TRIAMTERENE AND AMILORIDE: INHIBIT DISTAL H^+ SECRETION	H^+ EXCRETION ACCELERATED	H^+ EXCRETION LITTLE AFFECTED (SOME INCREASE IN HCO_3^- EXCRETION)
EFFECT ON RENAL HEMODYNAMICS	NO EFFECT ON RPF OR GFR	LITTLE EFFECT ON RPF OR GFR	MAY DEPRESS RPF AND GFR	SPIRONOLACTONE: NO EFFECT ON RPF TRIAMTERENE AND AMILORIDE: MAY DEPRESS GFR	LITTLE EFFECT AT LOW DOSES; LARGE DOSES MAY INCREASE RPF AND GFR	RPF AND GFR INCREASED
SITUATIONS IN WHICH DRUG IS PARTICULARLY USEFUL	PATIENTS WITH DILUTIONAL HYPONATREMIA; MODERATE TO EXTENSIVE EDEMA	PATIENTS WITH METABOLIC ALKALOSIS; COR PULMONALE	MILD TO MODERATE EDEMA	PATIENTS WITH HYPERALDOSTERONISM (CIRRHOSIS WITH ASCITES, NEPHROSIS, SEVERE CARDIAC FAILURE)	PATIENTS WITH PULMONARY EDEMA; EDEMA COMPLI–CATED BY AZOTEMIA, ELECTROLYTE OR ACID–BASE DISORDERS	PRERENAL AZOTEMIA; CEREBRAL EDEMA; POISONINGS
SIDE EFFECTS WHICH MAY BE PRODUCED BY DIURESIS	HYPOKALEMIA AND HYPOCHLOREMIC ALKALOSIS; NEPHROTOXICITY IN PATIENTS WITH RENAL DISEASE; HYPERSENSITIVITY REACTIONS	HYPERCHLOREMIC ACIDOSIS; HYPOKALEMIA ©CIBA	HYPOKALEMIA; HYPOCHLOREMIA, METABOLIC ALKALOSIS; DILUTIONAL HYPO–NATREMIA; PRERENAL AZOTEMIA; HYPERURICEMIA	HYPERKALEMIA; METABOLIC ACIDOSIS; AZOTEMIA	HYPOKALEMIA, HYPOCHLOREMIA; METABOLIC ALKALOSIS; MAY LEAD TO EXTRA–CELLULAR FLUID DEPLETION; OTOTOXICITY IN PATIENTS WITH RENAL DISEASE; HYPERURICEMIA	MAY PRODUCE PULMONARY EDEMA IN CARDIAC PATIENTS; CELLULAR DEHY–DRATION; EXTRACELLULAR FLUID DEPLETION; HYPONATREMIA IF URINARY LOSSES ARE INSUFFICIENTLY REPLACED

Diuretics

Continued from page 255

GFR through as yet undefined mechanisms. The presence of poorly reabsorbable solute in the glomerular filtrate retards tubular reabsorption of water which, directly or indirectly, retards sodium and chloride reabsorption in the proximal tubules, loop of Henle, and distal nephron. Potassium and hydrogen ion excretion rates may increase during diuresis, and with chronic therapy, supplemental potassium may be needed.

Adverse reactions may be related to the rate of infusion of the osmotic diuretic, the total volume given, or both. For instance, circulatory overload may result from excessive volume, whereas excessive shrinking of brain cells with cerebral hemorrhage may occur because of hypertonicity of extracellular fluid. Depletion of extracellular fluid volume and a proportionately greater loss of sodium, which produces hyponatremia, may result from insufficient replacement of urinary losses of fluid and salt which occur during an osmotic diuresis.

The use of urea is contraindicated in patients with liver or kidney failure, while mannitol is contraindicated in patients with oliguria who fail to respond to a test dose. □

Dietary Management of Renal Failure

In patients with chronic renal failure, amelioration of the symptoms of uremia, anorexia, nausea, vomiting, diarrhea, anemia, dyspnea, and fatigue can be obtained by lowering the protein intake and thus reducing the blood urea nitrogen (BUN) level.

Selected low protein diets have been designed to provide the daily requirements of the essential amino acids with the minimal amount of high biologic value proteins. By these diets nitrogen balance may be maintained with the lowest possible nitrogen intake. If less than the minimal requirements of the essential amino acids are ingested, it is likely that negative nitrogen balance will develop. Consequently, the load of nitrogen to be excreted will rise from the minimum of 3 to 6 gm; higher BUN levels, persistence of symptoms of uremia, and muscle wasting will result. In addition, if there is inadequate caloric intake, gluconeogenesis from protein vitiates the purpose of the diet and produces similar results.

Composition of Diet. Giovanetti and Maggiore suggested an egg diet. The minimal daily requirements of the essential amino acids in conjunction with minimal nitrogen intake are found in egg and milk proteins. One egg and 200 ml of milk contain the necessary essential amino acids and a total protein level of about 18 to 20 gm, enough to make the caloric intake palatable. Low protein calories may be obtained from some glucose polymers, low protein bread, low protein spaghetti and biscuits, and from fat as double cream or oil, or alcoholic distilled spirits such as brandy, whiskey, vodka, and gin (five to seven calories per gram of alcohol).

An 18- to 20-gm protein diet should never be given to a patient who has not experienced the gastrointestinal symptoms of uremia. A suggested schedule for the protein intake based upon the glomerular filtration rate (GFR) is as follows:

GFR	Daily Protein
10 ml/min	Free protein intake
5 ml/min	25 to 30 gm
3 ml/min	18 gm initially then 25 gm
2 ml/min	18 gm
<2 ml/min	No strict diet to be given

The success of the diet depends on a rigid adherence to the low protein intake. The services of a dietitian are thus essential.

Response to Diet. Clinically, there is abatement of gastrointestinal symptoms together with a feeling of well-being and a sensation of hunger as the BUN decreases, a process which takes about 2 to 4 weeks. However, dialysis may be required initially to lower the BUN sufficiently before the diet can be undertaken.

The response to the diet is good if the GFR is 3 ml/minute or more. If the GFR is less than this amount, *complete* biochemical normality will not ensue, but lesser, varying degrees of improvement may occur. Improvement is not to be expected if the GFR is less than 2 ml/minute. Nevertheless, once a patient is established on the diet and there is

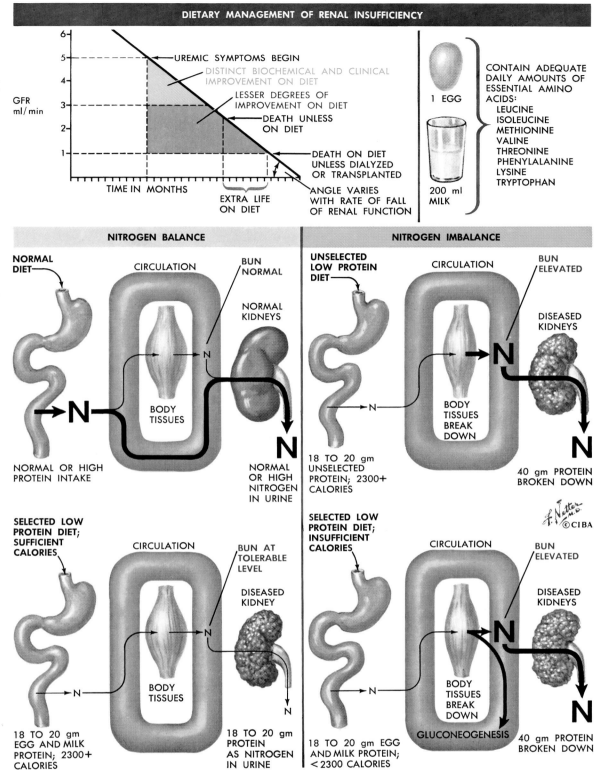

DIETARY MANAGEMENT OF RENAL INSUFFICIENCY

GFR ml/min — TIME IN MONTHS

UREMIC SYMPTOMS BEGIN
DISTINCT BIOCHEMICAL AND CLINICAL IMPROVEMENT ON DIET
LESSER DEGREES OF IMPROVEMENT ON DIET
DEATH UNLESS ON DIET
DEATH ON DIET UNLESS DIALYZED OR TRANSPLANTED
EXTRA LIFE ON DIET
ANGLE VARIES WITH RATE OF FALL OF RENAL FUNCTION

CONTAIN ADEQUATE DAILY AMOUNTS OF ESSENTIAL AMINO ACIDS:
LEUCINE
ISOLEUCINE
METHIONINE
VALINE
THREONINE
PHENYLALANINE
LYSINE
TRYPTOPHAN

1 EGG
200 ml MILK

NITROGEN BALANCE

NORMAL DIET — CIRCULATION — BUN NORMAL — NORMAL KIDNEYS — BODY TISSUES
NORMAL OR HIGH PROTEIN INTAKE
NORMAL OR HIGH NITROGEN IN URINE

SELECTED LOW PROTEIN DIET; SUFFICIENT CALORIES — CIRCULATION — BUN AT TOLERABLE LEVEL — DISEASED KIDNEY — BODY TISSUES
18 TO 20 gm EGG AND MILK PROTEIN; 2300+ CALORIES
18 TO 20 gm PROTEIN AS NITROGEN IN URINE

NITROGEN IMBALANCE

UNSELECTED LOW PROTEIN DIET — CIRCULATION — BUN ELEVATED — DISEASED KIDNEYS — BODY TISSUES BREAK DOWN
18 TO 20 gm UNSELECTED PROTEIN; 2300+ CALORIES
40 gm PROTEIN BROKEN DOWN

SELECTED LOW PROTEIN DIET; INSUFFICIENT CALORIES — CIRCULATION — BUN ELEVATED — DISEASED KIDNEYS — BODY TISSUES BREAK DOWN — GLUCONEOGENESIS
18 TO 20 gm EGG AND MILK PROTEIN; <2300 CALORIES
40 gm PROTEIN BROKEN DOWN

clinical improvement, it is likely that life can be maintained comfortably even though the GFR ultimately decreases to levels ordinarily not compatible with "nondialyzed" life, *i.e.,* 1 ml/minute. Additional decrease in the GFR will cause death, however, and dialysis or renal transplant is necessary.

As renal disease progresses, the rate of fall of the GFR largely determines the duration of survival on the diet. Rapid destruction of glomeruli occurs in patients with malignant hypertension and has a bad prognosis. In contrast, slowly progressive, normotensive renal disease, such as is found in Fanconi syndrome or polycystic disease, has a much better prognosis. Survival for more than 4 years after the start of dietary therapy has been noted.

Diet prolongs life sufficiently for hyperkalemia, acidosis, and metastatic calcification to become serious problems. Metastatic calcification occurs when the serum calcium-phosphorus product is greater than 70, usually because of the hyperphosphatemia which occurs in renal failure. The sites affected are the subcutaneous tissues and bursae around the joints, the arteries, and the eyes (see pages 113-122). Metastatic calcification at some sites can be reversed by oral administration of aluminum hydroxide which binds phosphate in the gut. Consequently, serum phosphate levels are lower, and the serum calcium-phosphorus product is less than 70.

Another major problem is salt and water imbalance which causes either heart failure or salt depletion (see pages 113-122).

It should be noted that dietary therapy does not compete with dialysis or transplantation. Instead, it offers a possibility of palliation in patients with advanced renal failure when no other facilities can be extended to the individual patient. □

Hemodialysis

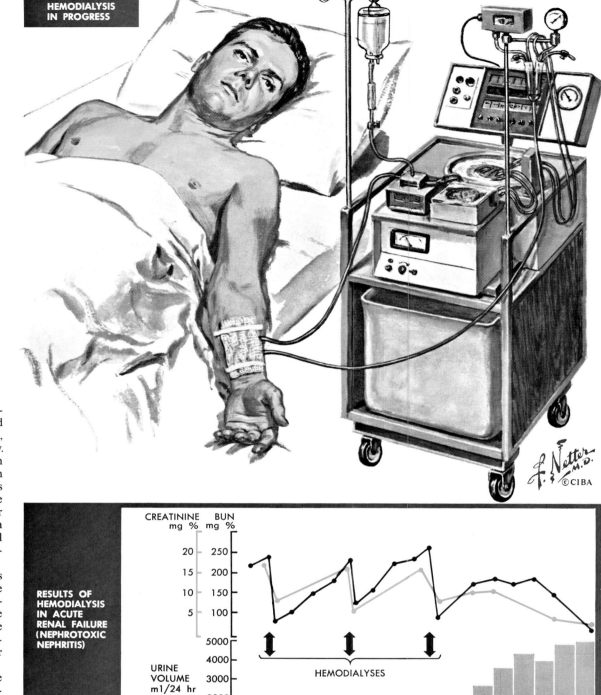

HEMODIALYSIS IN PROGRESS

RESULTS OF HEMODIALYSIS IN ACUTE RENAL FAILURE (NEPHROTOXIC NEPHRITIS)

CREATININE mg %   BUN mg %

URINE VOLUME ml/24 hr

HEMODIALYSES

DAYS 3   6   9   12   15   18

Any comprehensive review of great therapeutic strides in the 20th century would have to include, in a prominent position, the development of the artificial kidney. Thousands of individuals depend each day on the artificial kidney to maintain life, while uremic patients selected as candidates for transplant surgery are maintained by dialysis in the hospital or home until a suitable donor kidney can be found. Consequently, the artificial kidney has helped make kidney transplantation both possible and practical.

In addition, the artificial kidney has saved thousands of patients in acute renal failure from untimely death because of hyperkalemia or uremia (see page 111) and has been valuable in the treatment of patients who have accidentally or intentionally ingested poisons or overdoses of drugs.

The use of the artificial kidney in the terminal uremic patient may also be considered a valuable research tool; it has permitted investigators to observe patients passing in and out of clinical uremia, as well as to observe and study the pathogenesis of many uremic complications. Such complications include peripheral neuropathy and renal osteodystrophy which were previously seen only in a transient, early stage in the preterminal patient. Furthermore, through the use of an almost infinite variety of biochemical materials in the dialysis bath, much has been learned concerning the biochemistry of important intermediates in the uremic state.

The Principles of Dialysis

The fundamental physiologic principle in dialysis—that of a solute moving across a semipermeable membrane in a direction and at a rate consistent with concentration gradients—has been known since the early days of biochemistry. A classic example of the use of the concept is the technic by which protein-bound solutes are separated from nonprotein-bound ones in the experimental laboratory.

This fundamental and basically simple physiologic principle is the foundation for the operation of today's artificial kidney, or extracorporeal dialysis device. Blood or plasma, ideally in an extremely thin, well-stirred, uniform layer, flows along on one side of a semipermeable membrane. A wash solution, resembling normal extracellular fluid, flows with turbulence on the other side of the membrane, preferably countercurrent to the flow of blood.

Any solute which has a higher concentration in the blood than in the dialysate flows "down" its concentration gradient and so leaves the blood. Conversely, any solute which is in higher concentration in the dialysate (e.g., sodium, glucose, or bicarbonate) will leave the dialysate and cross the semipermeable membrane into the blood. The reconstituted and purified blood is then returned to the patient's circulation.

The circulation of the blood through the artificial kidney during the clinical dialysis of the uremic patient not only reverses acidosis and corrects electrolyte abnormalities but also provides nutrients such as glucose. The clinical benefits that accrue to the patient are the direct result of the arteriovenous difference in noxious solutes that is created while the blood is in the artificial kidney.

Which of the almost infinite number of metabolites removed constitutes the uremic "toxin" (or "toxins") is still unknown, and the search for this toxin continues. Nevertheless, empiric treatment with the artificial kidney has been an extraordinary success.

At the present time, over 10,000 individuals with chronic renal conditions are being maintained for long periods of time by the use of artificial kidneys. The actuarial figure for appropriate candidates seems

Hemodialysis

Continued

STRUCTURE AND FUNCTION OF TWIN-COIL HEMODIALYZER

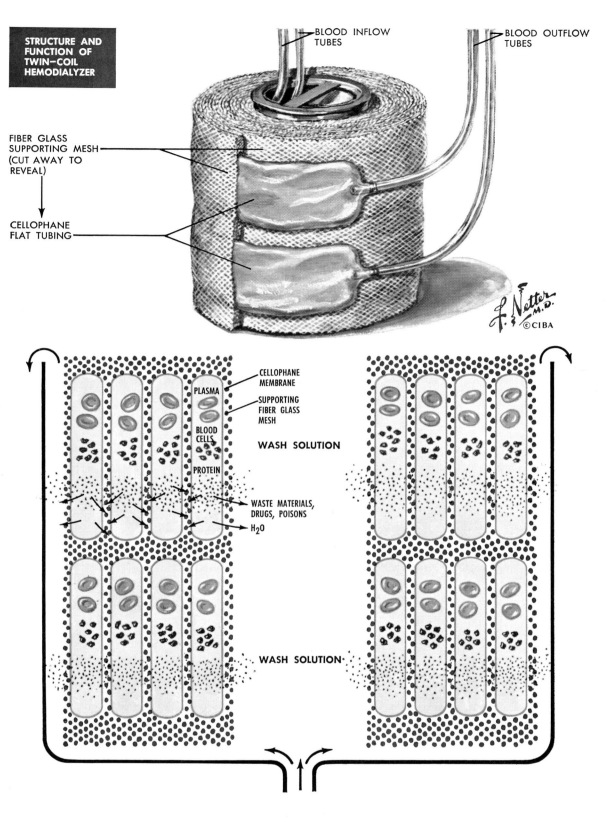

to be around 50 to 60 per million population per year. Dialysis is performed two or three times weekly for 4 to 12 hours each time, depending on the engineering configuration of the particular artificial kidney in use. Hundreds of other individuals who are awaiting the availability of a suitable donor kidney for transplant are maintained by dialysis. After the transplant is performed, patients can, if necessary, be returned to dialysis and be maintained for short periods of time through bouts of renal shutdown, or for longer periods in instances of transplant rejection. In no other complicated organ system has the ingenuity of man been so successful in replacing nature.

The History of Dialysis

The idea of supporting a living organism through a period of crisis by providing spare parts had intrigued man for many years. The greatest modern impetus for this idea came when man achieved the ability to transfer blood, a living organ, from one individual to another. It is surprising, however, that the highly complex kidney was the first organ for which man was able to devise a satisfactory functional replacement.

The era of extracorporeal dialysis began in 1913 when Abel, Rountree, and Turner devised the first artificial kidney, an apparatus made of celloidin tubes branching out in such a way that the last tubes through which the blood ran were parallel. This branching system was surrounded with a jacket filled with isotonic saline. Hirudin, obtained from leeches, was used as an anticoagulant. Foreseeing the possible application of dialysis in the treatment of acute renal failure, these pioneers also demonstrated the removal of sodium salicylate from the blood, thereby laying the groundwork for the dialysis of poisons. Subsequent workers, in attempts to improve hemodialysis, used defibrinated blood,

refined the apparatus, and tried membranes of a variety of materials including chicken intestine, fish bladder, and peritoneum treated with gelatin bichromate. Thalheimer, in 1937, was the first to use cellophane as the membrane and heparin as the anticoagulant. During and immediately after World War II, Kolff developed and constructed the first practical dialyzer in a rotating drum suitable for clinical application. He set up this equipment at the bedside and demonstrated that, with hemodialysis, most of the manifestations of uremia would disappear within 24 hours. In the postwar period, Kolff brought his apparatus to the United States where it was gradually introduced into clinical medicine.

Types of Artificial Kidneys

At present, two types of dialysis machinery are in common use. These are the *coil* and *flat-plate* systems.

The most frequently used coil dialyzer is the Kolff *twin-coil* system. This consists of two coils of flat cellophane tubing, supported by a fiberglass or crisscross polypropylene mesh and wound around a central core. The entire coil system is immersed in a canister through which dialysis fluid is pumped. The blood circulates through the cellulose coils, and waste materials, drugs, or poisons are washed out into the dialysate. (Plate 7 illustrates the *twin-coil* hemodialyzer.)

Because of resistance in the coils, a blood pump is needed to maintain an adequate blood flow throughout the twin-coil apparatus. A large reservoir of dialysis fluid—some 100 to 300 liters—is needed.

The prototype of the *flat-plate* system is the Skeggs-Leonards artificial kidney which is composed of flat sheets of cellophane clamped between solid, ridged, metal plates. *Continued on page 260*

Hemodialysis

Continued from page 259

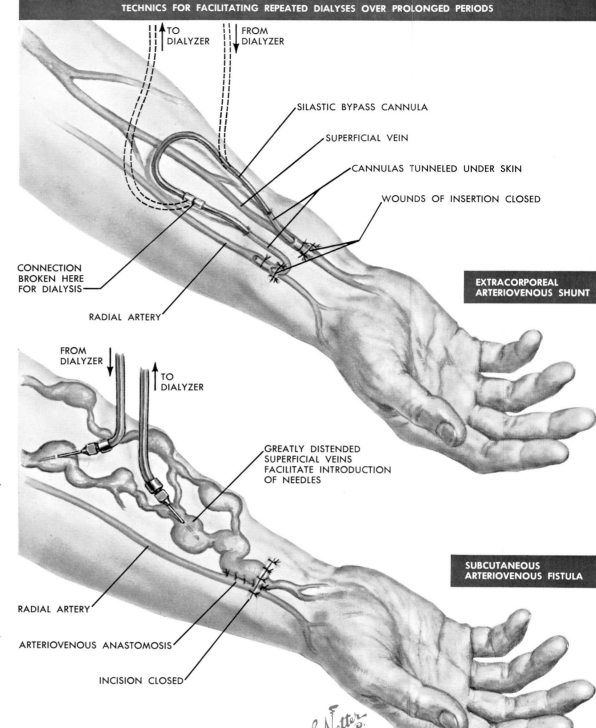

Blood flows in channels between the cellophane sheets, countercurrent to the dialysate, which flows in grooves between the cellophane sheets and the plates.

The Kiil dialyzer is a modification of the Skeggs-Leonards kidney, using different materials, *i.e.,* cuprophane instead of cellophane membranes, and polypropylene instead of metal plates.

The flat-plate type of apparatus provides a system with low resistance. Consequently, unlike the situation with the twin-coil kidney, adequate blood flow can generally be maintained by blood pressure alone, virtually obviating the need for a blood pump. However, as with the twin-coil kidney, a large reservoir of dialysate fluid is required.

A common reservoir of dialysis fluid is widely used in many dialysis centers, with 8 to 10 dialyzers supplied from one central fluid supply. Fortunately, the dialysate does not have to be kept bacteriologically sterile during dialysis runs, but aseptic technics must be followed whenever there is contact with blood.

The *capillary kidney* is a smaller, but apparently equally effective, hemodialyzer that is now undergoing active clinical trial. The use of rolled coils or extruded tubes has made possible a reduction in size, but perhaps most importantly, the capillary kidney does not require priming with blood prior to use.

Long-Term Dialysis

In the early days of hemodialysis, the repeated use of the procedure was restricted by: (1) the limited number of blood vessels available for cannulation and (2) the frequent occurrence of scar tissue at cutdown sites which precludes the multiple use of any given vessel.

The development of indwelling plastic arteriovenous shunts (as illustrated in Plate 8) has now made possible repeated

dialysis over a prolonged period and offers the added advantage of making it a painless procedure.

Cannulas are placed surgically in an artery and a vein of an arm or a leg. The arterial cannula can be attached to the inflow end of an artificial kidney and the venous cannula to the outflow end. When dialysis is not in progress, the two cannulas can be connected with a plastic loop, creating an external arteriovenous fistula.

Despite their utility, however, extracorporeal shunts of this type do present two major problems, *clotting* and *infection.*

Even in the most experienced dialysis centers, clotting has limited average shunt survival to anywhere from 4 to 9 months. If safe declotting procedures are not immediately successful, new shunts must be inserted. In a rare patient, frequent shunt troubles may lead to exhaustion of shunt sites, and vascular

grafting may become necessary to provide other sites.

Shunt infections occur frequently and are also potentially serious in that they may lead to thrombosis or even, on occasion, to septicemia.

To reduce these hazards, many dialysis centers have been turning to the surgical establishment of a subcutaneous arteriovenous fistula. This procedure has the advantage of eliminating the extracorporeal shunt, with its inherent dangers of infection and clotting, but has the disadvantage of requiring percutaneous punctures each time dialysis is instituted.

Other Problems in Long-Term Dialysis. A continuing problem in repeated dialysis is the volume of bank blood needed to prepare the artificial kidney and its connecting lines prior to use. Anywhere from 300 to 800 ml of blood is needed to prime different types of hemodialyzers. Repeated transfusions of such volumes of blood may result in the formation of multiple

Hemodialysis
Continued

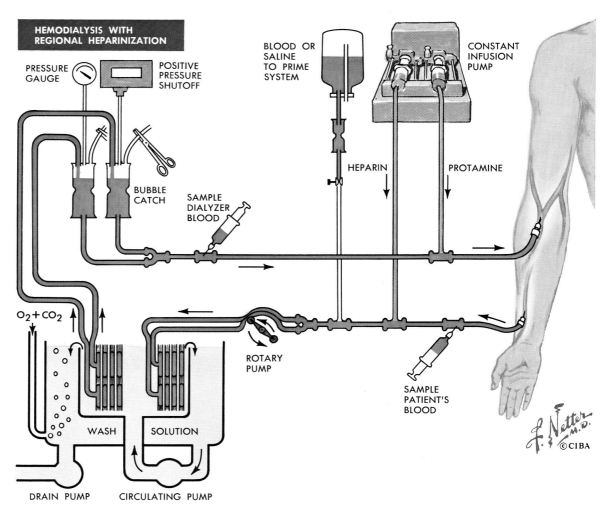

HEMODIALYSIS WITH REGIONAL HEPARINIZATION

PRESSURE GAUGE

POSITIVE PRESSURE SHUTOFF

BUBBLE CATCH

SAMPLE DIALYZER BLOOD

BLOOD OR SALINE TO PRIME SYSTEM

CONSTANT INFUSION PUMP

HEPARIN

PROTAMINE

O_2+CO_2

ROTARY PUMP

SAMPLE PATIENT'S BLOOD

WASH

SOLUTION

DRAIN PUMP

CIRCULATING PUMP

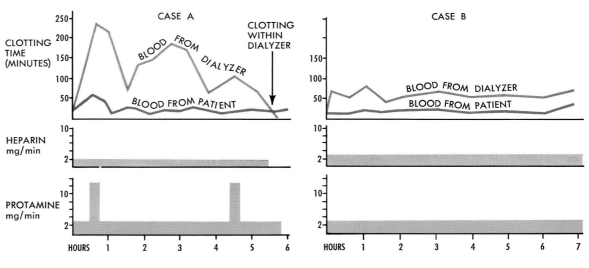

EXAMPLES DEMONSTRATING EFFECT OF REGIONAL HEPARINIZATION ON CLOTTING TIME

CASE A

CLOTTING WITHIN DIALYZER

CLOTTING TIME (MINUTES)

BLOOD FROM DIALYZER

BLOOD FROM PATIENT

HEPARIN mg/min

PROTAMINE mg/min

HOURS

CASE B

BLOOD FROM DIALYZER

BLOOD FROM PATIENT

red blood cell antibodies which may make future typing and cross-matching extremely difficult. Also, potential kidney donors may be eliminated if the recipient develops such antibodies. The development of antibodies to the recently discovered white blood cell antigens may also confuse the patient's blood profile and may disqualify even more donors who are otherwise satisfactory.

Perhaps the greatest single risk in long-term hemodialysis is the development of hepatitis. Outbreaks of hepatitis have occurred in virtually all dialysis units operating for more than 2 or 3 years. In a single outbreak, over half the patients—and half the staff as well —may contract the disease. The high incidence is probably related to frequent contact between the same group of patients and the same staff over protracted periods of time.

The major barrier to the effective use of maintenance dialysis is not the physiologic problems described but financial considerations. The inordinately high cost of hemodialysis runs to many thousands of dollars per patient every year and is the main factor limiting its widespread use.

Home Dialysis. The successful use of artificial kidneys in the home has been an important advance in the successful rehabilitation of patients with chronic and debilitating renal disease. In many instances, it has facilitated the return of these patients to a nearly normal life. For example, in the home, as opposed to in dialysis centers, patients can schedule their treatments to suit their convenience, such as in the evening after work.

Despite the increased convenience and independence that home dialysis offers a patient, certain factors limit its widespread use. Cost is again a limiting factor, for although the maintenance cost of

home dialysis is less than that in hospitals, the initial cost for home dialysis is far higher because each person must purchase his own dialysis equipment.

Furthermore, the patient must possess a suitable degree of intelligence and must be sufficiently motivated to cooperate in all aspects of his treatment. A responsible spouse, close relative, or partner is also necessary.

Psychologic stability of both the patient and his immediate family must be considered before home dialysis is instituted. Psychiatric problems associated with this type of therapy not only may arise in the patients themselves but have been reported in as many as 25 percent of their family members.

Regional Heparinization

Systemic heparinization is generally a precondition for hemodialysis. Therefore, in patients in whom

there is a contraindication to the prolongation of clotting time (*e.g.*, recent trauma, surgery, burns, or a history of bleeding ulcers), peritoneal dialysis is usually employed (see page 262). If rapid dialysance is necessary, the technic of regional heparinization may permit use of an artificial kidney. Some centers even use the regional heparinization technic routinely for all hemodialysis patients to eliminate possible risks of systemic heparinization.

As shown in Plate 9, regional heparinization involves the addition of heparin to the input or arterial side of the artificial kidney, followed by countertitration with protamine on the return or venous side. In this way, the clotting time of the blood in the machine is continuously prolonged from one half hour to infinity, whereas the clotting time of the person connected to the machine is maintained within normal limits by the protamine titration. *Continued on page 262*

Hemodialysis

Continued from page 261

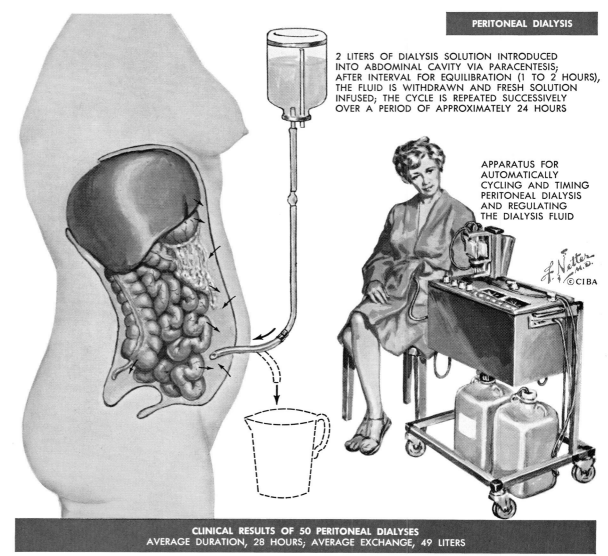

2 LITERS OF DIALYSIS SOLUTION INTRODUCED INTO ABDOMINAL CAVITY VIA PARACENTESIS; AFTER INTERVAL FOR EQUILIBRATION (1 TO 2 HOURS), THE FLUID IS WITHDRAWN AND FRESH SOLUTION INFUSED; THE CYCLE IS REPEATED SUCCESSIVELY OVER A PERIOD OF APPROXIMATELY 24 HOURS

APPARATUS FOR AUTOMATICALLY CYCLING AND TIMING PERITONEAL DIALYSIS AND REGULATING THE DIALYSIS FLUID

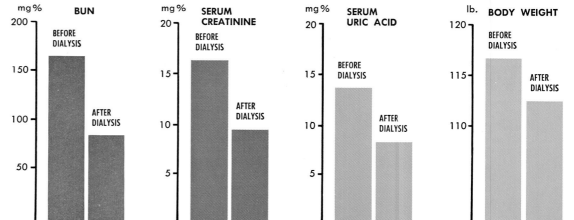

CLINICAL RESULTS OF 50 PERITONEAL DIALYSES
AVERAGE DURATION, 28 HOURS; AVERAGE EXCHANGE, 49 LITERS

The effectiveness of this technic depends on matching the rates of heparin and protamine administration to the rate of blood flow through the kidney. Since these two drugs have different distribution spaces in the body, it is possible that heparin returning to the bloodstream via the lymph may exert an anticoagulant effect several hours after the dialysis has ceased. This possibility should be kept in mind and counteracted, if necessary, by the administration of additional doses of protamine.

Peritoneal Dialysis

Peritoneal dialysis and hemodialysis are based on the same physiologic principle. They differ mainly in that peritoneal dialysis makes use of an *in vivo* biologic membrane and is generally less effective.

During peritoneal dialysis, 2 to 4 liters of dialysate is inserted into the peritoneal cavity through an indwelling catheter (Plate 10) or through a large-bore needle. The peritoneum then acts as the semipermeable membrane; the noxious solutes in the blood pass across the peritoneal membrane into the dialysis fluid. After a suitable interval to allow for equilibration, generally about 1 to 2 hours, the dialysate fluid, along with its harvest of harmful substances, is removed from the abdomen, either through the indwelling catheter, as illustrated, or through a polyvinyl catheter introduced with a trocar. The entire process is repeated frequently over a period of approximately 24 hours.

The membrane of the capillary wall seems to be the major cellular barrier in the delivery of blood-borne solutes to the peritoneal cavity. As a result, the rate of diffusion becomes a function of splanchnic blood flow, the concentration differences of solutes between the blood and dialysate fluid, and the degree of mixing of solutes which takes place dur-

ing the period of equilibration in the peritoneal cavity.

Many drugs have been used in an attempt to enhance splanchnic blood flow or change the qualities of the biologic membrane. Thus far these have met with little success.

With respect to the removal of poisons and the major chemicals studied in uremia, a good peritoneal dialysis can be considered approximately one sixth as efficient as hemodialysis, per unit of time. Nevertheless, the procedure is of value in patients with special conditions, such as myocardial infarction, in whom sudden changes of blood pressure are undesirable. In addition, peritoneal dialysis is helpful in conditions that preclude the use of systemic heparinization. (However, the technic of regional heparinization, as described on page 261, may be a suitable alternative.) Peritoneal dialysis can also be used to maintain patients with chronic renal failure until they can enter

a program of chronic dialysis with an artificial kidney.

Recirculation peritoneal dialysis involves the use of two cannulas. In a continuous stream, the dialysate is pumped into the peritoneal cavity through one cannula and returned, via the other, to an ultrafiltration dialyzer. This device not only removes noxious solutes *from* the dialysis fluid but concentrates, *within* the dialysate, the protein normally lost during the procedure. When the dialysate is then recycled through the patient, the increased concentration of protein minimizes further protein losses.

The peritoneal route has been used only sparingly for patients requiring chronic dialysis, because it is difficult to achieve nutritional balance with the protein losses that are commonly encountered. Moreover, infection after 6 or 8 months has been the rule in all but a few patients, even when the most meticulous care has been given to proper sterile technic. □

Dialysis of Drugs and Poisons

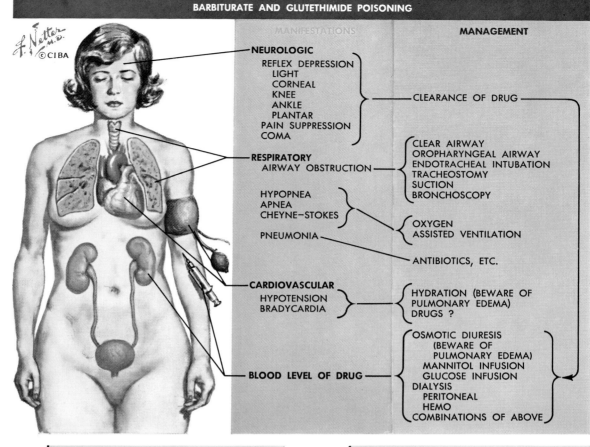

BARBITURATE AND GLUTETHIMIDE POISONING

MANIFESTATIONS	MANAGEMENT

NEUROLOGIC
REFLEX DEPRESSION
LIGHT
CORNEAL
KNEE
ANKLE
PLANTAR
PAIN SUPPRESSION
COMA

CLEARANCE OF DRUG

RESPIRATORY
AIRWAY OBSTRUCTION

CLEAR AIRWAY
OROPHARYNGEAL AIRWAY
ENDOTRACHEAL INTUBATION
TRACHEOSTOMY
SUCTION
BRONCHOSCOPY

HYPOPNEA
APNEA
CHEYNE-STOKES

OXYGEN
ASSISTED VENTILATION

PNEUMONIA

ANTIBIOTICS, ETC.

CARDIOVASCULAR
HYPOTENSION
BRADYCARDIA

HYDRATION (BEWARE OF
PULMONARY EDEMA)
DRUGS ?

BLOOD LEVEL OF DRUG

OSMOTIC DIURESIS
(BEWARE OF
PULMONARY EDEMA)
MANNITOL INFUSION
GLUCOSE INFUSION
DIALYSIS
PERITONEAL
HEMO
COMBINATIONS OF ABOVE

Thousands of patients die each year as a result of overdoses of drugs or poisons. Intentional overdose is a frequent method of suicide in women and nonviolent individuals, while accidental overdose is most frequent in alcoholics, and young, senile, and drug-addicted patients. Sedatives, analgesics, and alcohol are the agents most often responsible for suicide.

By rapid reversal of the concentration gradient, the bloodstream which carries a drug or poison from the site of absorption to the site of action can also be used to transport the agent *away* from the site of action. This reversal is best accomplished by peritoneal dialysis and hemodialysis, although osmotic diuresis might be appropriate for certain drugs.

Peritoneal clearance or dialysance may be calculated by the simple formula $C \text{ (ml/min)} = \dfrac{S_D \times V_D}{S_B \times t}$ in which S_D equals concentration of solute in dialysate drainage (change from zero), V_D is the dialysate volume, S_B is the concentration of solute in serum, and t is the time of the total exchange.

In hemodialysis, dialysance is calculated by the equation $D = a\,(1 - e^{-\frac{PS}{a}})$ in which D is dialysance, a is blood flow, P is the membrane permeability, S is the surface area, and e is the natural logarithm.* Therefore, *dialysance* is the rate of removal of a solute from the blood per unit concentration difference between arterial blood and bath fluid.

In 1958, this author formulated the standard criteria for judging the applicability of dialysis in the removal of drugs. These criteria are: (1) The drug molecule should be able to be diffused from plasma water through the dialyzing membrane, whether it be cellophane or peritoneum, at a reasonable removal rate or dialysance. (2) The drug must be sufficiently well distributed in accessible body fluid compartments. (3) The ultimate clinical toxicity should be dependent on the concentration of the drug in blood and the duration of the body's exposure to the circulating drug; this is often described as the "time-dose-cytotoxic" relationship. (4) The amount of drug dialyzed should be a significant addition to the amount of the drug metabolized and excreted

*See Glossary

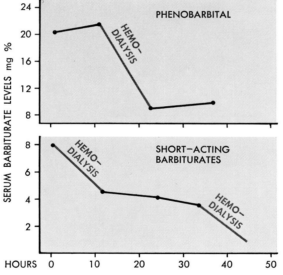

EFFECT OF HEMODIALYSIS ON BLOOD
LEVEL IN PHENOBARBITAL POISONING AND
IN SHORT-ACTING BARBITURATE POISONING

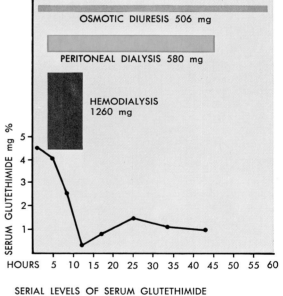

SERIAL LEVELS OF SERUM GLUTETHIMIDE
PLOTTED IN RELATION TO QUANTITIES
REMOVED BY DIALYSIS AND BY DIURESIS

by the body in lung, liver, kidney, and bowel.

The first drug dialysis was performed by Abel in 1913 with the removal of salicylic acid; the modern era of dialysance of drugs and poisons began in the 1950s. (See glossary for table of currently known dialyzable substances.)

The clinical indications for extracorporeal dialysis in acute drug poisonings are any of the following: (1) severe clinical intoxication with abnormalities of vital signs, (2) ingestion and probable absorption of a dose that is potentially lethal, (3) a blood level of drug that is known to be potentially fatal, (4) a degree of intoxication that impairs a major excretory pathway for that particular drug, (5) the presence of significant quantities of a circulating solute that will be metabolized to a more toxic substance, (6) progressive clinical deterioration of the patient despite other forms of medical treatment, (7) prolonged coma, (8) the presence of an

underlying disease that increases the hazards of coma, and (9) the development of significant complications.

As shown in the illustration, the blood level of phenobarbital can be lowered from the fatal to the nonfatal range in a matter of hours. Similar data are provided for short-acting barbiturates and glutethimide. In the case of the latter agent, hemodialysis is capable of removing significant quantities from the serum.

It must be emphasized, however, that dialysis is never a substitute for an adequate airway. Adequate ventilation by oropharyngeal airway insertion, endotracheal intubation, or tracheostomy is necessary. Oxygen and assisted ventilation are required in severe hypopnea or apnea. Nevertheless, all other things being equal, the best treatment for an overdose of a drug or poison is its removal from the body as rapidly as possible. □

Kidney Transplantation

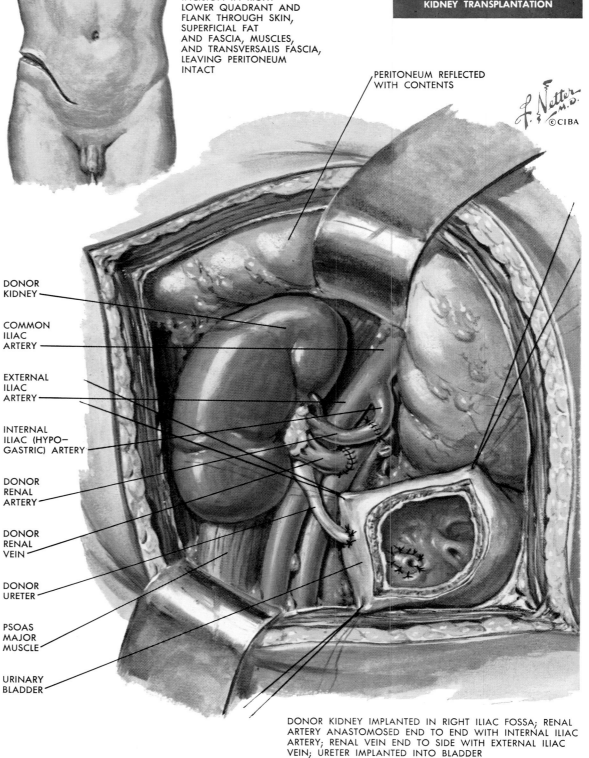

INCISION IN RIGHT LOWER QUADRANT AND FLANK THROUGH SKIN, SUPERFICIAL FAT AND FASCIA, MUSCLES, AND TRANSVERSALIS FASCIA, LEAVING PERITONEUM INTACT

PERITONEUM REFLECTED WITH CONTENTS

DONOR KIDNEY

COMMON ILIAC ARTERY

EXTERNAL ILIAC ARTERY

INTERNAL ILIAC (HYPO—GASTRIC) ARTERY

DONOR RENAL ARTERY

DONOR RENAL VEIN

DONOR URETER

PSOAS MAJOR MUSCLE

URINARY BLADDER

DONOR KIDNEY IMPLANTED IN RIGHT ILIAC FOSSA; RENAL ARTERY ANASTOMOSED END TO END WITH INTERNAL ILIAC ARTERY; RENAL VEIN END TO SIDE WITH EXTERNAL ILIAC VEIN; URETER IMPLANTED INTO BLADDER

Once considered revolutionary surgical procedure, the transplantation of the human kidney from one individual to another is now acceptable clinical treatment for chronic end-stage renal failure. Nevertheless, the problem of graft rejection still plagues the transplant operation, and efforts to determine the exact nature of the rejection mechanisms and to defeat these mechanisms continue.

The success of a kidney transplant is directly related to the source of the donated kidney. Kidneys are available from two types of donors. The first of these is the living, related donor who must be of the same blood type as the recipient. A survey published in April, 1973, showed the survival rate over an 8-year period for kidneys transplanted between siblings to be almost 90 percent. Kidneys transplanted from parent to child had a survival rate of approximately 84 percent. The success rate for the second type of donor, the unrelated, cadaver donor, was considerably less—approximately 68 percent for the same 8-year period.

Transplant Technic. When a living donor is available, the surgical procedure begins with the removal of the donor's left kidney, which is then rotated and placed in the recipient's right hemipelvis. Next, the renal artery is anastomosed end to end to the internal iliac (hypogastric) artery, and the renal vein end to side to the external iliac vein. The ureter of the donor kidney is implanted in the bladder through a submucosal tunnel. Alternatively, the recipient ureter may be anastomosed to the renal pelvis of the donor kidney, but the first procedure is considered more satisfactory and is more commonly employed.

Kidneys from cadaver donors are transplanted in much the same way. In this case, the right kidney may be utilized as well in another recipient. This second kidney is rotated and put in the left hemipelvis. Perfusion of the cadaver kidney and cooling by immersion in iced heparin-Ringer's solution usually permits successful transplantation for as long as 6 to 8 hours after the kidney has left the donor.

To suppress the immunologic reaction which causes graft rejection, azathioprine in a dosage of 2 to 3 mg/kg is administered to the patient for 24 hours before transplantation. Decreasing doses are given as renal function resumes. Corticosteroids, usually prednisone (2 mg/kg), are also prescribed on the day of the operation and are similarly tapered following surgery according to the return of renal function. Parenthetically, it is not uncommon for a cadaver kidney, which may have been ischemic for some hours, to remain anuric for a period of days, or even weeks, and then recover normal renal function. The immunosuppressive efficacy of antilymphocyte serum, or of the globulin recently derived from it, has not been established thus far in man.

The rejection process results from the immunization of the recipient by antigens of the donor kidney. The host forms both antibody globulin and sensitized lymphocytes, which seek to destroy the graft largely by acting upon the vasculature, including the glomerulus. *Clinically,* symptoms of rejection are a general feeling of lassitude, malaise, and anorexia. Fever is common, as is leukocytosis. Elevation of the blood pressure is frequent and indicates the involvement of the renal vasculature. Indeed, elevation of the blood pressure may be one of the first signs of chronic rejection. At an early stage, abnormalities in the renal blood flow and urine output may be reflected in the

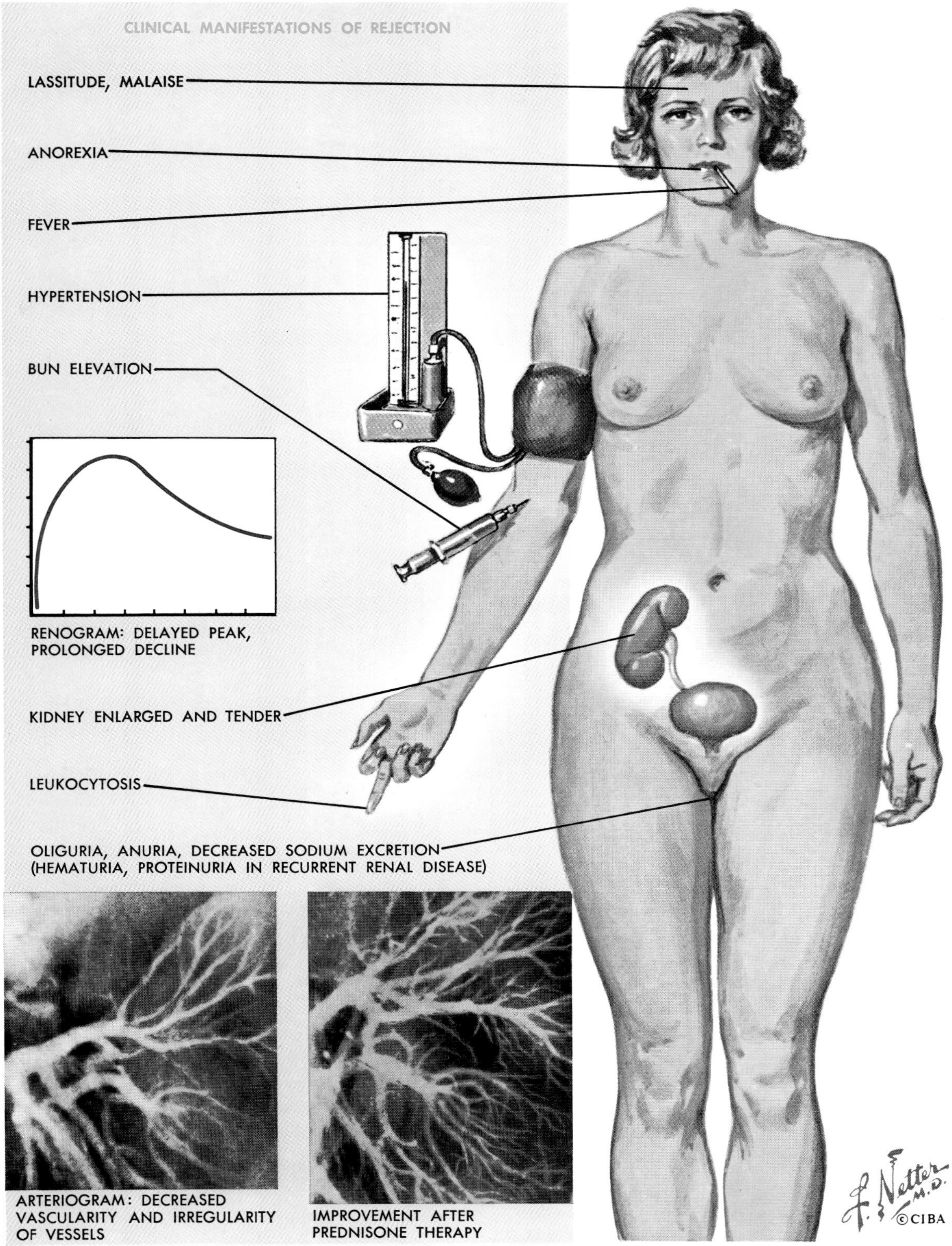

Kidney Transplantation

Continued

CLINICAL MANIFESTATIONS OF REJECTION

LASSITUDE, MALAISE

ANOREXIA

FEVER

HYPERTENSION

BUN ELEVATION

RENOGRAM: DELAYED PEAK, PROLONGED DECLINE

KIDNEY ENLARGED AND TENDER

LEUKOCYTOSIS

OLIGURIA, ANURIA, DECREASED SODIUM EXCRETION (HEMATURIA, PROTEINURIA IN RECURRENT RENAL DISEASE)

ARTERIOGRAM: DECREASED VASCULARITY AND IRREGULARITY OF VESSELS

IMPROVEMENT AFTER PREDNISONE THERAPY

radioisotope renogram. A decrease in both the height and the promptness of the early phase or peak (delayed) of the renogram, with a prolonged decline representing failure of urinary washout, indicates decreased renal blood flow and declining urinary output. Elevation of the blood urea nitrogen and creatinine, with decreasing urine volume, is also common. Examination of the urine may show an increase in red cells and proteinuria and, occasionally, clumps of lymphocytes.

In an individual with previously normal renal function, a first indication of rejection may be an increase in urine osmolality with a decreased sodium concentration, again reflecting vascular effects similar to those of renal arterial stenosis (see page 85). A renal angiogram obtained at this time would show a marked decrease in the visualization of the cortical vessels. The vascular effects may be reversed by adequate prednisone therapy.

Because the kidney frequently becomes enlarged, tender, and painful during the rejection episode, it may be difficult to differentiate between rejection, obstruction to the ureter, and severe pyelonephritis.

Pathology. To understand the pathologic picture, it is necessary to review the immunologic events which culminate in rejection. As has been stated, immunization of the host results from contact with antigens contained in the grafted kidney. The severity of this process varies with the antigenic differences between the tissues of the donor and those of the recipient. Immunization of the host results in the production of both antibody globulin

and sensitized lymphocytes. Antibody in both of these forms can be seen in and around the vessels of the graft in early stages. The combination of the antigen of the graft and the antibody of the host causes the activation of the complement sequence. The sequence, in turn, gives rise to leukotaxic factors which attract polymorphonuclear leukocytes and may denude the basement membrane of its endothelium. Subsequently, release of lysosomes from the polymorphonuclear leukocytes results in increased permeability and destruction of the wall of the vessel. The denuded basement membrane stimulates platelet deposition and aggregation which then release platelet factor 3. Platelet factor 3 facilitates the precipitation of fibrinogen, with subsequent deposition of fibrin and, ultimately, the organization of fibroblasts. A migration inhibitory factor (MIF) is also released by the activation of the complement sequence. MIF, as a result of the

increased vascular permeability created by the preceding events, encourages the aggregation of monocytes at the vessel wall and their migration through the vessel into the renal interstitium. The speed and severity with which the pathologic events occur determine the final picture.

Early biopsy of rat kidney allografts demonstrates the first event in the immunologic rejection of a transplanted kidney. Kidneys are transplanted from one inbred strain of a rat to another to create a constant tissue-type difference. The events noted in the experiments are thus predictable chronologically and can be carefully studied and recorded. The first event seen in the acute rejection of the rat kidney is the deposition of gamma globulin in the walls of the small veins. Cells producing gamma globulin (probably sensitized lymphocytes) approximate the vein wall and some migrate through it into the *Continued on page 266*

Kidney Transplantation

Continued from page 265

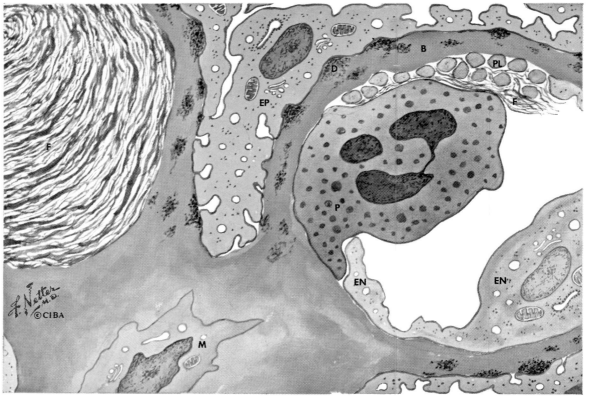

A: DIAGRAM OF ELECTRON PHOTOMICROGRAPHIC FINDINGS IN ACUTE REJECTION OF AN ALLOGRAFT: IN ONE CAPILLARY OF THE GLOMERULUS A PSEUDOPOD OF A POLYMORPHONUCLEAR LEUKOCYTE (P) IS UNDERMINING AND LIFTING OFF THE ENDOTHELIUM (EN); PLATELET (PL) AND FIBRIN (F) DEPOSITS ARE PRESENT; ELECTRON−DENSE DEPOSITS (D) APPEAR IN BASEMENT MEMBRANE (B); THE OTHER CAPILLARY IS COMPLETELY OBLITERATED BY FIBRIN. EP=EPITHELIUM, M=MESANGIAL CELL

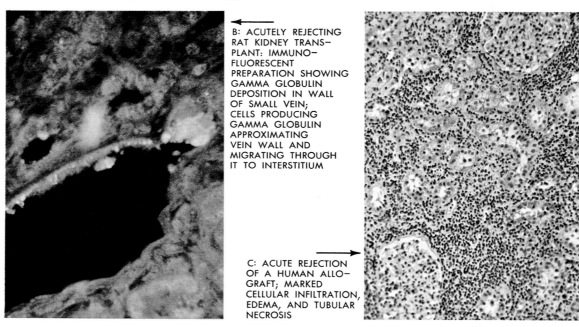

B: ACUTELY REJECTING RAT KIDNEY TRANS−PLANT: IMMUNO−FLUORESCENT PREPARATION SHOWING GAMMA GLOBULIN DEPOSITION IN WALL OF SMALL VEIN; CELLS PRODUCING GAMMA GLOBULIN APPROXIMATING VEIN WALL AND MIGRATING THROUGH IT TO INTERSTITIUM

C: ACUTE REJECTION OF A HUMAN ALLO−GRAFT; MARKED CELLULAR INFILTRATION, EDEMA, AND TUBULAR NECROSIS

renal interstitium. Similarly, acute rejection of the human renal allograft is accompanied by both the vascular and the interstitial phenomenon. The photomicrograph in Plate 14 depicts the marked interstitial cellular infiltration with edema and the varying amount of tubular necrosis which accompanies rejection. The early events recorded in the human kidney which correspond to those in transplant rejection in the rat are shown in Plate 15. Here, a human renal transplant, which has been biopsied soon after transplantation and stained with fluorescein-tagged human globulin, is pictured. The immunofluorescent study shows the deposits of gamma globulin on the basement membrane of the human renal allograft.

Because patients awaiting kidney transplantation frequently rely on artificial kidney dialysis for long periods of time and so require transfusions, they are exposed to human antigen in the form of human white cells and platelets in the transfused blood (see page 258). Consequently, such patients may be immunized against a number of human antigens among which may be those contained on the surface of the donor kidney. When the kidney is transplanted and the arterial anastomosis opened, the organ may be perfused with blood containing preformed antibodies against the graft antigens. In this case, violent rejection of the kidney occurs. Necrosis of vessels and glomeruli is typical of the rejection as the immune process is accelerated. This so-called hyperacute rejection, caused by preformed antibodies, is characterized by thrombosis of the afferent arteriole of the glomerulus in as-

sociation with interstitial edema and hemorrhage.

The rejection process may also be a slow, gradually progressive change. In all probability, the steps in the rejection of longer duration are immunologic attacks upon vessel walls, including the glomeruli, subsequent abortion of the rejection, and then healing of the inflammatory process by scarring. Over a period of years, therefore, despite the absence of evidence of acute rejection, slowly progressive degeneration of the vasculature of the graft may occur. The gradual attack may be characterized, in the case of the glomerulus, by typical glomerular lesions, including proliferative changes in the glomerular tuft, hyalinization of the glomeruli, and eventual obliteration of the glomerular tuft. The clinical sequence of events accompanying these changes may mimic, in every way, those seen in naturally occurring glomerulonephritis, including the nephrotic syndrome.

Similarly, over a period of years, changes in other renal vessels, including the small arteries, may cause scarring and replacement of the intima, disruption of the elastica, and narrowing or even obliteration of the lumen of the vessel. The net result is nephrosclerosis, hypertension, and, eventually, ischemic changes in the glomeruli, leading to functional failure.

In Plate 14, the diagram of an electron photomicrograph illustrates the early changes and the sequence of events. Note the polymorphonuclear leukocyte with a pseudopod projecting under the endothelium of the basement membrane. The basement membrane itself is uncovered. This denuding of the basement membrane stimulates platelet deposition, and platelet thrombi can be seen on the vessel wall. There is apparent deposition of fibrin, with the typical fibrin-strand forms. Subsequent changes in the glomerulus consist of fusion of the foot process, the

Kidney Transplantation

Continued

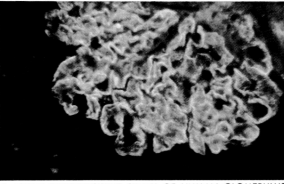

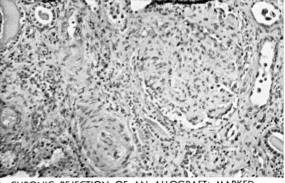

A: IMMUNOFLUORESCENT STUDY OF HUMAN GLOMERULUS IN CHRONIC REJECTION OF AN ALLOGRAFT: LINEAR DEPOSIT OF GAMMA GLOBULIN ON BASEMENT MEMBRANE

B: CHRONIC REJECTION OF AN ALLOGRAFT: MARKED MEMBRANOUS INVOLVEMENT OF A GLOMERULUS

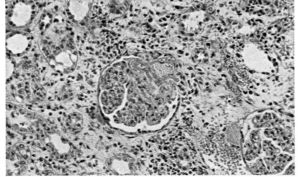

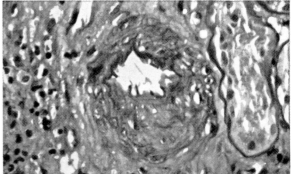

C: HYPERACUTE REJECTION: THROMBOSIS OF AFFERENT ARTERIOLE OF GLOMERULUS WITH INTERSTITIAL EDEMA AND HEMORRHAGE

D: CHANGES IN A SMALL RENAL ARTERY 2½ YEARS AFTER TRANSPLANTATION: DISRUPTION OF ELASTICA AND THICKENING OF INTIMA BY PAS—STAINING MATERIAL

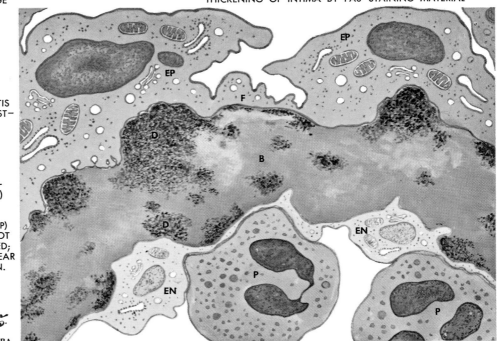

E: DIAGRAM OF ELECTRON PHOTO-MICROGRAPHIC FINDINGS IN GLOMERULUS IN RECURRENT GLOMERULONEPHRITIS MANY MONTHS POST-TRANSPLAN-TATION IN AN ISOGRAFT: BASEMENT MEM-BRANE (B) THICK-ENED AND DIS-RUPTED; ELECTRON-DENSE DEPOSITS (D) WITHIN BASEMENT MEMBRANE; EPITHELIAL CELLS (EP) SWOLLEN AND FOOT PROCESSES (F) FUSED; POLYMORPHONUCLEAR CELLS (P) IN LUMEN. EN=ENDOTHELIAL CELL

deposition of electron-dense deposits in the basement membrane, and eventual destruction of the glomerulus by fibrous tissue.

Rejection in Identical Twins. A striking and tragic early discovery in transplantation was the recurrence of glomerulonephritis in kidney grafts between identical twins. Since identical twins contain identical tissue antigens, no rejection process should occur. However, it is apparent that the immune process which originally caused the glomerular lesion may remain active and facilitate development of new glomerular lesions in the glomerular isograft. Plate 15 shows a photomicrograph of the glomerular changes which occurred in an identical twin recipient. Of 24 identical twin recipients studied, half developed glomerulonephritis. In all these recipients, glomerulonephritis was the original disease which necessitated nephrectomy and transplant. However, glomerular lesion did not occur after transplantation in five patients who had no history of glomerulonephritis.

Trends for the Future. Control of the rejection response lies in the knowledge of the immune process which has already been outlined. It may be possible, for instance, to interfere with the antigen-antibody reaction after antigen and antibody have combined but before the polymorphonuclear leukocytes have been mobilized and cause destruction.

It has already been shown that in experimental nephritis, cyclophosphamide, which destroys polymorphonuclear leukocytes, may prevent the lesion in spite of antigen-antibody combination. The recent use of antilymphocyte globulin (ALG) also shows promise. ALG is produced by using human lymphocytes to immunize a horse; the resulting horse serum, which contains antibodies against human lymphocytes, may be injected into humans. In this way, it is believed that circulating lymphocytes, capable of producing antibody, are destroyed, and that the antibody reaction is modified. Animals treated with preparations of ALG show marked depletion of lymphocytes in lymph nodes and spleen and decreased cellular infiltration of the allograft.

Of greatest promise, perhaps, is the technic of presurgical injection of donor antigen in the prospective recipient. In the animal, at least, this injection, usually made in subcellular fractions, and the use of immunosuppressive agents combine to produce tolerance to the donor kidney. Furthermore, the antibody itself need not be harmful. In fact, the presence of antibody seems to encourage allograft growth. Thus, carefully selected antibody, administered in correct dosage, and perhaps combined with small amounts of antigen, may coat the wall of the graft or the surface of the lymphocyte and so cover or block the antigen against the action of specific antibody. Thus, it might well be that immunofluorescent globulin could be made to block the action of a more effective and destructive antibody.

Although these methods of dealing with rejection have not yet been proved in the human, they are of unquestioned validity in the experimental animal. Were the described technics to become established therapeutic procedures in the human, the use of large doses of toxic immunosuppressive agents might be eliminated. Then the recipient could retain the graft and still reject infective microorganisms, which so often cause death in human kidney transplants. □

Renal Revascularization

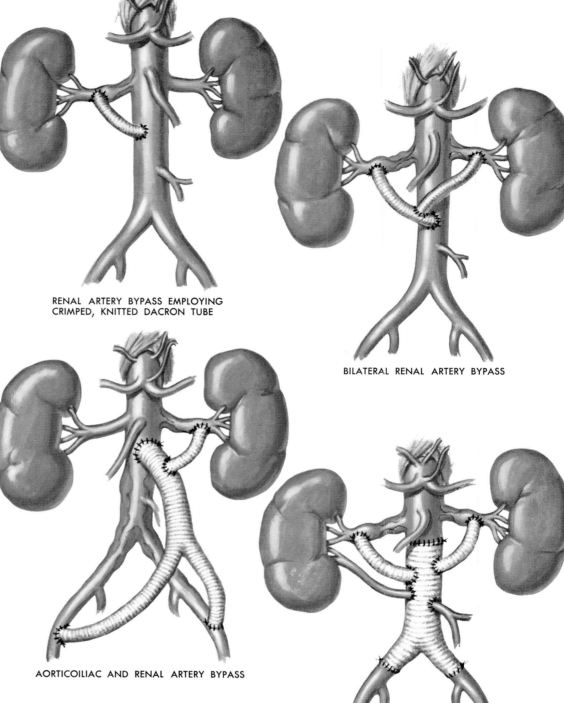

RENAL ARTERY BYPASS EMPLOYING
CRIMPED, KNITTED DACRON TUBE

BILATERAL RENAL ARTERY BYPASS

AORTICOILIAC AND RENAL ARTERY BYPASS

AORTIC GRAFT REPLACEMENT WITH BILATERAL
RENAL ARTERY BYPASS AND PRESERVATION OF
AN ACCESSORY RENAL ARTERY

Renovascular hypertension resulting from narrowing of one or both renal arteries is usually secondary to atherosclerosis. Among less common causes are fibromuscular hyperplasia, renal artery aneurysm, kinks, bands, congenital or developmental defects, traumatic deformities, and inflammatory lesions. The hypertension is often amenable to cure by a wide variety of surgical technics (also see pages 85, 86, and 156).

The first criterion in the selection of patients for operation is the existence of diastolic hypertension. On the excretory pyelogram, a delayed excretion from one kidney and a discrepancy of more than 2 cm in size between the two kidneys are suggestive of renovascular disease. Because of the high incidence of false-positive results, abnormal findings on renography have limited diagnostic value.

More specialized diagnostic tests are required to define precisely the cause of the hypertension. These tests include translumbar aortography if renovascular hypertension is suspected (see page 101). specific hormonal assays if an endocrine cause is suspected, percutaneous renal biopsy (see page 107) if bilateral primary renal disease is suspected but not established, and retrograde urography if obstruction or unilateral renal disease is suspected (see page 96). During surgery, the pressures in the aorta and distal renal artery should be measured simultaneously to confirm the physiologic significance of renal arterial disease.

The presence of cerebrovascular disease, coronary artery disease, and advanced age contraindicate surgical treatment.

The principal objective in the surgical treatment of renal hypertension resulting from an occlusive lesion of a renal artery is the restoration of normal pulsatile blood flow to the renal arterial bed. The restoration may be achieved by any of several basic surgical methods, and the choice depends on the nature and extent of the occlusive processes in the artery. These methods include the bypass graft and endarterectomy, with or without patch-graft angioplasty.

Technical Procedures. The *bypass graft procedure* has been found, in our experience, to be the most commonly used. The procedure lends itself to the most frequently encountered patterns of occlusive disease, and the technic is relatively simple. As illustrated, it may be used in a variety of ways.

The following technic is used for *unilateral lesions*

of the renal arteries. After the abdominal aorta and renal arteries have been exposed, a partial occluding clamp is applied to the anterior lateral aspect of the abdominal aorta about 4 to 5 cm below the origin of the renal artery. A longitudinal incision is made in the occluded portion of the aorta, and a 5- or 6-mm knitted *DeBakey Dacron®* graft is attached to this opening by end-to-side anastomosis. Occluding clamps are then applied to the renal artery just distal to the occlusive lesion, and a longitudinal incision is made in the renal artery. The Dacron graft is then tailored to fit this opening in the renal artery and is attached to the opening by an end-to-side anastomosis. Just before this anastomosis is closed, but after the procedure is otherwise completed, the occluding clamps are *temporarily* released to permit flushing of the artery and the graft; this removes any clots. The closing suture on the anastomosis is then completed, and all the

Renal Revascularization

Continued

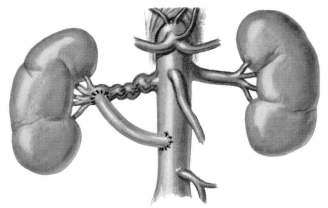

BYPASS TO DISTAL EXTREMITY OF RENAL ARTERY BEYOND EXTENSIVE FIBROMUSCULAR HYPERPLASIA, EMPLOYING SEGMENT OF SAPHENOUS VEIN

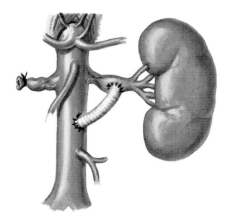

RENAL ARTERY BYPASS PLUS CONTRALATERAL NEPHRECTOMY

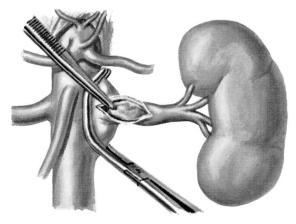

ENDARTERECTOMY

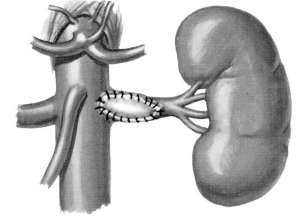

PATCH GRAFT WITH OR WITHOUT ENDARTERECTOMY

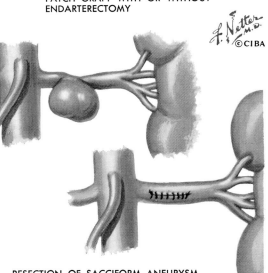

RENAL ARTERY BYPASS PLUS PATCH GRAFT TO ACCESSORY RENAL ARTERY

RESECTION OF SACCIFORM ANEURYSM OF RENAL ARTERY AND PRIMARY REPAIR

occlusive clamps are removed so that blood flows into the renal artery.

In patients with *bilateral lesions,* the bypass graft may be used on each side, as for patients with unilateral lesions. However, the graft on one side may be attached to the graft which extends from the aorta to the other renal artery, as shown.

If patients also have arterial insufficiency to the lower limbs because of aorticoiliac occlusive disease, treatment may be directed toward both the renal artery and aorticoiliac lesions. An end-to-side anastomosis of a *DeBakey knitted bifurcation graft* from the abdominal aorta to the external iliac artery or to the femoral arteries will bypass the aorticoiliac obstruction. A second graft is then anastomosed end-to-side to the bifurcation graft, and end-to-side to the renal artery.

In the presence of an associated aneurysm of the abdominal aorta, the aneurysm may need to be resected and replaced with a Dacron graft. The renal arteries may be revascularized by bypass grafts *to both renal arteries,* as shown in the illustration. Should the occasion arise, an *accessory renal artery* may also be attached by end-to-side anastomosis to an opening in the Dacron graft.

In the treatment of *fibromuscular hyperplasia,* the bypass graft is also particularly useful. Usually, in this type of occlusive disease, the lesions extend throughout most of the renal artery. However, the renal artery is generally relatively normal at the origin of its major branches. Accordingly, after the graft has

been anastomosed to the abdominal aorta, the distal end of the graft should be attached to an opening in the renal artery near or at the origin of its major branches. In relatively young patients, it has been found desirable to use a segment of autogenous saphenous vein for this purpose, as shown.

If a patient has bilateral vascular disease and virtual destruction of one kidney with no possibility of restoration of its blood supply, unilateral nephrectomy and the application of a bypass graft to the other side, as depicted, may be necessary.

Endarterectomy is indicated in patients who have localized lesions that are often found at the origin of the renal artery or in its proximal segment. In this procedure, a partial occluding clamp is applied to the abdominal aorta at the origin of the renal artery. A longitudinal incision is then made in the renal artery and extended across the origin of the artery into the

abdominal aorta. Next, a cleavage plane is forced between the occlusive lesion and the outer medial-adventitial layer of the artery. Care must be taken to prevent dissection of the media distally. After completion of the endarterectomy, the incision in the artery may be closed by simple continuous sutures or, preferably, by a partial graft which prevents constriction of the lumen. Under some circumstances, particularly if the occlusive lesion is smooth and firm and is confined to only a small portion of the circumference of the artery, it may be possible to perform simple *patch-graft* angioplasty without endarterectomy.

Sacciform aneurysms of the renal artery sometimes produce partial obstruction in blood flow, as a result of distal kinking of the artery. These lesions, which usually have a relatively narrow neck, can be excised and repaired by simple suture or, if necessary, by use of patch-graft angioplasty. □

Nephrectomy

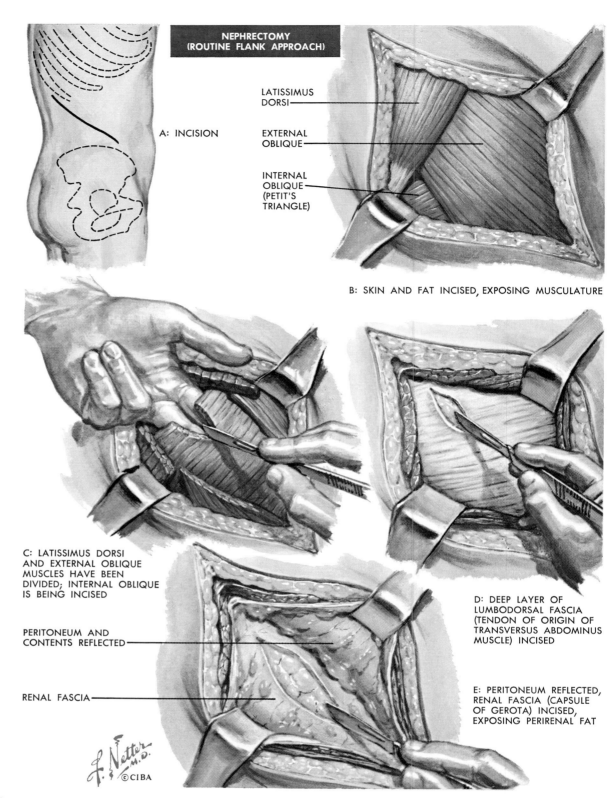

NEPHRECTOMY
(ROUTINE FLANK APPROACH)

A: INCISION

LATISSIMUS DORSI

EXTERNAL OBLIQUE

INTERNAL OBLIQUE (PETIT'S TRIANGLE)

B: SKIN AND FAT INCISED, EXPOSING MUSCULATURE

C: LATISSIMUS DORSI AND EXTERNAL OBLIQUE MUSCLES HAVE BEEN DIVIDED; INTERNAL OBLIQUE IS BEING INCISED

PERITONEUM AND CONTENTS REFLECTED

RENAL FASCIA

D: DEEP LAYER OF LUMBODORSAL FASCIA (TENDON OF ORIGIN OF TRANSVERSUS ABDOMINUS MUSCLE) INCISED

E: PERITONEUM REFLECTED, RENAL FASCIA (CAPSULE OF GEROTA) INCISED, EXPOSING PERIRENAL FAT

Although the first nephrectomy apparently was performed by Erastus Bradley Wolcott, an American surgeon, the method was perfected and popularized by Gustav Simon, Professor of Surgery at the University of Heidelberg. Less than 100 years ago, Simon wrote an impressive monograph on renal surgery, including his work on nephrectomy. Simon's success with the technic encouraged numerous other clinicians to perform nephrectomies, so that by the early 1900s Schmieben was able to collect reports of over 1,000 such procedures.

The indications for *unilateral nephrectomy* are now fewer because of the introduction of antibiotics and the development of other surgical technics. However, the procedure is still important and at times imperative. Patients with renal ma-

lignancies and, in some instances, patients with hypertension, renal infection, hydronephrosis, or renal calculi are candidates for nephrectomy. Of course, unilateral nephrectomies continue to be performed to obtain donor organs for transplants (see pages 264-267).

Bilateral nephrectomy is now being performed in certain patients with chronic renal failure who are under consideration for transplantation or chronic dialysis. The primary indication for bilateral nephrectomy in the chronic dialysis patient has been severe diastolic hypertension which cannot be normalized by volume regulation and which is associated with elevated circulating renin levels. In the patient who has received kidney transplants, bilateral nephrectomy has been most frequently performed when intractable renal infection appears to be a contraindication to immunosuppressive therapy. The surgical approach in

such cases is a matter of choice. The bilateral flank incision is preferred in some instances, while a transperitoneal approach is used in others.

Regardless of the indications, before unilateral nephrectomy is performed, the presence of an adequately functioning, contralateral kidney must be determined. While intravenous urography is useful in assessing morphologic aspects of the excretory system, it is not always an accurate index of renal function. The simplest, most accurate method of assessing renal function is by rapid scintillation scanning or renography, utilizing ^{131}I-labeled iodohippurate. In patients with intraabdominal trauma who require emergency surgical procedures, one should evaluate the functional status of both kidneys whenever feasible, thereby facilitating a proper decision concerning the advisability of unilateral nephrectomy in case of renal injury (see pages 213-214).

Nephrectomy
Continued

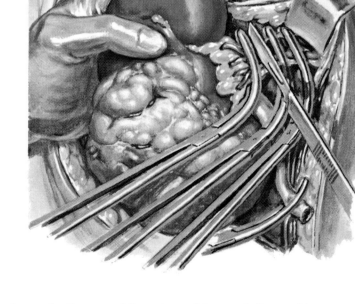

F: KIDNEY DELIVERED INTO WOUND

G: URETER ISOLATED, DOUBLY CLAMPED, DIVIDED, AND LIGATED

H: VASCULAR PEDICLE CLAMPED, DIVIDED, AND LIGATED; WOUND CLOSED IN LAYERS

The decision to perform a unilateral nephrectomy must be based on the reasonable certainty that a more conservative approach would be futile. Important considerations are the functional status of the other kidney, the age of the patient, and the surgical risk involved. While it is obvious that any normal renal parenchyma should be preserved whenever possible, it must be recognized that infection in one kidney may carry the risk of subsequent involvement of the other kidney. Particularly in older patients, attempts to preserve a diseased kidney via conservative surgery often increases morbidity and may entail more risk than nephrectomy.

The surgical approach depends on the patient's age and the nature of the renal disease. Although nephrectomy is often a simple procedure, it can be extremely complicated. Because the routine flank approach does not necessitate entering the peritoneal cavity, this exposure is probably the most widely employed and is definitely preferred when infection is present. This procedure can also be modified in many ways to gain better access to the upper portion of the kidney.

The flank approach, however, has severe limitations when nephrectomy is performed because of renal cancer, since considerable manipulation of the kidney is inevitable before the renal pedicle can be clamped. Moreover, in older patients, particularly those with decreased vital capacity, the flank position often leads to hypotension, thereby increasing the chances of cardiac or cerebral ischemia.

In patients with renovascular hypertension, the flank approach is not advisable because the choice between a nephrectomy or a renal artery repair often cannot be made until surgical exposure is complete. Also, in patients who have had spinal fusion or who have vertebral column deformities, this exposure cannot be used because of the required positioning.

An alternate procedure is the *anterior approach.* If necessary, a thoracoabdominal incision can be made as, for instance, when large tumors are present, particularly in the upper pole, or when exploration of the vena cava is required because of a tumor extending from the renal vein. In older patients who do not tolerate the flank position and in other patients in whom a retroperitoneal approach is desirable, an incision can be made through the rectus muscle. The peritoneum then can be carefully swept toward the midline thus permitting nephrectomy without the necessity of entering the peritoneal cavity. □

Glossary

allograft — literally a graft which has been reversed; refers to the usual method in renal transplantation of placing a left donor kidney in the right iliac fossa; the anterior surface of the donor kidney thus comes to lie posteriorly in the recipient

B₁C — beta-1 component of complement

carbamate reaction — the reversible reaction in which CO_2 is combined directly with the amino groups of HHb or other proteins; the reaction involving HHb is more important than that involving protein because it is also associated with the transport and exchange of oxygen

DPN — diphosphopyridine nucleotide; now called nicotinamide adenine dinucleotide (NAD)

DPNH — diphosphopyridine nucleotide, reduced; now called nicotinamide adenine dinucleotide, reduced (NADH)

e — the natural logarithm which has a numerical value of 2.7

enzymes — the following enzymes have been mentioned in this volume (Enzyme Catalogue Reference Number in parentheses):
AP: alkaline phosphatase (E.C. 3.1.3.1)
CA: carbonic anhydrase (E.C. 4.2.1.1)
G-6-PDH: glucose-6-phosphate dehydrogenase (E.C. 1.1.1.49)
GLDH: glutamate dehydrogenase (E.C. 1.4.1.2)
GOT: glutamate oxaloacetate transaminase (aspartate aminotransferase) (E.C. 2.6.1.1)
GPT: glutamate pyruvate transaminase (alanine aminotransferase) (E.C. 2.6.1.2)
ICDH: isocitrate dehydrogenase (E.C. 1.1.1.42)
LAP: leucine aminopeptidase (E.C. 3.4.1.1)
LDH: lactate dehydrogenase (E.C. 1.1.1.27)
MDH: maleate dehydrogenase (E.C. 1.1.1.37)

HHb — nonionized hemoglobin; also used to indicate that hemoglobin acts as an acid

IgE — immune globulin E (gamma E globulin)

IgG — immune globulin G (gamma G globulin)

IgM — immune globulin M (gamma M globulin)

insudate — from *in*, in + *sudare*, to sweat, literally sweating inward; used to refer to the passage of material into vessel walls

insudation — the act of insudating; from the verb *insudate (qv)*

IU — international units

JG — juxtaglomerular

LA — leucinamide

L-forms — forms of bacteria often produced in cultures if the normal formation of the bacterial cell wall is partially or completely inhibited; may occur as a result of the action of certain agents such as penicillin; if the bacteria have partial cell walls, they are called spheroplasts; if they have no cell walls, they are designated protoplasts

LPNA — leucine-p-nitroanilide

NAD — nicotinamide adenine dinucleotide

NADH — nicotinamide adenine dinucleotide, reduced

NZB mice — New Zealand Black mice

PAMS — periodic acid–methenamine silver stain

Currently Known Dialyzable Substances

Alcohols

Ethanol*
Ethylene glycol
Isopropanol
Methanol*

Analgesics

Acetophenetidin
Acetylsalicylic acid*
Dextropropoxyphene
Methylsalicylate*
Paracetamol

Antidepressants

Amphetamine
Isocarboxazid
Methamphetamine
Monomine oxidase inhibitors
Pargyline
Phenelzine
Tranylcypromine
Tricyclic secondary amines
Tricyclic tertiary amines

Antimicrobials

Ampicillin
Bacitracin
Carbenicillin
Cephalosporins
Chloramphenicol
Cycloserine
Isoniazid
Kanamycin
Neomycin
Nitrofurantoin
Penicillin
Polymyxin
Quinine
Streptomycin
Sulfonamides
Tetracycline
Vancomycin

Barbiturates*

Amobarbital
Barbital
Butabarbital
Butalbital
Cyclobarbital
Pentobarbital
Phenobarbital
Secobarbital

Depressants, Sedatives, and Tranquilizers

Chloral hydrate
Diphenhydramine
Diphenylhydantoin
Ethchlorvynol*
Ethinamate
Gallamine triethiodide
Glutethimide*
Heroin
Meprobamate
Methaqualone
Methyprylon
Paraldehyde
Primidone

Halides

Bromide*
Chloride*
Fluoride
Iodide

Metals

Arsenic
Calcium
Copper
Iron
Lead
Lithium
Magnesium
Mercury
Potassium
Sodium
Strontium
Zinc

Miscellaneous Substances

Amanita phalloides
Aniline
Boric acid
Camphor
Carbon monoxide
Carbon tetrachloride
Chlorpropamide
Chromic acid
Cyclophosphamide
Digoxin
Dinitro-ortho-cresol
Ergotamine
Eucalyptus oil
5-Fluorouracil
Mannitol
Methotrexate
Potassium chlorate
Potassium dichromate
Sodium chlorate
Sodium citrate
Thiocyanate*
Thiol
Trichlorethylene

*Kinetics of dialysis thoroughly studied and/or clinical experience extensive

Based upon Schreiner, GE and Teehan, BP: Dialysis of poisons and drugs—annual review, Trans. Amer. Soc. Artif. Intern. Organs 17:513, 1973
(For complete details and supporting data the reader is advised to consult the original reference.)

Selected References

Section I

General References

ALLEN, AC: *The Kidney, Medical and Surgical Diseases,* Grune & Stratton, Inc., New York, 1951

GOSS, CM, Editor: *Gray's Anatomy of the Human Body,* Lea & Febiger, Philadelphia, 1966

International Anatomical Nomenclature Committee: *Nomina Anatomica,* 3rd ed., Excerpta Medica Foundation, Amsterdam, 1968

KRIZ, W: *Der architektonische und funktionelle Aufbau der Rattenniere,* Z. Zellforsch. 82:495, 1967

OLIVER, J: *Nephrons and Kidneys,* Hoeber Medical Division, Harper and Row, New York, 1968

RHODIN, JAG: *Structure of the kidney* in *Diseases of the Kidney* ed. by Strauss, MB and Welt, LG, Little, Brown and Company, Boston, 1963

ROMANES, GJ, Editor: *Cunningham's Textbook of Anatomy,* 10th ed., Oxford University Press, London, 1964

SMITH, HW: *The Kidney, Structure and Functions in Health and Disease,* Oxford University Press, Inc., New York, 1951

SPERBER, I: *Studies on the mammalian kidney,* Zool. Bidrag. Uppsala, 22:249, 1944

	Plate
ABDEL-MALEK, ET: *Early development of the urinogenital system in the chick,* J. Morph. 86:599, 1950	28
ADACHI, B: *Das Arteriensystem der Japaner,* Vol. 2, Maruzen Co., Kyoto, 1928	14, 16
ADACHI, B: *Das Venensystem der Japaner,* Vol. 2, Kenkyusha, Tokyo, 1940	16
ANSON, BJ: *An Atlas of Human Anatomy,* W. B. Saunders Company, Philadelphia, 1963	14, 16
AREY, LB: *Developmental Anatomy: A Textbook and Laboratory Manual of Embryology,* 7th ed., W. B. Saunders Company, Philadelphia, 1965	33
BABICS, A AND RENYI-VAMOS, F: *Das Lymphgefässsystem der Niere und seine Bedeutung in der Nierenpathologie und Chirurgie,* Verlag der Ungarischen Akademie der Wissenschaften, Budapest, 1957	24
BARAJAS, L AND LATTA, H: *A three-dimensional study of the juxtaglomerular apparatus in the rat. Light and electron microscopic observations,* Lab. Invest. 12:257, 1963	6
BEGG, RC: *The urachus; its anatomy, histology and development,* J. Anat. 64:170, 1930	32
BERGLAS, B AND RUBIN, IC: *Histologic study of the pelvic connective tissue,* Surg. Gynec. Obstet. 97:277, 1953	19-20
BLOOM, W AND FAWCETT, DW: *A Textbook of Histology,* 9th ed., W. B. Saunders Company, Philadelphia, 1968	5, 15, 22
BRAITHWAITE, JL: *The arterial supply of the male urinary bladder,* Brit. J. Urol. 24:64, 1952	23
BULGER, RE et al: *Human renal ultrastructure. II. The thin limb of Henle's loop and the interstitium in healthy individuals,* Lab. Invest. 16:124, 1967	11
CAMERON, G AND CHAMBERS, R: *Direct evidence of function in kidney of an early human fetus,* Amer. J. Physiol. 123:482, 1938	29
DARNTON, SJ: *A possible correlation between ultrastructure and function in the thin descending and ascending limbs of the loop of Henle of rabbit kidney,* Z. Zellforsch. 93:516, 1969	11
DIETERICH, HJ: *Die Ultrastruktur der Gefässbündel im Mark der Rattenniere,* Z. Zellforsch. 84:350, 1968	11
FARQUHAR, MG AND PALADE, GE: *Functional evidence for the existence of a third cell type in the renal glomerulus,* J. Cell Biol. 13:55, 1962	6
FISHEL, A: *Entwicklung des Menschen,* Springer-Verlag, Berlin, 1929	28
FRASER, EA: *The development of the vertebrate excretory system,* Biol. Rev. 25:159, 1950	29
GERSH, I: *The correlation of structure and function in the developing mesonephros and metanephros,* Contr. Embryol. Carneg. Instn. 26:33, 1937	29
GLENISTER, TW: *The development of the penile urethra in the pig,* J. Anat. 90:461, 1956	32
GRIFFITH, LD, BULGER, RE, AND TRUMP, BF: *The ultrastructure of the functioning kidney,* Lab. Invest. 16:220, 1967	9
GRUENWALD, P: *The normal changes in the position of the embryonic kidney,* Anat. Rec. 85:163, 1943	31
GYLLENSTEEN, L: *Contributions to the embryology of the urinary bladder: the development of the definitive relations between the openings of the Wolffian ducts and the ureters,* Acta Anat. 7:305, 1949	32
HOLLINSHEAD, WH: *Anatomy for Surgeons,* Vol. 2, Hoeber Medical Division, Harper and Row, New York, 1956	3, 14-16, 19-20, 23
HUNTER, RH: *Observations on the development of the human genital tract,* Contr. Embryol. Carneg. Instn. 22:91, 1930	32
JOHNSON, FR AND DARNTON, SJ: *Ultrastructural observations on the renal papilla of the rabbit,* Z. Zellforsch. 81:390, 1967	13
JOKELAINEN, P: *An electron microscope study of the early development of the rat metanephric nephron,* Acta Anat. 52 (Suppl. 47), 1963	31
LANGMAN, J: *Medical Embryology,* 2nd ed., The Williams and Wilkins Company, Baltimore, 1963	29
LATTA, H, MAUNSBACH, AB, AND MADDEN, SC: *The centrolobular region of the renal glomerulus studied by electron microscopy,* J. Ultrastruct. Res. 4:455, 1960	6
LJUNGQVIST, A AND LAGERGREN, C: *Normal intrarenal arterial pattern in adult and ageing human kidney. A microangiographical and histological study,* J. Anat. 96:285, 1962	18
MACCALLUM, DB: *Arterial blood supply of mammalian kidney,* Amer. J. Anat. 38:153, 1926	18
MICHAELS, JP: *Study of ureteral blood supply and its bearing on necrosis of the ureter following the Wertheim operation,* Surg. Gynec. Obstet. 86:36, 1948	23
MILLER, F: *Hemoglobin absorption by the cells of the proximal convoluted tubule in mouse kidney,* J. Biophys. Biochem. Cytol. 8:689, 1960	9
MITCHELL, GAG: *Anatomy of the Autonomic Nervous System,* E. & S. Livingstone Ltd., Edinburgh, 1953	25-27
MITCHELL, GAG: *Cardiovascular Innervation,* The Williams and Wilkins Company, Baltimore; E. & S. Livingstone Ltd., Edinburgh, 1956	25-27
MOELLENDORFF, WV: *Handbuch der Mikroskopischen Anatomie des Menschen,* Vol. VII/1, Springer-Verlag, Berlin, 1930	22
MOFFAT, DB: *The fine structure of the blood vessels of the renal medulla with particular reference to the control of the medullary circulation,* J. Ultrastruct. Res. 19:532, 1967	17
MUELLER, CB: *The structure of the renal glomerulus,* Amer. Heart J. 55:304, 1958	6
OSVALDO, L: *Interstitial cells of renal medulla,* J. Ultrastruct. Res. 15:589, 1966	13
OSVALDO, L AND LATTA, H: *The thin limbs of the loop of Henle,* J. Ultrastruct. Res. 15:144, 1966	11
PATTEN, BM: *Human Embryology,* 2nd ed., Blakiston Co., New York, 1953	30
PATTEN, BM: *Human Embryology,* 3rd ed., Blakiston Division, McGraw-Hill Inc., New York, 1968	33
PEASE, DC: *Electron microscopy of tubular cells of the kidney cortex,* Anat. Rec. 121:723, 1955	9
PEIRCE, EC: *Renal lymphatics,* Anat. Rec. 90:315, 1944	24
PICK, JW AND ANSON, BJ: *Renal vascular pedicle; an anatomical study of 430 body-halves,* J. Urol. 44:411, 1940	14-15
POTTER, EL: *Development of the human glomerulus,* Arch. Path. 80:241, 1965	31
RAWSON, AJ: *Distribution of the lymphatics of the human kidney as shown in a case of carcinomatous permeation,* Arch. Path. 47:283, 1949	24
RHODIN, JAG: *Correlation of ultrastructural organization and function in normal and experimentally changed proximal convoluted tubule cells of the mouse kidney,* Thesis, Karolinska Institutet, Stockholm, 1954	9
RHODIN, JAG: *Anatomy of kidney tubules,* Int. Rev. Cytol. 7:485, 1958	9
RHODIN, JAG: *Electron microscopy of the kidney,* Amer. J. Med. 24:661, 1958	12

Continued on page 276

ROJO-ORTEGA, JM, HATT, PY, AND GENEST, J: *A propos de l'innervation des cellules juxtaglo-mérulaires. Etude au microscope électronique dans diverses conditions expérimentales chez le rat,* Path. Biol. 16:497, 1968 — 6

ROLLHÄUSER, H, KRIZ, W, AND HEINKE, W: *Das Gefäss-system der Rattenniere,* Z. Zellforsch. 64:381, 1964 — 17

SAKAGUCHI, H AND SUZUKI, Y: *Fine structure of renal tubule cells,* Keio J. Med. 7:17, 1958 — 11

SUZUKI, Y: *An electron microscopy of renal differentiation; II. Glomerulus,* Keio J. Med. 8:129, 1959 — 30

THORBURN, GD et al: *Intrarenal distribution of nutrient blood flow determined with krypton*[85] *in the unanesthetized dog,* Circ. Res. 13:290, 1963 — 17

TOBIN, CE: *The renal fascia and its relation to the transversalis fascia,* Anat. Rec. 89:295, 1944 — 3

TOBIN, CE AND BENJAMIN, JA: *Anatomical and surgical restudy of Denonvilliers' fascia,* Surg. Gynec. Obstet. 80:373, 1945 — 16

TORREY, TW: *Development of the urogenital system of the albino rat. I. The kidney and its ducts,* Amer. J. Anat. 72:133, 1943 — 28

TRUETA, J et al: *Studies of the Renal Circulation,* Blackwell, Oxford, 1947 — 17

WAUGH, D, PRENTICE, RS, AND YADAV, D: *The structure of the proximal tubule: a morphological study of basement membrane cristae and their relationships in the renal tubule of the rat,* Amer. J. Anat. 121:775, 1967 — 9

WEYRAUCH, HM, Jr: *Anomalies of renal rotation,* Surg. Gynec. Obstet. 69:183, 1939 — 33

YAMADE, E: *The fine structure of the renal glomerulus of the mouse,* J. Biophys. Biochem. Cytol. 1:551, 1955 — 6

YOUNG, D AND WISSIG, SL: *A histologic description of certain epithelial and vascular structures in the kidney of the normal rat,* Amer. J. Anat. 115:43, 1946 — 12

ZAMBONI, L AND DE MARTINO, C: *Embryogenesis of the human renal glomerulus,* Arch. Path. 86:279, 1968 — 31

ZIMMERMANN, KW: *Ueber den Bau des Glomerulus der menschlichen Niere,* Z. Mikr. Anat. Forsch. 18:520, 1929 — 6

ZIMMERMANN, KW: *Ueber den Bau des Glomerulus der menschlichen Niere,* Z. Mikr. Anat. Forsch. 32:176, 1933 — 30

Section II

BERLINER, RW: *Renal mechanisms for potassium excretion,* Harvey Lect. 55:141, 1961 — 8–12

BLACK, DAK, Editor: *Renal Disease,* 2nd ed., F. A. Davis Co., Philadelphia, 1967 — 1–7

GIEBISCH, G: *Functional organization of proximal and distal tubular electrolyte transport,* Nephron 6:260, 1969 — 8–12

GIEBISCH, G: *Renal potassium excretion* in *The Kidney: Morphology, Biochemistry, Physiology,* Vol. 3, ed. by Rouiller, C and Muller, AF, Academic Press, Inc., New York, 1971 — 8–12

GIEBISCH, G AND WINDHAGER, EE: *Renal tubular transfer of sodium, chloride and potassium,* Amer. J. Med. 36:643, 1964 — 8–12

GLICK, D: *Quantitative Chemical Techniques of Histo- and Cytochemistry,* Wiley-Interscience, Inc., New York, 1962 and 1963 — 23–24

GORDON, AS, Editor: *Regulation of Hematopoiesis,* Vol. 1, Appleton-Century-Crofts, Inc., New York, 1970 — 22

GORDON, AS, COOPER, GW, AND ZANJANI, ED: *The kidney and erythropoiesis,* Seminars Hemat. 4:337, 1967 — 22

GOTTSCHALK, CW: *Renal tubular function: lessons from micropuncture,* Harvey Lect. 58:99, 1963 — 8–12

GREGOIRE, F AND GEPTS, W: *Qualitative and quantitative histoenzymology of long surviving human renal homotransplants,* Nephron, 7:203, 1970 — 23–24

HEALY, JK AND GRAEME, ER: *Clinical assessment of glomerular filtration rate by different forms of creatinine clearance and a modified*

urinary phenolsulphonphthalein excretion test, Amer. J. Med. 44:348, 1968 — 1–7

MALNIC, G, KLOSE, RM, AND GIEBISCH, G: *Micropuncture study of renal potassium excretion in the rat,* Amer. J. Physiol. 206:674, 1964 — 8–12

MATTENHEIMER, H: *Clinical Enzymology, Principles and Applications,* Ann Arbor-Humphrey Science Publishers, Ann Arbor, 1970 — 23–24

MATTENHEIMER, H: *Enzymology of kidney tissue* in *Enzymes in Urine and Kidney* ed. by Dubach, UC, Huber, Berne, 1968 — 23–24

MATTENHEIMER, H: *Micromethods for the Clinical and Biochemical Laboratory,* Ann Arbor-Humphrey Science Publishers, Ann Arbor, 1970 — 23–24

MOUNTCASTEL, VB, Editor: *Medical Physiology,* 12th ed., C. V. Mosby Company, St. Louis, 1968 — 18–21

MÜLLER-BEISSENHIRTZ, P et al: *Early structural and metabolic changes during rejection in untreated homologous kidney transplants in the cat,* Abstract, XVth Congress, International Society of Urology, Tokyo, 1970 — 23–24

PAPPENHEIMER, JR: *Passage of molecules through capillary walls,* Physiol. Rev. 33:387, 1953 — 1–7

PITTS, RF: *Physiology of the Kidney and Body Fluids,* Year Book Medical Publishers, Inc., Chicago, 1963 — 1–7

PITTS, RF: *Physiology of the Kidney and Body Fluids,* 2nd ed., Year Book Medical Publishers, Inc., Chicago, 1968 — 8–12, 18–21, 23–24

RECTOR, FC: *Renal secretion of hydrogen* in *The Kidney: Morphology, Biochemistry, Physiology,* Vol. 3, ed. by Rouiller, C and Muller, AF, Academic Press, Inc., New York, 1971 — 18–21

RECTOR, FC: *Role of the kidney in the homeostatic control of hydrogen ion concentration in body fluids* in *Proceedings of the XXIII International Congress of Physiological Science,* Tokyo, Excerpta Medica International Congress Series No. 87, 1965 — 18–21

SMITH, HW: *Principles of Renal Physiology,* Oxford University Press, Inc., New York, 1956 — 1–7

STRAUSS, MB AND WELT, LG, Editors: *Diseases of the Kidney,* Little, Brown and Company, Boston, 1971 — 1–7

THURAU, K: *Renal hemodynamics,* Amer. J. Med. 36:698, 1964 — 1–7

VANDER, AJ: *Control of renin release,* Physiol. Rev. 47:359, 1967 — 8–12

VIEIRA, FL AND MALNIC, G: *Hydrogen ion secretion by rat renal cortical tubules as studied by an antimony microelectrode,* Amer. J. Physiol. 214:710, 1968 — 18–21

WHITTEMBURY, G AND PROVERBIO, F: *Two modes of Na extrusion in cells from guinea-pig cortex slices,* Pflueger Arch. 316:1, 1970 — 8–12

WINDHAGER, EE, LEWY, JE, AND SPITZER, A: *Intrarenal control of proximal tubular reabsorption of sodium and water,* Nephron 6:247, 1969 — 8–12

Section III

ABRAMS, H: *Angiography,* Little, Brown and Company, Boston, 1961 — 18–23

AXELROD, DR: *Phenolsulfonphthalein excretion for estimating residual urine,* Arch. Intern. Med. 117:74, 1966 — 13

BAILEY, RR AND LITTLE, PJ: *Suprapubic bladder aspiration in diagnosis of urinary tract infection,* Brit. Med. J. 1:293, 1963 — 1

BEALL, AC, Jr et al: *Translumbar aortography. Present indications and techniques,* Ann. Intern. Med. 60:843, 1964 — 29–30

BECKER, EL et al: *Kidney and Urinary Tract Infections,* Lilly Research Laboratories, Indianapolis, 1971 — 10–11

BENJAMIN, JA et al: *Cinefluorographic studies of bladder and urethral function,* J. Urol. 73:525, 1955 — 26

BERLINER, RW et al: *Dilution and concentration of the urine and the action of antidiuretic hormone,* Amer. J. Med. 24:730, 1958 — 11

BIRCHALL, R, BATSON, HM, Jr, AND BRANNAN, W: *Contribution of differential renal studies to diagnosis of renal arterial hypertension*

with emphasis on the value of U sodium/U creatinine, Amer. J. Med. 32:164, 1962 — 14–15

BLAHD, WH, Editor: *Nuclear Medicine,* Blakiston Division, McGraw-Hill Inc., New York, 1965 — 32–35

BLONDHEIM, SH, MARGOLIASH, E, AND SHAFRIR, E: *A simple test for myohemoglobinuria (myoglobinuria),* J.A.M.A. 167:453, 1958 — 3

BOEHM, JJ AND HAYNES, JL: *Bacteriology of "midstream catch" urines. Studies in newborn infants,* Amer. J. Dis. Child. 111:366, 1966 — 10–11

BORS, E: *Bladder disturbances and management of patients with injury to spinal cord,* J. Int. Coll. Surgeons 21:513, 1954 — 17

BOURGOIGNIE, J et al: *Renal venous renin in hypertension,* Amer. J. Med. 48:332, 1970 — 14–15

BOYD, JF AND NEDELKOSKA, N: *Inclusion-bearing cells in urinary sediment in infectious diseases,* J. Path. Bact. 88:115, 1964 — 6–8

BRODY, L, WEBSTER, MC, AND KARK, RM: *Identification of elements of urinary sediment with phase-contrast microscopy. A simple method,* J.A.M.A. 206:1777, 1968 — 5

BRODY, LH, SALLADAY, JR, AND ARMBRUSTER, K: *Urinalysis and the urinary sediment,* Med. Clin. N. Amer. 55:243, 1971 — 6–8

CAMERON, JS: *Estimating selectivity of proteinuria,* Lancet 1:729, 1967 — 2

CASTALDI, PA, EDWARDS, KDG, AND WHYTE, HM: *Urinary specific gravity as a measure of renal function,* Med. J. Aust. 1:847, 1960 — 11

COHEN, SN AND KASS, EH: *A simple method for quantitative urine culture,* New Eng. J. Med. 277:176, 1967 — 10–11

CONNOR, TB et al: *Unilateral renal disease as a cause of hypertension: Its detection by ureteral catheterization studies,* Ann. Intern. Med. 52:544, 1960 — 14–15

CROCKETT, AT, MAXWELL, M, AND KAUFMANN, JJ: *Delayed appearance time of intravenous urographic contrast media in renal ischemic hypertension,* J. Urol. 87:799, 1962 — 24

CUMMACK, DH: *Gastro-intestinal X-ray Diagnosis. A Descriptive Atlas,* E. & S. Livingstone Ltd., Edinburgh, 1969 — 29–30

DAUGHADAY, WH: *Hydrogen ion metabolism in diabetic acidosis. Disturbances before and after treatment,* Arch Intern. Med. 107:63, 1961 — 3

DAVIS, LA AND HOWERTON, LW: *Ureteral reflux,* Radiol. Clin. N. Amer. 3:583, 1963 — 26

DAYSOG, A, Jr AND DOBSON, HL: *Observations on the maltese cross phenomenon (anisotropic fat crystals) in sediments from normal and abnormal urine,* Techn. Bull. Regist. Med. Techn. 33:37, 1963 — 5

DEWEERD, JH: *Percutaneous aspiration of selected expanding renal lesions,* J. Urol. 87:303, 1962 — 31

DEYTON, WE et al: *Differential renal function evaluation by minute sequence pyelography,* J. Urol. 90:611, 1963 — 18–23

DOOLAN, PD, ALPEN, EL, AND THEIL, GB: *A clinical appraisal of the plasma concentration and endogenous clearance of creatinine,* Amer. J. Med. 32:65, 1962 — 12

EDELMANN, CM et al: *The renal response of children to acute ammonium chloride acidosis,* Pediat. Res. 1:452, 1967 — 16

EDWARDS, KDG AND WHYTE, HM: *Plasma creatinine level and creatinine clearance as tests of renal function,* Aust. Ann. Med. 8:218, 1959 — 12

ELKINGTON, JR et al: *The renal excretion of hydrogen ion in renal tubular acidosis. I. Quantitative assessment of the response to ammonium chloride as an acid load,* Amer. J. Med. 29:554, 1960 — 16

EMMETT, JL: *Clinical Urography,* 2nd ed., W. B. Saunders Company, Philadelphia, 1964 — 18–23

EMMETT, JL AND WITTEN, DM: *Clinical Urography,* W. B. Saunders Company, Philadelphia, 1971 — 25

EVANS, JA, DUBILIER, W, Jr, AND MONTEITH, JC: *Nephrotomography: A preliminary report,* Amer. J. Roentgen. 71:213, 1954 — 27

EVANS, JA, MONTEITH, JC, AND DUBILIER, W, Jr: *Nephrotomography,* Radiology, 64:655, 1955 — 18–23

FAJANS, SS: *Diagnostic tests for diabetes mellitus* in *Diabetes* ed. by Williams, RH, Hoeber Medical Division, Harper and Row, New York, 1960 — 3

FLOCKS, RH et al: *Diagnostic radiology in Encyclopedia of Urology*, Vol. 1, Springer-Verlag, Berlin, 1962 — 18-23

FOOT, NC et al: *Exfoliative cytology of urinary sediments. A review of 2,829 cases*, Cancer 11:127, 1958 — 6-8

FROESCH, ER AND RENOLD, AE: *Specific enzymatic determination of glucose in blood and urine using glucose oxidase*, Diabetes 5:1, 1956 — 3

GAULT, MH et al: *The plasma phenolsulfonphthalein index (PSPI) of renal function: II. Correlation with other parameters of renal function and indications for use*, Canad. Med. Ass. J. 94:68, 1966 — 13

GAULT, MH, KOCH, B, AND DOSSETOR, JB: *Phenolsulfonphthalein (PSP) in assessment of renal function*, J.A.M.A. 200:871, 1967 — 13

GRABSTALD, H: *Catheterization of renal cyst for diagnostic and therapeutic purposes*, J. Urol. 71:28, 1954 — 31

GRAHAM, RC AND KARNOVSKY, MJ: *Glomerular permeability. Ultrastructural cytochemical studies using peroxidases as protein tracers*, J. Exp. Med. 124:1123, 1966 — 2

GUTTMANN, D AND NAYLOR, GRE: *Dip-slide: An aid to quantitative urine culture in general practice*, Brit. Med. J. 3:343, 1967 — 10-11

HALPERN, M: *Percutaneous transfemoral arteriography: An analysis of the complications in 1,000 consecutive cases*, Amer. J. Roentgen. 92:918, 1964 — 29-30

HARRISON, JF et al: *Proteinuria in multiple myeloma*, Clin. Sci. 31:95, 1966 — 2

HARRISON, JF et al: *Urinary lysozyme, ribonuclease, and low-molecular-weight protein in renal disease*, Lancet 1:371, 1968 — 2

HEALY, JK, EDWARDS, KDG, AND WHYTE, HM: *Simple tests of renal function using creatinine, phenolsulphonphthalein, and pitressin*, J. Clin. Path. 17:557, 1964 — 13

HÖFFLER, D, OFFERMANN, G, AND FRENZ, H: *The intravenous PSP (phenol-red) test. II. Clinical application and interpretation*, German Med. Monthly 13:286, 1968 — 13

HUNTER, JA, WILCOX, HG, AND KARK, RM: *Problems in the management of renovascular hypertension*, Surg. Clin. N. Amer. 47:91, 1967 — 14-15

JOHNSON, RE, PASSMORE, R, AND SARGENT, F, II: *Multiple factors in experimental human ketosis*, Arch. Intern. Med. 107:43, 1961 — 3

KARK, RM: *Renal biopsy*, J.A.M.A. 205:220, 1968 — 36-37

KARK, RM AND BUENGER, RE: *Television-monitored fluoroscopy in percutaneous renal biopsy*, Lancet 1:904, 1966 — 36-37

KARK, RM et al: *A Primer of Urinalysis*, 2nd ed., Hoeber Medical Division, Harper and Row, New York, 1963 — 1

KARK, RM AND MUEHRCKE, RC: *Biopsy of kidney in prone position*, Lancet 1:1047, 1954 — 36-37

KASS, EH: *Bacteriuria and the diagnosis of infections of the urinary tract. With observations on the use of methionine as a urinary antiseptic*, Arch. Intern. Med. 100:709, 1957 — 10-11

KINCAID, OW, Editor: *Renal Angiography*, Year Book Medical Publishers, Inc., Chicago, 1966 — 18-23

KLEEMAN, CR, ADAMS, DA, AND MAXWELL, MH: *An evaluation of maximal water diuresis in chronic renal disease*, J. Lab. Clin. Med. 58:169, 1961 — 11

KONG, TQ et al: *Safety of selective renal arteriography*, Amer. J. Med. Sci. 246:527, 1963 — 29-30

KOROBKIN, MT, KIRKWOOD, R, AND MINAGI, H: *The nephrogram of hypotension*, Radiology 98:129, 1971 — 31

KREBS, HA: *The biochemical lesion in ketosis*, Arch. Intern. Med. 107:51, 1961 — 3

KUNIN, CM: *The natural history of recurrent bacteriuria in schoolgirls*, New Eng. J. Med. 282:1443, 1970 — 10-11

KUNIN, CM AND MCCORMACK, RC: *Prevention of catheter-induced urinary-tract infections by sterile closed drainage*, New Eng. J. Med. 274:1155, 1966 — 1

LANDES, RR AND RANSOM, CL: *Technique for the use of carbon dioxide in presacral retroperitoneal pneumography*, Surg. Gynec. Obstet. 105:268, 1957 — 28

LANG, EK: *A survey of the complications of percutaneous retrograde arteriography. Seldinger technique*, Radiology 51:257, 1963 — 29-30

LANG, EK: *The differential diagnosis of renal cysts and tumors. Cyst puncture, aspiration, and analysis of cyst content for fat as diagnostic criteria for renal cysts*, Radiology 87:883, 1966 — 18-23, 31

LANGWORTHY, QR, KOLB, LC, AND LEWIS, LG: *Physiology of Micturition*, The Williams and Wilkins Company, Baltimore, 1940 — 17

LAPIDES, J: *Cystometry*, J.A.M.A. 201:618, 1967 — 17

LAPIDES, J et al: *Denervation supersensitivity as a test for neurogenic bladder*, Surg. Gynec. Obstet. 114:241, 1962 — 17

LEADBETTER, GW, Jr AND MARKLAND, C: *Evaluation of technics and complications of renal arteriography*, New Eng. J. Med. 266:10, 1962 — 29-30

LECOCQ, FR, MCPHAUL, JJ, AND ROBINSON, RR: *Fixed and reproducible orthostatic proteinuria. V. Results of a 5-year follow-up evaluation*, Ann. Intern. Med. 64:557, 1966 — 2

LEONARDS, JR: *Evaluation of enzyme tests for urinary glucose*, J.A.M.A. 163:260, 1957 — 3

LEUALLEN, EC: *Efficacy of a urine preservative used by insurance companies*, Western Med. 7:51, 1966 — 1

LINDBLOM, K: *Percutaneous puncture of renal cysts and tumors*, Acta Radiol. 27:66, 1946 — 31

LIPPMAN, RW: *Urine and the Urinary Sediment. A Practical Manual and Atlas*, 2nd ed., Charles C Thomas, Springfield, Ill. 1969 — 4, 9

LÖFGREN, S AND SNELLMAN, B: *Instrument and technique of kidney biopsy*, Acta Med. Scand. 157:93, 1957 — 36-37

LONSTAM, GR: *Paper chromatography, a simple method for the differentiation of sugar in the urine*, Diabetes 7:36, 1958 — 3

LOWMAN, RM AND DELUCA, JT: *Nephrotomography: Its role in routine urographic studies*, J. Urol. 83:308, 1960 — 27

MANUEL, Y, REVILLARD, JP, AND BETUEL, H: *Proteins in Normal and Pathological Urine*, University Park Press, Baltimore, 1970 — 2

MARBLE, A: *The diagnosis of the less common melliturias including pentosuria and fructosuria*, Med. Clin. N. Amer. 31:313, 1947 — 3

MARTIN, JF, DEYTON, WE, AND GLENN, JF: *The minute sequence pyelogram*, Amer. J. Roentgen. 90:55, 1963 — 24

MAXWELL, MH, LUPU, AN, AND KAUFMAN, JJ: *Individual kidney function tests in renal arterial hypertension*, J. Urol. 100:384, 1968 — 14-15

MCAFEE, JG: *A survey of complications of abdominal aortography*, Radiology 68:825, 1957 — 29-30

MCLELLAND, R, LANDES, RR, AND RANSOM, CL: *Retroperitoneal pneumography: A safe method using carbon dioxide*, Radiol. Clin. N. Amer. 3:113, 1965 — 28

MCQUEEN, EG AND SYDNEY, MB: *Composition of urinary casts*, Lancet 1:397, 1966 — 4, 9

MØLLER, E, MCINTOSH, JF, AND VAN SLYKE, DD: *Studies of urea excretion; relationship between urine volume and rate of urea excretion by normal adults*, J. Clin. Invest. 6:427, 1928 — 12

MONZON, OT et al: *A comparison of bacterial counts of the urine obtained by needle aspiration of the bladder, catheterization and midstream-voided methods*, New Eng. J. Med. 259:764, 1958 — 1

MÖRSTAD, KS: *On the demonstration of Bence Jones proteinuria*, Acta Med. Scand. 182:457, 1967 — 2

MUEHRCKE, RC, KARK, RM, AND PIRANI, CL: *Technique of percutaneous renal biopsy in the prone position*, J. Urol. 74:267, 1955 — 36-37

NASH, J, LISTER, J, AND VOBES, DH: *Clinical tests for ketonuria*, Lancet 1:801, 1954 — 3

OLSSON, O: *Diagnostic radiology: retroperitoneal pneumography in Encyclopedia of Urology*, Springer-Verlag, Berlin, 1962 — 28

PAPANICOLAOU, GN: *Cytology of the urine sediment in neoplasms of the urinary tract*, J. Urol. 57:375, 1947 — 6-8

PFISTER, RC AND SHEA, TE: *Nephrotomography. Performance and interpretation*, Radiol. Clin. N. Amer. 9:41, 1971 — 27

PILLAY, VKG: *Clinical testing of renal function*, Med. Clin. N. Amer. 55:231, 1971 — 12

PIRANI, CL AND SALINAS-MADARGALI, L: *Evaluation of percutaneous renal biopsy in Pathol-*

ogy Annual, Appleton-Century-Crofts, Inc., New York, 1968 — 36-37

POTOLSKY, AI AND FRIEDMAN, EA: *Comparative value of refractometer and hydrometer in predicting urine osmolality. Normal and abnormal urines*, New York J. Med. 65:2126, 1965 — 11

PRESCOTT, LF AND BRODIE, DE: *A simple differential stain for urinary sediment*, Lancet 2:940, 1964 — 6-8

PRYLES, CV AND STEG, NL: *Specimens of urine obtained from young girls by catheter versus voiding. A comparative study of bacterial cultures, gram stains and bacterial counts in paired specimens*, Pediatrics 23:441, 1959 — 1

QUINN, JL, III, Editor: *Scintillation Scanning in Clinical Medicine*, W.B.Saunders Company, Philadelphia, 1964 — 32-35

RAPOPORT, A: *Modification of the "Howard Test" for the detection of renal-artery obstruction*, New Eng. J. Med. 263:1159, 1960 — 14-15

RATHE, JC: *Differential "nephropacification" screening procedure for unilateral renal artery occlusion*, Radiology 76:629, 1961 — 24

RELMAN, AS: *Some clinical aspects of chronic pyelonephritis in Biology of Pyelonephritis* ed. by Quinn, EL and Kass, EH, Little, Brown and Company, Boston, 1960 — 10-11

RENNIE, ID: *Proteinuria*, Med. Clin. N. Amer. 55:213, 1971 — 2

ROBERTSON, PW, DYSON, ML, AND SUTTON, PD: *Renal angiography. A review of 1750 cases*, Clin. Radiol. 20:401, 1969 — 29-30

ROGOFF, SM: *Lumbar aortography in Angiography*, Vol. 2, ed. by Abrams, HL, Little, Brown and Company, Boston, 1961 — 29-30

RUBINI, ME AND WOLF, AV: *Refractometric determination of total solids and water of serum and urine*, J. Biol. Chem. 225:869, 1957 — 11

SACCHAROW, L AND PRYLES, CV: *Further experience with the use of percutaneous suprapubic aspiration of the urinary bladder. Bacteriologic studies in 654 infants and children*, Pediatrics 43:1018, 1969 — 10-11

SCHENCKER, B, MORCURE, RW, AND MOODY, DL: *Simplified nephrotomography: The drip infusion technique*, Amer. J. Roentgen. 95:283, 1965 — 27

SCHLEGEL, JU AND BAKULE, PT: *A diagnostic approach in detecting renal and urinary tract disease*, J. Urol. 104:2, 1970 — 32-35

SCHWARTZ, WB et al: *A syndrome of renal sodium loss and hyponatremia probably resulting from inappropriate secretion of antidiuretic hormone*, Amer. J. Med. 23:529, 1957 — 11

SCOTT, WC: *Infusion pyelography in perspective*, Clin. Radiol. 19:83, 1968 — 18-23

SELDINGER, SI: *Catheter replacement of the needle in percutaneous arteriography; new technique*, Acta Radiol. 39:368, 1953 — 29-30

SELMAN, J: *The Fundamentals of X-ray and Radium Physics*, 4th ed., Charles C Thomas, Springfield, Ill., 1965 — 18-23

SHOPFNER, CE: *Cystourethrography: An evaluation of method*, Amer. J. Roentgen. 95:468, 1965 — 26

SHOPFNER, CE: *Cystourethrography: Methodology, normal anatomy and pathology*, J. Urol. 103:92, 1970 — 26

SIMON, N et al: *Clinical characteristics of renovascular hypertension*, J.A.M.A. 220:1209, 1972 — 14-15

STAMEY, TA et al: *Functional characteristics of renovascular hypertension*, Medicine 40:347, 1961 — 14-15

TAPLIN, GV et al: *The radioisotope renogram. An external test for individual kidney function and upper urinary tract patency*, J. Lab. Clin. Med. 48:886, 1956 — 32-35

TILLOTSON, PM AND HALPERN, M: *Selective renal arteriography*, Amer. J. Roentgen. 90:124, 1963 — 29-30

VESTBY, GW: *Percutaneous needle-puncture of renal cysts. New method in therapeutic management*, Invest. Radiol. 2:449, 1967 — 31

WAGNER, HN, Jr, Editor: *Principles of Nuclear Medicine*, W. B. Saunders Company, Philadelphia, 1968 — 32-35

WHITLEY, JE: *Renal arteriography*, Radiol. Clin. N. Amer. 3:224, 1965 — 29-30

Continued on page 278

WILHELM, SF: *Gas insufflation through the lumbar and presacral routes*, Surg. Gynec. Obstet. 99:319, 1954 — 28

WILLIAMS, GL, CAMPBELL, H, AND DAVIES, KJ: *Urinary concentrating ability in women with asymptomatic bacteriuria in pregnancy*, Brit. Med. J. 3:212, 1969 — 11

WILLIAMS, RH: *Ketosis. Summarization*, Arch. Intern. Med. 107:69, 1961 — 3

WINTER, CC: *Radioisotope Renography*, The Williams and Wilkins Company, Baltimore, 1963 — 32-35

WITTEN, DM, GREENE, LF, AND EMMETT, JL: *An evaluation of nephrotomography in urologic diagnosis*, Amer. J. Roentgen. 90:115, 1963 — 27

WOLF, AV AND PILLAY, VKG: *Renal concentration tests. Osmotic pressure, specific gravity, refraction and electrical conductivity compared*, Amer. J. Med. 46:837, 1969 — 11

WOLSTENHOLME, GEW AND CAMERON, MP, Editors: *Renal Biopsy*, Ciba Foundation Symposium, J. & A. Churchill, Ltd., London, 1961 — 36-37

WOODBURNE, RT: *Structure and function of the urinary bladder*, J. Urol. 84:79, 1960 — 17

WRONG, O AND DAVIES, HE: *The excretion of acid in renal disease*, Quart. J. Med. 28:259, 1959 — 2, 16

ZIMMER, JG et al: *The origin and nature of anisotropic urinary lipids in the nephrotic syndrome*, Ann. Intern. Med. 54:205, 1961 — 5

Section IV

BACANI, RA et al: *Rapidly progressive (nonstreptococcal) glomerulonephritis*, Ann. Intern. Med. 69:463, 1968 — 22-23, 25

BALDWIN, DS AND MCCLUSKEY, RT: *Renal involvement in systemic lupus erythematosus, periarteritis nodosa, scleroderma, and cryoglobulinemia* in *Structural Basis of Renal Disease* ed. by Becker, EL, Hoeber Medical Division, Harper and Row, New York, 1968 — 28-29

BALDWIN, DS et al: *Renal failure and interstitial nephritis due to penicillin and methicillin*, New Eng. J. Med. 279:1245, 1968 — 30

BARTTER, FC, Editor: *Clinical Use of Aldosterone Antagonists*, Charles C Thomas, Springfield, Ill., 1960 — 12-15

BECKER, EL, Editor: *Structural Basis of Renal Disease*, Hoeber Medical Division, Harper and Row, New York, 1968 — 12-15, 22-23, 25

BERMAN, LB AND SCHREINER, GE: *Clinical and histologic spectrum of the nephrotic syndrome*, Amer. J. Med. 24:249, 1958 — 12-15

BLACK, DAK, Editor: *Renal Disease*, 2nd ed., F. A. Davis Co., Philadelphia, 1967 — 3-11

BLAINEY, JD, HARDWICKE, J, AND LANNIGAN, R: *Focal glomerulonephritis* in *Structural Basis of Renal Disease* ed. by Becker, EL, Hoeber Medical Division, Harper and Row, New York, 1968 — 26

BRUN, C: *Acute anuria*, Thesis, Munksgaard, Copenhagen, 1954 — 1-2

BRUN, C AND MUNCK, O: *Lesions of the kidney in acute renal failure following shock*, Lancet 1:603, 1957 — 1-2

BRUN, C AND MUNCK, O: *Pathophysiology of the kidney in shock and in acute renal failure* in *Progress in Surgery*, Vol. 4, ed. by Allgöwer M, S. Karger, Basle, 1964 — 1-2

BURKHOLDER, PM: *Immunology and immunohistopathology of renal diseases* in *Structural Basis of Renal Disease* ed. by Becker, EL, Hoeber Medical Division, Harper and Row, New York, 1968 — 19-21

CAMERON, JS et al: *Membranoproliferative glomerulonephritis and persistent hypocomplementemia*, Brit. Med. J. 4:7, 1970 — 24

CHURG, J: *Pathology of glomerulonephritis*, Bull. N. Y. Acad. Med. 46:761, 1970 — 24

CHURG, J et al: *Structure of glomerular capillaries in proteinuria*, Arch. Intern. Med., 109:97, 1962 — 22-23, 25

COUNCILMAN, WT: *Acute interstitial nephritis*, J. Exp. Med. 3:393, 1898 — 30

DIXON, FJ: *The pathogenesis of glomerulonephritis*, Amer. J. Med. 44:493, 1968 — 22-23, 25

DIXON, FJ, FELDMAN, JD, AND VASQUEZ, JJ: *Experimental glomerulonephritis. The pathogenesis of a laboratory model resembling the spectrum of human glomerulonephritis*, J. Exp. Med. 113:899, 1961 — 16-18

DODGE, WF et al: *The relationship between the clinical and pathologic features of poststreptococcal glomerulonephritis. A study of the early natural history*, Medicine 47:227, 1968 — 19

EARLE, DP AND JENNINGS, RB: *Focal glomerular lesions*, Trans. Amer. Clin. Climat. Ass. 72:24, 1960 — 26

EDGINGTON, TS, GLASSOCK, RJ, AND DIXON, FJ: *Autologous immune-complex pathogenesis of experimental allergic glomerulonephritis*, Science 155:1432, 1967 — 16-18

GAIRDNER, D: *The Schönlein-Henoch syndrome (anaphylactoid purpura)*, Quart. J. Med. 17:95, 1948 — 27

HALL, PW, III et al: *Investigation of chronic endemic nephropathy in Yugoslavia. II. Renal pathology*, Amer. J. Med. 39:210, 1965 — 31

HALL, PW, III et al: *Renal function studies in individuals with the tubular proteinuria of endemic Balkan nephropathy*, Quart. J. Med. XLI:385, 1972 — 31

HEPTINSTALL, RH: *Pathology of the Kidney*, Little, Brown and Company, Boston, 1966 — 12-15, 22-23, 25

HEYMANN, W et al: *Production of nephrotic syndrome in rats by Freund's adjuvants and rat kidney suspensions*, Proc. Soc. Exp. Biol. Med. 100:660, 1959 — 16-18

JOACHIM, GR et al: *Selectivity of protein excretion in patients with nephrotic syndrome*, J. Clin. Invest. 43:2332, 1964 — 12-15

JONES, DB: *Glomerulonephritis*, Amer. J. Path. 29:33, 1953 — 22-23, 25

KARK, RM et al: *The nephrotic syndrome in adults: a common disorder with many causes*, Ann. Intern. Med. 49:751, 1958 — 12-15

KASSIRER, JP AND SCHWARTZ, WB: *Acute glomerulonephritis*, New Eng. J. Med. 265:686, 1961 — 19

KOFFLER, D, SCHUR, PH, AND KUNKEL, HG: *Immunological studies concerning the nephritis of systemic lupus erythematosus*, J. Exp. Med. 126:607, 1967 — 28-29

KRISHNAN, C AND KAPLAN, MH: *Immunopathologic studies of systemic lupus erythematosus II. Antinuclear reaction of γ-globulin eluted from homogenates and isolated glomeruli of kidneys from patients with lupus nephritis*, J. Clin. Invest. 46:569, 1967 — 28-29

LERNER, RA AND DIXON, EJ: *Transfer of ovine experimental allergic glomerulonephritis (EAG) with serum*, J. Exp. Med. 124:431, 1966 — 16-18

LUETSCHER, JA, Jr: *The nephrotic syndrome* in *Transactions of the Fifth Conference on Renal Function*, Josiah Macy, Jr. Foundation, New York, 1953 — 12-15

LUETSCHER, JA, Jr AND JOHNSON, BB: *Chromatographic separation of the sodium-retaining corticoid from the urine of children with nephrosis, compared with observations on normal children*, J. Clin. Invest. 33:276, 1954 — 12-15

LUETSCHER, JA, Jr et al: *Isolation of crystalline aldosterone from urine of a child with the nephrotic syndrome*, J. Biol. Chem. 217:505, 1955 — 12-15

LUETSCHER, JA, Jr, NEHER, R, AND WETTSTEIN, A: *Isolation of crystalline aldosterone from the urine of a nephrotic patient*, Experientia 10:456, 1954 — 12-15

MAXWELL, MH AND KLEEMAN, CR: *Clinical Disorders of Fluid and Electrolyte Metabolism*, 2nd ed., McGraw-Hill Inc., New York, 1972 — 3-11

MCCLUSKEY, RT AND BALDWIN, DS: *Natural history of acute glomerulonephritis*, Amer. J. Med. 35:213, 1963 — 19

MCCLUSKEY, RT AND VASSALLI, P: *Experimental glomerular diseases* in *The Kidney, Morphology, Biochemistry, Physiology*, Vol. 2, ed. by Rouiller, C and Muller, AF, Academic Press, Inc., New York, 1969 — 16-18

MICHAEL, AF et al: *Studies on chronic membranoproliferative glomerulonephritis with hypo-*

complementemia, J. Exp. Med. 134:208s, 1971 — 24

MUEHRCKE, RC et al: *Primary renal amyloidosis with nephrotic syndrome studied by serial biopsies of kidney*, Guy Hosp. Rep. 104:295, 1955 — 12-15

OLDSTONE, MBA AND DIXON, FJ: *Lymphocytic choriomeningitis; production of antibody by "tolerant" infected mice*, Science 158:1193, 1967 — 16-18

OLSEN, TS: *Ultrastructure of the renal tubules in acute renal insufficiency*, Acta Path. Microbiol. Scand. 71:203, 1967 — 1-2

OLSEN, TS AND SKJOLDBORG, H: *The fine structure of the renal glomerulus in acute anuria*, Acta Path. Microbiol. Scand. 70:205, 1967 — 1-2

PITTS, RF: *Physiology of the Kidney and Body Fluids*, 2nd ed., Year Book Medical Publishers, Inc., Chicago, 1968 — 3-11

RADONIC, M: *Epidemiologie, clinique, histologie et etiologie de la nephrite endemique en Yougoslavie* in *Proceedings of the First International Congress on Nephrology*, S. Karger, Basle, 1960 — 31

RASMUSSEN, H: *Thyroxine metabolism in the nephrotic syndrome*, J. Clin. Invest. 35:792, 1956 — 12-15

RECANT, L AND RIGGS, DS: *Thyroid function in nephrosis*, J. Clin. Invest. 31:789, 1952 — 12-15

RICH, AR: *Visceral hazards of hypersensitivity to drugs*, Trans. Amer. Clin. Climat. Ass. 72:46, 1960 — 30

ROGERS, J AND ROBBINS, SL: *Intercapillary glomerulosclerosis: a clinical and pathological study. I. Specificity of the clinical syndrome*, Amer. J. Med. 12:688, 1952 — 12-15

ROGERS, J, ROBBINS, SL, AND JEGHERS, H: *Intercapillary glomerulosclerosis: a clinical and pathological study. II. A clinical study of 100 anatomically proven cases*, Amer. J. Med. 12:692, 1952 — 12-15

ROUILLER, C AND MULLER, AF, Editors: *The Kidney*, Vol. 3, Academic Press, Inc., New York, 1971 — 3-11

SCHREINER, GE: *The glomerular membrane in the nephrotic syndrome* and *The use of diuretics in edema of renal origin* in *Edema, Mechanisms and Management* ed. by Moyer, JH and Fuchs, M, W. B. Saunders Company, Philadelphia, 1960 — 12-15

SCHREINER, GE AND MAHER, JF: *Uremia: The Biochemistry, Pathogenesis and Treatment*, Charles C Thomas, Springfield, Ill., 1961 — 3-15

SEEGAL, BC et al: *Studies on the pathogenesis of acute and progressive glomerulonephritis in man by immunofluorescein and immunoferritin techniques*, Fed. Proc. 24:100, 1965 — 19-21

SIMENHOFF, ML, GUILD, WR, AND DAMMIN, GJ: *Acute diffuse interstitial nephritis*, Amer. J. Med. 44:618, 1968 — 30

SQUIRE, JR: *The nephrotic syndrome*, Advances Intern. Med. 7:201, 1956 — 12-15

SQUIRE, JR: *The nephrotic syndrome*, Brit. Med. J. 2:1389, 1953 — 12-15

SQUIRE, JR, BLAINEY, JD, AND HARDWICKE, J: *The nephrotic syndrome*, Brit. Med. Bull. 13:43, 1957 — 12-15

STEBLAY, RW: *Glomerulonephritis induced in sheep by injections of heterologous glomerular basement membrane and Freund's complete adjuvant*, J. Exp. Med. 116:253, 1962 — 16-18

STICKLER, GB, BURKE, EC, AND MCKENZIE, BF: *Electrophoretic studies of the nephrotic syndrome in children: preliminary report*, Mayo Clin. Proc. 29:555, 1954 — 12-15

STRAUSS, MB AND WELT, LG, Editors: *Diseases of the Kidney*, 2nd ed., Little, Brown and Company, Boston, 1971 — 3-11

UNANUE, ER AND DIXON, FJ: *Experimental glomerulonephritis: immunological events and pathogenetic mechanisms*, Advances Immun. 6:1, 1967 — 27

VERNIER, RL et al: *Anaphylactoid purpura. I. Pathology of the skin and kidney and frequency of streptococcal infection*, Pediatrics 27:181, 1961 — 27

VIVIEN, P, GOUFFAULT, J, AND GUILLON, M: *Peculiar etiological circumstances of the nephrotic syndrome in adults*, Bull. Soc. Med. Hop. Paris, 75:323, 1959 — 12-15

VOLHARD, F AND FAHR, T: *Die Brightsche*

Nierenkrankheit, Springer-Verlag, Berlin, 1914   19-21

WELT, LG, Editor: *Symposium on uremia*, Amer. J. Med. 44:653, 1968   3-11

WEST, CD et al: *Hypocomplementemic and normocomplementemic persistent (chronic) glomerulonephritis: clinical and pathological characteristics*, J. Pediat. 67:1089, 1965   24

WOLSTENHOLME, GEW AND KNIGHT, J, Editors: *The Balkan Nephropathy*, Ciba Foundation Study Group 30, J. & A. Churchill, Ltd., London, 1967   31

Section V

ALLEN, AC: *The Kidney, Medical and Surgical Diseases*, 2nd ed., Grune & Stratton, Inc., New York, 1962   30

AVIOLI, LV et al: *Early effects of radiation on renal function in man*, Amer. J. Med. 34:329, 1963   12-13

BAGGENSTOSS, AH AND ROSENBERG, EF: *Visceral lesions associated with chronic infectious (rheumatoid) arthritis*, Arch. Path. 35:503, 1943   17

BANSON, BB AND LACY, PE: *Diabetic microangiopathy in human toes: with emphasis on the ultrastructural change in dermal capillaries*, Amer. J. Path. 45:41, 1964   1-3

BARGER, AC: *Renal hemodynamic factors in congestive heart failure*, Ann. N.Y. Acad. Sci. 139:276, 1966   25

BECKER, EL, Editor: *Structural Basis of Renal Disease*, Hoeber Medical Division, Harper and Row, New York, 1968   1-3

BELL, ET: *Renal vascular disease in diabetes mellitus*, Diabetes 2:376, 1953   1-3

BIAVA, CG et al: *Kaliopenic nephropathy. A correlated light and electron microscopic study*, Lab. Invest. 12:443, 1963   28

BRAIN, MC, DACIE, JV, AND HOURIHANE, DO: *Microangiopathic hemolytic anemia: the possible role of vascular lesions in pathogenesis*, Brit. J. Haemat. 8:358, 1962   10-11

BRANDT, K, CATHCART, ES, AND COHEN, AS: *A clinical analysis of the course and prognosis of 42 patients with amyloidosis*, Amer. J. Med. 44:955, 1968   14-16

BRICKER, NS AND SCHULTZE, RG: *Renal function: general concepts* in *Clinical Disorders of Fluid and Electrolyte Metabolism* ed. by Maxwell, MH and Kleeman, CR, McGraw-Hill Inc., New York, 1972   25

CARONE, FA et al: *The effects upon the kidney of transient hypercalcemia induced by parathyroid extract*, Amer. J. Path. 36:77, 1960   29

CAULFIELD, JB AND SCHRAG, BA: *Electron microscopic study of renal calcification*, Amer. J. Path. 44:365, 1964   29

CHURG, J et al: *Hemolytic-uremic syndrome as a cause of postpartum renal failure*, Amer. J. Obstet. Gynec. 108:253, 1970   10-11

COHEN, AS: *Amyloidosis*, New Eng. J. Med. 277:522, 574, and 628, 1967   14-16

COHEN, AS: *Constitution and genesis of amyloid* in *International Review of Experimental Pathology*, Vol. 4, ed. by Richter, CW and Epstein, MA, Academic Press, Inc., New York, 1965   14-16

CRAIG, JM AND GITLIN, D: *The nature of the hyaline thrombi in thrombotic thrombocytopenic purpura*, Amer. J. Path. 33:251, 1957   10-11

DACHS, S et al: *Diabetic nephropathy*, Amer. J. Path. 44:155, 1964   1-3

DAVSON, J, BALL, J, AND PLATT, R: *The kidney in periarteritis nodosa*, Quart. J. Med. 17:175, 1948   27

DEODHAR, SD, HAAS, E, AND GOLDBLATT, H: *Production of antirenin to homologous renin and its effect on experimental renal hypertension*, J. Exp. Med. 119:425, 1964   9

DUFFY, JL, SUZUKI, Y, AND CHURG, J: *Acute calcium nephropathy. Early proximal tubular changes in the rat kidney*, Arch. Path. 91:340, 1971   29

EARLE DP et al: *Symposium on epidemic hemorrhagic fever*, Amer. J. Med. 16:617, 1954   31

EYLER, WR et al: *Angiography of renal areas including comparative study of renal arterial stenoses in patients with and without hypertension*, Radiology, 78:879, 1962   7

FAHEY, JL et al: *Wegener's granulomatosis*, Amer. J. Med. 17:168, 1954   18

FARQUHAR, MG, HOPPER, J, JR, AND MOON, HD: *Diabetic glomerulosclerosis: electron and light microscopic studies*, Amer. J. Path. 35:721, 1959   1-3

FARQUHAR, MG AND PALADE, GE: *Functional evidence for the existence of a third cell type in the renal glomerulus: phagocytosis of filtration residues by a distinctive "third" cell*, J. Cell Biol. 13:55, 1962   1-3

FENNELL, RH, JR, REDDY, CRRM, AND VASQUEZ, JJ: *Progressive systemic sclerosis and malignant hypertension. Immunohistochemical study of renal lesions*, Arch. Path. 72:209, 1961   17

FISHER, ER, PEREZ-STABLE, E, AND ZAWADSKI, ZA: *Ultrastructural renal changes in multiple myeloma with comments relative to the mechanism of proteinuria*, Lab. Invest. 13:1561, 1964   30

FISHER, ER AND ZAWADSKI, SA: *Ultrastructural features of plasma cells in patients with paraproteinemias*, Amer. J. Clin. Path. 54:779, 1970   30

FRANKLIN, EC: *The immune-globulins—their structure and function and some techniques for their isolation* in *Progress in Allergy*, Vol. 8, ed. by Kallos, P and Waksman, B, S. Karger, Basle, 1964   30

FRIEDERICI, HHR, TUCKER, WR, AND SCHWARTZ, TB: *Observations on small blood vessels of skin in normal and in diabetic patients*, Diabetes 15:233, 1966   1-3

GASSER, VC et al: *Hämolytisch-urämische Syndrome: bilaterale Nierenrindennekrosen bei akuten erworbenen hämolytischen Anämien*, Schweiz. Med. Wschr. 85:905, 1955   10-11

GELLMAN, DD et al: *Diabetic nephropathy: a clinical and pathologic study based on renal biopsies*, Medicine 38:321, 1959   1-3

GILCHRIST, GS et al: *Heparin therapy in the haemolytic-uraemic syndrome*, Lancet 1:1123, 1969   10-11

GOLDBLATT, H: *Hypertension of renal origin: historical and experimental background*, Amer. J. Surg. 107:21, 1964   9

GOODPASTURE, EW: *The significance of certain pulmonary lesions in relation to the etiology of influenza*, Amer. J. Med. Sci. 158:863, 1919   27

GREENWALD, HP, BRONFIN, GJ, AND AUERBACH, O: *Needle biopsy of the kidney. A report of 5 cases of multiple myeloma*, Amer. J. Med. 15:198, 1953   30

HABIB, R, MATHIEU, H, AND ROYER, P: *Le syndrome hémolytique et urémique de l'enfant*, Nephron 4:139, 1967   10-11

HAMBURGER, J et al: *Nephrology*, tr. by Walsh, A, W. B. Saunders Company, Philadelphia, 1968   27

HANSEN, RØ: *A quantitative estimate of the peripheral glomerular basement membrane in recent juvenile diabetics*, Diabetologia 1:97, 1965   1-3

HEPTINSTALL, RH: *Pathology of the Kidney*, Little, Brown and Company, Boston, 1966   1-3

KIMMELSTIEL, P: *Diabetic nephropathy* in *The Kidney* ed. by Mostofi, FK and Smith, DE, The Williams and Wilkins Company, Baltimore, 1966   1-3

KIMMELSTIEL, P: *The nature of chronic pyelonephritis*, Geriatrics 19:145, 1964   1-3

KIMMELSTIEL, P, KIM, OJ, AND BERES, J: *Studies on renal biopsy specimens, with the aid of the electron microscope. 1. Glomeruli in diabetes*, Amer. J. Clin. Path. 38:270, 1962   1-3

KIMMELSTIEL, P, OSAWA, G, AND BERES, J: *Glomerular basement membrane in diabetics*, Amer. J. Clin. Path. 45:21, 1966   1-3

KIMMELSTIEL, P AND WILSON, C: *Intercapillary lesions in the glomeruli of the kidney*, Amer. J. Path. 12:83, 1936   1-3

KINCAID-SMITH, P, MCMICHAEL, J, AND MURPHY, EA: *The clinical course and pathology of hypertension with papilloedema (malignant hypertension)*, Quart. J. Med. 27:117, 1958   6

KOBERNICK, SD AND WHITESIDE, JH: *Renal glomeruli in multiple myeloma*, Lab. Invest. 6:478, 1957   30

KOFFLER, D AND PARONETTO, F: *Fibrinogen deposition in acute renal failure*, Amer. J. Path. 49:383, 1966   10-11

KOSS, LG: *Hyaline material with staining reaction of fibrinoid in renal lesions in diabetes mellitus*, Arch. Path. 54:528, 1952   1-3

KUSSMAUL, A AND MAIER, R: *Ueber eine bisher nicht beschriebene eigentümliche Arterienerkrankung (Periarteritis Nodosa) die mit Morbus Brightii und rapid fortschreitender allgemeiner Muskellahmung einhergeht*, Dtsch. Arch. klin. Med. 1:484, 1866   18

LARAGH, JH: *Aldosteronism and arterial hypertension*, Med. Clin. N. Amer. 45:321, 1961   8

LECOMPTE, PM: *Vascular lesions in diabetes mellitus*, J. Chronic Dis. 2:178, 1955   1-3

LEVITT, M AND ALTCHEK, A: *Hypertension and toxemia of pregnancy* in *Medical, Surgical, and Gynecologic Complications of Pregnancy*, 2nd ed., ed. by Rovinsky, J and Guttmacher, AF, The Williams and Wilkins Company, Baltimore, 1965   22

LINTON, AL et al: *Microangiopathic haemolytic anaemia and the pathogenesis of malignant hypertension*, Lancet 1:1277, 1969   10-11

LUXTON, RW: *Effects of irradiation on the kidney* in *Diseases of the Kidney* ed. by Strauss, MB and Welt, LG, Little, Brown and Company, Boston, 1963   12-13

LUXTON, RW: *Radiation nephritis*, Acta Radiol. (Ther.) 1:397, 1963   12-13

LUXTON, RW AND KUNKLER, PB: *Radiation nephritis*, Acta Radiol. (Ther.) 2:169, 1964   12-13

MANDEMA, E et al, Editors: *Proceedings of the Symposium on Amyloidosis*, Excerpta Medica Foundation, Amsterdam, 1968   14-16

MARBLE, A: *Diabetic nephropathy* in *Diseases of the Kidney* ed. by Strauss, MB and Welt, LG, Little, Brown and Company, Boston, 1963   1-3

MASUGI, M AND YÄ, S: *Die diffuse Sklerodermie und ihre Gefässveränderung*, Virchow. Arch. (Path. Anat.) 302:39, 1938   17

MAUTNER, W et al: *Preeclamptic nephropathy; an electron microscopic study*, Lab. Invest. 11:518, 1962   22

MCCORMACK, LJ: *Occlusive disease of main renal artery* in *The Ciba Collection of Medical Illustrations*, Vol. 5 by Netter, FH, ed. by Yonkman, FF, CIBA Pharmaceutical Company, Summit, 1969   7

MCFARLAND, JB: *Renal venous thrombosis in children*, Quart. J. Med. 34:269, 1965   23

MORITZ, AR AND OLDT, MR: *Arteriolar sclerosis in hypertensive and non-hypertensive individuals*, Amer. J. Path. 13:679, 1937   4

MOSTOFI, FK: *Radiation effects on the kidney* in *The Kidney* International Academy of Pathology, Monograph No. 6 ed. by Mostofi, FK, The Williams and Wilkins Company, Baltimore, 1966   12-13

MOSTOFI, FK AND BERDJIS, CC: *The Kidney* in *Pathology of Irradiation* ed. by Berdjis, CC, The Williams and Wilkins Company, Baltimore, 1971   12-13

MOSTOFI, FK, PANI, KC, AND ERICSSON, J: *Effects of irradiation on canine kidney* in *Pathology of Irradiation* ed. by Berdjis, CC, The Williams and Wilkins Company, Baltimore, 1971   12-13

MUEHRCKE, RC AND ROSEN, S: *Hypokalemic nephropathy in rat and man. A light and electron microscopic study*, Lab. Invest. 13:1359, 1964   28

OSAWA, G, KIMMELSTIEL, P, AND SEILING, V: *Thickness of glomerular basement membranes*, Amer. J. Path. 45:7, 1966   1-3

OSSERMAN, EF AND TAKATSUKI, K: *Plasma cell myeloma: gamma globulin synthesis and structure. A review of biochemical and clinical data, with the description of a newly-recognized and related syndrome, "H$^{\gamma-2}$-chain (Franklin's) disease,"* Medicine 42:357, 1963   30

Continued on page 280

PAGE, IH: *Eyegrounds in hypertension* in *The Ciba Collection of Medical Illustrations*, Vol. 5 by Netter, FH, ed. by Yonkman, FF, CIBA Pharmaceutical Company, Summit, 1969   5

PAPPER, S: *The role of the kidney in Laennec's cirrhosis of the liver*, Medicine, 37:299, 1958   26

PAPPER, S AND VAAMONDE, CA: *Renal failure in cirrhosis—role of plasma volume*, Ann. Intern. Med. 68:958, 1968   26

PARKIN, TW et al: *Hemorrhagic and interstitial pneumonitis with nephritis*, Amer. J. Med. 18:220, 1955   27

PERERA, GA: *Hypertensive vascular disease; description and natural history*, J. Chronic Dis. 1:33, 1955   5

POLLAK, VE et al: *The kidney in rheumatoid arthritis: studies by renal biopsies*, Arthritis Rheum. 5:1, 1962   17

RAYER, P: *Traites des maladies des reins*, Balliere, Paris, 1840   23

RICH, AR AND GREGORY, JE: *The experimental demonstration that periarteritis nodosa is a manifestation of hypersensitivity*, Bull. Johns Hopk. Hosp. 72:65, 1943   18

RITCHIE, S AND WAUGH, D: *The pathology of Armanni-Ebstein diabetic nephropathy*, Amer. J. Path. 33:1035, 1957   1-3

ROBBINS, SL: *The reversibility of glycogen nephrosis in alloxan-treated diabetic rats*, Amer. J. Med. Sci. 219:376, 1950   1-3

ROBINSON, G: *Researches into the connection existing between an unnatural degree of compression of the blood contained in the renal vessels and the presence of certain abnormal matters in the urine*, Med. Chir. 26:51, 1843   23

RODNAN, GP: *A review of recent observations and current theories on the etiology and pathogenesis of progressive systemic sclerosis (diffuse scleroderma)*, J. Chronic Dis. 16:929, 1963   17

ROSEN, S et al: *Radiation nephritis, light and electron microscopic observations*, Amer. J. Clin. Path. 41:487, 1964   12-13

ROSENMANN, E, POLLAK, VE, AND PIRANI, CL: *Renal vein thrombosis in the adult: a clinical and pathologic study based on renal biopsies*, Medicine 47:269, 1968   23

RUSBY, NL AND WILSON, C: *Lung purpura with nephritis*, Quart. J. Med. 29:501, 1960   27

SCHOTTSTAEDT, MF AND SOKLOW, M: *The natural history and course of hypertension with papilledema (malignant hypertension)*, Amer. Heart J. 45:331, 1953   6

SCHREINER, GE: *Toxic nephropathy* in *Diseases of the Kidneys* ed. by Beeson, PB and McDermott, W, W. B. Saunders Company, Philadelphia, 1971   19-21

SCHREINER, GE: *Toxic nephropathy* in *Structural Basis of Renal Disease* ed. by Becker, EL, Hoeber Medical Division, Harper and Row, New York, 1968   19-21

SCHWARTZ, WB AND RELMAN, AS: *Effects of electrolyte disorders on renal structure and function*, New Eng. J. Med. 276:383, 1967   28

SCHWARTZ, WB AND RELMAN, AS: *Effects of electrolyte disorders on renal structure and function (concluded)*, New Eng. J. Med. 276:452, 1967   29

SIPPERSTEIN, MD, UNGER, RH, AND MADISON, LL: *Studies of muscle capillary basement membranes in normal subjects, diabetic, and prediabetic patients*, J. Clin. Invest. 47:1973, 1968   1-3

SPARGO, B, MCCARTNEY, CP, AND WINEMILLER, R: *Glomerular capillary endotheliosis in toxemia of pregnancy*, Arch. Path. 68:593, 1959   22

SPEAR, GS: *Glomerular alterations in cyanotic congenital heart disease*, Bull. Johns Hopk. Hosp. 106:347, 1960   24

SORENSON, GD, HEEFNER, WA, AND KIRKPATRICK, JE: *Experimental amyloidosis* in *Methods and Achievements in Experimental Pathology*, Vol. 1, ed. by Bajusz, E and Jasmin, G, Year Book Medical Publishers, Inc., Chicago, 1966   14-16

SPEAR, GS AND KIHARA, I: *The glomerulus and serum sickness in experimental hypoxia*, Brit. J. Exp. Path. 53:265, 1972   24

SPEAR, GS: *Implications of the glomerular lesions of cyanotic congenital heart disease*, J. Chronic Dis. 19:1083, 1966   24

SPEAR, GS AND VITSKY, BH: *Hyalinization of afferent and efferent glomerular arterioles in cyanotic congenital heart disease*, Amer. J. Med. 41:309, 1966   24

STANTON, MC AND TANGE, JD: *Goodpasture's syndrome (pulmonary haemorrhage associated with glomerulonephritis)*, Aust. Ann. Med. 7:132, 1958   27

STRAUSS, MB AND WELT, LG, Editors: *Diseases of the Kidney*, Little, Brown and Company, Boston, 1963   1-3

SUZUKI, Y et al: *The mesangium of the renal glomerulus: electron microscopic studies of pathologic alterations*, Amer. J. Path. 43:555, 1963   1-3

TEILUM, G AND LINDAHL, A: *Frequency and significance of amyloid changes in rheumatoid arthritis*, Acta Med. Scand. 149:449, 1954   17

VENKATACHALAM, MA, JONES, DB, AND NELSON, DA: *Microangiopathic hemolytic anemia in rats with malignant hypertension*, Blood 32:278, 1968   10-11

VERTES, V, GOLD, H, AND LEB, D: *Renovascular hypertension* in *Structural Basis of Renal Disease* ed. by Becker, EL, Hoeber Medical Division, Harper and Row, New York, 1968   4

VERTES, V, GRAUEL, JA, AND GOLDBLATT, H: *Renal arteriography, separate renal-function studies and renal biopsy in human hypertension*, New Eng. J. Med. 270:656, 1964   7

VITSKY, BH et al: *The hemolytic-uremic syndrome: a study of renal pathologic alterations*, Amer. J. Path. 57:627, 1969   10-11

WARREN, S, LECOMPTE, PM, AND LEGG, MA: *The Pathology of Diabetes Mellitus*, 4th ed., Lea & Febiger, Philadelphia, 1966   1-3

WEGENER, F: *Über eine eigenartige rhinogene Granulomatose mit besonderer Beteiligung des Arteriensystems und der Nieren*, Beitr. Path. Anat. 102:36, 1939   18

WESTCOTT, RN: *Heart disease in hypertension* in *The Ciba Collection of Medical Illustrations*, Vol. 5 by Netter, FH, ed. by Yonkman, FF, CIBA Pharmaceutical Company, Summit, 1969   5

ZEEK, PM: *Periarteritis nodosa and other forms of necrotizing angiitis*, New Eng. J. Med. 248:764, 1953   18

ZUCKER-FRANKLIN, D: *Multiple myeloma. II. Structural features of cells associated with the paraproteinemias*, Seminars Hemat. 1:165, 1964   30

Section VI

ABRAHAMS, C AND LEVIN, NW: *Experimentally induced analgesic nephropathy*, J. Med. Proceedings 13:506, 1967   10

ALKEN, CE et al, Editors: *Encyclopedia of Urology*, Vols. V/1, VI, VIII, IX/1, IX/2, X, XI/1, XII, and XV, Springer-Verlag, New York   1-4, 11-12, 16-19, 21-36

ANDERSEN, BR AND JACKSON, GG: *Persistent pyelitis and pyelonephritis from retrograde urinary tract infection with a strain of Klebsiella in rats*, J. Lab. Clin Med. 60:457, 1962   5-9

AOKI, S et al: *"Abacterial" and Bacterial Pyelonephritis*, New Eng. J. Med. 281:1375, 1969   5-9

BECKER, EL, Editor: *Structural Basis of Renal Disease*, Hoeber Medical Division, Harper and Row, New York, 1968   5-9

BEESON, PB: *Factors in pathogenesis of pyelonephritis*, Yale J. Biol. Med. 28:81, 1955   5-9

BENGTSSON, H: *A comparative study of chronic non-obstructive pyelonephritis and renal papillary necrosis*, Acta Med. Scand. 172:1, 1962   10

BENGTSSON, U: *Analgesic nephropathy—chronic pyelonephritis* in *Proceedings of 3rd International Congress of Nephrology*, Vol. 2, *Morphology, Immunology, Urology* ed. by Heptinstall, RH, S. Karger, Basle, 1967   10

BROD, J: *Chronic pyelonephritis* in *Renal Disease* ed. by Black, DA, F. A. Davis Co., Philadelphia, 1962   5-9

BRUN, C AND RAASCHOU, F: *Percutaneous renal biopsy in pyelonephritis* in *Renal Biopsy: Clinical and Pathological Significance* in *Ciba Foundation Symposium* ed. by Wolstenholme, GEW and Cameron, MP, Little, Brown and Company, Boston, 1961   5-9

CAMPBELL, MF, Editor: *Urology*, W. B. Saunders Company, Philadelphia, 1963   1-4, 11-12, 16-19, 21-36

CLAUSEN, E: *Renal damage following long-term administration of phenacetin and acetylsalicylic acid*, Thesis, Århus University, Munksgaard, Copenhagen, 1967   10

DELIVELIOTIS, A, KEHAYAS, P, AND VARKARAKIS, M: *The diagnostic problem of the hydatid disease of the kidney*, J. Urol. 99:139, 1968   13

DIAZ-ESQUIVEL, J AND FARMER, S: *The effect of phenacetin on experimental ascending pyelonephritis*, Arch. Path. 85:129, 1968   10

EKSTRÖM, T et al: *Medullary Sponge Kidney*, Almqvist & Wiksell, Stockholm, 1959   20

EMMETT, JL: *Clinical Urography*, W. B. Saunders Company, Philadelphia, 1964   1-4, 11-12, 16-19, 21-36

FUWA, M AND WAUGH, D: *Experimental renal papillary necrosis. Effects of diuresis and antidiuresis*, Arch. Path. 85:404, 1968   10

GILMAN, A: *Analgesic nephrotoxicity*, Amer. J. Med. 36:167, 1964   10

GLOOR, F: *Pathologische Anatomie der Pyelonephritis* in *Die Pyelonephritis* ed. by Losse, H and Kienitz, M, Georg Thieme Verlag, Stuttgart, 1966   10

GLOOR, F: *Some morphologic features of chronic interstitial nephritis (chronic pyelonephritis) in patients with analgesic abuse* in *Progress in Pyelonephritis* ed. by Kass, EH, F. A. Davis Co., Philadelphia, 1965   10

HARVALD, B: *Renal papillary necrosis: a clinical survey of sixty-six cases*, Amer. J. Med. 35:481, 1963   10

HEPTINSTALL, RH: *Pathology of the Kidney*, Little, Brown and Company, Boston, 1966   1-12, 16-19, 21-36

JACKSON, GG AND GRIEBLE, HG: *Pathogenesis of renal infection*, Arch. Intern. Med. 100:692, 1957   5-9

JACKSON, GG et al: *Profiles of pyelonephritis*, Arch. Intern. Med. 110:663, 1962   5-9

JACKSON, GG, POIRIER, KP, AND GRIEBLE, HG: *Concepts of pyelonephritis: experience with renal biopsies and long-term clinical observations*, Ann. Intern. Med. 47:1165, 1957   5-9

JACOBSON, MH AND NEWMAN, W: *Study of pyelonephritis using renal biopsy material*, Arch. Intern. Med. 110:211, 1962   5-9

JORDAN, P AND WEBBE, G: *Human Schistosomiasis*, Charles C Thomas, Springfield, Ill., 1969   14-15

KARK, RM et al: *The clinical value of renal biopsy*, Ann. Intern. Med. 43:807, 1955   5-9

KASS, EH: *Bacteriuria and pyelonephritis of pregnancy*, Arch. Intern. Med. 105:194, 1960   5-9

KASS, EH: *Hormones and host resistance to infection*, Bact. Rev. 24:177, 1960   5-9

KEEFER, CS: *Pyelonephritis—its natural history and course*, Bull. Hist. Med. 100:107, 1957   5-9

KIMMELSTIEL, P et al: *Chronic pyelonephritis*, Amer. J. Med. 30:589, 1961   5-10

KIMMELSTIEL, P: *Diabetic nephropathy* in *The Kidney* ed. by Mostofi, FK and Smith, DE, The Williams and Wilkins Company, Baltimore, 1966   10

KIMMELSTIEL, P: *The nature of chronic pyelonephritis*, Geriatrics, 19:145, 1964   5-9

KINCAID-SMITH, P: *Analgesic nephropathy and papillary necrosis*, Postgrad. Med. 44:807, 1968   10

KINCAID-SMITH, P: *Analgesic nephropathy in perspective*, Med. J. Aust. 2:320, 1967   10

KINCAID-SMITH, P: *Pathogenesis of the renal lesion associated with the abuse of analgesics*, Lancet 1:859, 1967   10

KIPNIS, GP et al: *Renal biopsy in pyelonephritis; correlative study of kidney morphology, bacteriology, and function in patients with chronic urinary infections*, Arch. Intern. Med. 95:445, 1955   5-9

KLEEMAN, CR, HEWITT, WL, AND GUZE, LB: *Pyelonephritis*, Medicine 39:3, 1960   5-9

KLEEMAN, SE AND FREEDMAN, LR: *The finding of chronic pyelonephritis in males and females at autopsy*, New Eng. J. Med. 263:988,1960   5-9

KUNIN, CM AND HALMAGYI, NE: *Urinary-tract infections in schoolchildren. II. Characterization of invading organisms*, New Eng. J. Med. 266:1297, 1962   5-9

KUNIN, CM, ZACHA, E, AND PAQUIN, AJ, Jr: *Urinary-tract infections in schoolchildren. I. Prevalence of bacteriuria and associated urologic findings*, New Eng. J. Med. 266:1287,1962   5-9

LEHMAN, JS, Jr et al: *Hydronephrosis, bacteriuria, and maximal urine concentration in urinary schistosomiasis*, Ann. Intern. Med. 75:49, 1971   14-15

LEHMAN, JS, Jr et al: *Renal function in urinary schistosomiasis*, Amer. J. Trop. Med. 19:1001, 1970   14-15

LOWSLEY, OS AND KIRWIN, TJ: *Clinical Urology*, The Williams and Wilkins Company, Baltimore, 1956   1-4, 11-12, 16-19, 21-36

LUPTON, CH AND McMANUS, JF: *The nature of chronic pyelonephritis*, Lab. Invest. 11:860, 1962   5-9

MAKAR, N: *Urologic Aspects of Bilhariasis in Egypt*, Societe Orientale de Publicite Press, Cairo, 1955   14-15

MARTIN, CM AND BOOKRAJIAN, EN: *Bacteriuria prevention after indwelling urinary catheterization*, Arch. Intern. Med. 110:703, 1962   5-9

MOSTOFI, FK AND SMITH, DE: *The Kidney*, The Williams and Wilkins Company, Baltimore, 1966   1-4, 11-12, 16-19, 21-36

NEUMANN, CG AND PRYLES, CV: *Pyelonephritis in infants and children. Autopsy experience at the Boston City Hospital 1933-1960*, Amer. J. Dis. Child. 104:215, 1962   5-9

NORDENFELT, O AND RINGERTZ, N: *Phenacetin takers dead with renal failure—27 men and 3 women*, Acta Med. Scand. 170:385, 1961   10

O'SULLIVAN, DJ et al: *Urinary tract infection. A comparative study in the diabetic and general populations*, Brit. Med. J. 1:786, 1961   5-9

PALUBINSKAS, AJ: *Medullary sponge kidney*, Radiology 76:911, 1961   20

PAQUIN, AJ, Jr. MARSHALL, VF, AND McGOVERN, JH: *The megocystic syndrome*, J. Urol. 83:634, 1960   5-9

PAWLOWSKI, JM, BLOXDORF, JW, AND KIMMELSTIEL, P: *Chronic pyelonephritis: a morphologic and bacteriologic study*, New Eng. J. Med. 268:965, 1963   5-9

PEARSON, HH: *Residual renal defects in nonfatal phenacetin nephritis*, Med. J. Aust. 2:308, 1967   10

PRESCOTT, LF: *Effects of acetylsalicylic acid, phenacetin, paracetamol, and caffeine on renal tubular epithelium*, Lancet 2:91, 1965   10

PUTSCHAR, W: *Die entzündlichen Erkrankungen der ableitenden Harnwege und der Nierenhüllen, einschliesslich der Pyelonephritis und der Pyonephrose* in *Handbuch der Speziellen Pathologischen Anatomie und Histologie*, Vol. 6, Part II, ed. by Henke, F and Lubarsch, O, Springer-Verlag, Berlin 1934   5-9

ROSS, JH AND ROSS, IP: *The value of renal biopsy*, Lancet 2:559, 1957   5-9

SANJURJO, LA: *Parasitic diseases of the genitourinary system* in *Urology*, 3rd ed., ed. by Campbell, MF and Harrison, JH, W. B. Saunders Company, Philadelphia, 1970   13

SARMA, KP: *Tumors of the Urinary Bladder*, Appleton-Century-Crofts, Inc., New York, 1969   1-4, 11-12, 16-19, 21-36

SCHREINER, GE: *Clinical and histological spectrum of pyelonephritis*, Arch. Intern. Med. 102:32, 1958   5-9

SCHREINER, GE: *The nephrotoxicity of analgesic abuse*, Ann. Intern. Med. 57:1047, 1962   10

SHELLEY, JH: *Phenacetin, through the looking glass*, Clin. Pharmacol. Ther. 8:427, 1967   10

SMITH, JF: *The diagnosis of scars of chronic pyelonephritis*, J. Clin. Path. 15:522, 1962   5-9

SORENSEN, AW: *Is the relation between analgesics and renal disease coincidental and not causal?* Nephron 3:366, 1966   10

SPÜHLER, von O AND ZOLLINGER, HU: *Die Chronisch-interstitielle Nephritis*, Z. klin. Med. 151:1, 1953   10

STRAUSS, MB: *Microcystic disease of the renal medulla* in *Diseases of the Kidney*, 2nd ed., ed. by Strauss, MB and Welt, LG, Little, Brown and Company, 1971   20

SZÜCS, S et al: *The relation between diabetes mellitus and infections of the urinary tract*, Amer. J. Med. Sci. 240:186, 1960   5-9

THELEN, A, ROTHER, K, AND SARRE, H: *Experimental studies on the pathogenesis of pyelonephritic contracted kidney*, Urol. Int. 3:359, 1956   5-9

THOMSEN, A: *The significance of renal biopsy for the diagnosis of pyelonephritis in diabetic patients* in *Renal Biopsy: Clinical and Pathological Significance* in *Ciba Foundation Symposium* ed. by Wolstenholme, GEW and Cameron, MP, Little, Brown and Company, Boston, 1961   5-9

VERNIER, RL: *Kidney biopsy in the study of renal disease*, Pediat. Clin. N. Amer. 7:353, 1960   5-9

VIVALDI, E: *Effect of chronic administration of analgesics on resistance to experimental infection of the urinary tract in rats*, Nephron, 5:202, 1968   10

VIVALDI, E et al: *Experimental pyelonephritis consequent to induction of bacteriuria in Biology of Pyelonephritis*, Henry Ford Hospital Symposium, 1960   5-9

WALLACE, DM et al: *Tumours of the Bladder*, E. & S. Livingstone Ltd., Edinburgh, 1959   1-4, 11-12, 16-19, 21-36

WEISS, S AND PARKER, F, Jr: *Pyelonephritis; its relation to vascular lesions and to arterial hypertension*, Medicine 18:221, 1939   5-9

WEISS, S AND PARKER, F, Jr: *Relation of pyelonephritis and other urinary-tract infections to arterial hypertension*, New Eng. J. Med. 223:959, 1940   5-9

Section VII

AAS, TN: *Ureterocele: a clinical study of sixty-eight cases in fifty-two adults*, Brit. J. Urol. 32:133, 1960   14

ABESHOUSE, BS AND ABESHOUSE, GA: *Calyceal diverticulum: report of sixteen cases and review of the literature*, Urol. Int. 15:329, 1963   11

ABESHOUSE, BS AND BHISITKUL, I: *Crossed renal ectopia with and without fusion*, Urol. Int. 9:63, 1959   10

ALBERS, DD, GEYER, JR, AND BARNES, SE: *Blind-ending branch of bifid ureter: report of three cases*, J. Urol. 99:160, 1968   13

ALKEN, CE et al, Editors: *Encyclopedia of Urology*, Vols. XV and VII/1, Springer-Verlag, New York   5-6

AMAR, AD AND SCHEER, CW: *Ureterocele with associated vesicoureteral reflux*, J. Urol. 92:197, 1964   12

AMBROSE, SS AND NICOLSON, WP: *Ureteral reflux in duplicated ureters*, J. Urol. 92:439, 1964   12

AMESUR, NR AND SINGH, JP: *Crossed renal ectopia*, Brit. J. Urol. 35:11, 1963   9

ANDERSON, EE AND HARRISON, JH: *Surgical importance of the solitary kidney*, New Eng. J. Med. 273:683, 1965   1

ANNAMUNTHODO, H: *Multicystic disease of the kidney in the newborn: report of two cases*, Brit. J. Urol. 32:34, 1960   4

ASHLEY, DJ AND MOSTOFI, FK: *Renal agenesis and dysgenesis*, J. Urol. 83:211, 1960   1, 3

BÄCKLUND, L, GROTTE, G, AND REUTERSKIÖLD, A: *Functional Stenosis as a cause of pelviureteric obstruction and hydronephrosis*, Arch. Dis. Child. 40:203, 1965   11

BAIN, AD AND SCOTT, JS: *Renal agenesis and severe urinary tract dysplasia: a review of 50 cases, with particular reference to the associated anomalies*, Brit. Med. J. 1:841, 1960   3

BARNETT, JS AND STEPHENS, FD: *The role of the lower segmental vessel in the aetiology of hydronephrosis*, Aust. New Zeal. J. Surg. 31:201, 1962   11

BARTMAN, J AND BARRACLOUGH, G: *Cystic dysplasia of the kidneys studied by micro-

dissection in a case of 13-15 trisomy*, J. Path. Bact. 89:233, 1965   4

BAURYS, W AND WENTZELL, RA: *Bifid blind-ending ureter*, Amer. J. Surg. 94:499, 1957   13

BERDON, WE et al: *Ectopic ureterocele*, Radiol. Clin. N. Amer. 6:205, 1968   14

BERLIN, HS, STEIN, J, AND POPPEL, MH: *Congenital superior ectopia of the kidney*, Amer. J. Roentgen. 78:508, 1957   9

BERNSTEIN, J: *Development abnormalities of the renal parenchyma—renal hypoplasia and dysplasia*, Pathol. Annu. 3:213, 1968   3

BERNSTEIN, J AND MEYER, R: *Parenchymal maldevelopment of the kidney* in *Brennemann's Practice of Pediatrics*, Vol. 3, Hoeber Med. Div., Harper and Row, Hagerstown, 1967   3

BERNSTEIN, J AND MEYER, R: *Some speculations on the nature and significance of developmentally small kidneys (renal hypoplasia)*, Nephron 1:137, 1964   2

BLUNDON, KE: *The treatment of retrocaval ureter in the solitary kidney*, J. Urol. 88:29, 1962   15

BODIAN, M: *Some observations on the pathology of congenital idiopathic bladder-neck obstruction*, Brit. J. Urol. 29:393, 1957   19

BOISSANAT, P: *What to call hypoplastic kidney?* Arch. Dis. Child. 37:142, 1962   2

BOYDEN, EA: *Congenital absence of the kidney*, Anat. Rec. 52:325, 1932   1

BUCKALEW, VM, Jr et al: *Incomplete renal tubular acidosis*, Amer. J. Med. 45:32, 1968   26-27

BURKE, EC, WENZL, JE, AND UTZ, DC: *The intrathoracic kidney. Report of a case*, Amer. J. Dis. Child. 113:487, 1967   9

BURNS, E, CUMMINS, H, AND HYMAN, J: *Incomplete reduplication of bladder with congenital solitary kidney; report of case*, J. Urol. 57:257, 1947   20

BURWELL, RG AND KENT, SG: *The solitary ectopic pelvic kidney: case report with a review*, Brit. J. Urol. 31:254, 1959   1, 9

CAMPBELL, JE: *Ureteral peristalsis in duplex renal collecting systems*, Amer. J. Roentgen. 99:577, 1967   13

CAMPBELL, M: *Primary megalo-ureter*, J. Urol. 68:584, 1952   18

CAMPBELL, MF: *Anomalies of the kidney* in *Urology*, Vol. 2, 3rd ed., ed. by Campbell, MF and Harrison, JH, W. B. Saunders Company, Philadelphia, 1970   8, 10, 13, 17, 19-20

CAMPBELL, MF, Editor: *Urology*, W. B. Saunders Company, Philadelphia, 1963   5-6

CARLSON, HE: *Supernumerary kidney: summary of 51 reported cases*, J. Urol. 64:224, 1950   1

CHERRY, JW: *Patent urachus; review and report of case*, J. Urol. 63:693, 1950   17

CONSIDINE, J: *Retrocaval ureter: a review of the literature, with a report on two new cases followed for fifteen years and two years, respectively*, Brit. J. Urol. 38:412, 1966   15

CORBUS, BC, ESTREM, RD, AND HUNT, W: *Retro-iliac ureter*, J. Urol. 84:67, 1960   15

COX, CE AND HUTCH, JA: *Bilateral single ectopic ureter: a report of two cases and review of the literature*, J. Urol. 95:493, 1966   12

CRAIG, RD: *Unilateral multicystic disease of the kidney*, Brit. J. Urol. 34:19, 1962   4

CRAWHALL, JC et al: *Cystinosis; plasma cystine and cysteine concentrations and the effect of D-penicillamine and dietary treatment*, Amer. J. Med. 44:330, 1968   25

DAJANI, AM: *Horseshoe kidney: a review of twenty-nine cases*, Brit. J. Urol. 38:388, 1966   10

DOROSHOW, LW AND ABESHOUSE, BS: *Congenital unilateral solitary kidney: report of 37 cases and a review of the literature*, Urol. Survey 11:219, 1961   1

DORST, JP, CUSSEN, GH, AND SILVERMAN, FN: *Ureterocele in children, with emphasis on the frequency of ectopic ureteroceles*, Radiology 74:88, 1960   14

DOUGLAS, AW: *The ectopic ureter: a cause of female urinary incontinence*, New Zeal. Med. J. 61:487, 1962   12

EKSTRÖM, T: *Renal Hypoplasia: a clinical study of 179 cases*, Acta Chir. Scand., Suppl. 203, 1955   2

Continued on page 282

EKSTRÖM, T, AND NILSON, AE: *Retrocaval ureter; two roentgenographically diagnosed and surgically corrected cases*, Acta Chir. Scand. 118:53, 1959 — 15

ELKINGTON, JR et al: *The renal excretion of hydrogen ion in renal tubular acidosis. I. Quantitative assessment of the response to ammonium chloride as an acid load*, Amer. J. Med. 29:554, 1960 — 26-27

ELLERKER, AG: *The extravesical ectopic ureter*, Brit. J. Surg. 45:344, 1958 — 12

ERICSSON, NO: *Ectopic ureterocele in infants and children; clinical study*, Acta Chir. Scand. (suppl. 197) 1954 — 14

ERICSSON, NO, RUDHE, U, AND LIVADITIS, A: *Hydronephrosis associated with aberrant renal vessels in infants and children*, Surgery 50:687, 1961 — 11

FALKINBURG, LW, KAY, MN, AND KLUTZ, WS: *Crossed renal ectopia without fusion; report of a case in a seven-month-old female infant, with review*, Amer. J. Dis. Child. 99:86, 1960 — 9

FINE, MG AND BURNS, E: *Unilateral multicystic kidney: report of six cases and discussion of the literature*, J. Urol. 81:42, 1959 — 4

GLENN, JF: *Analysis of 51 patients with horseshoe kidney*, New Eng. J. Med. 261:684, 1959 — 10

GOLDBLOOM, RB et al: *Hereditary renal disease associated with nerve deafness and ocular lesions*, Pediatrics 20:241, 1957 — 22

GRUENWALD, P: *Normal changes in position of embryonic kidney*, Anat. Rec. 85:163, 1943 — 8

HARVARD, BM AND THOMPSON, GJ: *Congenital exstrophy of urinary bladder; late results of treatment by Coffey-Mayo method of ureterointestinal anastomosis*, J. Urol. 65:223, 1951 — 21

HEPTINSTALL, RH: *Pathology of the Kidney*, Little, Brown and Company, Boston, 1966 — 5-6

HIGGINS, CC: *Exstrophy of the bladder: review of 156 cases*, J.A.M.A. 171:1922, 1959 — 21

HILL, JE AND BUNTS, RC: *Thoracic kidney: case report*, J. Urol. 84:460, 1960 — 9

HILSON, D: *Malformation of ears as sign of malformation of genito-urinary tract*, Brit. Med. J. 2:785, 1957 — 1

HIROOKA, M, KUBOTA, N, AND OHNO, T: *Congenital nephropathy associated with hearing loss, ocular abnormalities, mental retardation, convulsions and abnormal E.E.G.*, Tohoku J. Exp. Med. 98:329, 1969 — 22

HUTCH, JA, HINMAN, F, Jr, AND MILLER, ER: *Reflux as a cause of hydronephrosis and chronic pyelonephritis*, J. Urol. 88:169, 1962 — 11

JOHNSTON, JH: *Hydro-ureter and mega-ureter* in *Paediatric Urology* ed. by Williams, DI, Appleton-Century-Crofts, Inc., New York, 1968 — 18

JOHNSTON, JH: *Urinary tract duplication in childhood*, Arch. Dis. Child. 36:180, 1961 — 12

KANASAWA, M et al: *Dwarfed kidneys in children. The classification, etiology, and significance of bilateral small kidneys in 11 children*, Amer. J. Dis. Child. 109:130, 1965 — 2

KJELLBERG, SR, ERICSSON, NO, AND RUDHE, U: *The lower urinary tract in childhood: some correlated clinical and roentgenologic observations* in *Ectopic Ureter and Ureterocele*, Year Book Medical Publishers, Inc., Chicago, 1957 — 12

KRON, SD AND MERANZE, DR: *Completely fused pelvic kidney*, J. Urol. 62:278, 1949 — 10

LANE, V: *The ectopic ureter: an elusive cause of urinary incontinence in the female*, Lancet 1:937, 1962 — 12

LATTIMER, JK AND SMITH, MJV: *Exstrophy closure: a followup on 70 cases*, J. Urol. 95:356, 1966 — 21

LEADBETTER, GW, Jr AND LEADBETTER, WF: *Diagnosis and treatment of congenital bladder-neck obstruction in children*, New Eng. J. Med. 260:633, 1959 — 19

LEIBOWITZ, S AND BODIAN, M: *A study of the vesical ganglia in children and the relationship of the megaureter megacystis syndrome and Hirschsprung's disease*, J. Clin. Path. 16:342, 1963 — 18

LENAGHAN, D: *Bifid ureters in children: an anatomical, physiological and clinical study*, J. Urol. 87:808, 1962 — 12

LICH, R, Jr: *The obstructed ureteropelvic junction*, Radiology 68:337, 1957 — 11

LICH, R, Jr AND BARNES, ML: *A clinicopathologic study of ureteropelvic obstruction*, J. Urol. 77:382, 1957 — 11

LJUNGQVIST, A AND LAGERGREN, C: *The Ask-Upmark kidney: a congenital renal anomaly studied by micro-angiography and histology*, Acta Path. Microbiol. Scand. 56:277, 1962 — 3

LONGENECKER, CG, RYAN, RF, AND VINCENT, RW: *Malformations of the ear as a clue to urogenital anomalies; report of six additional cases*, Plast. Reconstr. Surg. 35:303, 1965 — 1

LOWSLEY, OS AND KIRWIN, TJ: *Clinical Urology*, The Williams and Wilkins Company, Baltimore, 1956 — 5-6

LYON, RP AND SMITH, DR: *Distal urethral stenosis*, J. Urol. 89:414, 1963 — 19

LYON, RP AND TANAGHO, EA: *Distal urethral stenosis in little girls*, J. Urol. 93:379, 1965 — 19

MARQUARDT, CR AND PICK, JW: *True supernumerary, accessory or third kidney: report of a case*, Proc. N. cent. Sect. Amer. urol. Ass. p. 49, 1957 — 1

MARSHALL, VF AND MUECKE, EC: *Variations in exstrophy of the bladder*, J. Urol. 88:766, 1962 — 21

MATHE, CP: *Diminutive kidney, congenital hypoplasia and atrophic pyelonephritis*, Calif. Med. 84:110, 1956 — 2

MATHIESON, AJM: *Calyceal diverticulum: case with discussion and review of condition*, Brit. J. Urol. 25:147, 1953 — 11

McCRORY, WW et al: *Symposium on disorders in growth arising from renal tubular dysfunctions; introduction and commentary on renal rickets*, J. Pediat. 57:1, 1960 — 24-27

McCRORY, WW, SHIBUYA, M, AND WORTHEN, HG: *Hereditary renal glomerular disease in infancy and childhood*, Advances Pediat. 14:253, 1966 — 22

MITCHELL, JP: *Association of valves in the posterior urethra with bladder-neck obstruction*, Acta Urol. Belg. 31:507, 1963 — 19

MORRIS, RC, Jr: *Renal tubular acidosis. Mechanisms, classification and implications*, New Eng. J. Med. 281:1405, 1969 — 26-27

MUECKE, EC: *The role of the cloacal membrane in exstrophy: the first successful experimental study*, J. Urol. 92:659, 1964 — 21

MULROW, PJ et al: *Hereditary nephritis. Report of a kindred*, Amer. J. Med. 35:737, 1963 — 22

NESBIT, RM AND LABARDINI, MM: *Urethral valves in the male child*, J. Urol. 96:218, 1966 — 19

NIXON, HH: *Hydronephrosis in children: clinical study of 78 cases with special reference to role of aberrant renal vessels and results of conservative operations*, Brit. J. Surg. 40:601, 1953 — 11

NUNN, IN AND STEPHENS, FD: *The triad syndrome: a composite anomaly of the abdominal wall, urinary system and testes*, J. Urol. 86:782, 1961 — 16

OLSSON, O AND WHOLEY, M: *Vascular abnormalities in gross anomalies of kidneys*, Acta Radiol. (Diagn) 2:420, 1964 — 10

PAQUIN, AJ, Jr: *Ureterovesical anastomosis: the description and evaluation of a technique*, J. Urol. 82:573, 1959 — 18

PARKER, RA AND PEIL, CF: *The nephrotic syndrome in the first year of life*, Pediatrics 25:967, 1960 — 23

PERKOFF, GT et al: *A follow-up study of hereditary chronic nephritis*, Arch. Intern. Med. 102:733, 1958 — 22

PHOKITIS, P: *The supernumerary kidney*, Urol. Int. 17:265, 1964 — 1

PITT, DC: *Retrocaval ureter: a case diagnosed preoperatively by intravenous and retrograde pyelography*, Radiology 84:699, 1965 — 15

POTTER, EL: *Bilateral absence of ureters and kidneys: report of 50 cases*, Obstet. Gynec. 25:3, 1965 — 1

POTTER, EL: *Facial characteristics of infants with bilateral renal agenesis*, Amer. J. Obstet. Gynec. 51:885, 1946 — 1

PRESMAN, D AND FIRFER, R: *Diagnostic method for retrocaval ureter*, Amer. J. Surg. 92:628, 1956 — 15

QURESHI, MA AND MULVANEY, WP: *Retrocaval ureter: report of two cases*, Amer. Surg. 31:50, 1965 — 15

ROWLAND, HS, BUNTS, RC, AND IWANO, JH: *Operative correction of retrocaval ureter: a report of four cases and review of the literature*, J. Urol. 83:820, 1960 — 15

ROYER, P et al: *L'Hypoplasie renale bilaterale avec oligonephronie*, Arch. Franc. Pediat. 24:249, 1967 — 3

RUBENSTEIN, M, MEYER, R, AND BERNSTEIN, J: *Congenital abnormalities of the urinary system. I. A postmortem survey of developmental anomalies and acquired congenital lesions in children's hospital*, J. Pediat. 58:356, 1961 — 2-3

SAINT-YVES, IF: *Problems associated with the diagnosis of solitary kidney: congenital or acquired?* Brit. J. Urol. 36:347, 1964 — 1

SCHAFER, IA, SCRIVER, CR, AND EFRON, ML: *Familial hyperprolinemia, cerebral dysfunction and renal anomalies occurring in a family with hereditary nephropathy and deafness*, New Eng. J. Med. 267:51, 1962 — 22

SCHNEIDER, JA, BRADLEY, K, AND SEEGMILLER, JE: *Increased cystine in leukocytes from individuals homozygous and heterozygous for cystinosis*, Science 157:1321, 1967 — 25

SCHNEIDER, JA, WONG, V, AND SEEGMILLER, JE: *The early diagnosis of cystinosis*, J. Pediat. 74:114, 1969 — 25

SCHULMAN, JD, BRADLEY, KH, AND SEEGMILLER, JE: *Cystine: compartmentalization within lysosomes in cystinotic leukocytes*, Science 166:1152, 1969 — 25

SELBY, GW AND PARMALEE, AH, Jr: *Bilateral renal agenesis and oligohydramnios*, J. Pediat. 48:70, 1956 — 1

SENGER, FL AND SANTARE, VJ: *Congenital multilocular bladder: case report*, J. Urol. 68:283, 1952 — 20

SHILLER, WR AND WISWELL, OB: *A fused pelvic (cake) kidney*, J. Urol. 78:9, 1957 — 10

SIBLEY, WL: *Cyst of urachus*, Amer. J. Surg. 79:465, 1950 — 17

SLUNGAARD, RK AND JAECK, JL: *Bilateral dwarfed kidneys*, Amer. J. Dis. Child. 97:575, 1959 — 2

SPENCE, HM: *Congenital unilateral multicystic kidney: entity to be distinguished from polycystic kidney disease and other cystic disorders*, J. Urol. 74:693, 1955 — 4

SPENCE, HM: *Ureterosigmoidostomy for exstrophy of bladder: Results in personal series of thirty-one cases*, Brit. J. Urol. 38:36, 1966 — 21

SPENCE, HM AND ALLEN, T: *Congenital absence of abdominal musculature. Urologic aspects*, J.A.M.A. 187:814, 1964 — 16

STEINER, MM AND OECONOMOPOULOS, CT: *Double lower genitourinary system in a child*, J. Urol. 85:540, 1961 — 20

STEPHENS, FD: *Intramural ureter and ureterocele*, Postgrad. Med. J. 40:179, 1964 — 14

STRAUSS, MB: *Clinical and pathological aspects of cystic disease of the renal medulla: an analysis of eighteen cases*, Ann. Intern. Med. 57:373, 1962 — 7

STRAUSS, MB: *Microcystic disease of the renal medulla* in *Diseases of the Kidney*, 2nd ed., ed. by Strauss, MB and Welt, LG, Little, Brown and Company, Boston, 1971 — 7

STRAUSS, MB AND SOMMERS, SC: *Medullary cystic disease and familial juvenile nephronophthisis: clinical and pathological identity*, New Eng. J. Med. 277:863, 1967 — 7

SWENSEN, O, FISHER, JH, AND CENDRON, J: *Megaloureter: investigation as to the cause and report on the results of newer forms of treatment*, Surgery 40:223, 1956 — 18

TAUBER, J AND BLOOM, B: *Infected urachal cysts*, J. Urol. 66:692, 1951 — 17

THOMPSON, GJ, AND KELALIS, PP: *Ureterocele: clinical appraisal of 176 cases*, J. Urol. 91:488, 1964 — 14

THOMPSON, RF: *Renal hypoplasia*, Trans. S. cent. Sect. Amer. urol. Ass., p. 10, 1957 — 2

TRACKLER, RT AND McALISTER, WH: *Obstruction of the lower ureter by the distal hypogastric (umbilical) artery*, Amer. J. Roentgen. 98:160, 1966 — 15

UEHLING, D AND BARBER, KE: *Unilateral multicystic kidney*, J. Urol. 96:286, 1966 — 4

USON, CU, LATTIMER, JK, AND MELICOW, MM:

Ureteroceles in infants and children: a report based on 44 cases, Pediatrics 27:971, 1961   14

VELLIOS, F AND GARRETT, RA: Congenital unilateral multicystic disease of the kidney, Amer. J. Clin. Path. 35:244, 1961   4

VICTOR, I AND SU, CT: Horseshoe kidney associated with tumor: review of literature and case report of resection of inferior vena cava, J. Urol. 93:669, 1965   10

WARD, JN, NATHANSON, B, AND DRAPER, JW: The pelvic kidney, J. Urol. 94:36, 1965   9

WATERHOUSE, K AND HAMM, FC: The importance of urethral valves as a cause of vesical neck obstruction in children, Trans. Amer. Ass. Genitourin. Surg. 53:138, 1961   19

WEHRBEIN, HL: Double kidney and ureter, and bilocular bladder in child, J. Urol. 43:804, 1940   20

WEYRAUCH, HM, Jr: Anomalies of renal rotation, Surg. Gynec. Obstet. 69:183, 1939   8

WHALEN, RE et al: Hereditary nephropathy, deafness and renal foam cells, Amer. J. Med. 31:171, 1961   22

WILLIAMS, DI: Agenesis of the abdominal muscles in Paediatric Urology, ed. by Williams, DI, Appleton-Century-Crofts, Inc., New York, 1968   16

WILLIAMS, DI: Mega-ureter, Postgrad. Med. J. 34:159, 1958   18

WILLIAMS, DI: Reflux in double ureters, Proc. Roy. Soc. Med. 55:423, 1962   12

WILLIAMS, DI AND BURKHOLDER, GV: The prune belly syndrome, J. Urol. 98:244, 1967   16

WILLIAMS, DI, CHIR, M, AND KARLAFTIS, CM: Hydronephrosis due to pelvi-ureteric obstruction in the newborn, Brit. J. Urol. 38:138, 1966   11

WILLIAMS, DI AND MININBERG, DT: Hydrocalycosis: report of three cases in children, Brit. J. Urol. 40:541, 1968   11

WILLIAMS, DI AND WOODARD, JR: Problems in the management of ectopic ureteroceles, J. Urol. 92:635, 1964   14

WITZLEBEN, CL: Complete frontal septum of the bladder, J. Urol. 94:427, 1965   20

WORTHEN, HG: Renal tubular disorders in Brennemann-Kelley Practice of Pediatrics, Vol. 3, W. F. Prior Company, Hagerstown, 1966   24-27

WORTHEN, HG AND GOOD, RA: The de Toni-Fanconi syndrome with cystinosis; clinical and metabolic study of two cases in a family and a critical review on the nature of the syndrome, Amer. J. Dis. Child. 95:653, 1958   25

WORTHEN, HG, VERNIER, RL, AND GOOD, RA: Infantile nephrosis; clinical, biochemical, and morphologic studies of the syndrome, Amer. J. Dis. Child. 98:73!, 1959   23

Section VIII

ABEL, JJ, ROUNTREE, LG, AND TURNER, BB: On the removal of diffusible substances from the circulating blood of living animals by dialysis, J. Pharmacol. Exp. Ther. 5:275, 1914   6-10

ALKEN, CE et al, Editors: Encyclopedia of Urology, Vol. XIII/1, Springer-Verlag, New York   18-19

BANK, N: Physiological basis of diuretic action, Ann. Rev. Med. 19:103, 1968   1-4

BARTTER, FC, Editor: Clinical Use of Aldosterone Antagonists, Charles C Thomas, Springfield, Ill., 1960   1-4

BERLINER, RW AND ORLOFF, J: Carbonic anhydrase inhibitors, Pharmacol. Rev. 8:137, 1956   1-4

BERLYNE, GM AND HOCKEN, AG: Dietary therapy of chronic renal failure in Nutrition in Renal Disease ed. by Berlyne, GM, E. & S. Livingstone Ltd., London, 1968   5

CANNON, PJ et al: Ethacrynic acid: effectiveness and mode of diuretic action in man, Circulation 31:5, 1965   1-4

CLAPP, JR, NOTTEBOHM, GA, AND ROBINSON, RR: Proximal site of action of ethacrynic acid—importance of filtration rate, Amer. J. Physiol. 220:1355, 1971   1-4

CROSLEY, AP, Jr et al: Triamterene, a new natriuretic agent. Preliminary observations in man, Ann. Intern. Med. 56:241, 1962   1-4

DAMMIN, GJ AND MERRILL, JP: Transplantation, tissue rejection, and the kidney in Structural Basis of Renal Disease ed. by Becker, EL, Hoeber Medical Division, Harper and Row, New York, 1968   12-15

DEBAKEY, ME AND MORRIS, GC, Jr: Conservative vascular surgery in renal hypertension, in Scientific Foundations in Surgery ed. by Wells, C and Kyle, J, American Elsevier Publishing Company, Inc., New York, 1967   16-17

DEBAKEY, ME et al: Coarctation of the abdominal aorta with renal arterial stenosis: surgical considerations, Ann. Surg. 165:830, 1967   16-17

DIRKS, JH, CIRKSENA, WJ, AND BERLINER, RW: Micropuncture study of the effect of various diuretics on sodium reabsorption by the proximal tubules of the dog, J. Clin. Invest. 45:1875, 1966   1-4

GIORDANO, C et al: Dietary treatment in renal failure in Proceedings of 3rd International Congress of Nephrology, Vol. 3, Clinical Nephrology ed. by Becker, EL, S. Karger, Basle, 1967   5

GIOVANNETTI, S: Diet in chronic uremia in Proceedings of International Congress of Nephrology, Vol. 3, Clinical Nephrology ed. by Becker, EL, S. Karger, Basle, 1967   5

GLASSROCK, RJ et al: Human renal isografts: a clinical and pathologic analysis, Medicine 47:411, 1968   12-15

GLENN, JF AND BOYCE, WH: Urologic Surgery, Hoeber Medical Division, Harper and Row, New York, 1969   18-19

KOLFF, WJ: New Ways of Treating Uremia: The Artificial Kidney, Peritoneal Lavage, Intestinal Lavage, J. & A. Churchill, Ltd., London, 1947   6-10

LARAGH, JH: The mode of action and use of chlorothiazide and related compounds, Circulation 26:121, 1962   1-4

LINDQUIST, RR et al: Human renal allografts. Interpretation of morphologic and immunohistochemical observations, Amer. J. Path. 53:851, 1968   12-15

LOWRIE, EG et al: Survival of patients undergoing chronic hemodialysis and renal transplantation, New Eng. J. Med. 288:863, 1973   12-15

MERRILL, JP: Biologic problems raised by the observations of organ transplants in Advance in Transplantation ed. by Dausset, J, Hamburger, J, and Mathe, G, Proc. First Int. Cong. of Transpl. Soc., The Williams and Wilkins Company, Baltimore, 1968   12-15

MERRILL, JP: What the family physician should know about transplantation, Sandoz Panorama, 7:12, 1969   12-15

MERRILL, JP et al: Successful homotransplantation of the human kidney between identical twins, J.A.M.A. 160:277, 1956   12-15

MERRILL, JP et al: Successful homotransplantation of the kidney between nonidentical twins, New Eng. J. Med. 262:1251, 1960   12-15

MORRIS, GC, Jr AND DEBAKEY, ME: Renal arterial hypertension in Cardiovascular Disorders ed. by Brest, AN and Moyer, JH, F. A. Davis Co., Philadelphia, 1968   16-17

MORRIS, GC, Jr, DEBAKEY, ME, AND ZANGER, LCC: Renovascular hypertension, Surg. Clin. N. Amer. 46:931, 1966   16-17

SCHREINER, GE: Dialysis of poisons and drugs—annual review, Trans. Amer. Soc. Artif. Intern. Organs 16:544, 1970   11

SCHREINER, GE AND MAHER, JF: Uremia: Biochemistry, Pathogenesis, and Treatment, Charles C Thomas, Springfield, Ill., 1961   6-10

SELDIN, DW et al: Localization of diuretic action from the pattern of water and electrolyte excretion, Ann. N. Y. Acad. Sci. 139:273, 1966   1-4

STASON, WB et al: Furosemide: a clinical evaluation of its diuretic action, Circulation 34:910, 1966   1-4

Subject Index

(Numerals refer to pages, not plates. Boldface numerals indicate major emphasis.)

Cheyne-Stokes breathing, 263
Chinard theory of glomerular filtration, 39
chloride, 40
  and diuretics, 253, 255
  reabsorption of, **48**, 53, 55, 57, 59, 115, 116, 246, 254
  in renal tubular acidosis, 249
  in sodium pump, 47, 48
chloride shift, 62
chlormerodrin, 103, 106, 206, 207, 214
chlorothiazide, 246, 254, 256
cholesterol esters, 124, 125
chromatography, paper, 73, 74
chromogens, 45, 120
cineroentgenography, 97
circulation
  antibody, 129-130
  systemic, 39
circulation time, 98
circulatory diseases, 123
cirrhosis, *see* liver
claudication, 149
clearance
  calculation of, 43
  concept of, 40
  filtration, 111
  hydrogen ion, 87
  inulin, 39, 40
  osmolar, 82
  PAH, 42, 43, 156, 157, 247
  test protein and transferrin, 124
  urea/creatinine, 40, **44, 45, 83**, 84, 120-121, 122
clearance tests, 83
clitoris, 22, 34
  divided, 243
cloaca, 30, 31, 34
  exstrophy of, 243
clotting; clotting time, 260, 261
coagulation, 159-160
coil dialyzer, 259
"cold spots," 105, 106, 186, 207
collagen, 14, 150, 166
collagen disorders, 76, 113
collaterals, 25
collecting ducts, 31, 33, 53, 64
Colles' fascia, *see* fascia, Colles'
collimator, 103, 104, 105
colloid osmotic pressure, 39, 175
colon, 2, 3, 4, 35
columns, renal, of Bertin, 5
coma, 176, 263
complement, 128, 129, 130, 131, 133, 136, 137
complement sequence, 265
complexes
  antigen-antibody, 127, 133, 139, 142, 143
  circulating immune, 129-130
concentration gradient, 46, 47, 48, 62, 63, 64, 248
concentration test, 82
concussion, spinal, 220
conduit obstruction, 84
conjunctival plaques, 164
conjunctivitis, 119
connective tissue, retroperitoneal, 99
contrast media, 89, 91-96, 97, 98, 100, 101, 102, 108
  introduction of, 96
  reactions to, 91, 92-93
convolutions, renal tubular, 13, 33
convulsions, 121
cord, spinal, 28, 29, 101, 220
cornea, cystine deposition in, 247
coronary artery disease, 154
cor pulmonale, 254, 256
corpus cavernosum, 20
corpuscles, renal, of Malpighi, 6, **7**, 8, **9**, 19, 33
corpus spongiosum, 20, 22
cortex, renal, 5, 6, 18, 44
  blood supply, 19
  in congestive heart failure, 175
  in cystinosis, 247
  enzyme activity in, 67
  in glomerulonephritis, 135
  in hemolytic-uremic syndrome, 159

cortex, renal—*continued*
  lymph vessels, 26
cortex, suprarenal, 49, 65, 116, 157, 158, 254
corticosteroids, 141, 142, 264
countercurrent mechanism, 51-55
  exchange (diffusion), 51, 54-55
  multiplication, 12, 13, 51, 52-53, 54, 55, 56
Cowper's gland, *see* glands, bulbourethral
creatinine, 83, 121, 122, 169, 176, 258, 262, 265
  in renal artery stenosis, 85, 86
  in renal failure, 120-121
creatinine clearance, **45, 83**, 84, 120-121, 122
crescent formation, 127, 128, 132, 133, 135, 137, 141, 142, 143
crest, iliac, 2, 3, 4
crush kidney, 111
cryptorchidism, 238, 243
crystals
  cholesterol ester, 124
  sodium iodide, 104, 105
  in urine, 80
Cushing's syndrome, 72, 74, 178
cyclophosphamide, 267
cylindroids, 75
cylindruria, 122, 131, 134, 164, 169, 176, 178, 244
cystine, 247
cystine calculi, 72, 200, 201
cystine crystals, 80
cystinosis, 178, 247
cystinuria, 80, 200
cystitis, 187-188, 190, 210, 211
  acute hemorrhagic, 188
  "bullous," 188
  chronic interstitial, 188
  from foreign bodies, 219
  glandular or cystic, 188, 209
  honeymoon, 191
  polypoid, 188
  ulcerative, 188
cystitis emphysematosa, 188
cystography, 97, 217, 218
cystometry, 88
cystoscopy, 96, 210, 211
cystotomy, 203, 211
cystourethrography, 97, 238
cysts
  benign, 102
  calyceal, 233
  and cystic disease, 227-228, 229
  distinguished from neoplasms, 94, 98, 100, 106
  hydatid, 197
  in renal dysplasia, 225, 226
  and renal osteodystrophy, 117
  in sponge kidney, 204
  urachal, 239
cytoplasm, 162, 172

D

dartos fascia, *see* fascia, dartos
deafness, 163
  nerve, 244
DeBakey grafts, 268, 269
defects (*see also* anomalies)
  acidification, 116
  filling, 93, 169, 170, 199, 208, 210
  generalized capillary, 125, 127
  glomerular, 180
  intrinsic tubular, 82
  tubular reabsorptive, 125, 127
defibrination syndrome, 159
dehydration, 82, 111, 173, 249, 256
  hypertonic, 246
  and IVP, 91, 92, 94, 95
  and renal failure, 116
  in uremia, 121
dementias, 163
demineralization
  bone, 229
  skull, 118
Denonvilliers, fascia of, *see* fascia, rectovesical
dense deposits ("humps"), 129, 130

desmosomes, 14
de Toni-Fanconi syndrome, *see* Fanconi syndrome
dextran, 112
diabetes, 139, 220
  and cystitis, 187
  hereditary and nonhereditary, 151
  nodular glomerulosclerosis of, 136
diabetes insipidus, 82, 240, **246**
  nephrogenic, **246**, 247
diabetes mellitus, 41, 73, 74, 77, 123, 163, 164, 178, 189
diabetic nephropathy, 149-152
diabetic nephropathy, 149-152
dialysance, 263
dialysis, 112, 121, 122, 159, 170, 257, 270
  for drugs and poisons, 263
  hemodialysis, 169, 258-262
  peritoneal, 169, 261, 262, 263
diaphragm, 2, 3, 197
  urogenital, 20, 21, 22, 29
diatrizoate sodium, 97, 98
dichlorphenamide, 256
diet
  acid-ash, 61
  high or low potassium, 50
  management of, in renal failure, 257
Dietl's crisis, 186
diffusion
  back, 19, 38, 44
  countercurrent, 54-55
"diffusion trapping," 64
digitalis intoxication, 254
digitalization, 112
dilatation
  bladder, 188, 238, 240
  collecting ducts, 204
  renal pelvis, 92
  ureteral, 92, 202, 238, 240, 241
dilution test, 82
dimercaprol, 169
diphtheria, 144
dipstick tests, 72, 73, 74, 81
disequilibrium syndrome, 121
distal RTA (renal tubular acidosis), 115, 116
diuresis, 44, 58, 95, 112, 121, 127, 131, 178
  in hemorrhagic fever, 181
  isotonic or hypotonic, 253, 254
  osmotic, 114, 116, 121, 263
diuretics, 246, 253-256
  carbonic anhydrase inhibitors, 253-254
  ethacrynic acid and furosemide, 255
  mercurials, 253
  osmotic, 255-256
  potassium-retaining, 254-255
  and PSP test, 84
  thiazides, 254
diverticula
  bladder, **218**, 242
  congenital calyceal, 233
  urachal, 239, 242
  ureteric, 235
diverticulitis, 185, 187
DNA (deoxyribonucleic acid), 143
donors, kidney, 264, 267
dose calibrator, 105
double-contrast study, 102
drainage
  lymphatic, 26
  by suprapubic tube, 203
  urinary, 217, 220
drip-infusion pyelography, **94**, 98
dropsy, *see* edema
drugs (*see also* specific drugs)
  analgesic, 169-170, 194, 263
  antibacterial, 187-188, 189
  anticoagulant, 128, 259, 262
  antimicrobial, 81
  antioxidant, 209-210, 211
  dialysis for, 263
  diuretic, 246, 253-256
  intoxication with, 254, 255
  and PSP test, 84
  reactions to, 144, 167
  and toxic nephropathy, 168

ducts
  collecting, 31, 33, 53, 64
  in dysplasia, 225
  ejaculatory, 234
  lymph, 26
  in medullary cystic disease, 229
  mesonephric (wolffian), 22, 30, 31, 34, 235
  metanephric, 30, 31, 34, 235
  müllerian, 34
  papillary (of Bellini), 5, 6, 14
  pronephric, 30
ductus deferens, *see* vas deferens
duodenum, 2, 4, 23
dyes, and tests of renal ischemia, 84, 86
dyscrasias, blood, 75
dysphagia, 164
dysplasia, renal, 225-226
dyspnea, 131, 164, 177

E

ecchymoses, 92, 122
echinococcus disease, 197
Echinococcus granulosus, 197
eclampsia, 159, 172
ectoderm, 30
ectopia, 231
  with fusion, 232
  ureteral, **235**, 236
edema
  in acute diffuse interstitial nephritis, 144
  in acute renal failure, 112
  in anaphylactoid purpura, 140
  bullous, 187, 188
  in diabetic nephropathy, 149
  diuretics for, 253-256
  in essential hypertension, 154
  in glomerulonephritis, 131, 134, 135, 244
  in hemorrhagic fever, 181
  in infantile nephrosis, 245
  interstitial, 173, 267
  in liver disease, 176
  nephrotic, 125-127
  in nephrotic syndrome, 123, 124, 125, 127
  pulmonary, 255, 256
  with renal allograft, 266
  in toxemia of pregnancy, 172
egg protein, 257
elastica interna, 19
electrical potential, 47, 48, 50
electrolytes, 246, 247, 253
electron microscopy, 112, 132-133
electrophoresis, 72, 73
embryology, 17, 22, 30, 31-33, 35
encephalopathy, 121, 131, 167
endarterectomy, 269
endocarditis, 75, 139, 141
endothelium, 7, 32, 128, 129, 130
  destruction of, 265, 266
  fenestrated, 19
  in glomerulonephritis, 132, 135, 136
  in nephroglomerulosis, 162
  in renal vein thrombosis, 173
energy, 11, 13
enteritis, 123
enzyme-dependent reactions, 62
enzymes, 11, 157, 158
  activity of, in nephron, 66-67
eosin methylene blue agar, 81
eosinophilis, 132, 140, 144, 167, 180
epispadias, 243
epithelium, 7, 128, 129, 130, 162, 266
  in acute renal failure, 111, 112
  columnar, 225
  cuboidal, 204, 225
  in glomerulonephritis, 132, 135
  multilayered, 204
  neoplasms of, 208
  transitional, 24
  vacuolization of, 178
erythroblasts, 65
erythrocytes, 65, 133, 138, 139
erythrocytosis, 65
erythrogenin, 65
erythropoiesis, 65

erythropoiesis-stimulating factor (ESF or erythropoietin), 7, 65, 121
Escherichia coli, 76, 81, 190
esophagus, 2, 15
estimated renal plasma flow (ERPF), 43
estrogens, 65
ethacrynic acid, 47, 48, 50, 127, 254 **255**, 256
ethylene glycol poisoning, 170
event (gamma radiation), 105
excretion test (PSP), 84
exogenous antigen disease, 129
exstrophy, bladder, 243
extracellular transport paths, 48-49
extravasation
    intra- and extraperitoneal, 217
    venous, 92

F

Fanconi syndrome, 72, 84, 113, 116, 178, 247
fascia
    Buck's, 20
    Camper's, 20, 21
    Colles', 20, 22
    dartos, 20
    Denonvilliers', 20
    diaphragmatic, 4
    Gerota's, 4
    levator ani, 21
    lumbodorsal, 3, 270
    obturator, 21
    prostatic, 20, 22
    rectal, 20
    renal, **4**, 99, 270
    Scarpa's, 20, 21
    spermatic, 20
    transversalis, 4, 20, 21
    umbilical prevesical, 20, 21, 22
    vesical, 20, 22
fat
    free, 75, 77
    perirenal and pararenal, 4
fat bodies, 75, 76, 77, 123, 124, 125, 126
feedback mechanisms, 65
fenestration, 19
Ferrein's rays, see rays, medullary
fever, 191,194, 246, 253, 264, 265
    catheterization, 190
    epidemic hemorrhagic, 181
    of pyelonephritis, 189
fibers
    afferent and efferent, 28-29
    autonomic, 29
    collagenous, 14
    muscle; 22, 24
    parasympathetic, 28, 29
    sympathetic, 27, 28, 29
fibrin, 128, 133, 155, 160, 265, 266
fibrinogen, 160, 265
fibrinoid, 128, 141, 142, 155
fibroblasts, 265
fibroelastosis, 155, 241
fibroma, 205
fibroplasia, intimal, 155
fibrosarcoma, 206
fibrosis
    generalized, 225
    glomerular, 177, 193
    interstitial, 133, 136, 137, 145, 173, 178, 194, 244, 247
    intertubular and periglomerular, 179
    intimal, 153
    in polyarteritis nodosa, 167
    renal, 78
    retroperitoneal, 113
Fick principle, 43
filling defects, 93, 169, 170, 199, 208, 210
filtration, see glomerular filtration
filtration clearances, 111
filtration permeability factor, 39
fistula, arteriovenous, 100, 101, 260
flat-plate hemodialyzer, 259-260
flexure
    duodenojejunal, 4
    hepatic, of colon, 2
    splenic, of colon, 2

fluid
    accumulation of, in hemorrhagic fever, 181
    extracellular, 175, 256
    interstitial, 60, 125, 127, 175, 255
    tubular, 46, 47, 48, 49, 50, 51, 56, 58
fluoroscopy, 97, 100, 101, 102, 108
folds
    interureteric, 22
    mucosal, 24
    sacrogenital, 20
    umbilical, 21, 25
    urorectal, 34
    uterosacral, 23
foot-process disease, 123, 125, 126, 127
foot processes
    epithelial, 112
    glomerular capillary, 129, 130
    fused, 126, 127, 133, 136, 137, 141, 160, 162, 165, 173, 180, 245, 266, 267
foramen, obturator, 21
foregut, 30
foreign bodies in bladder, 187, 219
foreskin, 20
fossa
    intersigmoid, 23
    navicular, 20
    paravesical, 20
    rectovesical, 20
    renal, 2
    supravesical, 21
fractures, 117, 118
Franklin-Silverman needle, 107, 108
Frost method, 79
fructosuria, 73
furosemide, 50, 127, 254, **255**, 256
fusion
    of foot processes, see foot processes
    renal, 232

G

galactosuria, 73
gamma globulin
    in glomerulonephritis, 127, 128, 129, 130, 131, 133, 136, 137
    in kidney transplant, 265, 266, 267
    in lipoid nephrosis, 127
    in lupus nephritis, 141, 143
    in scleroderma, 166
gamma globulinemia, Waldenström's, 73
gamma scintillation camera, 103, 104-105
gammopathy, monoclonal, 165
ganglia
    aorticorenal, 27, 28, 29
    autonomic nervous system, 2
    celiac, 27, 29
    dorsal root, 28, 29
    mesenteric, 29
    renal, 27, 28, 29
    sympathetic, 27
    ureteric nerves, 27
gangrene, 149
gas insufflation, 99
Gerota's capsule; Gerota's fascia, see capsule; fascia
GFR (glomerular filtration rate), 40, **41**, 45, 49, 50, 175, 176, 178, 257
    and creatinine clearance, 83, 120-121
    in cystinosis, 247
    with diuretics, 253, 254, 255, 256
    in glomerulonephritis, 131, 134
    with myeloma, 180
    with nephron hypertrophy, 113, 114
    in nephrotic syndrome, 123, 127
    in renal insufficiency, 115, 116, 117, 119, 121
glands
    bulbourethral (Cowper's), 20
    cephalic, 198
    parathyroid, 229
    paraurethral, 34
    pituitary, 181, 246
    prostate, see prostate
    suprarenal, 2, 4, 5, 15, 207, 223, 224, 229

glands—continued
    thyroid, 65, 207
    urethral, 34
glans penis, 20, 71, 243
glaucoma, 163
globulins (see also gamma globulin)
    antibody, 264, 265
    antilymphocyte (ALG), 267
    immunofluorescent, 267
    in urine, 72
glomerular disease, 84, 113, **127-130**
glomerular filtration, 38, **39**, 41, 45
    in ischemia, 86
    and timed pyelography, 95
glomerular filtration rate, see GFR
glomerular selectivity, 124-125
glomeruli, 6, 7, 18 **19**, 56
    in acute renal failure, 111, 112
    amyloid deposit in, 165
    in analgesic abuse, 169
    in anti-GBM disease, 127, 128
    in congestive heart failure, 175
    in cyanotic congenital heart disease, 174
    in cystinosis, 247
    degenerating, 18
    development, 30, 32-33
    enzyme activity in, 66, 67
    hyalinization of, 161
    in infantile nephrosis, 245
    juxtamedullary, 6, 18, 19
    in kidney transplant, 266, 267
    lymph capillaries surrounding, 26
    in medullary cystic disease, 229
    in myeloma, 180
    in nephroglomerulosis, 162
    in polyarteritis nodosa, 167
    in pyelonephritis, 192
    in renal dysplasia, 225
    in renal vein thrombosis, 173
    in toxemia of pregnancy, 172
    with use of diuretics, 253, 254, 255
glomerulitis, 154
glomerulonephritis, 75, 92, 127-128, 129, 130, 172, 193, 267
    acute, 111, **131-132**, 173
    chronic, 124, 125, 126, **134-137**, 138, 153, 154, 174
    and chronic renal failure, 113
    diffuse, 132, 138
    exudative, 132
    focal, 123, 134, 137, 138, **139**, 174
    hereditary, 244
    lupus, 139
    matrix deposition in, 150, 151
    membranoproliferative (mesangio-capillary or lobular), 123, 127, 130, 135, 174
    membranous, 123, 124, 125, 126, 127, 136-137, 173
    and nephrotic syndrome, 123
    poststreptococcal, 130, 132, 133, 134, 139, 140
    proliferative, 124, 125, 126, 132
    rapidly progressive (extracapillary), 133
    recurrent, 139
glomerulonephropathy, membranous, 166
glomerulosclerosis, 128, 145, 176
    diabetic, 136, **149-151**, 152
    diffuse, 150-151
    focal and segmental, 127, 137
    intercapillary, 113, 124, 152
    lipoid nephrosis with, 123
    nodular, 136, 149-150, 151, 152
gluconeogenesis, 257
glucose, 255, 263
    glomerular filtration of, 41
    metabolism of, in renal failure, 122
    in urine, 41, **73-74**, 112
glucose-6-phosphate dehydrogenase (G-6-PDH), 66, 67
glutamate dehydrogenase (GLDH), 66, 67
glutamate oxaloacetate transaminase (GOT), 66, 67
glutamate pyruvate transaminase (GPT), 66, 67

glutaminase I and II, 66
glutamine, 60, 64, 66, 248
glutethimide, 263
glycinuria, 200
glycolysis, 67
glycoproteins, 150
glycosuria, 41, 73, 74, 247
Golgi apparatus, 10, 11, 12, 13, 14
gonorrhea, 81
Goodpasture's syndrome, 113, 130, 177
gout, 113, 168, 200
gradient (distal) RTA, 115, 116
graft (see also transplantation)
    bypass, 268-269
    patch, 269
    rejected, 264-265, 266, 267
granules, 7, 10, 11, 14
granulocytes, 112
granulomatosis, Wegener's, 167, 177
guanidosuccinate, 121
gut, primitive, 30

H

hamartoma, 205
Hank's solution, 77, 79
hay fever, 167
heart
    calcium deposits in, 119
    in hemorrhagic fever, 181
    metastases to, 207
heart disease, cyanotic congenital, 174
heart failure, 84, 123, 134, 149, 154, 155, 175, 255, 256
heat and acetic acid protein test, 72, 73
heavy metal poisoning, 113
hemangioma, 205
hematemesis, 140, 164
hematocrit level, 181
hematoma, 213, 220
hematoxylin bodies, 141, 143
hematoxylin and eosin (H. and E.) stain, 7, 10, 151
hematuria, 74, 75, 76, 78, 79, 94, 96, 101, 129
    in acute diffuse interstitial nephritis, 144
    with adenocarcinoma, 206
    in amyloidosis, 164
    in anaphylactoid purpura, 140
    in calcium nephropathy, 179
    with calculi, 201, 202, 203
    in echinococcus disease, 197
    in glomerulonephritis, 131, 134, 136, 138, 139, 244
    with hemangioma, 205
    in hydronephrosis, 233
    in lung purpura with nephritis, 177
    in lupus nephritis, 141, 142, 143
    in obstructive uropathy, 185, 186
    in papillary necrosis, 194
    in renal failure, 112, 122
    with renal transplant, 265
    in renal tuberculosis, 196
    in renovascular hypertension, 154
    with sponge kidney, 204
    in tóxic nephropathy, 170
    with tumors, 208, 210
hemecasts, 111, 112
hemodialysis, 121, 137, 169, 170 258-262, 263
    home, 261
    long-term, 260-261
    principles and history of, 258-259
    with regional heparinization, 261-262
hemoglobin, 62, 74
hemoglobinuria, 74
hemolysis, 159, 160
hemolytic-uremic syndrome (HUS), 159-160
hemoptysis, 164, 177
hemorrhage
    in carbon tetrachloride poisoning, 170
    cerebral, 140
    in essential hypertension, 154, 155
    in hemorrhagic fever, 181
    interstitial, 162

nicotinamide adenine dinucleotide (NAD), 67
"nil" disease, 123, 136
niridazole, 199
nitrazine paper, 72
nitrogen
  in blood, *see* azotemia
  and renal failure, 120, 121
  retention of, 140, 144
nitrogen balance, maintenance of, 257
nocturia, 178, 227, 246
nonstreptococcal infection, 138, 139
notching, pelvic or ureteral, 93-94
nuclear inclusion bodies, 168
nuclei
  dorsal vagal, 28
  renal tubular, 10, 12, 13, 14
  solitary tract, 28
  supraoptic, 51

O

obliterative vascular disease, 155
obstruction
  airway, 263
  causing diverticulum, 218
  conduit, 84
  congenital bladder outlet, 241
  intestinal, 72
  renal, 103, 191
  renal artery, 85-86, 157
  and renal dysplasia, 225
  ureteropelvic junction, 233
  urinary tract, 84, 111, 185-186, 201
obstructive arterial disease, 157
obstructive diseases, 113
obstructive uropathy, 121, 185-186, 211
oculocerebrorenal disease (Lowe's syndrome), 67
oligemia, 116, 121
oligohydramnios, 223, 238
oliguria, 82, 101, 253, 255, 265
  in glomerulonephritis, 131, 133, 244
  in hemorrhagic fever, 181
  in interstitial nephritis, 144
  in polyarteritis nodosa, 167
  in renal failure, 111, 121, 176
  in renovascular hypertension, 155
orifices, ureteral, 20, 21, 22, 23, 96, 196, 209, 218, 234, 235, 240, 243
ortho-amino-phenols, 209
orthopnea, 131
orthotolidine, 74
oscilloscope, 105
osmolality, 51, 52, 53, 54, 55, 56, 58, 82, 114, 121
osmolar ratio, urine-to-serum, 82
osmometer, 82
osmoreceptors, 51
osmotic diuretics, 255-256
osmotic gradients, 51, 52-53, 54, 56, 58
osteitis fibrosa, 118, 119, 120, 229
osteocytes, 118
osteodystrophy, renal, 117, 224, 226, 229, 258
osteomalacia, 117, 119, 120
osteomyelitis, 163, 165
osteosclerosis, 117
ototoxicity, 255
ouabain, 47, 50
oval fat bodies, 75, 76, 77, 123
ovary, 65
overdose of drugs, 113, 263
overhydration, 112
oxidative phosphorylation, 67
oxygen
  consumption of, in acute renal failure, 111
  diffusion of, 62
  extraction of, 175
  and REF concentration, 65
oxyhemoglobin, 62

P

Paget's disease, 179
PAH (para-aminohippurate), 40, 42, 43, 86, 111, 113, 156, 157, 247
pancreas, 2, 4, 164

pancreatitis, 112
Papanicolaou smear, 79, 80, 102
paper chromatography, 73, 74
paper electrophoresis, 72
papillae, renal, 5, 66, 67, 194, 202
papilledema, 167
papillitis, necrotizing, 185
papilloma, 145, 185, 199, 208, 209, 210, 211
Pappenheimer theory, 39
para-aminohippurate, *see* **PAH**
para-aminosalicylic acid, *see* **PAS**
paracentesis, 176, 262
paracolon bacilli, 190
paralysis agitans, 220
paraproteinemias, 180
parasympathetic nervous system, 28, 29, 220
parathyroidectomy, 120
parathyroid hormone, 115, 117, 118, 119, 120
parenchyma, renal, 5, 18, 19
  compression of, 186
  damage to, 192, 201, 214, 234
  diseases of, 82, 253, 255
parenchymatous acute renal failure, 111
paresthesia, 164
PAS (para-aminosalicylic acid), 136, 151
pCO₂, 61, 62, 63, 116
pelvis, renal, 5, 31, 35, 181
  anomalies of, 93, 233
  bifid or duplicated, 233, 234
  dilatation of, 92
  in dysplasia, 225
  extrarenal, 233
  tumors of, 208
  wounds to, 214
penicillamine, 201
penicillin, 84, 135, 144
penis, 20, 34
  duplicated, 242
  rudimentary, 243
pentosuria, 73
periarteritis, *see* **polyarteritis nodosa**
pericapsulitis, 141
pericarditis, 121, 122, 141
pericytes, 150, 151
periglomerulitis, 142
perinephritis, 195
perineum, 20, 34
peristalsis, 24
peritoneal dialysis, 261, 262, 263
peritoneum, 2, 4, 20, 21, 22, 207, 264, 270
pes cavus, 163
petechiae, 140, 155, 162
Petit's triangle, *see* **triangle, lumbar**
pH
  blood, 114, 115, 116
  urine, 61, 63, 64, 66, **72**, 87, 115, 116, 248, 249
phagocytes, 247
phase microscopy, 76, **77**, 81
phenacetin, 113, 116, 168, 169
phenobarbital, 263
phenolsulfonphthalein (PSP) test, 84
phenylalanine, 257
phenylketonuria, 72
pheochromocytoma, 74, 101, 163
phimosis, 185
phlebography, 102, 173
phosphate buffers, 64
phosphate crystals, 80
phosphate levels, 115, 116, 122, 247, 248, 249, 257
phosphorus-calcium disturbances, 117-120
phosphorylation, oxidative, 67
photomultiplier tubes, gamma camera, 104, 105
pitressin test, 246
pK, 61, 64
plain films, 96, 98
planigraphy, *see* **tomography**
plaques, 100
  arteriosclerotic, 155
  conjunctival, 164

plasma
  amino acids in, 247
  bicarbonate in, 62, 64, 115, 116
  bilirubin in, 74
  chloride concentration in, 48
  creatinine in, 83, 120-121, 122
  glucose in, 41
  inulin in, 39
  ketone levels in, 74
  PAH in, 42, 43
  protein in, 128, 129, 130
  renin levels in, 155, 156, 157, 158
  sodium concentration in, 46, 49
plasma oncotic pressure, 125, 127
platelets, 128, 265, 266
plating method, 81
pleura, 3
pleuritis, 141
plexuses
  aortic (intermesenteric), 27, 28, 29, 220
  capsular, 18, 19
  celiac, 2, 27, 28
  embryonic, 17
  endopelvic venous, 25
  extramuscular, 26
  hypogastric, 27, 28, 29, 220
  medullary capillary, 18
  prostatic, 27, 29
  pudendal venous, 20, 21, 22, 25
  rectal, 25, 27, 28, 29, 220
  renal, 27, 28, 29
  sacral, 27, 28, 29
  subcapsular, 26
  urogenital arterial rete, 35
  vesical, 25, 27, 28, 29, 220
plica interureterica, 22
plumbism, 168
pneumography, 4, **99**
pneumonia, 263
pneumonitis, uremic, 122
podocytes, 7, 32
poisoning, 168-170
  dialysis for, 263
  ethylene glycol, 170
  heavy metal, 113
  mercury, 168-169, 171
  methyl alcohol, 72
pole, urinary; vascular, 6
poliomyelitis, 220
polkissen, 19
polyarteritis nodosa, 75, 111, 123, 138, 139, **167**, 177
polycystic disease, 227-228
polycythemia, 122, 206
polydipsia, 178, 179, 226, 246
polyuria, 114, 178, 179, 226, 229, 246, 249
Ponceau-S stain, 77, 78
"pore" theory, 39
porphyrinuria, 71
postrenal factors in acute renal failure, 111
poststreptococcal glomerulonephritis, 130, 132, 133, 134, 139, 140
potassium
  depletion of, 72, 82, 113, 178, 247, 248, 253, 254, 255, 256
  disturbed balance of, in renal failure, 115, 116, 122
  interaction of hydrogen and, 48, 61, 254, 255
  levels of, in serum, 112
  reabsorption and secretion of, 50
  in sodium-potassium exchange pump, 47, 48, 50
potassium antimony tartrate, 199
potassium intoxication, 112
potassium-retaining diuretics, 254-255, 256
Potter syndrome, 223
prednisone, 177, 264, 265
pre-eclampsia, 172
pregnancy
  asymptomatic bacteriuria of, 82
  bacteriuria or pyuria in, 191
  clearances found in, 83
  glycosuria in, 74
  and hemolytic-uremic syndrome, 159

pregnancy—*continued*
  lactosuria of, 73, 74
  and nephrotic syndrome, 123
  pyelonephritis in, 189
  toxemia of, 172
prerenal factors in acute renal failure, 111
presacral technic, 99
Prescott-Brodie stain, 76, 77, 78
primary atrophy, 223
primary glomerular disease, 193
primary hyperaldosteronism, 72, 120, 157, 158, 178
primary vascular diseases, 193
proctodeum, 34
proerythroblasts, 65
proESF (erythropoietinogen), 65
progressive renal insufficiency, 131-132
progressive vascular disease, 153
proline, 244
prominence, nuclear, 12
pronephros, 30
properdin, 127
proptosis, 164
prostate, 20, 22, 34
  enlarged, 113
  fibroelastosis of, 241
  hypertrophied, 218
  in obstructive uropathy, 185
prostatitis, 185
protamine, 261, 262
proteins
  abnormal, in serum, 180
  and albuminuria, 172
  Bence Jones, 72, 73, **180**
  binding of calcium by, 118
  and BUN, 120, 121
  in dialyzer, 259, 262
  low, in diet, 257
  plasma, 128, 129, 130
proteinuria
  in amyloidosis, 164
  in Balkan nephropathy, 145
  Bence Jones, 72, 73, **180**
  in calcium nephropathy, 179
  in cyanotic heart disease, 174
  in diabetic nephropathy, 149
  in glomerular disease, 128, 129, 130
  in glomerulonephritis, 131, 134, 138, 244
  heavy, 73, 134, 136, 141, 143
  in hemorrhagic fever, 181
  in hypokalemic nephropathy, 178
  with kidney radiation, 161, 162
  with kidney transplant, 265
  in lung purpura with nephritis, 177
  in lupus nephritis, 141, 142, 143
  of nephrotic syndrome, 123, 124-125, 127
  postural, 73
  in pyelonephritis, 192
  in renal dysplasia, 226
  with renal failure, 112, 122
  with renal vein thrombosis, 173
  in renovascular hypertension, 154
  in rheumatoid arthritis, 166
  testing for, 72-73
  in toxic nephropathy, 169
  transient, orthostatic, and persistent, 73
Proteus, 72, 81, 190
proton secretion, 115
protoplasts, 190, 192
proximal RTA (renal tubular acidosis), 115, 116
"prune-belly" syndrome, 238
pruritus, 122
pseudofenestrations, 7
pseudofractures, 117, 118, 119
Pseudomonas, 81
pseudotubercles, 198
psychotherapy, 170
ptosis, 185, 231
pulmonary opacities, 177
purpura, 122, 164
  Henoch-Schönlein (anaphylactoid), 138, 140
  lung, with nephritis, 177
  in lupus nephritis, 141

veins—*continued*
  stellate, 5, 16, 18, 19
  studies of, 102
  subcardinal and supracardinal, 17, 237
  suprarenal, 15
  testicular or ovarian, 2, 15, 207
  thrombosis of, 173
  ureteric, 25
  vesical, 25, 198
vena cava, 2, 4, 15, 17, 25, 100, 206, 207, 237
vena cavography, 102
venography, selective renal, 102
venulae rectae, 18, 19
verumontanitis, 185
verumontanum, 241

vesicles
  apical, 14
  metanephric, 31, 33
  seminal, 20, 34, 234
vestibule, 34, 234
Vim-Silverman needle, 107, 108
virus, lymphocytic choriomeningitis, 129
vitamin D, 117, 118-119, 120, 179, 249
voiding cystourethrography, 97, 238
voiding reflex, 220

W

Waldenström's gamma globulinemia, 73
water
  and acid-loading tests, 87

water—*continued*
  back diffusion of, 38
  excessive intake of, 246 (*see also* **polydipsia**)
  excreted in renal insufficiency, 113-114
  reabsorption of, 47, 48-49, 51, 53, 54, 55, 56, 57, 58, 59, 85, 86, 95
  in renal ischemia, 85, 86
  retention of, 125, 127, 131, 157, 158, 176, 253
  transfer of, 47, 175
  transmission of infection by, 198
  use of, in cystometry, 88
Wegener's granulomatosis, 167, 177
Wilm's tumor, 186, 206, **212**
"wire loop" lesions, 141, 142, 143

wounds (*see also* **trauma**)
  nonpenetrating, 213
  penetrating, 213-214

X

X-linked inheritance, 244, 246

Y

Y-V plasty of bladder neck, 240

Z

zona glomerulosa, 229
zones
  renal, 33
  subcapsular, 18
zonula occludens, 10

Information on
CIBA COLLECTION
Volumes

THE CIBA COLLECTION OF MEDICAL ILLUSTRATIONS is accepted by members of the medical community the world over as a unique work of medical scholarship. The remarkable illustrations by Frank H. Netter, M.D. and text discussions by select specialists make these books unprecedented in their educational, clinical, and scientific value.

Volume 1	**NERVOUS SYSTEM**
	"…a beautiful bargain…and handsome reference work."
	Psychological Record
Volume 2	**REPRODUCTIVE SYSTEM**
	"…a desirable addition to any nursing or medical library."
	American Journal of Nursing
Volume 3/I	**DIGESTIVE SYSTEM (Upper Digestive Tract)**
	"…a fine example of the high quality of this series."
	Pediatrics
Volume 3/II	**DIGESTIVE SYSTEM (Lower Digestive Tract)**
	"…a unique and beautiful work, worth much more than its cost."
	Journal of the South Carolina Medical Association
Volume 3/III	**DIGESTIVE SYSTEM (Liver, Biliary Tract and Pancreas)**
	"…a versatile, multipurpose aid to clinicians, teachers, researchers, and students…" *Florida Medical Journal*
Volume 4	**ENDOCRINE SYSTEM and Selected Metabolic Diseases**
	"…another in the series of superb contributions made by CIBA…"
	International Journal of Fertility
Volume 5	**HEART**
	"The excellence of the volume…is clearly deserving of highest praise."
	Circulation
Volume 6	**KIDNEYS, URETERS, AND URINARY BLADDER**
	"…a model of clarity of language and visual presentation…"
	Circulation
Volume 7	**RESPIRATORY SYSTEM**
	5 years in preparation, a book as vital as the lungs themselves.

In the United States, copies of all CIBA COLLECTION books may be purchased from the Medical Education Division, CIBA Pharmaceutical Company, Division of CIBA-GEIGY Corporation, Summit, New Jersey 07901. In other countries, please direct inquirers to the nearest CIBA-GEIGY office.